Radioguided Surgery

Ken Herrmann • Omgo E. Nieweg
Stephen P. Povoski
Editors

Radioguided Surgery

Current Applications and Innovative Directions in Clinical Practice

Springer

Editors
Ken Herrmann
Department of Nuclear Medicine
Universitätsklinikum Würzburg
Würzburg
Germany

Omgo E. Nieweg
Melanoma Institute Australia and
The University of Sydney
Sydney
New South Wales
Australia

Stephen P. Povoski
Division of Surgical Oncology
Department of Surgery
The Ohio State University
Comprehensive Cancer Center –
Arthur G. James Cancer Hospital and
Richard J. Solove Research Institute
Columbus, OH
USA

ISBN 978-3-319-26049-5 ISBN 978-3-319-26051-8 (eBook)
DOI 10.1007/978-3-319-26051-8

Library of Congress Control Number: 2016933448

Springer Cham Heidelberg New York Dordrecht London

Printed on acid-free paper

Springer International Publishing AG Switzerland is part of Springer Science+Business Media (www.springer.com)

We would like to dedicate this book to our families and loved ones, not only for their understanding and sacrifice during the writing of this book but also for their endearing and endless support throughout our entire medical careers.

Ken Herrmann
Omgo E. Nieweg
Stephen P. Povoski

Foreword

My own journey into radioguided surgery began in the late 1970s. Two principles were the basis for further developing this technology. First, surgery should be based upon more science and less emotion. Second, it is not what is removed at the time of cancer surgery that is important, but it is what is left behind (residual cancer) that is most impactful. Based upon these two principles, I have spent the past 40 years attempting to improve surgical outcomes. Therefore, it is most apropos that Chapter 1 of this book succinctly professes "radioguided surgery provides the surgeon with critical and real-time information regarding the exact location of disease and the overall extent of disease burden, as well as allowing the surgeon to minimize the degree of surgical invasiveness associated with many commonplace diagnostic and therapeutic surgical procedures, while still maintaining maximum treatment-directed benefits to the patient."

Radioguided surgery requires a significant amount of technology for its implementation. Surgeons and nuclear medicine physicians should have knowledge and expertise relevant to this technology that extends beyond standard training. Likewise, nuclear medicine technologists, operating room personnel, and pathologists should be very familiar with this technology. Therefore, appropriate resources are needed that adequately describe all aspects of radioguided surgery. This book fully addresses all of the basic principles of radioguided surgery and provides a comprehensive overview of the technical details of various radioguided surgical procedures for a variety of malignancies. As a resource, this book is invaluable.

This book includes 29 chapters written and edited by well-known experts in the field of radioguided surgery. Chapter 2 provides essential knowledge for understanding the basic principles of radiodetection. The terminology and explanations target a wide array of audiences. The contents of this chapter should prove intelligible and understandable.

Complete resection of all tumor-containing tissues is critical for the best survival potential for cancer patients. During radioguided surgery, radiodetection with handheld gamma detection probes can provide the surgeon with real-time information regarding the location of the target lesions and helps confirm accurate lesion resection. With limitations to handheld gamma detection probes, intraoperative gamma cameras have been designed to further facilitate radioguided surgery. These gamma camera imaging systems must meet several requirements to be employed in the operating room: (1) a portable and mobile design, (2) no delay between image acquisition and display, and (3) the possibility for continuous monitoring, spatial orientation on screen, real-time quantification, and display of radioactive count data. Such systems should also have an adequate spatial resolution, sensitivity, and field of view. Chapter 3 provides an in-depth description of this technology.

The proper use and handling of radioactive substances for radioguided surgery requires adherence to strict principles of radiation safety in order to limit the risk to patients and staff, including those in the nuclear medicine department, the operating room, and the pathology department. The knowledge of proper disposal of radioactive waste is of utmost importance. Chapter 6 stresses the importance of all these principles.

The histologic status of the axillary lymph nodes remains one of the most important prognostic indicators in breast cancer and impacts recommendations for adjuvant therapies. Axillary lymph node dissection, once considered the standard of care for diagnostic axillary staging in all breast cancer patients, has been largely replaced by sentinel lymph node biopsy in patients with a clinically negative axilla and in a select group of patients with node-positive breast cancer. This has reduced the extensive morbidity of full axillary lymph node dissection. Chapter 7 reviews the lymphatic drainage patterns of the breast, the technical aspects of sentinel lymph node biopsy (with particular attention to the radioguided surgical aspects), and the clinical implications of the findings. The development of radioguided sentinel lymph node biopsy is truly one of the greatest success stories in contemporary surgical oncology.

The role of surgery in the treatment of cancer has not changed appreciably over the past 100 years. With cancer being the second leading cause of death, it is clear that there is a need for a more scientific approach to the removal of cancer. Updated technology in the operating room is needed to enhance the surgeon's ability to identify the extent of disease and perform a more complete resection of the cancer. Staging and grading of malignant disease plays a significant role in determining prognosis. Chapter 24 nicely describes the history of radioimmunoguided surgery and its invaluable role in improving the ability to accurately stage tumors. Hopefully, as we continue to learn how to better integrate this technology into future radioguided surgical approaches, it will become a more recognizable method for improving our ability to forecast prognosis.

As discussed in this book, fully integrated whole body preoperative nuclear medicine imaging and intraoperative radioguided detection of a radiotracer (using a single injection dose) is the most effective way to perform radioguided surgery. This allows the nuclear medicine physician and surgeon to jointly generate a virtual navigation roadmap regarding the location of the expected and unexpected lesions, including locations of distant metastatic disease. The navigation concept can provide the operating specialist with information regarding the location and margins of target lesions during surgery and as such can help improve the accuracy of the surgical procedure. This enhanced radioguided surgery technology has the potential to significantly impact upon the success of cancer operations and improve long-term survival for our patients.

It is very evident that radioguided surgery has a long history dating back to the late 1940s, with significant groundbreaking contributions from many individuals. Therefore, the collective expectations of this book are to show exactly how the wide variety of current applications and future innovative directions of radioguided surgery can impact all disciplines within the clinical practice of surgery. Clearly, the co-editors of this book, Prof. Ken Herrmann, Prof. Omgo E. Nieweg, and Dr. Stephen P. Povoski, have fully met these expectations. As radioguided surgery moves forward through the twenty-first century, we envision further growth of its current technological platforms along with the development of other innovative methods.

Edward W. Martin Jr.
Division of Surgical Oncology, Department of Surgery
Arthur G. James Cancer Hospital and Richard J. Solove Research
Institute and Comprehensive Cancer Center
The Ohio State University
Columbus, USA

Preface

Radioguided surgery, a concept dating back to the late 1940s, is simply a surgical procedure which incorporates the use of some sort of radiation detection device, in a real-time fashion, for the identification of a radioisotope that has been administered to a patient prior to the time of attempted detection and for the sole purpose of guiding the successful performance of the surgical procedure. Its successful undertaking requires a collaborative interplay of the disciplines of surgery and nuclear medicine, and its clinical application has dramatically impacted upon our current surgical management of cancer patients.

The purpose of this book is to provide the readership (including surgeons, surgical technologists, nuclear medicine physicians, nuclear medicine technologists, and various trainees) with a comprehensive overview of the state-of-the-art practice of radioguided surgery. This includes chapters devoted to discussing the basic physics principles for detection and imaging, radiation detection device technology, principles of surgical navigation, radionuclides and radiopharmaceuticals, and radiation safety. Likewise, this includes chapters devoted to discussing a wide range of clinical applications of radioguided surgery for a variety of malignancies, including breast cancer, melanoma and other cutaneous malignancies, gynecologic malignancies, head and neck malignancies, thyroid cancer, urologic malignancies, colon cancer, gastroesophageal cancer, lung cancer, bone tumors, parathyroid adenomas, and neuroendocrine tumors. The editors have enlisted the talents of over 65 authors, each considered an expert in his or her own field. For each clinical application, the recommended methodological approaches are discussed, and the available cumulative clinical experiences of investigators from across the globe are reviewed. A conscious effort is made to bring forth and highlight recent developments and innovative approaches within each clinical area. Interesting cases and novel approaches are further highlighted by the presentation of a series of selected case reports at the end of the book.

It is our hopes that the information provided in this book will allow surgeons and nuclear medicine physicians alike to gain a broad-based understanding of the basic yet essential procedural skills and clinical acumens that are necessary for incorporating radioguided surgery technologies into the care of their cancer patients.

Würzburg, Germany — Ken Herrmann
North Sydney, NSW, Australia — Omgo E. Nieweg
Columbus, OH, USA — Stephen P. Povoski

Acknowledgments

We wish to acknowledge the collective dedicated efforts of over 65 contributing authors for the successful writing of all of the chapters included within this book, as well as the expert and sometimes frank advice provided by many of them along the way. In particular, we are deeply indebted and forever grateful to Dr. Christina Blümel for her commitment and dedication of untold hours to the development and successful execution of this book, from researching potential relevant authors to reviewing and revising numerous chapters, and with keeping the book writing process on track whenever the editorial focus seemed to be misplaced. Likewise, we would very much like to offer a special thanks to Prof. Sergi Vidal-Sicart, without whom several essential chapters within the book would have never been realized without his personal and expert intervention in the writing process. Additionally, we would also like to thank Petra Thomas and Christina Racke-Nestler for providing administrative assistance, as well Rick Mills for providing copyediting assistance on several chapters.

Lastly, we would like to recognize and acknowledge all of the past and present pioneers and iconic figures in the field of radioguided surgery, and for whom without their innovative thinking, this integrated surgical and nuclear medicine discipline would have never been developed. In similar regard, we are hopeful that all those who have contributed to the field of radioguided surgery over the past seven decades have been appropriately recognized and acknowledged within the pages of this book.

Ken Herrmann
Omgo E. Nieweg
Stephen P. Povoski

Contents

Part I

Introduction

1 The History of Radioguided Surgery: Early Historical Milestones and the Development of Later Innovative Clinical Applications

Stephen P. Povoski

Contents

S.P. Povoski, MD
Division of Surgical Oncology,
Department of Surgery, Arthur G. James Cancer Hospital and Richard J. Solove Research Institute and Comprehensive Cancer Center,
The Ohio State University, Columbus,
OH 43210, USA
e-mail: stephen.povoski@osumc.edu

Abstract

Radioguided surgery involves utilizing a radiation detection device within the operating room in a real-time fashion to identify a radioisotope that has been administered to a patient prior to the time of attempted detection and for the sole purpose of guiding the successful performance of the surgical procedure. Since its first description in the late 1940s, radioguided surgery has expanded tremendously and has become a well-established discipline within the practice of surgery. It has been investigated and applied to the surgical management of numerous solid malignancies and has most significantly impacted upon the surgical management of breast cancer, melanoma, and parathyroid disease. Radioguided surgery provides the surgeon with critical and real-time information regarding the exact location of the disease and the overall extent of disease burden, as well as allows the surgeon to minimize the degree of surgical invasiveness associated with many commonplace diagnostic and therapeutic surgical procedures, while still maintaining maximum treatment-directed benefits to the patient. As we move forward through the twenty-first century, we envision further growth of the current technological platforms of radioguided surgery, with a continued emphasis upon promoting integration of handheld radiation detection devices and advanced nuclear medicine molecular imaging

K. Herrmann et al. (eds.), *Radioguided Surgery: Current Applications and Innovative Directions in Clinical Practice*, DOI 10.1007/978-3-319-26051-8_1

for guiding and optimizing the intraoperative detection and resection of conditions affecting both cancer and noncancer patients.

1.1 Overview: Conceptualization and Realization of Radioguided Surgery

Radioguided surgery is simply the general concept of utilizing a radiation detection device within the operating room in a real-time fashion to identify a radioisotope that has been administered to a patient prior to the time of attempted detection and for the sole purpose of guiding the successful performance of the surgical procedure. Since its first description in the late 1940s, the use of radioguided surgery has expanded tremendously and has evolved into a well-established discipline within the practice of surgery [1]. Its use has been investigated and applied to the surgical management of numerous solid malignancies and has most significantly revolutionized the surgical management of breast cancer, melanoma, and parathyroid disease. Radioguided surgery has proven impactful on many levels in the surgical management of various disease entities and has most significantly contributed to providing the surgeon with critical and real-time information regarding the exact location of the disease and the overall extent of disease burden. Furthermore, radioguided surgery allows the surgeon to minimize the degree of surgical invasiveness associated with many commonplace diagnostic and therapeutic surgical procedures, while still maintaining maximum treatment-directed benefits to the patient.

1.2 The Early Years: Historical Milestones in Radioguided Surgery

The first reported description in the literature of utilizing a radiation detection device within the operating room to identify a radioisotope administered to a patient dates back to 1949 and comprises the work performed by Bertram Selverstone and his colleagues from Massachusetts General Hospital and Harvard Medical School (Boston, Massachusetts, USA) [1–3]. The radiation detection device utilized in this first reported description of radioguided surgery [2, 3] was a Geiger-Müller counter, a device that non-discriminately detects ionizing radiation, including alpha, beta, and gamma radiation, and for which the development of this practical electron counting tube (i.e., Geiger-Müller tube) was first realized in 1928 by Hans Geiger and Walther Müller at the University of Kiel (Kiel, Germany) [4].

In their initial published reports, Selverstone et al. [1–3] from Massachusetts General Hospital and Harvard Medical School (Boston, Massachusetts, USA) utilized a portable handheld gas-filled Geiger-Müller counter device to intraoperatively detect ionizing radiation during brain tumor surgery emitted from phosphorus-32 (^{32}P), a pure beta-emitting radionuclide with a physical half-life of 14.3 days. The characteristic constraining feature of beta emissions, such as those from ^{32}P, is their ability to only travel a few millimeters within biologic tissues. In their cumulative reported experience, Selverstone et al. [3] described a series of 33 patients with suspected brain tumors (as determined preoperatively by neurologic examination, electroencephalography, and ventriculography) that were intravenously injected with 0.95–4.2 millicuries (35.2–155.4 megabecquerels) of ^{32}P in a buffered sodium phosphate solution at a time interval of 1.8–186.8 h prior to the surgical procedure. They utilized a prototype sterilizable handheld argon-ethyl acetate gas-filled Geiger-Müller counter device (possessing a 2 or 3 mm diameter cannula-like shaft containing the radiation-sensitive portion of the device for more easily penetrating the brain tissue) which was connected to either a pre-amplifier and a standard binary scaling unit or an analog-display counter ratemeter located outside of the sterile surgical field. At surgery, after the appropriate area of the cerebral cortex was exposed by way of a craniotomy, the cannula-like shaft of the handheld Geiger-Müller counter device was then placed on the surface of the brain in the area of the suspected brain tumor and advanced at successive 1 cm increments beneath the surface, to a maximum depth of up to approximately 6 cm, with count data (corrected counts per minute) taken at the location. A similar process for count data collection was performed on an area of presumed normal brain tissue away from the location of the suspected brain tumor. In selected cases, following successful location of the brain tumor, attempts were made to demarcate its tumor boundaries using the Geiger-Müller counter. Of 33 evaluated patients, 28 brain tumors (including 14 glioblastomas, 4 astrocytomas, 3 unclassified gliomas, 2 metastatic carcinomas, 1 medulloblastoma, 1 astroblastoma, 1 oligodendroglioma, 1 ependymoma, and 1 angiosarcoma) were localized using the handheld Geiger-Müller counter device, of which 23 brain tumors were located beneath the surface of the brain. In 12 patients, the handheld Geiger-Müller counter device was used to attempt to demarcate the tumor boundaries in order to facilitate total extirpation of tumor. In four patients, tumor was not localized by means of the handheld Geiger-Müller counter device, including two false-negative results that were attributed to the inability to correctly place the handheld Geiger-Müller counter device in close proximity to the tumor, one patient with diffuse infiltration of the entire cerebral hemisphere with tumor that precluded distinguishing it from normal adjacent tissue, and one patient in which no tumor was correctly identified.

Shortly thereafter in 1950–1951, Selverstone and his colleagues from Massachusetts General Hospital and Harvard Medical School (Boston, Massachusetts, USA) [5–7] also applied this technique of radioguided brain mapping during brain tumor surgery not only to ^{32}P in 114 presumed brain tumor patients but also to potassium-42 (^{42}K) in 36 presumed brain tumor patients. The radionuclide ^{42}K has a physical half-life of 12.4 h, and its emission profile was described by Selverstone et al. [6] as including "more energetic beta particles" that could "theoretically be detected at distances of up to 1.8 cm through the brain," as well as gamma emissions that were relatively inefficient in being counted by their handheld Geiger-Müller counter device. Sweet [7], who noted that ^{42}K not only had a propensity to accumulate in brain tumors but also avidly accumulated in the muscle surrounding the calvarium, emphasized that the gamma emission capabilities of ^{42}K "permits external localization through the intact skull in many cases."

It was then not until 1956, when C. Craig Harris and his colleagues at the Oak Ridge National Laboratory and Oak Ridge Institute of Nuclear Studies Medical Hospital (Oak Ridge, Tennessee, USA) reported the first description in the literature of radioguided surgery utilizing a gamma scintillation detection device, and, most specifically, a portable handheld gamma detection probe system, with the specific application of the identification of thyroid tissue [1, 8]. This system described by Harris et al. [8] consisted of a handheld gamma detection probe, utilizing a thallium-activated cesium iodide (CsI(TI)) scintillation crystal. There were two separate nickel probe head configurations which were designed with platinum collimation, including one probe head measuring 1/4 in. in diameter and 3 5/8 in. in length and containing a CsI(TI) scintillation crystal of 0.22 in. in diameter and 3/8 in. in length and another probe head measuring 1/8 in. in diameter and 3 1/2 in. in length and containing a CsI(TI) scintillation crystal of 0.10 in. in diameter and 1/4 in. in length. These two probe head designs were mounted to a handheld photomultiplier-preamplifier and connected by a coaxial cable to a metal box unit containing the power supply, an analog-display counter ratemeter, and speaker/volume control to elicit an audible signal (i.e., "howler"). In their published report, Harris et al. [8] described the evaluation of a patient with a history of thyroid cancer who had previously undergone a total thyroidectomy some 3 years earlier and who had persistent iodine uptake in the neck region. The patient was intravenously injected with 0.25 millicuries (9.25 megabecquerels) of iodine-131 (^{131}I), a radionuclide gamma emitter with a physical half-life of 8.04 days, which has a minority of gamma emissions (representing approximately 10 % of its energy, with 81 % of gamma emissions being at 364 keV) and which has a majority of beta emissions (representing approximately 90 % of its energy, which travel only up to 2 mm in biologic tissue, and are responsible for its tissue damage effect as a form of radiotherapy). At surgery, using this handheld gamma detection probe, they were able to localize a discrete solitary area of significant radioactivity situated along the left side of the trachea, and this allowed for the successful identification and successful excision of a 5 × 5 × 2 mm nodule near the entrance of the left recurrent laryngeal nerve that was subsequently histologically proven to represent an area of residual thyroid tissue.

Then, in the late 1950s, the principles of radioguided surgery using gamma detection devices were first applied in the development of techniques for continuous monitoring of systemic leakage during performance of regional isolated perfusion for locally advanced and unresectable malignancies [1, 9–12]. Early on in the development of regional isolated perfusion technologies, John Stehlin and his colleagues at the University of Texas M.D. Anderson Hospital and Tumor Institute (Houston, Texas, USA) recognized two important considerations in achieving the highest possible dose of chemotherapeutic agent for attaining maximum clinical efficacy from regional isolated perfusion [9–12]. These considerations were (1) "local tissue tolerance" (i.e., the maximum amount of chemotherapy agent which normal tissues can tolerate without being permanently damaged) and (2) the "leakage factor" (i.e., the extent of "cross-circulation" between the isolated circuit of the perfused region and the systemic circulation). John Stehlin and his colleagues believed that the "leakage factor" represented the most serious limitation to achieving a successful regional isolated perfusion procedure, and were the first to recognize the potential beneficial utility of radioguided technologies for monitoring of systemic leakage during regional isolated perfusion, and investigated radioguided monitoring techniques during regional isolated perfusion for locally advanced and unresectable malignancies, such as malignant melanoma, sarcoma, squamous cell carcinoma, basal cell carcinoma, and adenocarcinoma, which were confined to the extremities, as well as a small number of cases which were confined to the pelvic region and head region. Stehlin et al. [10, 11] injected 2–10 microcuries (0.074–0.370 megabecquerels) of ^{131}I-labeled human serum albumin intravenously into the patient for determination of a calibration count baseline and injected approximately tenfold more ^{131}I-labeled human serum albumin, consisting of 20–100 microcuries (0.74–3.70 megabecquerels) of ^{131}I-labeled human serum albumin into the arterial line leading from the perfusion pump to the isolated perfusate circuit for eventual calculation of the percentage systemic leakage factor. For monitoring of the systemic leakage during the regional isolated perfusion procedure, they utilized a single, small field-of-view scintillation crystal detector probe unit with a built-in photomultiplier tube and preamplifier and with 1.25 in. thickness of lead side shielding for detection of gamma emissions. The single, small field-of-view scintillation detector unit was mounted overhead on a wheel-based pole tower apparatus for easy mobility and positioning during the regional isolated perfusion procedure and was positioned over the heart for lower extremity cases or positioned over the groin for upper extremity cases. The single, small field-of-view scintillation detector unit was connected by way of a 30 ft coaxial cable to an analog-display counter ratemeter and a rectilinear pen recorder for quantifying and recording the results of the systemic leakage of ^{131}I-labeled human serum albumin from the isolated perfusate circuit.

Although some 30 years later, the same principles of radioguided monitoring of systemic leakage during regional isolated perfusion, which were first established by John Stehlin [10–12] using an overhead-mounted small field-of-view scintillation detector unit, were later adapted to the use of a handheld semiconductor gamma detection system [1, 13]. This system, described in 1989 by Sardi et al. [13] at the Ohio State University (Columbus, Ohio, USA), consisted of two commercially available handheld gamma probes, each consisting of a Neoprobe® 1000 gamma detection probe (formerly Neoprobe Corporation, Dublin, Ohio, USA), which each employed a cadmium zinc telluride (CdZnTe) semiconductor crystal of 11 mm in diameter and 15 mm in length. One of the handheld gamma probes was positioned over the precordial area, and the other handheld gamma probe was positioned over the distal aspect of the thigh. Patients received 0.8 millicuries (29.6 megabecquerels) of technetium-99 m (^{99m}Tc) pentetate through the isolated perfusate circulation. ^{99m}Tc is a radionuclide gamma emitter with a physical half-life of 6.04 h, which has a predominant gamma emission at 140 keV. The percentage of ^{99m}Tc pentetate leakage was calculated by a simultaneous reading of the two gamma detection probes at 1 min intervals, as well as determined by the standard method of intermittent simultaneous blood sampling from the isolated perfusate and systemic circulations at 15 min intervals using a gamma well counter. An essentially identical percentage of systemic leakage was detected by the minute-by-minute monitoring of the two handheld gamma probe system as compared to that determined by the intermittent (every 15 min) blood sampling method from the isolated perfusate and systemic circulations. Nevertheless, the minute-by-minute monitoring of the two handheld gamma probe system provided the surgeon with a more instantaneous and real-time indication of any fluctuations in the percentage of systemic leakage than did the intermittent (every 15 min) blood sampling method from the isolated perfusate and systemic circulations, thus allowing the surgeon to make more immediate intraoperative decision-making during regional isolated perfusion procedure.

1.3 Innovative Clinical Applications of Radioguided Surgery in the 1980s

During most of the 1960s and 1970s, the application of radiation detection devices for guiding surgical procedures within the operating room fell into some level of dormancy. However, starting in the early 1980s, successful clinical application of innovative radioguided surgery techniques began to develop at a more accelerated rate. This included the development of clinical applications of radioguided surgery directed toward the biopsy and resection of suspicious bone lesions, the identification of parathyroid tissue, and the development of antigen-directed intraoperative radioimmunodetection for the radioguided localization and resection of tumors (i.e., radioimmunoguided surgery) [1].

It was in 1981 that the application of radioguided surgery was first applied to the biopsy and resection of suspicious bone lesions [1, 14, 15]. At that time, Harvey et al. [14] at the Presbyterian Hospital of Dallas (Dallas, Texas, USA) first reported the application of a sterilizable prototype handheld scintillation gamma detection probe for intraoperative radioguided biopsy of benign and metastatic bone lesions in four patients using an intravenous injection of 2–20 millicuries (74–740 megabecquerels) of ^{99m}Tc-methylene diphosphonate in three cases and 5 millicuries (185 megabecquerels) of gallium-67 (^{67}Ga) citrate in one case. ^{67}Ga is a radionuclide gamma emitter with a physical half-life of 78.3 h, which has predominant gamma emissions at 93 keV (37.8 % abundance), 184 keV (20.1 % abundance), and 300 keV (16.8 % abundance). This system consisted of a prototype handheld gamma detection probe containing a 0.64 × 2.54 cm thallium-activated sodium iodide (NaI(TI)) scintillation crystal housed in a stainless steel housing (16.5 cm in length × 1.5 cm diameter) with 2 mm of lead side shielding for collimation (formerly Harshaw Chemical Company, Solon, Ohio) and which was coupled to a 38 mm bialkali (antimony reacted with potassium and cesium) photomultiplier tube (Hamamatsu Photonic K.K., Hamamatsu City, Shizuoka Prefecture, Japan), via a flexible fiberoptic cable which was attached to an audible count-rate indicator. Additionally, in 1981, Ghelman et al. [15] at the Hospital for Special Surgery (New York, New York, USA) also reported the application of another prototype handheld scintillation gamma detection probe for intraoperative radioguided resection of a single patient with a benign bone tumor (i.e., osteoid osteoma) using an intravenous injection of 15 millicuries (555 megabecquerels) of ^{99m}Tc-methylene diphosphonate. This system consisted of a prototype handheld gamma detection probe containing a nonspecified thallium-activated sodium iodide (NaI(TI)) scintillation crystal housed in a stainless steel housing (18.2 cm in length × 1.6 cm diameter) and enveloped in a cylindrical lead shield for collimation measuring 20.5 cm in length and with an 8 mm distal end aperture (formerly Harshaw Chemical Company, Solon, Ohio, USA) and which was attached to a digital-/analog-display scaler/counter ratemeter (Lundlum Measurements, Inc., Sweetwater, Texas, USA) for count recording.

It was in 1984 that the application of radioguided surgery was first applied to the identification of parathyroid tissue [1, 16]. At that time, Ubhi et al. [16] at Queen's Medical Centre/University Hospital (Nottingham, England, UK) reported the application of a sterilizable handheld gamma semiconductor gamma detection probe for identification and radioguided resection of an ectopic mediastinal parathyroid adenoma within a patient undergoing neck exploration with the finding of two normal left neck parathyroid glands and only one normal right neck parathyroid gland after a 1.6 millicuries (60 megabecquerels) intravenous injection using of thallium-201 (^{201}Tl) thallous chloride. This system consisted of a handheld gamma detection probe containing a cadmium telluride (CdTe) semiconductor crystal connected to a digital-display counter ratemeter for count recording. ^{201}Tl has a physical half-life of 73.0 h, and decays predominantly by electron capture, emitting Hg X-rays (in the 70–80 keV range), and has gamma photon emission at 167 keV of 10 % abundance and at 135 keV of 3 % abundance.

However, it was not for another decade until further refinements in radioguided surgical techniques for the identification of parathyroid tissue were reported in the literature and thus subsequently leading to the adoption of this technology for the surgical management of primary hyperparathyroidism [1, 17, 18]. Specifically, in 1995, Martinez et al. at [17] the Ohio State University (Columbus, Ohio, USA) first reported the use of ^{99m}Tc-methoxyisobutylisonitrile (MIBI) for the radioguided surgical detection of parathyroid gland pathology in three patients. The patients were intravenously injected with 0.4–2.0 millicuries (14.8–74 megabecquerels) of ^{99m}Tc-MIBI. Then, approximately 2–6 h after ^{99m}Tc-MIBI administration, patients underwent intraoperative radioguided localization of abnormal parathyroid glands using the commercially available handheld Neoprobe® 1000 gamma detection probe (formerly Neoprobe Corporation, Dublin, Ohio). Then, in 1997, Norman and Chheda [18] at the University of South Florida (Tampa, Florida, USA) reported on their first series of 15 patients undergoing minimally invasive radioguided surgery using ^{99m}Tc-MIBI for the surgical management of primary hyperparathyroidism. This report by Norman and Chheda [18] was followed by many other publications by the Norman group, and led to the popularization and widespread application of minimally invasive radioguided parathyroidectomy using ^{99m}Tc-MIBI for the surgical management of primary hyperparathyroidism, and which today remains an important mainstay in parathyroid surgery.

The year 1984 also marked the inauguration of the radioguided surgical concept of radioimmunoguided surgery [1]. The idea of utilizing antibodies directed against cancer-specific antigens for intraoperative radioimmunodetection, localization, and resection of tumors was pioneered at the Ohio State University (Columbus, Ohio, USA) by a surgical oncologist, Dr. Edward W. Martin, Jr., and a professor emeritus of electrical engineering, Dr. Marlin O. Thurston [1]. Their initial experimental animal model testing and human application of intraoperative radioimmunodetection were first reported in 1984 by Aitken et al. [1, 19, 20]. In their initial experimental animal model testing, they grow subcutaneous tumor implants of CEA-producing human colonic adenocarcinoma cells (CX-1) on the flank in Swiss nude mice and demonstrated the feasibility of handheld gamma probe detection of ^{131}I-labeled baboon anti-CEA polyclonal antibody within these subcutaneous tumor implants, with greater sensitivity of the handheld gamma detection probe as compared to gamma camera imaging for small tumor implants [1, 19, 20]. In their first clinical application of intraoperative radioimmunodetection, they intravenously injected a single patient with rectal carcinoma with 1.9 millicuries (70.3 megabecquerels) of ^{131}I-labeled baboon anti-CEA polyclonal antibody at a time of 3 days prior to the planned surgical procedure and intraoperatively utilized a prototype handheld gamma detection probe system (consisting of a single CdTe semiconductor crystal housed within a 16 mm diameter lead collimator with a 4 mm aperture, and connected to a preamplifier, and an amplifier with a digital-display counter) for radioactive count recording [1, 20]. The prototype handheld gamma detection probe intraoperatively detected an increased level of the ^{131}I-labeled baboon anti-CEA polyclonal antibody in the rectal tumor as compared to normal sigmoid colon, ileum, abdominal wall, and anal verge. Shortly thereafter in 1985, Martin et al. [1, 21] reported the results of the first radioimmunoguided surgery clinical series involving 28 patients with primary ($n = 12$) and recurrent ($n = 16$) colorectal cancer and using the same prototype handheld gamma detection probe system. Each patient was intravenously injected with 2.2 millicuries (81.4 megabecquerels) of ^{131}I baboon anti-CEA polyclonal antibody at approximately 48–72 h prior to the planned surgical procedure. Preoperative whole-body scintillation imaging correctly localized tumor in only 33 % of the patients with primary colorectal cancer and only 64 % of patients with recurrent colorectal cancer. In contrast, intraoperative radioimmunodetection with the prototype handheld gamma detection probe was successful in all 28 patients, with a mean tumor-to-background ratio of 3.97:1 in primary lesions and 4.18:1 in recurrent lesions. Thereafter, nearly all subsequent radioimmunoguided surgery clinical trials conducted at the Ohio State University (Columbus, Ohio, USA) used various monoclonal antibodies targeted against tumor-associated glycoprotein-72 (TAG-72), a mucin-like, extracellular antigen overexpressed by many adenocarcinomas, which were radiolabeled with iodine-125 (^{125}I) [1].

1.4 Innovative Clinical Applications of Radioguided Surgery in the 1990s

Beginning in the early 1990s, there was a further acceleration in the development of successful clinical applications for radioguided surgery. This included the development of radioguided sentinel lymph node biopsy for melanoma and breast cancer, as well as radioguided lesion localization for the surgical excision of non-palpable breast lesions seen on breast imaging [1].

The generalized concept of a so-called "sentinel node" in our modern medical literature was first coined by Ernest A. Gould and his colleagues from the Washington Hospital Center (Washington, DC, USA) in 1960 in their description of a lymph node that was routinely "noted at the junction of the anterior and posterior facial vein" at the time of surgery for parotid gland cancer [1, 22]. In their landmark report, Gould et al. [22] stated "The lymph node that is now used routinely for frozen section assay is easily found. After the skin incision has been made and the flaps reflected, the inferior posterior surface of the parotid is separated from the anterior margin of the sternomastoid muscle. The anterior facial vein curves downward and posteriorly at the lower edge of the gland to meet the posterior facial vein to form the common facial truck. It is in the area of the angle formed by the junction of these 2 veins that this "sentinel node" is always found. It may be removed easily, and the parotid dissection may progress during the pathologist's study of the node". They concluded by remarking that "routine excision of this angular node be done for frozen section study." However, it was not until almost two decades later in 1977 that the "sentinel node" concept reappeared in the modern medical literature and was more notably attributed to the work of Ramón M. Cabañas at the National University of Asunción (Asunción, Paraguay) in the area of penile squamous cell carcinoma [1, 23]. This reappearance of the "sentinel node" concept was based upon the careful work and meticulous description of lymphadenography of the dorsal lymphatics of the penis which was previously published by Manuel Riveros, Ramiro Garcia, and Ramón M. Cabañas at the same university in 1967 [1, 24]. In his landmark report, Cabañas [23] stated "A 5-cm incision is made parallel to the inguinal ligament, two finger-breadths (4.5 cm) lateral and two finger-breadths (4.5 cm) distal to the pubic tubercle….. This lies over the greater sapheno-femoral junction. By inserting the finger under the upper flap towards the pubic tubercle, the SLN is encountered….. The SLN corresponds to the lymph nodes associated with the superficial epigastric vein..... The position of the SLN in relationship to the superficial epigastric vein may vary but never by a distance greater than 1 cm." Cabañas concluded by remarking that "Anatomically, clinically, and pathologically it was found that the SLN is the first site of metastasis and may be the only lymph node involved..... If SLN biopsies are negative for metastases, no further surgical therapy is immediately indicated." In their landmark reports, the strict definition of the "sentinel node" by both Gould in 1960 [1, 22] and Cabañas in 1977 [1, 23] was based solely upon its proximity to a static, predefined anatomical landmark (i.e., the angle of the confluence of the anterior and posterior facial veins, as described by Gould, and the superficial epigastric vein, as described by Cabañas), and this definition of the "sentinel node" was not based upon actual variations in the pattern of lymphatic drainage observed within patients undergoing any sort of individualized, real-time, intraoperative lymphatic mapping procedure at the time of surgery.

The actual concept of intraoperative lymphatic mapping for selective identification and removal of sentinel lymph nodes at the time of surgery was first introduced into the modern medical literature in 1992 for melanoma by Donald L. Morton and his colleagues at the John Wayne Institute for Cancer Treatment and Research (Santa Monica, California, USA) using intradermally injected vital blue dyes alone in a total of 223 melanoma patients [25]. Sentinel lymph nodes were successfully identified in 194 of the 237 lymph node basins evaluated. However, it was not until 1 year later in 1993 that David N. Krag, James C. Alex, and colleagues at the University of Vermont (Burlington, Vermont, USA) published the first reports of intraoperative radioguided identification of sentinel lymph nodes in both melanoma and breast cancer patients using ^{99m}Tc-sulfur colloid and a handheld gamma detection probe [26, 27]. Alex et al. [26] reported on ten melanoma patients who were intradermally injected with 0.4 millicuries (14.8 megabecquerels) ^{99m}Tc-sulfur colloid in 0.5 milliliters of normal saline, underwent preoperative lymphoscintigraphy between 10 min and 150 min after injection, and subsequently underwent a sentinel lymph node biopsy procedure approximately 2.5–5.0 h after injection utilizing a handheld gamma detection probe. The handheld gamma detection probe contained a NaI scintillation crystal coupled to a photomultiplier tube, and both contained within a tungsten-alloyed housing and connected to a preamplifier and a signal processor with a digital and analog readout for radioactive count recording (C-Trak, Care Wise Medical Products, Morgan Hill, California, USA). Sentinel lymph nodes were successfully identified in all ten patients. Krag et al. [27] reported on 22 breast cancer patients who were injected with 0.4 millicuries (14.8 megabecquerels) ^{99m}Tc-sulfur colloid in 0.5 milliliters of normal saline into the normal breast tissue adjacent to the lesion or the biopsy site and subsequently underwent a sentinel lymph node biopsy procedure approximately 1–9 h after injection utilizing the same previously described handheld gamma detection probe system. Sentinel lymph nodes were successfully identified in 18 of the 22 patients injected. It is realistic to assert that the introduction of radioguided sentinel lymph node biopsy to the surgical management of melanoma and breast cancer by Krag and Alex [26, 27] represents the single most impactful advancement that radioguided surgery has had on reshaping the surgical management of any given disease entity.

The concept of radioguided localization of non-palpable breast lesions was first introduced into the literature in 1996 by Charles E. Cox and colleagues from the H. Lee Moffitt Cancer Center and Research Institute (Tampa, Florida, USA) [28]. In their initial case report, Cox et al. [28] described a breast cancer patient intravenously injected 1 h prior to surgery with 18 millicuries (692 megabecquerels) of ^{99m}Tc-MIBI and subsequently performed radioguided excision of the breast cancer using a handheld gamma detection probe. This initial report laid the groundwork for the subsequent development of two variations in the technique of radioguided localization and excision of non-palpable breast lesions utilizing mammographic or ultrasound-guided placement of a radionuclides into the region of the non-palpable breast lesion. Starting in 1998, Alberto

Luini and Umberto Veronesi from the European Institute of Oncology (Milan, Italy) reported the first series of papers on the radioguided occult lesion localization (ROLL) technique, which involved an intratumoral injection (using prior-day mammographic or ultrasound guidance) of 0.1 millicuries (3.7 megabecquerels) of ^{99m}Tc-colloidal human serum albumin in 0.2–0.3 milliliters of normal saline, followed by next day radioguided excisional breast biopsy using various handheld gamma detection probes [29–31]. Their reported cumulative success rate was 99.5 % among 647 patients [31]. Similarly, starting in 1999, Emilia L. Dauway, Charles E. Cox, and Richard J. Gray from the H. Lee Moffitt Cancer Center and Research Institute (Tampa, Florida, USA) reported the first series of papers on the radioguided seed localization (RSL) technique, which involved placement of a 0.29 millicuries (10.7 megabecquerels) ^{125}I-labeled titanium seed (4.5 mm × 0.8 mm in dimension) up to 5 days prior to surgery, followed by radioguided excisional breast biopsy using a handheld gamma detection probe [32–34]. Their reported cumulative success rate was 100 % among 51 patients [34].

1.5 Concluding Remarks

It is very evident that radioguided surgery has a long and rich history dating back to the late 1940s, with significant groundbreaking contributions from many individuals and with far too many contributions of significance to even begin to be discussed within this introductory chapter alone. Therefore, the collective expectations of this current textbook are to show exactly how the many current applications and future innovative directions of radioguided surgery can impact upon all discipline within the clinical practice of surgery. As we move forward through the twenty-first century, we envision further growth of the current technological platforms of radioguided surgery, with a continued emphasis upon promoting integration of handheld radiation detection devices and advanced nuclear medicine molecular imaging for guiding and optimizing the intraoperative detection and resection of conditions affecting both cancer and noncancer patients.

References

1. Povoski SP, Neff RL, Mojzisik CM, O'Malley DM, Hinkle GH, Hall NC, Murrey Jr DA, Knopp MV, Martin Jr EW. A comprehensive overview of radioguided surgery using gamma detection probe technology. World J Surg Oncol. 2009;7:11.
2. Selverstone B, Solomon AK, Sweet WH. Location of brain tumors by means of radioactive phosphorus. J Am Med Assoc. 1949;140:277–8.
3. Selverstone B, Sweet WH, Robinson CV. The clinical use of radioactive phosphorus in the surgery of brain tumors. Ann Surg. 1949;130:643–51.
4. Geiger H, Müller W. Elektronenzählrohr zur messung schwächster aktivitäten. Naturwissenschaften. 1928; 16:617–8.
5. Selverstone B, Sweet WH, Ireton RJ. Radioactive potassium, a new isotope for brain tumor localization. Surg Forum. 1950;1:371–5.
6. Selverstone B, White JC. Evaluation of the radioactive mapping technic in the surgery of brain tumors. Ann Surg. 1951;134:387–96.
7. Sweet WH. The uses of nuclear disintegration in the diagnosis and treatment of brain tumor. N Engl J Med. 1951;245:875–8.
8. Harris CC, Bigelow RR, Francis JE, Kelly GG, Bell PR. A CsI(TI)-crystal surgical scintillation probe. Nucleonics. 1956;14:102–8.
9. Reemtsma K, Ryan RF, Krementz ET, Creech Jr O. Treatment of selected adenocarcinomas by perfusion technique. AMA Arch Surg. 1959;78:724–7; discussion 727–8.
10. Stehlin Jr JS, Clark Jr RL, White EC, Smith Jr JL, Griffin AC, Jesse Jr RH, Healey Jr JE. Regional chemotherapy for cancer: experiences with 116 perfusions. Ann Surg. 1960;151:605–69.
11. Stehlin Jr JS, Clark Jr RL, White EC, Healey Jr JE, Dewey WC, Beerstecher S. The leakage factor in regional perfusion with chemotherapeutic agents. Arch Surg. 1960;80:934–45.
12. Stehlin Jr JS, Clark Jr RL, Dewey WC. Continuous monitoring of leakage during regional perfusion. Arch Surg. 1961;83:943–9.
13. Sardi A, Minton JP, Mojzisik C, Nieroda CA, Ferrara PJ, Hinkle GH, Thurston MO, Martin Jr EW. The use of a hand-held gamma detector improves the safety of isolated limb perfusion. J Surg Oncol. 1989;41:172–6.
14. Harvey WC, Lancaster JL. Technical and clinical characteristics of a surgical biopsy probe. J Nucl Med. 1981;22:184–6.
15. Ghelman B, Thompson FM, Arnold WD. Intraoperative radioactive localization of an osteoid-osteoma. Case report. J Bone Joint Surg Am. 1981;63:826–7.

16. Ubhi CS, Hardy JG, Pegg CA. Mediastinal parathyroid adenoma: a new method of localization. Br J Surg. 1984;71:859–60.
17. Martinez DA, King DR, Romshe C, Lozano RA, Morris JD, O'Dorisio MS, Martin Jr E. Intraoperative identification of parathyroid gland pathology: a new approach. J Pediatr Surg. 1995;30:1306–9.
18. Norman J, Chheda H. Minimally invasive parathyroidectomy facilitated by intraoperative nuclear mapping. Surgery. 1997;122:998–1003; discussion 1003–4.
19. Aitken DR, Thurston MO, Hinkle Jr GH, Martin DT, Haagensen Jr DE, Houchens D, Tuttle SE, Martin Jr EW. Portable gamma probe for radioimmune localization of experimental colon tumor xenografts. J Surg Res. 1984;36:480–9.
20. Aitken DR, Hinkle GH, Thurston MO, Tuttle SE, Martin DT, Olsen J, Haagensen Jr DE, Houchens D, Martin Jr EW. A gamma-detecting probe for radioimmune detection of CEA-producing tumors, Successful experimental use and clinical case report. Dis Colon Rectum. 1984;27:279–82.
21. Martin DT, Hinkle GH, Tuttle S, Olsen J, Nabi H, Houchens D, Thurston M, Martin Jr EW. Intraoperative radioimmunodetection of colorectal tumors with a hand-held radiation detector. Am J Surg. 1985;150: 672–5.
22. Gould EA, Winship T, Philbin PH, Kerr HH. Observations on a "sentinel node" in cancer of the parotid. Cancer. 1960;13:77–8.
23. Cabanas RM. An approach for the treatment of penile carcinoma. Cancer. 1977;39:456–66.
24. Riveros M, Garcia R, Cabañas R. Lymphadenography of the dorsal lymphatics of the penis. Technique and results. Cancer. 1967;20:2026–31.
25. Morton DL, Wen DR, Wong JH, Economou JS, Cagle LA, Storm FK, Foshag LJ, Cochran AJ. Technical details of intraoperative lymphatic mapping for early stage melanoma. Arch Surg. 1992;127:392–9.
26. Alex JC, Weaver DL, Fairbank JT, Rankin BS, Krag DN. Gamma-probe-guided lymph node localization in malignant melanoma. Surg Oncol. 1993;2:303–8.
27. Krag DN, Weaver DL, Alex JC, Fairbank JT. Surgical resection and radiolocalization of the sentinel lymph node in breast cancer using a gamma probe. Surg Oncol. 1993;2:335–9; discussion 340.
28. Cox CE, Hyacinthe M, Berman C, Dupont EL, Wagner A. Localization of an occult primary breast cancer with technetium-99m sestamibi scan and an intraoperative gamma probe. Cancer Control. 1996;3:448–50.
29. Luini A, Zurrida S, Galimberti V, Paganelli G. Radioguided surgery of occult breast lesions. Eur J Cancer. 1998;34:204–5.
30. Luini A, Zurrida S, Paganelli G, Galimberti V, Sacchini V, Monti S, Veronesi P, Viale G, Veronesi U. Comparison of radioguided excision with wire localization of occult breast lesions. Br J Surg. 1999;86:522–5.
31. Gennari R, Galimberti V, De Cicco C, Zurrida S, Zerwes F, Pigatto F, Luini A, Paganelli G, Veronesi U. Use of technetium-99m-labeled colloid albumin for preoperative and intraoperative localization of nonpalpable breast lesions. J Am Coll Surg. 2000;190: 692–8; discussion 698–9.
32. Dauway EL, Sanders R, Friedland J, Berman C, Ku NN, Reintgen DS, Yeatman T, Falcone R, Crawford S, Cox CE. Innovative diagnostics for breast cancer: new frontiers for the new millennium using radioactive seed localization. Surg Forum. 1999;50:348–9.
33. Gray RJ, Giuliano R, Dauway EL, Cox CE, Reintgen DS. Radioguidance for nonpalpable primary lesions and sentinel lymph node(s). Am J Surg. 2001;182:404–6.
34. Gray RJ, Salud C, Nguyen K, Dauway E, Friedland J, Berman C, Peltz E, Whitehead G, Cox CE. Randomized prospective evaluation of a novel technique for biopsy or lumpectomy of nonpalpable breast lesions: radioactive seed versus wire localization. Ann Surg Oncol. 2001;8:711–5.

Part II

Detailed Methodology Part

Physics of Radioguided Surgery: Basic Principles and Methods of Radiation Detection

2

Thomas Wendler, Uta Eberlein, and Michael Lassmann

Contents

T. Wendler (✉)
Lehrstuhl für Informatikanwendungen in der Medizin & Augmented Reality, Technische Universität München, Munich, Germany

Nuklearmedizinische Klinik und Poliklinik, Klinikum rechts der Isar der Technischen Universität München, Munich, Germany
e-mail: wendler@tum.de

U. Eberlein • M. Lassmann
Klinik und Poliklinik für Nuklearmedizin, Universitätsklinikum Würzburg, Würzburg, Germany

Abstract

Radioguided surgery requires a significant amount of technology for its implementation. As a result, surgeons working in this field must have a basic know-how that extends beyond the standard surgical training and covers the relevant physics. Within this chapter we have tried to synthesize the background knowledge needed for a complete understanding of the most important aspects and processes. The terminology and the explanations target people just starting in the field, and the contents should prove readily intelligible as long as the complete chapter is read.

K. Herrmann et al. (eds.), *Radioguided Surgery: Current Applications and Innovative Directions in Clinical Practice*, DOI 10.1007/978-3-319-26051-8_2

2.1 Radioactivity

Radioactivity is a manifestation of the weak force or the weak nuclear force, one of the four fundamental physical interactions.[1] Radioactivity,[2] also known as radioactive decay or nuclear decay, is a process in which a nucleus of an unstable atom (the "parent") transforms into a more stable one (the "daughter") by releasing energy in the form of particles and/or γ rays. The way in which this energy is released depends on the internal structure of the parent nucleus. This structure is understood as the amount of protons and neutrons of the nucleus as well as its level of excitation. In order to distinguish atoms of the same chemical element with a different nuclear structure and energy content, reference is commonly made to *nuclides*.

The officially accepted nomenclature for nuclides is denoted by the mass number *A*, i.e., the sum of protons and neutrons, using one of the following forms:

- *Z-A*, e.g., In-111, F-18
- ^{A}Z, e.g., ^{68}Ga, ^{123}I

Commonly only one level of energy excitation of a nucleus exists; however, some atoms may have different so-called metastable levels of excitation (levels that are sufficiently stable to be detected). In order to refine the nomenclature just presented, such nuclides are designated by the letter "m" following their mass number *A*, e.g., Tc-99m is a different nuclide from Tc-99 since the former has a higher level energy. If there are several metastable levels of energy, then an integer is added to the "m," i.e., m^2, m^3, etc.

In general, nuclides that eventually undergo nuclear decay are termed *radioactive* or, in nuclear technology jargon, *radionuclides*. On the other hand, nuclides that do not decay for a significant amount of time are termed *stable*.

A common representation of stable and unstable nuclides is the mass/atomic number plot (Fig. 2.1), where all existing nuclides are plotted and marked according to the main decay modes. Normally the nuclides with a lower mass number than the stable nuclides are β^+ emitters, while those with a higher mass number than the stable nuclides are β^- emitters.

2.2 Half-Life

Radioactive decay is a random process, which, as such, cannot be predicted or triggered by any external condition.[3] According to quantum theory, the probability that a single radioactive atom will decay follows an exponential law. This means that independently of how long a radioactive atom has existed, the likelihood *p* that it will decay within a certain period doubles at constant time intervals. One of these intervals is called a half-life, denoted $T_{1/2}$:

$$2 \times p\left(T_{1/2}\right) = p\left(2 \times T_{1/2}\right)$$

In practice this means that for a given radionuclide, the number of radioactive atoms *N* will diminish on average by half within one half-life:

$$N\left(T_{1/2}\right) = \frac{N(0)}{2}$$

[1] Today's physics distinguishes four major independent interactions: gravitation, electromagnetism, and the two nuclear forces (the weak and the strong).

[2] The term "radioactivity" derives from Marie Curie [1], who discovered this process in radium, which was among the first elements to be discovered by her and her husband, Pierre, at the turn of the nineteenth century.

[3] As mentioned above, radioactivity is an independent fundamental interaction.

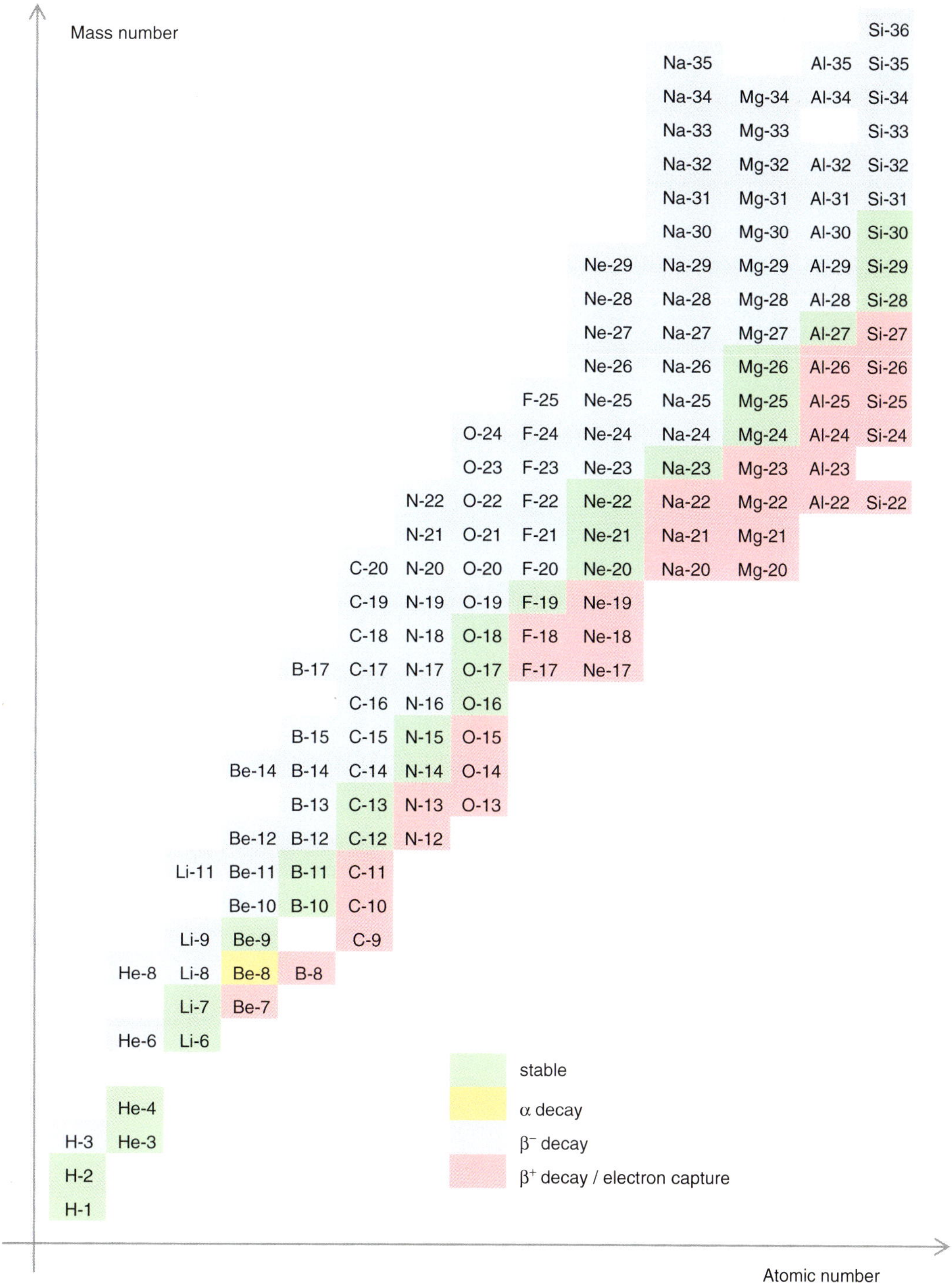

Fig. 2.1 Mass/atomic number plot for the first 15 elements of the periodic table. The *x*-axis shows the atomic number, which is the number of protons in the nucleus; the *y*-axis shows the mass number, the sum of protons and neutrons. The *color* indicates the main decay modes of the corresponding nuclide (Table generated using data extracted from [2])

In general the number of radioactive atoms $N(t)$ at a time t, with an amount $N(t_0)$ at a time point t_0, is given by

$$N(t) = N(t_0) \times e^{-\frac{ln2}{T_{1/2}}t} = N(t_0) \times e^{-\lambda t}$$

The rate of decays per second (λ) of a radioactive material is its radioactivity and is characteristic for each nuclide. The SI unit used to describe one decay per second is a *Becquerel*,[4] *Bq*. Some countries still use the unit *Curie*,[5] *Ci* and 1 Ci = 3.7×10^{10} Bq. Common radioactivity values in radioguided surgery are kBq to MBq or μCi to mCi.

2.3 Decay Modes

Depending on the nuclear structure and internal energy of a nuclide, different types of radioactive decay are likely. The most common or best known are α, β, and γ decay; however, these are not the only types. The types of decay most relevant to radioguided surgery are explained below.

2.3.1 β⁺ Decay

β⁺ decay (Fig. 2.2) is fundamental to the development of positron emission tomography (PET) and the use of PET nuclides in radioguided surgery. Within a β⁺ decay, a proton p in the nucleus of the decaying atom converts into a neutron, emitting a positively charged electron e^+ (also known as a positron or antielectron) and a neutrino ν:

$$p \rightarrow n + e^+ + \nu$$

An example of this decay is F-18, the workhorse for PET imaging, which emits a positron in 96.7 % of cases and converts into a negatively charged O-18:

$$^{18}F \rightarrow {}^{18}O^- + e^+ + \nu$$

[4]The unit Becquerel honors the discoverer of radioactivity, Henri Becquerel [1].

[5]In honor of Marie and Pierre Curie, pioneers in the understanding of radioactivity

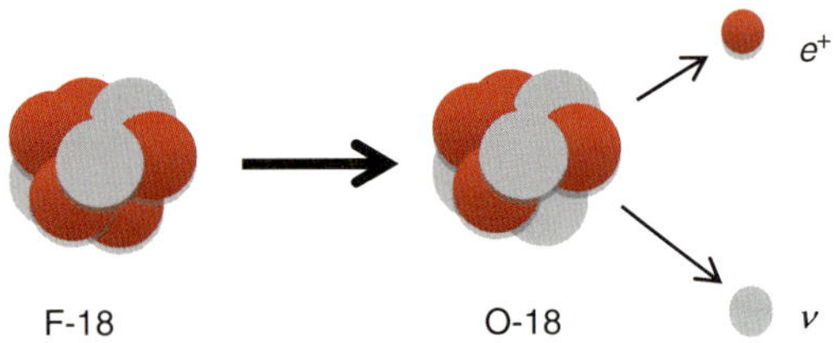

Fig. 2.2 Example of β⁺ decay: F-18 decays to 97 % in O-18 with a half-life of 109.77 min and a β⁺ maximum energy of 633.5 keV (Data from [2])

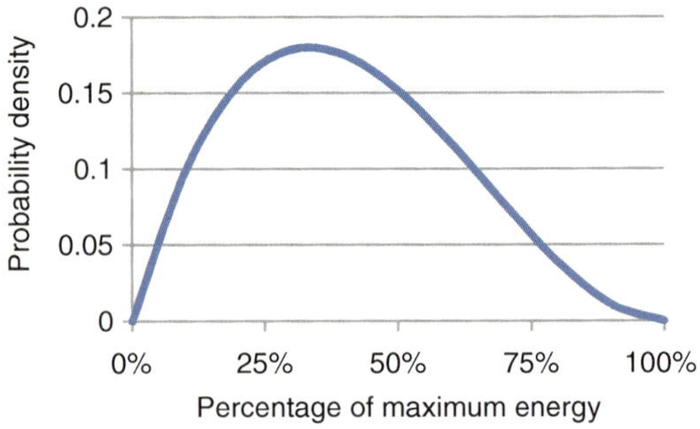

Fig. 2.3 Schematic shape of positron emission spectrum as a function of the energy of the emitted positron. The average energy of a positron is roughly two-thirds of the maximum energy

Following the law of conservation of energy, the energy released in this nuclear decay is divided between the positron, the neutrino and the daughter nuclide. As a result the positron has a continuous spectrum of energy with a fixed maximum [3] (Fig. 2.3). In the case of F-18, the maximum energy is 633.5 keV.

If the resulting nucleus after the decay is a short-lived metastable state, the β⁺ decay can be followed by a prompt (almost immediate) γ decay (see below, isomeric transition).

2.3.2 β⁻ Decay

β⁻ decay (Fig. 2.4) is commonly used in nuclear medicine for therapy as these particles deposit their energy very close to the place where they have been emitted. Nevertheless, secondary γ rays or bremstrahlung X-rays emitted can be used for radioguided surgery, as in the case of I-131, a nuclide used for therapy and imaging.

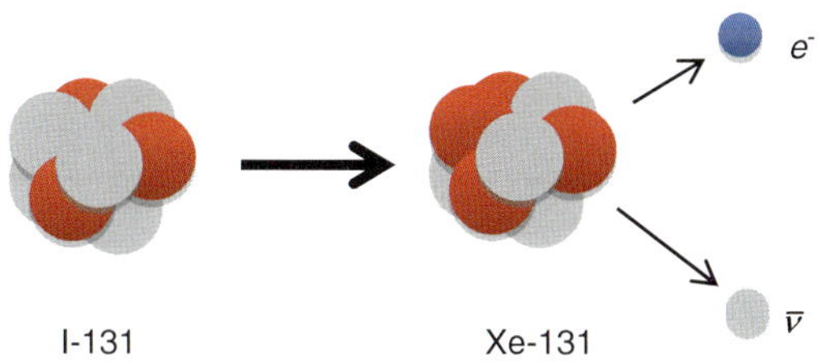

Fig. 2.4 Example of β– decay: I-131 decays to 89.9 % in Xe-131 with a half-life of 8.02 days and a β^- maximum energy of 606 MeV (Data from [2])

Similar to β^+ decay, where a charged particle is expelled from the nucleus, in β^- decay an electron e^- is emitted. During this process a neutron n transforms into a proton p, an electron e^-, and an antineutrino $\bar{\nu}$:

$$n \rightarrow p + e^- + \bar{\nu}$$

In I-131 different energy states are possible, resulting in a variety of β^- decays, each with a different maximum energy. The most frequent (89.9 % of all decays) maximum energy is 606 keV [2]:

$$^{131}I \rightarrow {}^{131}Xe^+ + e^- + \bar{\nu}$$

As in the β^+ decay, there is no rule for the distribution of energy between electron, antineutrino, and daughter nuclide, resulting in a spectrum with a similar bell shape to that in Fig. 2.3.

Also, it is possible for a β^- decay to be followed by an almost immediate (prompt) γ decay, as happens during the β^- decay of I-131, when several γ rays are emitted, the most relevant being at 364 keV.

2.3.3 Electron Capture

A more interesting and complex decay mode is the so-called electron capture [4] or inverse β decay (Fig. 2.5).

Nuclei like F-18 also may become more stable by capturing an electron from the inner orbits and making a neutron out of it and a proton. A neutrino is also emitted in this case:

$$p + e^- \rightarrow n + \nu$$

In the case of F-18, 3 % [2] of all decays are electron captures, which are described by

$$^{18}F \rightarrow {}^{18}O + \nu$$

The drop in energy of the nucleus in this process is emitted in the form of γ rays or is passed to an electron. In the particular case of F-18, there is one γ ray emission at 1.34 MeV.

Electron captures commonly result in additional radiation, since X-rays or light are also frequently emitted. The explanation for this is that the missing (captured) electron in the inner orbit will then cause higher orbit electrons to fall into the lower orbit, emitting characteristic X-rays or light (Fig. 2.5). Alternatively the energy may be passed to another outer shell electron, which is then expelled from the atom (Auger effect[6]) [5].

A relevant example of an electron capture in radioguided surgery is Co-57, used for the calibration of detectors, as described below:

$$^{57}Co \rightarrow {}^{57}Fe + \nu$$

The decay of Co-57 produces at least three γ rays of relevance and a wide spectrum of characteristic X-rays (Table 2.1).

2.3.4 γ Decay

The γ decay provides the foundation for single-photon emission computed tomography (SPECT).

There are two relevant types of γ emission in radioguided surgery. The simplest derives from an isomeric transition. In this case, a nucleus in an excited state releases energy in the form of γ rays but its nuclear structure remains unchanged. The excited state is normally denoted by a "*" to the right of the element symbol:

$$^{A}Z^* \rightarrow {}^{A}Z$$

In the particular case when the excited state does not generate a prompt emission but rather a

[6] Effect named after Pierre Auger, who in 1923 discovered it independently from Lise Meitner, who was the first to report on it shortly beforehand in 1922 [5]

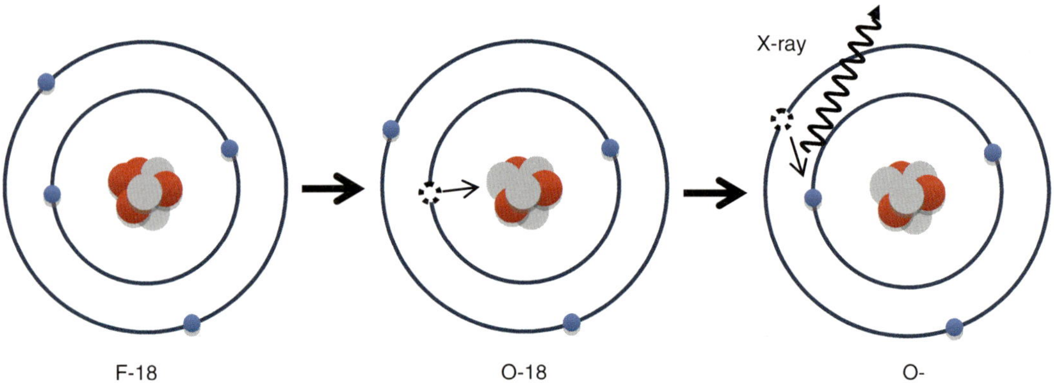

Fig. 2.5 Example of electron capture: F-18 decays to 3 % in O-18 [2], capturing an electron from the K shell. A neutrino is also emitted in the first step (not shown). The K shell electron hole is replaced by an L shell electron, resulting in the emission of a characteristic X-ray or an Auger electron

Table 2.1 The most frequent γ rays and characteristic X-rays of Co-57

γ rays		Characteristic X-rays		
E (keV)	*P* (%)	*E* (keV)	*P* (%)	X-ray
14.4	9.16	0.7	0.56	Fe $L_{\alpha 1}$
122.1	85.60	0.72	0.42	Fe $L_{\beta 1}$
136.5	10.68	6.39	16.40	Fe $K_{\alpha 2}$
692	0.16	6.4	32.60	Fe $K_{\alpha 1}$
		7.06	1.99	Fe $K_{\beta 3}$
		7.06	3.88	Fe $K_{\beta 1}$

Data taken from [2]

delayed emission, one speaks of a metastable state, which is denoted by an "m," as explained above:

$$^{Am}Z \rightarrow {}^{A}Z$$

Tc-99m is an example of a pure γ decay producing several γ rays, the 142-keV γ ray being the most relevant.

2.4 Nuclides Used in Radioguided Surgery

To close this section, Table 2.2 lists the most relevant nuclides in radioguided surgery.

2.5 Interaction of Radiation and Matter

After a radioactive decay, the emitted particles interact with matter. These interactions play a relevant role in the way in which the radioactive source is detected during the surgical procedure and also how and whether the radiation reaches the detector. Commonly a distinction is drawn between interactions of charged particles (β^+ and β^- particles) and γ or X-rays.

2.5.1 γ or X-Ray Interactions

When a γ or an X-ray (a photon) hits an atom, its energy can be transferred to the atom and in particular to its electrons. There are two major interactions that need to be considered at the levels of energy used in radioguided surgery.

The first interaction takes place when the energy of an incident photon is completely absorbed by an electron. In this case one speaks of the photoelectric effect[7] (Fig. 2.6). In the photoelectric effect, as the energy of the photon is completely transferred, the photon disappears (complete absorption). Further, the electron that has received this energy is expelled from the atom. This effect commonly occurs if the incident photon hits a lower shell electron.

The expelled electron is commonly called a photoelectron, and it carries the kinetic energy resulting from the energy of the incident photon minus the binding energy of the electron when it was in the atom. As a result a photoelectric effect can only happen if the incident photon has sufficient energy to free an electron in the given atom.

[7] The first explanation of the photoelectric effect in terms of currently accepted physics comes from Albert Einstein [6].

Table 2.2 Most frequent nuclides used in radioguided surgery for both intraoperative detection and calibration

Nuclide	Half-life	Main decay modes	γ, X, or max. β energy	Probability of emission (%)	Use
C-11	20.4 min	β^+	960 keV	100	PET
F-18	109.7 min	β^+	633 keV	97	PET
Na-22	2.60 a	EC (γ)	1.27 MeV	100	None
		β^+	546 keV	90	Calibration/QC
Co-57	271.8 days	EC (γ)	122 keV	86	Calibration/QC
		EC (γ)	136 keV	11	Calibration/QC
Ga-68	67.6 min	β^+	1.90 MeV	88	PET
		β^+	2.92 MeV	9	PET
Zr-89	78.4 h	EC (γ)	909 keV	100	None
		β^+	902 keV	23	PET
Tc-99m	6.01 h	IT	142 keV	89	SPECT
In-111	2.80 days	EC (γ)	171 keV	90	SPECT
		EC (γ)	245 keV	94	SPECT
I-123	13.3 h	EC (γ)	158 keV	83	SPECT
		EC (X)	27 keV	72	None
		EC (X)	31 keV	12	None
I-124	4.18 days	EC (γ)	602 keV	63	None
		EC (γ)	722 keV	10	None
		EC (γ)	1.69 MeV	11	None
		β^+	1.53 MeV	12	PET
		β^+	2.14 MeV	11	PET
I-125	59.4 days	EC (γ)	35 keV	7	Marker
		EC (γ)	27 keV	100	Marker
		EC (γ)	31 keV	20	Marker
I-131	8.02 days	IT	364 keV	82	SPECT
		IT	637 keV	7	None
		β^-	333 keV	7	Therapy
		β^-	606 keV	90	Therapy

Data taken from [2]
PET nuclides are used for direct β^+ detection or detection of annihilation photons. SPECT nuclides are used for γ detection. In particular I-125 is used for solid markers implanted in tissue interventionally to guide surgical resection
QC quality control, *EC* electron capture, *IT* isomeric transition

Of major relevance is the fact that if an electron expelled is from a low shell, it is common for a characteristic X-ray or light to be emitted, as described in the section on γ decay.

If a photon is not completely absorbed by an atom, one speaks of the Compton[8] effect (Fig. 2.7). Therein only part of the energy of a photon is transferred to an electron. As a result, a lower energy photon is scattered in a direction which can be calculated from its final energy. As in the photoelectric effect, the electron absorbing the energy is expelled from the atom. Commonly this electron is called a Compton recoil electron. This effect takes place with higher shell electrons that are loosely bound.

Given an energy E_0 of the incident photon, a final energy $E(\theta)$, and a scattering angle θ, one has

$$E(\theta) = \frac{E_0 m_e c^2}{m_e c^2 + E_0 (1 - \cos\theta)}$$

In the above formula, the constant m_e is the mass of an electron and c the speed of light. The constant $m_e c^2$ is commonly given as 511 keV.

[8] In honor of Arthur H. Compton, who first observed and reported this in 1923 [7]

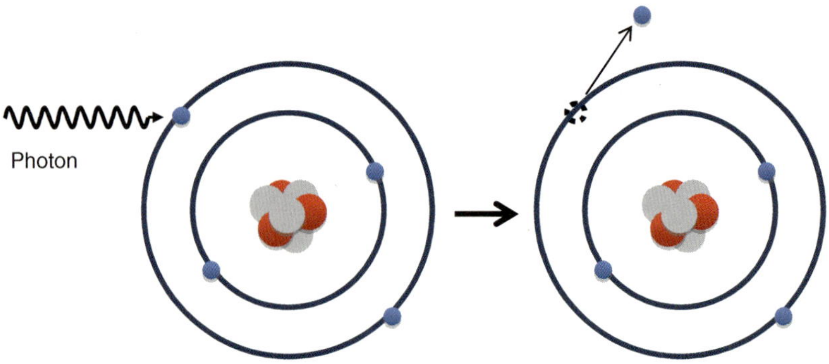

Fig. 2.6 Photoelectric effect, where a photon is completely absorbed by an atom. Its energy is transferred to an electron, which is then expelled from the atom

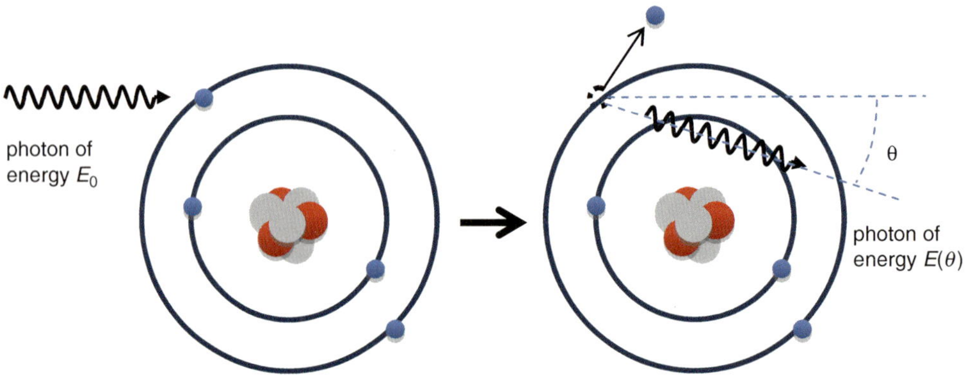

Fig. 2.7 The Compton effect, wherein a photon is scattered by a loosely bound electron of an outer shell, losing energy and freeing the electron with which it collided

Following this formula the scattering can be in any direction. Photons that are scattered by 180° or "backscattered" lose the most energy.

The likelihood that a photon will undergo a photoelectric or a Compton effect depends on its energy and the material through which it passes. A way to model this takes into account the fact that, given a certain path through a material, the likelihood that a photon will be absorbed follows an exponential law. An amount I_0 of gamma rays or X-rays passing a distance x of a material is absorbed, resulting in a diminished amount $I(x)$, as shown in Fig. 2.8:

$$I(x) = I_0 e^{-\tau_l x - \sigma_l x}$$

The coefficient τ_l is the linear attenuation coefficient due to the photoelectric effect, and σ_l is the linear attenuation coefficient due to the Compton effect.

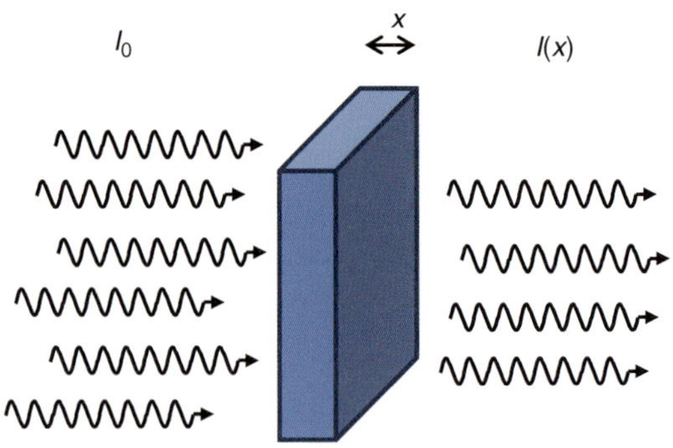

Fig. 2.8 Attenuation of intensity of γ rays crossing a distance x of a material

Commonly one uses the linear attenuation coefficient μ_l due to both interactions:

$$\mu_l = \tau_l + \sigma_l$$

The distribution between the photoelectric effect and the Compton effect depends on the material and the energy of the incident photons (see Fig. 2.9 as example for water).

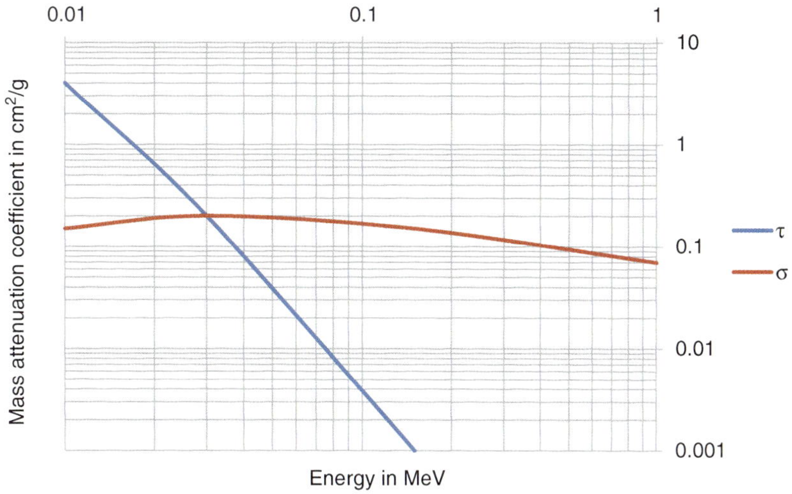

Fig. 2.9 Relative value of mass attenuation coefficient for the photoelectric and the Compton effect for water as a function of the energy of the incident photon (Data taken from [8])

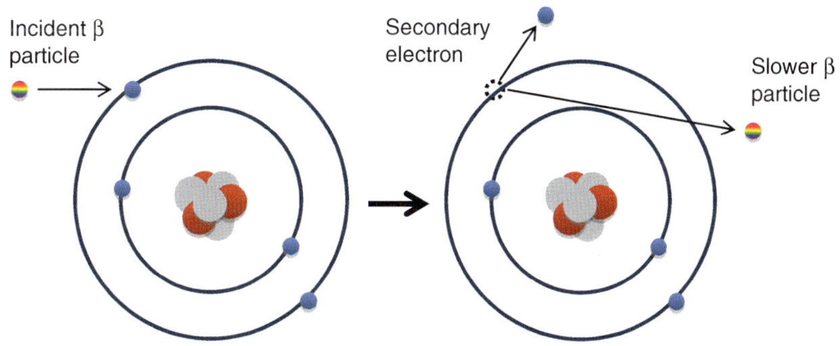

Fig. 2.10 Collision between a β particle and an electron, generating a secondary electron and slowing down the β particle

The quantity used in Fig. 2.9 is the mass attenuation coefficient μ_m, which can be derived from the linear attenuation coefficient μ_l and the density of the material ρ.

2.6 Interaction of β Particles

β^+ and β^- are charged particles. As a result, their interactions with matter are mainly dominated by their charge and the interaction of it with electrons or the nucleus. In these interactions the charged particles lose energy. Among these interactions, the particular case of β^+ annihilation plays an important role in radioguided surgery.

2.6.1 Interactions with Electrons

There are two main interactions of β particles with electrons: collision with an orbital electron and orbital electron excitation.

In the collision with an electron, the charged particle passes energy to the orbital electron, expelling it from its orbit. This expelled electron is frequently referred to as a secondary electron (Fig. 2.10). As explained in the section on γ decay, the fact that an electron is expelled can cause emission of a characteristic X-ray.

Even if the β particle does not collide with an orbital electron, it may still pass energy to it, bringing it to a higher excitation level. In this case, of course, the β particle still loses energy and slows down, but no secondary electron is generated.

2.6.2 Interactions with the Nucleus

A β particle can interact not only with electrons but also with the nuclei of the atoms in its path. This interaction normally results in a major change in the trajectory of the β particle and the emission of photons. These photons are known as bremsstrahlung, from the German "braking radiation" (Fig. 2.11).

The likelihood (percentage $P_{\text{Bremsstrahlung}}$) that bremsstrahlung will occur relative to collisions or excitation is roughly approximated by an equation involving the maximum energy of the β particle *(E_β)* and the atomic number *Z* of the material through which the β particle passes [9]:

$$P_{\text{Bremsstrahlung}} \approx \frac{ZE_\beta}{3000\ \text{MeV}}$$

2.6.3 β⁺ Annihilation

If a β^+ loses its complete kinetic energy (or comes close to doing so), it will combine with an electron in an atomic matter–antimatter reaction. This reaction will convert both particles to pure energy. Due to the law of conservation of energy and momentum, the energy will then be dissipated in the form of two 180° oriented photons, each with the energy equivalent to the mass of the electron/positron, i.e., 511 keV (Fig. 2.12).

If the positron has not been completely stopped, the two photons may display a small deviation from the 180° orientation, canonically explained in physics books.

2.6.4 Penetration of β Particles in Tissue

Unlike γ rays, β particles do not follow an exponential law in terms of penetration. Rather, owing to the complexity of the interactions and the fact that their emission energy is not a line but a spectrum, empirical formulas have to be used.

A common approach is the use of the formula given by Katz and Penfold [10], where the tissue-independent range *R* in g/cm² of a β particle of an energy *E* in MeV is given by

$$R = \begin{cases} 0.412E^{1.265-0.0945\ \ln E} & 0.01 < E < 2.5\ \text{MeV} \\ 0.530E - 0.106 & E < 2.5\ \text{MeV} \end{cases}$$

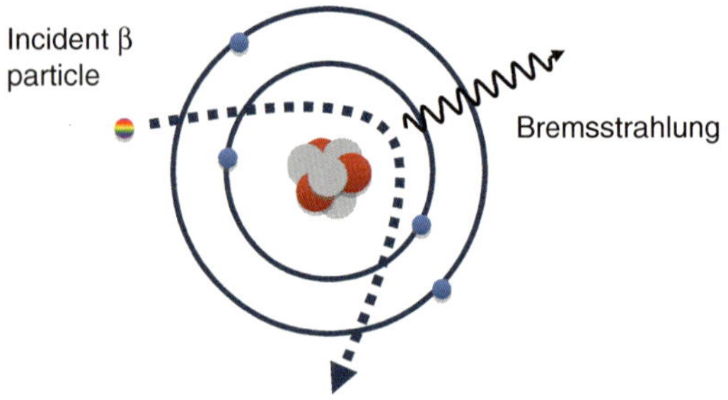

Fig. 2.11 Bremsstrahlung caused by a strong change in the trajectory of a β particle passing close to a nucleus

2.7 Detection of Radiation

In the previous sections, the basic principles of radioactivity and its interaction with matter have been discussed. These principles govern the way in which radiation is emitted and "comes out of the patient." They also explain the process of detection, a key part of radioguided surgery. Within this section, only the most relevant technologies for detection will be considered.

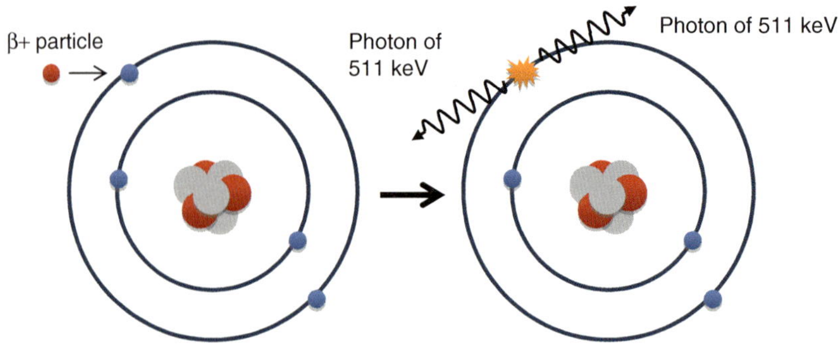

Fig. 2.12 Annihilation of β+ and orbital electron. The energy of the mass of both particles is emitted in the form of two photons at almost 180° to each other

2.7.1 Scintillator Crystals and Light Detection

During the early days of X-ray imaging, it was realized that some crystals will shine if they are placed close to a radioactive source. This effect was termed scintillation and crystals behaving in this way were called scintillators.

In scintillation, a γ ray or a β particle interacts with electrons by the effects described above in such a way that either free electrons or photons are emitted. They on their own interact again and eventually a significant amount of the energy is deposited in the material and then re-emitted in the form of light. The total generated light intensity is proportional to the energy deposited in the crystal. If the emitted light is visible, humans will be able to see the scintillation.

If used for detection of radiation, this effect is very convenient as photon-counting techniques are widely available. The ones most commonly used in radioguided surgery are explained below.

2.7.2 Photomultiplier Tubes

Photomultiplier tubes (PMTs) are still the most used technology in nuclear medicine for photon counting.

Their mechanism of action consists first in converting an incident light photon into an electron using a photocathode, a thin-layer vapor-deposited conducting material. The reason why a photocathode emits an electron is explained by the previously described photoelectric effect.

The photoelectron is amplified by the use of a strong electric field (voltages in the range of a few thousand volts) and so-called dynodes (Fig. 2.13). Dynodes are nothing more than electrodes each at a higher potential than the previous one. They enable an iterative process. In practice the first photoelectrons are accelerated to the first dynode, which they hit, generating secondary electrons. These are then accelerated to the next dynode, where they generate more secondary electrons as they arrive. After several steps the initial light and small amount of photoelectrons reaches several orders of magnitude so that when the last electrode (the anode) is hit, a clear electrical peak can be measured.

The amplification process of a PMT takes ~50 ns. A normal design of a PMT has ~10 dynodes, each generating ~5 secondary electrons per incident electron. As a result, a typical amplification factor is 10^7 [11].

It is important to note that due to variations in construction, voltages, temperature, inpurities, PMTs coupled to scintillators only reach energy resolutions in the range of 8.5–50 % at 122 keV [11]. On the other hand, due to the large differences in crystals, their area of application is wide.

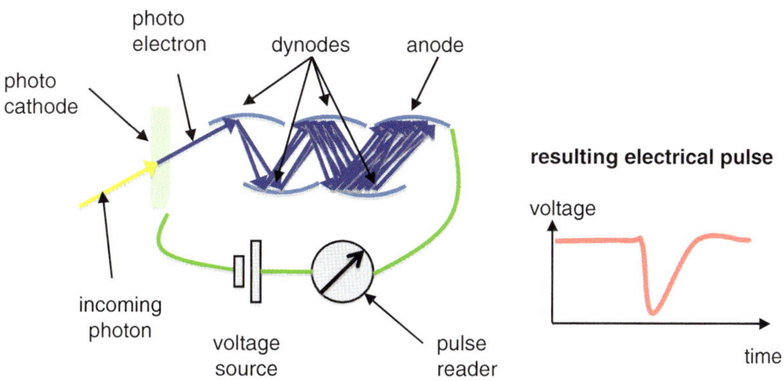

Fig. 2.13 Schematic representation of a PMT. The incoming photon is converted into a photoelectron in the photocathode. This is then accelerated to the first dynode. When the dynode is hit, several secondary electrons are generated. They are then accelerated to the next dynode and the process is repeated. Once the cascade of electrons reaches the anode, a pulse is detected

Table 2.3 The most relevant scintillating crystals in radioguided surgery: thallium-doped sodium and cesium iodine [NaI(Tl) and CsI(Tl)], sodium-doped cesium iodine [CsI(Na)], bismuth germanate (BGO), and lutetium-yttrium oxyorthosilicate (LYSO)

	NaI(Tl)	CsI(Tl)	CsI(Na)	BGO	LYSO
Density [g/cm^3]	3.67	4.51	4.51	7.13	7.15
Hygroscopic	Yes	Slightly	Yes	No	No
Light yield [photons/MeV γ]	38×10^3	54×10^3	41×10^3	9×10^3	32×10^3
Primary decay time [μs]	0.25	1	0.63	0.3	0.041

Data taken from [12]

2.7.3 Silicon Photomultipliers

Silicon photomultipliers (SiPMs) have been developed during the past two decades. They essentially combine several avalanche photodiodes (APDs) in arrays for linear light amplification. Their main advantages over PMTs are a reduced size, the need for significantly lower voltages (<100 V), a higher speed, and immunity to electromagnetic fields. Gains are in ranges similar to those achieved by PMTs [8].

A SiPM consists of up to 1000 APDs per square millimeter working in Geiger mode. This makes it possible to detect up to that amount of photons simultaneously per area unit. The moment a photon hits an APD, it will fire, resulting in a pulse. If more photons arrive at the same time, the pulse will be proportional to the amount of incident photons [8].

2.7.4 Scintillating Crystals

PMTs and SiPMs are only one way to convert light into electrical signals. They always require a scintillator, a scintillating crystal, to convert radiation to light. A commonly used nomenclature for crystals employs their chemical formula, e.g., NaI – sodium iodine, followed by any type of doping used to change their basic characteristics in parenthesis, e.g., NaI(Tl) – thallium-doped sodium iodine.

The most important characteristics of these crystals are

1. Density: The denser a crystal, the higher the likelihood that it will detect higher energy radiation. As a result, in order to detect the 511 keV annihilation photons, crystals like BGO or LYSO are commonly used, whereas for the 140 keV of Tc-99m, NaI(Tl) is normally sufficient. The thickness at which the crystal can be manufactured also plays an important role here.
2. Hygroscopic character: Some crystals tend to absorb moisture from the air, resulting in a deterioration of the crystal in the long term. NaI(Tl) is a material for which this property is problematic; as a result, NaI(Tl) crystals are only used when well sealed from the exterior world.
3. Light yield: The greater the light yield from a crystal, the higher will be the sensitivity and the better the energy resolution. As a result, crystals like CsI(Tl) and LYSO are preferred for SPECT and PET, respectively, as they have a better light yield than comparable materials.
4. Primary decay time: If many photons are to be detected simultaneously or if coincidences are to be measured, a fast response is desirable.

A list of the main characteristics of the most important scintillators is displayed in Table 2.3.

2.8 Direct Radiation Detection

Semiconductors can also be used for radiation detection. As radiation passes through a semiconductor, it ionizes the material, which can be measured directly (Fig. 2.14).

In radioguided surgery in particular, CdTe and CdZnTe (CZT) alloys are commonly used. These

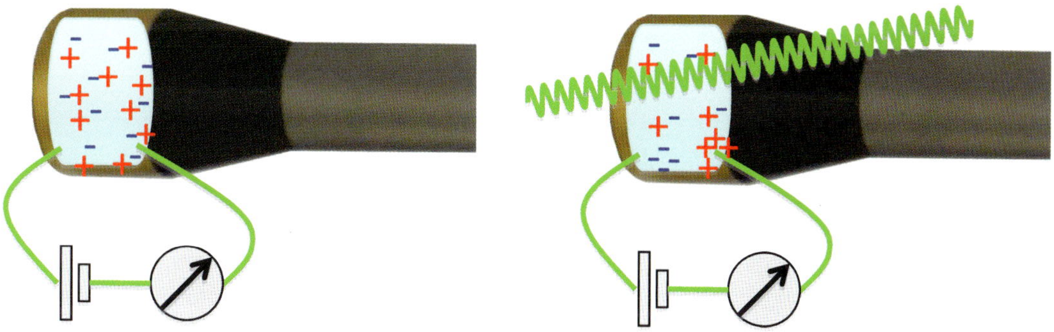

Fig. 2.14 Charges are distributed relatively homogeneously within the semiconductor; however, as a γ ray passes through it, negative and positive charges (electrons and holes) are separated and flow to the anode and cathode, respectively. This results in an electrical pulse, as explained in the section on PMTs

are very versatile and possess a major advantage over scintillator detectors in that they have a significantly higher energy resolution (~5 % versus ~9–10 % for properly tuned scintillator detectors [13]). In practice this plays a role in image quality and scatter rejection. A well-calibrated CZT detector will not detect much of a Co-57 source if it has been tuned for Tc-99m, while a scintillator detector will detect most γ rays emitted from Co-57 in its Tc-99m window.

2.9 Collimation and Radiation Shielding

Radiation detectors are not particularly useful for radioguided surgery if they are not properly shielded and collimated. Shielding entails surrounding part of the detector with a strong absorbing material such that no or only a little radiation is detected from regions at which the detector is not pointing.

For γ rays, the materials most commonly used for shielding are W (wolfram) and Pb (lead). The choice between these materials depends mainly on cost, weight, thickness, shape to be built, and the fact that Pb is toxic, so that it needs to be properly covered for use in medicine. Table 2.4 compares the two materials.

Shielding is much easier for β particles: only a few millimeters of Al (aluminium or aluminum) are sufficient to stop most β particles used in radioguided surgery.

Collimation is used to shape the radiation-sensitive region in front of a radiation detector.

Table 2.4 Comparison of *W* and Pb as shielding materials

	W	Pb
Density [g/cm^3]	19.25	11.34
Half-length [mm] @ 140 keV	0.23	0.3
Half-length [mm] @ 511 keV	2.6	3.7
Bulk modulus [GPa]	310	46

Data taken from [14, 15]

W has a stronger "stopping power"(as seen from the half-lengths in Table 2.4, a thinner layer of tungsten is needed to stop the same amount of γ rays than lead) than Pb; it is also harder and denser. However, it is significantly more expensive and harder to process. Half-length is the depth that a γ ray has to pass through the said material before losing half of its intensity

Depending upon whether the detector to be used is a single detector (a probe) or a 2D array of detectors (a camera), the collimation can have different shapes and different aspects need to be considered. Collimation is used in radioguided surgery in the context of the detection of γ rays, since β particles follow random paths and as such cannot be "collimated" (i.e., it is almost impossible to determine their origin, and shaping the region where they are detected is highly complex).

For gamma probes the choice of collimator entails a trade-off between sensitivity and spatial resolution. The sensitivity is commonly given as the counts per second (CPS) detected by the gamma probe from a source of 1 MBq situated at a certain distance. The spatial resolution is frequently given as the full-width half maximum

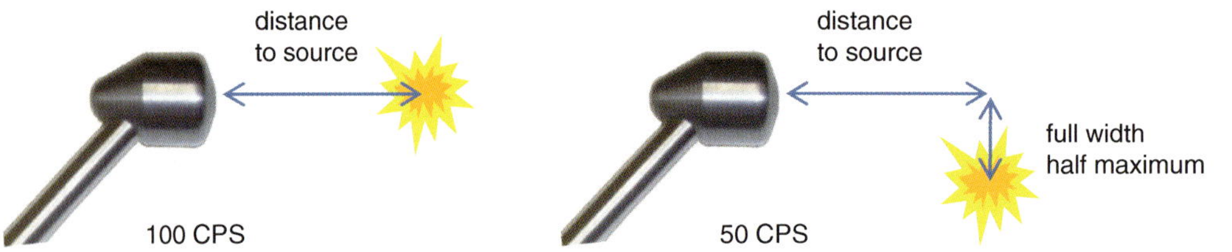

Fig. 2.15 Definition of spatial resolution in terms of full-width half maximum at a certain distance between source and probe

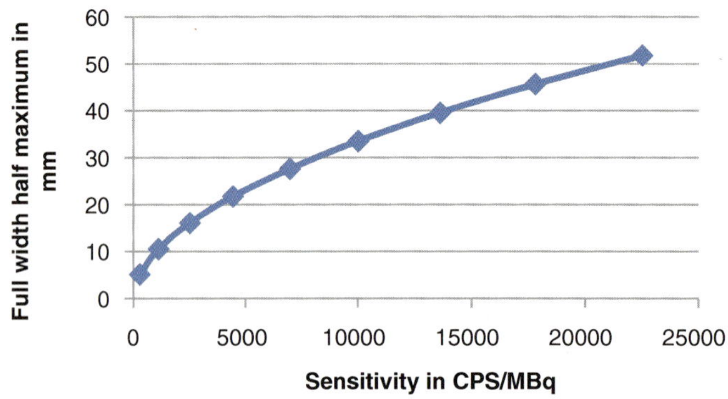

Fig. 2.16 Spatial resolution (in terms of full-width half maximum of a point source: the larger this number, the worse the resolution) as a function of sensitivity (the higher the better) for a standard gamma probe and a source at 30 mm. For this plot a cylindrical crystal of 6 mm diameter and 8 mm length and 2 mm tungsten shielding were assumed. If a high resolution is desired (e.g., 10 mm), the sensitivity is very poor, at 1000 CPS/MBq. On the other hand, a high sensitivity of 18,000 CPS/MBq yields a resolution of only 46 mm. A good trade-off (and common design in commercial gamma probes) would be a sensitivity of 10,000 CPS/MBq which generates a resolution of 33.5 mm

of a source at a certain distance, i.e., the displacement that the source has to have on the perpendicular axis for the detector to report half the counts (Fig. 2.15).

An example of the relation between spatial resolution and sensitivity for a standard gamma probe optimized for Tc-99m detection is given in Fig. 2.16.

In the case of gamma cameras, collimation is a far more complex issue owing to the availability of different collimator options. In general, two types are used: parallel hole collimators and pinhole collimators.

Pinhole collimators use the concept of a "camera obscura"; as a result, they produce high-resolution images of close objects and magnify them, while far objects are depicted as small spots (Fig. 2.17). The main problems with these collimators are their lack of sensitivity and the distortion effect, which may induce difficulties in interpretation.

Parallel hole collimators are used more frequently as they do not introduce any distortion. On the other hand, they have a limited field of view as only objects directly in front of them are seen, and these objects are "clipped" if they are partly outside this field of view (Fig. 2.18).

As with gamma probes, in gamma cameras, the collimator characteristics are also dependent on each other. Here, spatial resolution and sensitivity again play a role. In the particular case of parallel hole collimators, since only parallel incoming rays are considered, sensitivity is almost not a function of distance.

2.10 Measuring Radiation in the Human Body

In order to avoid injuries to incorrect structures and unnecessary extension of the search for hot lesions, it is vital that surgeons have an

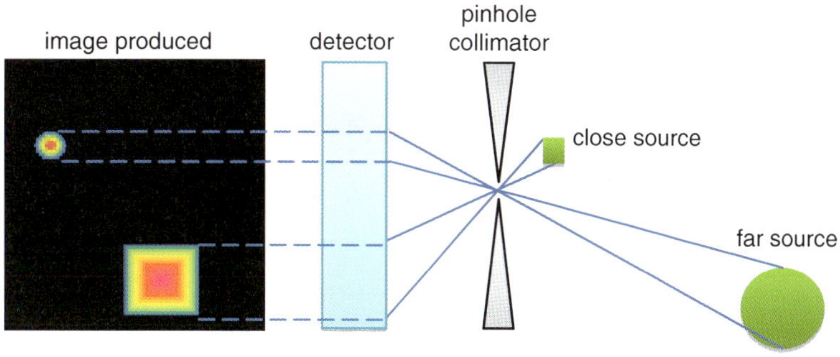

Fig. 2.17 Image produced by a gamma camera with a pinhole collimator. The close square object is depicted magnified as it is very close to the pinhole. The round object, on the other hand, is only a small dot in the camera image

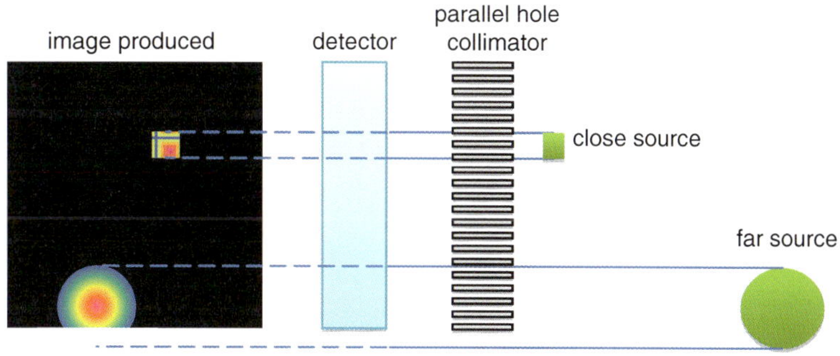

Fig. 2.18 Image produced by a gamma camera with a parallel hole collimator. The objects are depicted in their original shape, but there is clipping of the round object

understanding of the major effects of radiation in the body and the potential pitfalls arising from the underlying physics.

2.10.1 Interactions of Radiation with Tissue

As described in the section on the interactions of radiation with matter, different interactions may occur, primarily depending on the type of radiation. Since the task of radioguided surgery is to detect radioactive sources in the human body, the effects to be considered can be distinguished according to the type of emission traced.

The effect of geometry is, however, common for all types of radiation. Approximately, the amount I_D of radiation that a detector of diameter D receives from a source of intensity I_0 placed at a distance d is proportional to the quotient of their squares:

$$I_D \propto I_0 \times \frac{D^2}{d^2}$$

Put another way, the farther away the source is, the less radiation will be detected. It is still necessary for the surgeon to know approximately how deep he/she needs to go as small faint sources of activity may be detectable only at a close distance. This effect is purely geometric and is called, in the radioguided surgery jargon, the "solid angle effect."

2.10.2 γ or X-Ray Detection

Almost all radioguided procedures are based on γ or X-ray detection, since β particles have a short penetration in tissue. Independent of the origin of the γ or X-rays (γ decay, radioactive-related X-ray emissions, bremsstrahlung, or annihilation of β^+ particles) or the type of detector (γ probe or γ camera), the main interactions of γ or X-ray radiation with matter are absorption and scatter.

Absorption due to the photoelectric effect and geometry explains why sources in tissue farther away from the detector seem less active than closer sources with the same activity and solid angle. In tissue, attenuation due to this effect is not as high as in shielding material, collimators, or even the detector itself (the density of tissue is significantly lower than the densities of the

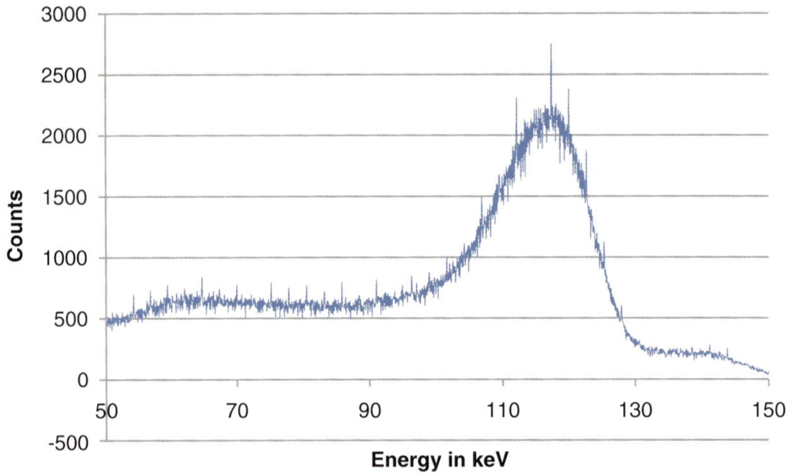

Fig. 2.19 Typical energy spectrum of a Co-57 source as seen by a CZT detector (here averaged over 256 pixels). The major peak consists mostly of "true" counts of the 122-keV peak of Co-57. Counts at lower energies result from electronic noise and, mainly, scatter (at lower energies). Counts at higher energy may also be attributable to electronic noise but mainly with the 136-keV peak of Co-57. An appropriate choice of the energy window would be to set the limits slightly below and slightly above the main peak to reduce most of the influence of electronic noise and scatter

collimator and detector materials), but it still exerts a major impact on the search for radioactive sources.

In tissue, Compton scatter is the predominant contributor to scatter in the energy range considered, causing photons to change trajectory and lose energy. In practice this means that if a γ detector is pointed at a structure which is not radioactive, it may still show a response to radiation due to photon scatter from a nearby structure. Appropriate choice of the energy window may reduce this effect but it cannot be completely eliminated (Fig. 2.19).

2.10.3 β Detection

If β particles are to be detected next to the solid angle effect, the sum of all interactions that the particle undergoes can be seen as the penetration. As mentioned in a previous section, penetration of β particles cannot be modeled easily in tissue, but a good approximation is the empiric formula of Katz and Penfold.

It needs to be borne in mind that β particles have a continuous energy spectrum. In most cases, this spectrum will have an average energy at approximately one-third of the maximum energy. As a consequence, for most relevant nuclides the penetration will be only a few millimeters. A thin layer of tissue can thus cover a radioactive source, so care should be taken not to overlook radioactive target tissue if a complete resection is needed.

2.11 Pitfalls during Radioguided Surgery

2.11.1 Fast Measurements, Fast Movements

First, there is one effect common to both γ or X-ray detection and β detection which influences detection, namely, the statistical nature of the radioactive decay coupled with the speed of detection (the speed of the electronics and especially the integration time of the detector).

As explained above, radioactive decays are random in nature and are independent of all physical effects around them. This forces to integrate measurements over a period of time, i.e., all

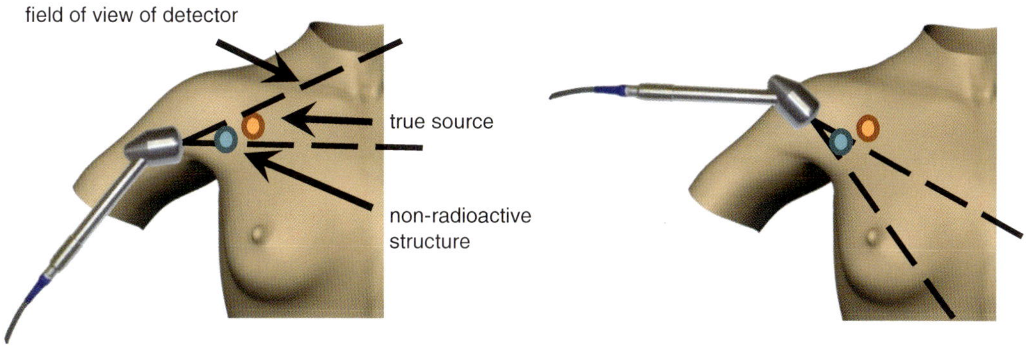

Fig. 2.20 Example of shine-through and how to avoid it. *Left*: Two structures are within the field of view of the detector, but only the deeper one is radioactive. *Right*: In order to avoid potential resection of a nonradioactive structure, the angle of the detector has to be changed such that it points away from potential sources, thereby ensuring that the structure is indeed radioactive

events detected within a sampling time are added. This is relevant to radioguided surgery as normally only minimal amounts of radioactivity are used and integration times are in the range of 0.5–10 s.

In practice, the structures for which the surgeon is looking commonly have count rates in the range of 10–30 CPS. In this case, a faint source can easily be overlooked if the detector is moved rapidly above it. For example, if a source emitting 30 CPS is pointed at the source for 1 s and there is a background activity of 20 CPS, there is an almost 50 % chance that a surgeon will miss it if he/she is using a discrimination threshold of 10 CPS. Even if the discrimination threshold is only 5 CPS, the likelihood of missing the source is about 15 %.

On top of this problem, it must be considered that rapid movement can also "smear" the radioactivity over an area, making it impossible for the user to distinguish a faint spot over a larger low-radioactivity area.

The solution is to move the detector slowly, if possible remaining for a few seconds above structures that potentially have activity. If it is expected that a low activity will be detected, then a longer integration time should be used and the detector should be held steady in the same position for the duration of this integration time.

2.11.2 Shine-Through

When performing a sentinel lymph node biopsy in a breast cancer patient, a procedure in which a radioactive lymph node is extracted from the axilla, it is not uncommon for the surgeon to remove a lymph node that he/she believes contains radioactivity only for measurement outside the body to reveal that this is not the case. Frequently the real radioactive lymph node lies directly behind it and slightly deeper.

This problem is called "shine-through." It is explained by the fact that due to improper handling of the detector, one structure is thought to be radioactive while the true radioactive structure is shining through it (Fig. 2.20).

The structure that shines through does not have to be the target structure. In procedures like sentinel lymph node biopsy, it is also possible for the injection site to be the source of the counts.

The way to avoid this pitfall is to try to point the gamma detector at the structure being analyzed from different angles so as to ensure that the radioactive structure is detected (cf. Fig. 2.20). Additionally, use of preoperative imaging, e.g., planar scintigraphy or SPECT/CT, or 3D intraoperative imaging such as freehand SPECT may help the surgeon to obtain a clearer view of the source of the radiation and thus avoid resection of a nonradioactive structure.

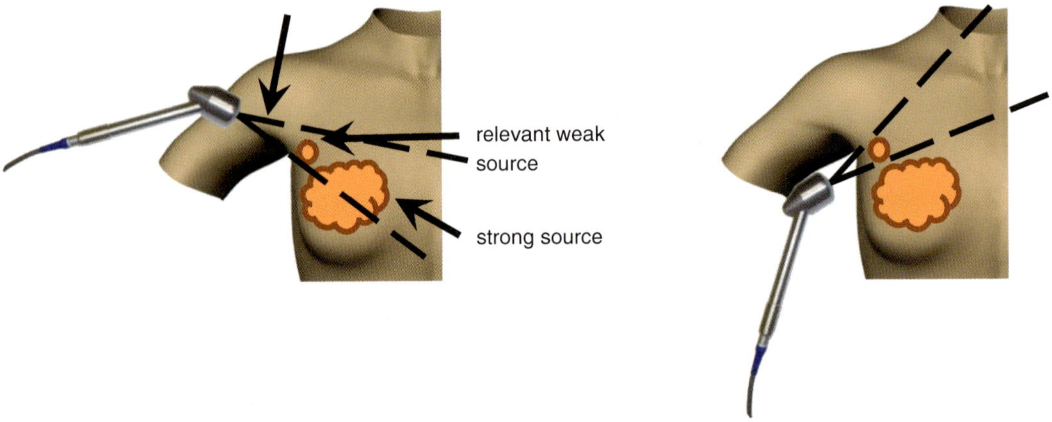

Fig. 2.21 Example of shadowing and how to avoid it. *Left*: Two structures are within the field of view of the detector, but only the closer, smaller one is relevant. *Right*: In order to avoid missing this structure, the angle of the detector has to be changed such that it points away from the strong source (the strong source should not be in the field of view of the detector) before abandoning scanning of the anatomy of interest

2.11.3 Shadowing

Almost the opposite effect of shine-through is the shadowing effect. Here, a faint radioactive source is missed by the surgeon since it is too close to a hot radioactive source which "shadows" it.

This is an extremely common occurrence in radioguided surgery as the biological uptake of structures such as the liver or activity at the injection site (in the case of sentinel lymph node biopsy) may disguise small structures that contain less radioactivity and are potentially of more importance than the shadowing structure.

In this case, proper use of the gamma detector, as well as the use of more highly collimated detectors, freehand SPECT, or preoperative information, may help the surgeon to avoid overlooking a structure of clinical relevance (Fig. 2.21).

Conclusions

Within this chapter we have tried to explain all relevant aspects of the physics underlying radioguided surgery to provide a sound basic understanding for users of γ probes, β probes, or γ cameras.

Pitfalls, recommendations, and content have been chosen based on our experience gained over many years in radioguided surgery in different organs, with different nuclides, and a wide variety of radiation detectors.

In general, a deeper understanding of the physics of radioguided surgery enables a good surgeon to become a good radioguided surgeon, ensuring excellent performance to the benefit of patients.

References

1. Curie E. Madame Curie: a biography. Reissue edition. Da Capo Press; 2001. ISBN-13 978-0306810381.
2. Ekström LP, Firestone RB. WWW table of radioactive isotopes. Database version 2/28/99 from URL http://ie.lbl.gov/toi (Nuclide Search).
3. Carsten J. Controversy and consensus: nuclear beta decay 1911–1934. Birkhäuser Verlag; 2000. ISBN: 3-7643-5313-9.
4. Alvarez LW. The capture of orbital electrons by nuclei. Phys Rev. 1938;54:486–97.
5. Duparc OH. Pierre Auger – Lise Meitner: comparative contributions to the Auger effect. Int J Mater Res. 2009;100(09):1162.
6. Einstein A. Über einen die Erzeugung und Verwandlung des Lichtes betreffenden heuristischen Gesichtspunkt. Ann Phys. 1905;17(6):132–48.
7. Compton AH. A quantum theory of the scattering of X-rays by light elements. Phys Rev. 1923;21(5): 483–502.
8. Knoll GF. Radiation detection and measurement. 4th ed. Wiley; 2010. ISBN-13 978-0470131480.

9. Bardach H, Wisnieff S. The evolution of a radiologic measuring technique – innovative metrology – key to progress. Standards Laboratory Conference; NBS Special Publication 1970;13:11–21.
10. Katz L, Penfold AS. Range-energy relations for electrons and the determination of beta-ray end-point energies by absorption. Rev Mod Phys. 1952;24:28.
11. Hakamata T, et al. Photomultiplier tubes, basics and applications – Hamamatsu Photonics KK. 3rd ed. 2007.
12. Datasheets of crystals taken from the website of Saint-Gobain Ceramics & Plastics, Inc. http://www.crystals.saint-gobain.com/.
13. Mestais C, Baffert N, Bonnefoy JP, Chapuis A, Koenig A, Monnet O, Ouvrier Buffet P, Rostaing JP, Sauvage F, Verger L. A new design for a high resolution, high efficiency CZT gamma camera detector. Nucl Inst Methods Phys Res A. 2001; 458(1–2):62–7.
14. Lide DR, editors. CRC handbook of chemistry and physics. 84th ed. Section 4: Properties of the elements and inorganic compounds; physical properties of the rare earth metals. Boca Raton: CRC Press; 2003.
15. Lombardi MH. Radiation safety in nuclear medicine. 2nd ed. CRC Press; 2006. ISBN-13 978-0849381683.

The Use of Intraoperative Small and Large Field of View Gamma Cameras for Radioguided Surgery

3

Daan Hellingman and Sergi Vidal-Sicart

Contents

D. Hellingman
Nuclear Medicine Department, The Netherlands Cancer Institute-Antoni van Leeuwenhoek Hospital, Amsterdam, The Netherlands
e-mail: d.hellingman@nki.nl

S. Vidal-Sicart (✉)
Nuclear Medicine Department, Hospital Clínic Barcelona, Institut d'Investigació Biomèdica August Pi I Sunyer (IDIBAPS), Barcelona, Spain
e-mail: svidal@clinic.ub.es

Abstract

Intraoperative small and large field of view gamma cameras and handheld gamma cameras, when used in conjuction with standard handheld gamma detection probes, can help further facilitate the successful performance of various radioguided surgery procedures. A variety of prototype and commercially available intraoperative gamma cameras have been clinically evaluated in radioguided surgery. Such intraoperative gamma cameras: (i) must be portable and stable in design; (ii) have no delay between image acquistion and display: (iii) provide continuous monitoring, spatial orientation on screen, real-time quantification, and display of the counts recorded; and (iv) have an adequate spatial resolution, sensitivity, and

K. Herrmann et al. (eds.), *Radioguided Surgery: Current Applications and Innovative Directions in Clinical Practice*, DOI 10.1007/978-3-319-26051-8_3

field of view. Intraoperative gamma cameras have been clinically applied to many disease entities, most commonly including breast canceer, melanoma, head and neck malignancies, parathyroid surgery, urogenital malignancies, and bone tumors. The application of intraoperative gammma cameras to radioguided sentinel lymph node (SLN) biopsy procedures is most advantageous in difficult SLN biopsy cases, such as: (i) when the SLNs are located near the primary injection site, (ii) when the SLNs are deeply located within the region of interest, or (iii) when SLNs have a relaively low level of radiotracer uptake.

3.1 Background

In most centers, radioguided surgery relies on preoperative imaging in combination with intraoperative handheld gamma probe guidance. A handheld gamma probe provides count rate display and variable-pitch audio output based on the local radioactivity concentration. Radioguided surgery requires rapid and precise detection, as is generally provided simply by handheld gamma detection probes. There are however several limitations: (1) gamma probes do not provide image documentation for the medical record, (2) its usefulness is dependent on correct gamma probe positioning and thus highly operator dependent, (3) deeply located sentinel lymph nodes (SLNs) may be missed due to low count statistics as a result of tissue attenuation, and (4) when SLNs are located in close proximity to the radiotracer injection site, the high radioactive background signal may hamper the ability to intraoperative distinguish the SLNs from the radiotracer injection site. This is referred to as the "shine-through" effect.

With these limitations to handheld gamma detection probes, intraoperative gamma cameras have been designed to facilitate radioguided surgery. These systems must meet several requirements to be employed in the operating room: (1) a portable and stable design, (2) no delay between image acquisition and display, and (3) the possibility for continuous monitoring, spatial orientation on screen, real-time quantification, and display of the counts recorded. Last, such systems should also have an adequate spatial resolution, sensitivity, and field of view [1].

Real-time imaging with an intraoperative gamma camera provides a larger field of view than a gamma probe can cover and visual assistance in localization and verification of resection of the targeted tissue. Its position can be adjusted to also show SLNs near the radiotracer injection site or to distinguish between two radiolabeled tissues, which can easily be overlooked by using a conventional handheld gamma probe. Still it is advised to use an intraoperative gamma camera in conjunction with a handheld gamma probe for most radioguided surgery procedures, because both systems have their added value.

Intraoperative maneuverability determined by the outer dimensions and weight of the detector head is one of the most important characteristics of such intraoperative gamma cameras. Intraoperative gamma cameras can be divided into two categories: handheld gamma cameras and portable/mobile gamma cameras. Small gamma cameras weighing about 1 kg or less can be physically held and positioned by the average person for the time necessary to achieve the required image, 10–60 s on average. These systems are referred to as handheld gamma camera. However, those gamma cameras weighing 2 kg or more cannot be easily held by the average person and need some sort of adjunct stabilization/support system. These systems are referred to as portable gamma cameras (PGCs). Finally, the term "small field of view" (SFOV) gamma camera applies to those systems having a field of view that is 5×5 cm^2 or smaller in size, while gamma cameras with a larger field of view are considered "large field of view" gamma cameras.

3.2 History

The first prototype handheld gamma camera, the "imaging probe," was patented by Soluri et al. in 1997 [2]. The imaging probe was a small gamma camera having a field of view of $22.8 \times 22.8\ mm^2$. Advancements in the development of position-sensitive photomultiplier tubes (PS-PMTs) allowed for new gamma cameras designs with improved high resolution (spatial resolution smaller than 4 mm). As example, a prototype gamma camera, "preoperative", compact imager (POCI), was developed by Menard et al. and the first clinical results of both systems in sentinel lymph node (SLN) procedures were published in 1999 [3, 4]. These early systems used conventional continuous thallium-doped cesium iodide CsI(Tl) or sodium-doped cesium iodide CsI(Na) scintillation crystals linked to a PS-PMT or PS-photodiode (PD). The main problems with these early units were their SFOV and the resulting large number of images required to scan the whole surgical field.

In 2001, Soluri et al. improved the spatial resolution and sensitivity of their imaging probe by integrating the crystals into the collimator holes [5]. A prototype large field of view PGC, 2020tc imager, based on CsI(Tl)-photodiode coupling, was tested in minimally invasive radioguided parathyroidectomy by Kitagawa et al. in 2002 [6]. Pitre et al. improved the POCI system by reducing the weight and increasing its detector field of view and sensitivity in 2003 [7]. In the same year, the first prototype solid-state cameras were presented by two different groups [8, 9]. These solid-state systems were based on crystal-photodiode coupling or semiconductors crystals, such as cadmium telluride (CdTe) or zinc cadmium telluride (CdZnTe).

Thereafter, commercially available SFOV gamma cameras were developed and clinically evaluated. While the first prototypes were heavy handheld devices, the newer commercially available SFOV gamma cameras were either lighter handheld gamma camera systems or were PGCs equipped with a stabilization/support system [10]. The pioneering of the commercially available systems has led to their commonplace application to many aspects of radioguided surgery, including radioguided parathyroidectomy, as well as radioguided SLN biopsy procedures for melanoma and breast cancer. Additionally, the clinical application of PGCs and handheld gamma cameras has been described for radioguided bone surgery [11] and for radioguided SLN biopsy procedures for head/neck cancers [12] and for urogenital cancers [13, 14].

3.3 Device Characteristics

Several prototype or commercially available intraoperative gamma cameras have been clinically evaluated in radioguided surgery. SFOV PGCs (Fig. 3.1) and handheld (Fig. 3.2) gamma cameras are optimized for the detection of technetium-99 m (^{99m}Tc), having an energy photopeak of 140 keV; however, such devices have a global energy range from 30 to 250 keV. This energy range enables detection of multiple other low- and medium-gamma photon energy-emitting radiotracers, such as cobalt-57 (^{57}Co), gallium-67 (^{67}Ga), indium-111 (^{111}In), iodine-123 (^{123}I), and ^{125}I. Nevertheless, the technology used for the different cameras is very heterogeneous (Table 3.1). Performance characteristics were obtained using widely differing

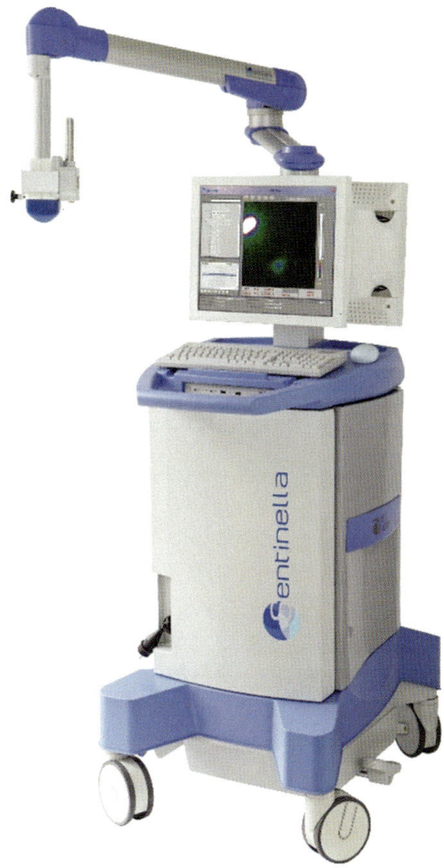

Fig. 3.1 Portable small field of view gamma camera "Sentinella S102" (Provided courtesy of Oncovision GEM Imaging S.A., Valencia, Spain)

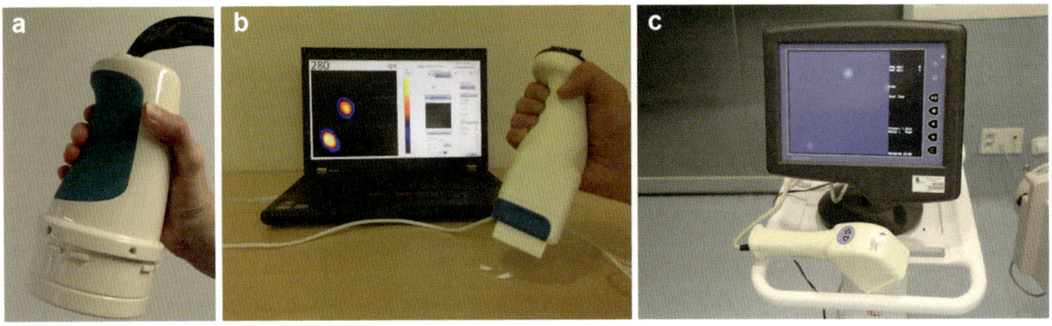

Fig. 3.2 Small field of view handheld gamma cameras; (**a**) compact gamma camera "CGC" (Provided courtesy of John E.W. Lees Space Research Centre, University of Leicester, Leicester, United Kingdom), (**b**) CrystalCam, (**c**) Minicam II (Provided courtesy of Dr. Juan I. Rayo, Complejo Hospitalario Universitario de Badajoz, Badajoz, Spain)

Table 3.1 Technical characteristics of portable and handheld gamma cameras

Camera (manufacturer)	Handheld or portable	Collimator	Detector	Size detector head (mm^3)	Weight (kg)
Small field of view					
Sentinella S102[a] [17] (Oncovision, Spain)	Portable	Pinhole (2.5 and 4.0 mm)	CsI (Na) PS-PMT	154 × 82 × 80	1.3
Minicam II[a] (Eurorad, France)	Handheld	Parallel hole	CdTe	70 × 170 × 250	0.7
CrystalCam [96] (Crystal Photonics, Germany)	Handheld	Parallel hole	CdZnTe	60 × 60 × 140	0.8
NODE VIEWTM[a] [97] (Intra-Medical Imaging, USA)	Handheld	Parallel hole	NaI(Tl) PS-PMT	64 × 64 × 76	1.1
IP Guardian II [98] (Li-Tech, Italy)	Handheld	Parallel hole	CsI (Tl) PS-PMT	–[b]	1.2
eZ-SCOPE [8] (Anzai Medical, Japan)	Handheld	Parallel hole	CdZnTe	77 × 73 × 212	0.8
CGC[a] [99] (Gamma Technologies, UK)	Handheld	Pinhole (0.5 mm)	CsI(Tl) CCD	Ø 95 × 200	1.0
GammaCAM/OR [34] (Gamma Medica, USA)	Portable	Parallel hole	NaI(Tl) PS-PMT	–[b]	10
CarolIReS [35] (prototype, France)	Portable	Parallel hole	Gd2SiO5 (Ce) PS-PMT	78 × 78 × 275	2.5
POCI [7] (Prototype, France)	Handheld	Parallel hole	CsI (Na) PS-PD	Ø 95 × 90	1.2
Large field of view					
Ergo[a] [81] (Digirad, USA)	Portable	Parallel hole	CsI(Tl) PS-PD	421 × 284 × 102	193
Mobile gamma camera [55] (prototype, USA)	Portable	Parallel hole	NaI(Tl) PS-PMT	–[b]	–[b]

[a]Updated information was obtained from commercial brochure or corresponding author
[b]Missing information

experimental designs, and therefore, a precise comparison is not always possible. For example, different source-to-collimator distances will affect the sensitivity and spatial resolution of each system. A uniform standard to examine performance characteristics is required for precise comparison. Existing National Electrical Manufacturers Association (NEMA) protocols for assessing the performance characteristics of conventional large field of view gamma cameras can be inappropriate and require modification for use with SFOV gamma camera systems [15, 16].

3.3.1 Detectors

The development of high-resolution gamma cameras resulted in four different detectors technologies: (1) scintillation crystals coupled with a PS-PMT, (2) scintillation crystals coupled with photodiodes, (3) scintillation crystals coupled with a CCD detector, and (4) semiconductor crystals (CdTe and CdZnTe, whose charge is directly read by dedicated electronics). Scintillation-based detection devices are cheaper than semiconductors-based detection devices. Semiconductors are direct converters of photons to energy, with no light conversion. Because of this, there is no spread of light and corresponding cross talk, as occurs with scintillating crystals. Semiconductors show less peripheral problems (e.g., reduced peripheral dead zones) than scintillation crystals coupled with a PS-PMT. The main difference is that semiconductors have a better energy resolution than most scintillators, while scintillators have a higher sensitivity. Photodiodes can offer the advantages of semiconductors, such as reduced peripheral dead zone and high energy resolution, and the benefits of the PS-PMTs, such as a high sensitivity. Finally, scintillators coupled with a CCD detector have naturally a better spatial resolution due to the smaller pixel size than the other detectors. Most of the cameras listed in Table 3.1 are built with scintillators.

3.3.2 Field of View

Another important feature is the detector's field of view, which is the actual patient region of interest that can be scanned in one image by the gamma camera. The field of view depends on the type of collimator and on the detector dimensions. Some systems are equipped with interchangeable collimators. It is important to choose an appropriate collimator for the specific surgical application, secondary to the trade-off between sensitivity and spatial resolution. If the field of view is too small, it may be difficult to completely encompass the targeted region of interest and multiple images will be needed. On the other hand, a large detector with a large field of view may not allow optimal maneuverability during any given surgical procedure. Systems using a parallel-hole collimator have a fixed field of view limited to the detector dimensions. A pinhole collimator enables imaging with a field of view larger than the detector dimensions, which is ideal for scanning the whole surgical field using only a small camera system. When the camera is moved further away from the patient, increasing the source-to-pinhole collimator distance, the image field of view will become larger. However, a larger source-to-pinhole collimator distance will drastically lower the spatial resolution and sensitivity of the system, reducing the overall image quality. Most of the cameras listed in Table 3.2 are SFOV systems (5×5 cm or smaller) even those using pinhole collimators, enabling larger field of view imaging, since the classification is based on the detector dimensions.

3.3.3 Sensitivity

Sensitivity is expressed as counts per second per unit activity (cps/Bq) and depends on the collimator-detector geometry (geometrical efficiency) multiplied by the detector efficiency. The sensitivity increases as the square of the collimator hole size and decreases as the square of the hole length. Source-to-collimator distance is inversely quadratic related to the sensitivity of pinhole collimators. The sensitivity of a parallel-hole collimator is in theory independent of source-to-collimator distances, but in reality a minimal decrease in sensitivity due to scattering will be detected at larger distances. A high sensitivity is important in the operating room to image low activities. Image acquisition times can be reduced using high-sensitivity systems, which means that the surgeon does not lose too much time looking for radiotracer tissue uptake in the areas of interest. All sensitivity values in Table 3.2 are based on ^{99m}Tc 140 keV measurements.

3.3.4 Spatial Resolution

The spatial resolution of a system can be expressed as intrinsic and extrinsic resolution. Intrinsic resolution refers to how well the detector localizes an interaction in the scintillator or semiconductor crystals. Extrinsic resolution is a combination of the intrinsic resolution and collimator

Table 3.2 Performance characteristics of portable and handheld gamma cameras

Camera (manufacturer)	Image matrix size	Detector field of view (mm^2)	Intrinsic resolution (FWHM in mm)	Extrinsic resolution (FWHM in mm)	Extrinsic sensitivity (cps/MBq)	Energy resolution (FWHM)
Small field of view						
Sentinella S102[a] [17] (Oncovision, Spain)	300 × 300	40 × 40	1.8	2.6–5.5[c] or 4.6–8.7[d] (at 13–50 mm)	145–59[c] or 345–150[d] (at 30–50 mm)	15.9 %
Minicam II[a] (Eurorad, France)	16 × 16	40 × 40	2.5	–[b]	250	5–7%
CrystalCam [96] (CrystalPhotonics, Germany)	16 × 16	40 × 40	1.9	3.8–4.9[e] (at 25–50 mm)	237[e] or 554[f]	5.2 %
NODE VIEWTM[a] [97] (Intra-Medical Imaging, USA)	29 × 29	50 × 50	1.8	1.8 (at 6 mm)	135	12 %
IP Guardian II [98] (Li-Tech, Italy)	18 × 18	44 × 44	2.2	2.5–2.9 (at 0–15 mm)	204	20 %
eZ-SCOPE [8] (Anzai Medical, Japan)	16 × 16	32 × 32	1.9	2.3–8.0[e] or 3.0–9.1[f] (at 10–50 mm)	184[e] or 477[f]	8.6 %
CGC[a] [99] (Gamma Technologies, UK)	125 × 125	8 × 8	0.6	1.28–2.9 (at 13–50 mm)	214 (at 3 mm)	58 %
GammaCAM/OR [34] (Gamma Medica, USA)	–[b]	125 × 125	–[b]	–[b]	61	–[b]
CarolIReS [35] (prototype, France)	50 × 50	50 × 50	3	10 (at 30 mm)	1000 (theoretical)	45 % (^{57}Co)
POCI [7] (prototype, France)	50 × 50	Ø 40	2.3	3.9–7.6 mm (at 10–50 mm)	290	32 %
Large field of view						
Ergo[a] [81] (Digirad, USA)	512 × 512	396 × 310	3.3	10.3 (at 100 mm)	113	7.9 %
Mobile gamma camera [55] (prototype, USA)	40 × 40	130 × 130	–[b]	–[b]	405	–[b]

All performance characteristics are measured using ^{99m}Tc (140 keV)
[a]Updated information was obtained from commercial brochure or corresponding author
[b]Missing information
[c]2.5 mm pinhole collimator
[d]4.0 mm pinhole collimator
[e]Low-energy high-resolution (LEHR) collimator
[f]Low-energy high-sensitivity (LEHS) collimator

resolution. In practice, the intrinsic resolution of a detector is small compared to the extrinsic resolution. For this reason, a comparison of extrinsic spatial resolution provides a better indication of how a camera will behave in clinical practice. Spatial resolution, expressed as the full width at half maximum (FWHM), is linear inversely related the source-to-collimator distance for both pinhole and parallel-hole collimators. At short distances, gamma camera systems fitted with a pinhole collimator have a higher resolution than when parallel collimators are used.

3.3.5 Energy Resolution

As mentioned above sensitivity partly defines the image acquisition time. But a good quality image is also related to the capacity of the detector to reject diffuse (scattered) photons whose trajectories do not point back to the initial source and therefore must be eliminated. This is done by applying a proper energy window that mainly selects the direct gamma photons coming from the source. The energy resolution of the detector is expressed as the FWHM of the ^{99m}Tc or ^{57}Co photopeak, 140 or 122 keV, respectively, and plays an important role: the lower (better) it is, the stricter the selection in photon energy can be. In conclusion, a large energy window is needed for detectors having a broad energy photopeak (large FWHM) to retain the sensitivity of the detector. However, a larger energy window will misinterpreted scattered photons for direct photons and therefore reduce the contrast and overall quality of your image.

3.3.6 Advanced Camera Features

The above mentioned technical performance characteristics are the major determinates for any given gamma camera in the clinical setting. However, there are some additional features that might influence the performance of any given radioguided surgery procedure. For example, the Sentinella S102 camera has evolved over the years from a handheld device to an articulated system with a stabilization/support arm, thus enabling stable imaging over longer image acquisition times [14, 17]. A laser pointer is included in the supporting structure and displays a red cross over the patient's skin (Fig. 3.3). The position of this red cross is virtually visible on the computer screen of the camera. If the virtual laser pointer matches the radioactive hotspot signal on screen, this indicates that the radiolabeled tissue has been precisely localized. The laser pointer facilitates the image interpretation for the surgeons, who must relate the output image of the portable gamma camera (PGC) to the visible surface of the surgical field. An additional advantage is that the camera can be easily positioned in the same position for comparing pre- and post-excision images.

All systems should have software tools for flexible display windowing, convenient region-of-interest definition, and rapid image analysis. These features should be readily available and be easily controlled by the individual positioning the camera. For example, the Sentinella S102 camera has copied some software tools (dynamic imaging, dual-isotope imaging, and virtually shielding the highly radioactive injection site) from conventional large field of view gamma cameras; however, these tools are still unique among the SFOV devices. Dynamic imaging can facilitate SLN detection by imaging directly after radiotracer injection in situations when an intraoperative injection is performed. Dual-isotope imaging can be helpful in those radioguided interventions using two different radioisotopes, such as in the simultaneous use of an ^{125}I seed to guide breast-conserving tumor excision and ^{99m}Tc-nanocolloid for SLN biopsy in breast cancer [18]. In the clinical scenario in which the SLNs are located near the radiotracer injection site, visualization of the SLNs can be hampered by the background radioactivity from radiotracer injection site, even when the PGC is pointing at the most optimal angle. Thus, in this difficult clinical scenario, covering the radiotracer injection site with a software tool that simulates a lead shield (masking the injection activity) can facilitate SLN visualization [19].

Up until recently, all SFOV PGCs and handheld gamma cameras have been based on just one single imaging modality (gamma imaging), which

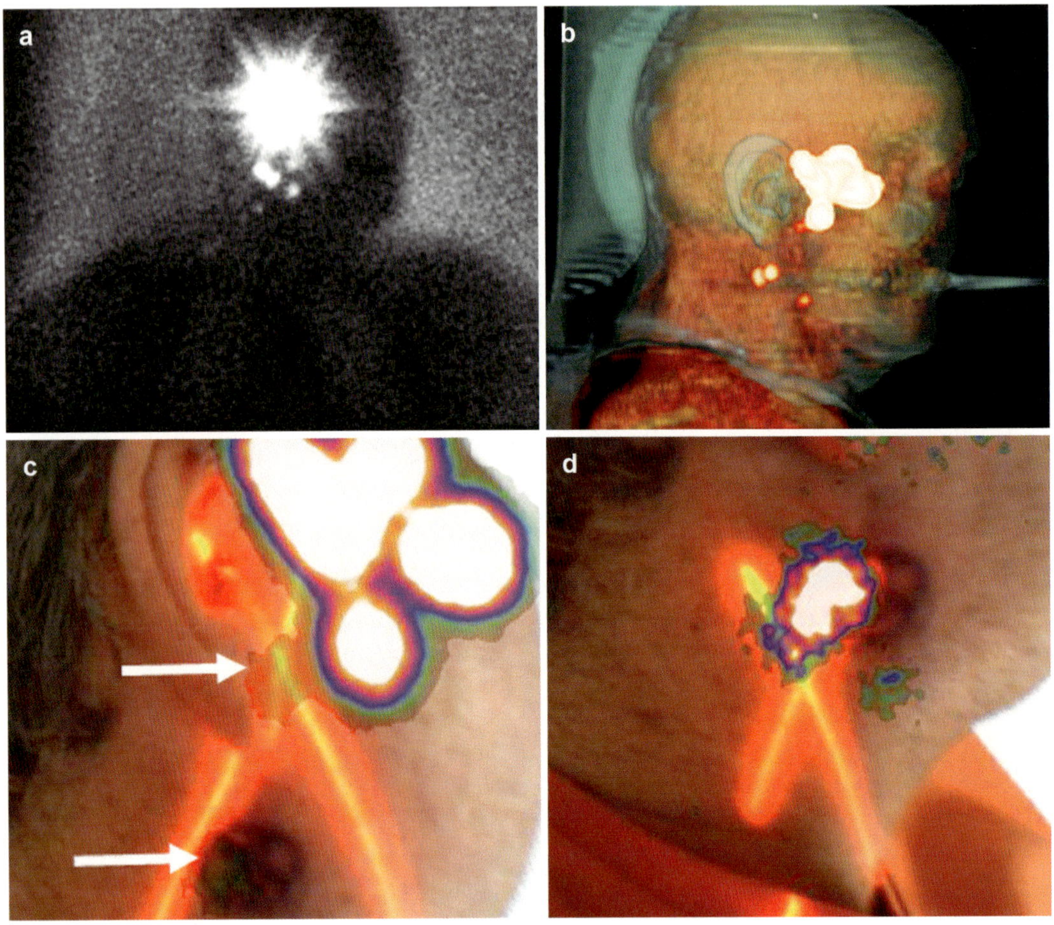

Fig. 3.3 Lateral (**a**) planar lymphoscintigraphic image showing SLNs caudal from the site of 99mTc-nanocolloid injection around a preauricular-located melanoma. These SLNS are displayed on 3D volume rendering SPECT/CT (**b**) for a better anatomical recognition. The PGC upgraded with an optical camera module was placed above the lymphatic field to obtain an image at a distance of approximately 12 cm. The red laser pointer cross is pointing towards a near the highly radioactive injection site located SLN. Combined optical and scintigraphic imaging visualizes the image field of view and two anatomical SLN locations (*white arrows*) (**c**). A second combined optical and scintigraphic image visualizes the SLN cluster in the lower part of the neck (**d**)

provides no correlative anatomical information, thus sometimes hampering image interpretation. In order to overcome this limitation, new multimodality system configurations have been described that combine optical and gamma imaging. Haneishi et al. were the first who proposed a parallel optical and gamma camera configuration [20, 21]. This portable hybrid camera system projects the obtained gamma image onto an optical image. Later Lees et al. described an optical camera upgrade for a handheld compact gamma camera enabling fused optical and gamma imaging with a matched image field of view [22, 23]. Hellingman et al. were the first who evaluated a prototype portable hybrid camera for preoperative lymphatic mapping in SLN procedures in 2015 [24]. Fused optical and gamma imaging makes it easier to relate the position of the radioactive hotspots and the image field of view with the real-life situation (Fig. 3.3).

Another interesting development is the navigation system called "declipseSPECT" (SurgicEye, München, Germany), which expands the applications of radioguided interventions. declipseSPECT

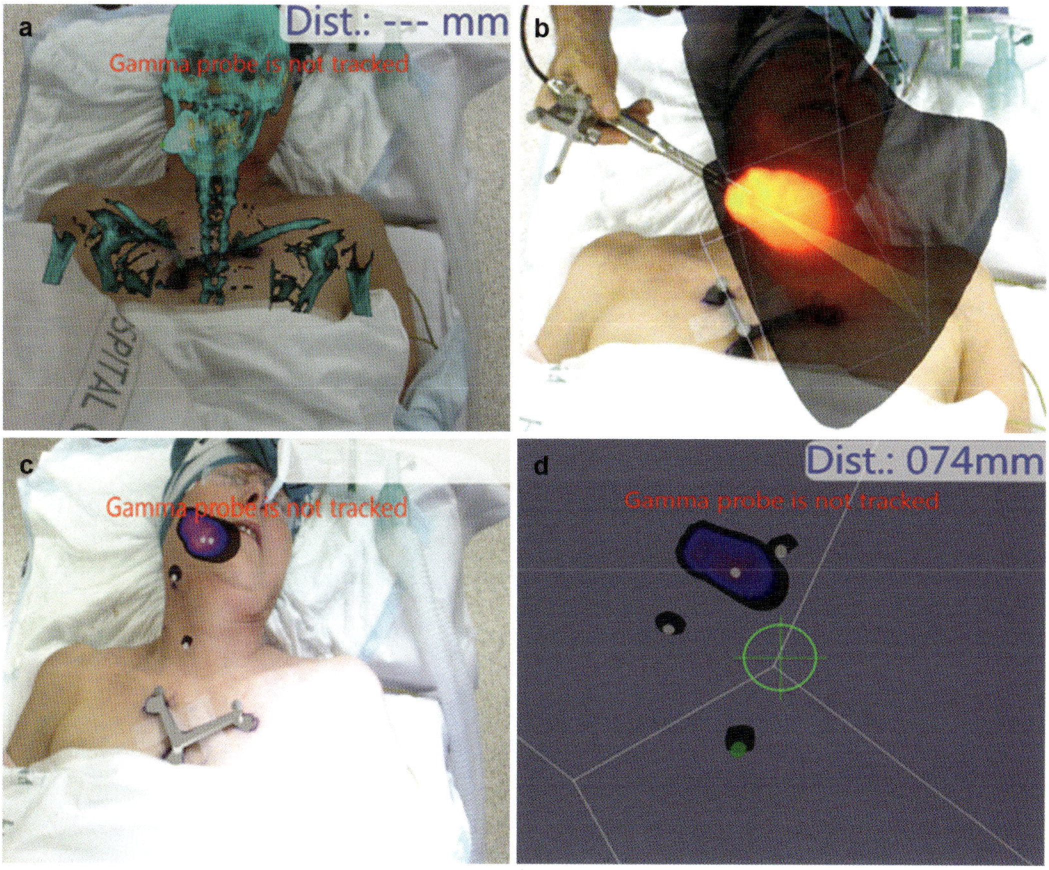

Fig. 3.4 Preoperative SPECT/CT scan of patient visualized as video overlay on the live video of the patient (**a**). Pre-incision freehand SPECT acquisition using a position-tracked gamma probe (**b**). Subsequently, the gathered data is reconstructed to visualize the radioactive foci projected onto the live video of the patient (**c**) and in a (**d**) 3D virtual reality view from the perspective of the gamma probe

is another type of imaging system that integrates a positioning system attached to a conventional gamma probe [25]. A freehand single-photon emission computed tomography (SPECT) scan, few minutes of manual scanning using an optically tracked gamma probe, can provide additional depth information using a 3D reconstruction of the radioactive target lesions (Fig. 3.4). The position of the gamma probe relative to the attached device is tracked by infrared technology, and the output of the gamma probe is co-registered in the surgical field (depicted by a video camera) and displayed on a monitor where the surgeon can easily check the location and depth of the foci of radioactivity. A unique feature of the "CrystalCam" is the possibility to integrate this SFOV handheld gamma camera into the declipseSPECT system. Freehand-SPECT scans can be made using the CrystalCam, which has a higher resolution and sensitivity than a conventional gamma probe. The first clinical reports of this feature were reported by Freesmeyer et al. in 2014 [26, 27].

3.4 Experiences in Breast Cancer

SFOV and large field of view PGCs and handheld gamma cameras have been widely utilized in radioguided breast cancer procedures. Part of these experiences has been reported in a recent review [28]. The use of these systems in the surgical management of breast cancer has included: preoperative and intraoperative lymphatic mapping in SLN procedures, radioguided occult lesion localization (ROLL), sentinel node and occult lesion localization (SNOLL), and breast cancer detection using ^{99m}Tc-mikusestamibi.

3.4.1 Sentinel Lymph Node Biopsy

In most centers, preoperative planar lymphoscintigraphy is performed using a large conventional gamma camera to visualize lymphatic drainage from the radiotracer injection site. Sequential planar images will show successive stages of drainage and thereby help to determine the number and location of SLNs. Goto and colleagues studied the ability to perform preoperative lymphatic mapping using a large field of view PGC and compared the results with conventional lymphoscintigraphy [29]. Concordant results were obtained in 15/19 patients with both cameras. In four (21 %) patients, axillary SLNs were correctly detected using the PGC whereas these hot spots could not be seen with the conventional lymphoscintigraphy. According to the authors, the better performance of the PGC is due to a combination of a close imaging distance and a better signal-to-noise ratio that allows the PGC to distinguish SLNs located near the injection site. Kerrou and colleagues were the first who compared a SFOV handheld gamma camera with conventional lymphoscintigraphy in 138 patients [30]. Multiple images were needed using this SFOV device to scan the whole axillary and extra-axillary region. Although the handheld gamma camera was used after conventional lymphoscintigraphy, benefiting from a longer radiotracer migration, fewer SLNs were detected with this handheld gamma camera in 34 of the 138 (25 %) patients. Concordant results were obtained in 54/138 patients and more SLNs were detected in 50/138 (36 %) patients using the handheld camera. Another study was performed using a SFOV PGC fitted with a pinhole collimator to overcome the need to make multiple images due to the limited field of view [31]. The PGC was placed at 18 cm distance to cover a 20×20 cm field of view. SLN visualization was seen in 39 of 52 patients (75 %) using the PGC, while conventional lymphoscintigraphy showed SLN visualization in 49 of 52 patients (94 %). When a lead shield was used to mask the injection activity, conventional lymphoscintigraphy and the PGC visualized a SLN in 41 of 43 patients (95 %) and 38 of 43 cases (88 %), respectively. The poor performance of the PGC was attributed to the low spatial resolution and sensitivity at this large source-to-collimator distance.

Scopinaro and colleagues published the first intraoperative breast cancer SLN studies including only a limited number of patients [32, 33]. The first validation of new portable and handheld gamma cameras generally occurs in breast cancer SLN procedures [7, 32, 34, 35]. In intraoperative setting, portable and handheld gamma cameras are often compared to conventional gamma probes to evaluate their clinical value. Although most studies include only a small number of patients (<20 patients), these reports describe clearly the usefulness of intraoperative imaging. Firstly, high-resolution imaging using portable or handheld gamma cameras facilitates the detection of near the injection site located SLNs which are missed by preoperative lymphoscintigraphy or gamma probe screening [14, 32, 36]. Secondly, they provide detection of SLNs (deeply located or low tracer uptake nodes) which were initially missed by gamma probe screening [7, 14, 36–40]. Thirdly, intraoperative imaging provides more confidence about SLN localization and excision using pre- and post-excision images [33, 34, 41]. Additionally, some studies demonstrated that intraoperative imaging reduces operating time since SLNs are faster found and excised compared to procedures in which only a gamma probe is used [42, 43]. In this sense, the application of intraoperative imaging in the parasternal area overcomes the problem of very faint uptake of these tiny nodes and helps the surgeon to precisely localize the correct intercostal space to make the incision [15]. Finally, Goñi and colleagues conducted a retrospective study using a prospective database of 754 patients who had undergone a SLN biopsy between January 2003 and December 2011 [44]. All patients were divided into two groups to analyze whether the introduction of the PGC, since October 2009, had improved the SLN identification rate. Group 1 consisted of 501 patients in which the procedure was performed using only a gamma probe (January 2003 to October 2009). Group 2 consisted of 253 patients in which the SLN biopsy was performed using both the PGC and a gamma probe (October 2009 to December 2011). In group 1 the SLN identification rate was 94.6 %, while in group 2 identification rate, it was 99.2 %. Chronologically, the improvement of the SLN identification rate during the study period has been observed. The authors concluded that this can be explained by the experience gained by the surgical team and that the introduction of the PGC played an important role as well.

One of the most important benefits of intraoperative imaging described for this surgical procedure is the assessment of remaining activity in the surgical field at the end of the procedure, in order to attempt to identify any missed SLNs. A strict intraoperative protocol is necessary to study how many additional SLNs are found by intraoperative imaging. First, the surgeon removes the SLNs by localizing them using only the gamma probe. When no further radioactive nodes are detected by the gamma probe (negative gamma probe screening), the surgical field is scanned using the portable or handheld gamma camera searching for possible "missed" radioactive lymph nodes. Olcott et al. found two additional SLNs in 11 patients [39]. Chondrogiannis et al. found five additional SLNs in 16 patients [40]. Of course the goal is not to harvest more nodes but to not miss tumor-positive nodes undetected by the gamma probe. SLN biopsy is a diagnostic procedure used to determine whether breast cancer has spread to those nodes. In the study of Chondrogiannis et al., one of the five additional SLNs was tumor positive and prevented a false-negative procedure in that patient. Finding an additional tumor-positive node, which was initially missed by gamma probe screening, using intraoperative imaging has been reported before [14, 37]. Unfortunately, these "true" additionally found SLNs and their pathology are often not described in studies; therefore, the benefit of intraoperative imaging in breast cancer SLN biopsy is still a matter of debate [45]. Larger prospective (multi)center studies are needed to access the real value of intraoperative imaging using portable or handheld gamma cameras in breast cancer. Based on the available evidence, it can be concluded that such systems are useful under the following conditions: (1) when no conventional gamma camera is available for preoperative lymphoscintigraphy, (2) in difficult cases when the SLN is located near the injection site (i.e., internal mammary chain (parasternal) or intramammary nodes), and (3) deeply located nodes or nodes with a low radiotracer uptake. The opportunity to obtain different images with such devices can solve the majority of these problems [46].

3.4.2 Radioguided Occult Lesion Localization and Concurrent Sentinel Node Biopsy

Radioguided occult lesion localization (ROLL) is an alternative to wire-guided localization for guiding surgical excision of non-palpable breast lesions and breast cancers. Paredes and colleagues were the first who evaluated the usefulness of a PGC to assess the resection of non-palpable breast lesions in 42 patients [47]. In this study, the major tool to guide the surgeon has been the handheld gamma probe, and the PGC was validated on the ex vivo specimens. Pathologic examination demonstrated tumor-free margins in 14/23 cases when radioactivity was found in the center of the breast specimen based on the PGC image. Involved margins were found in 11/19 non-centered cases (i.e., when radioactivity was observed near the specimen border). These results show a concordance of 60 % (25 of 42) between pathologic results and the PGC images.

SNOLL is a combination of two procedures, SLN biopsy and ROLL. Lombardi and colleagues studied 186 consecutive patients with breast cancer scheduled for SNOLL using a gamma probe and a handheld gamma camera [48]. Radioguided axillary SLN biopsy was possible in 184/186 patients (99 %). In 22 (12 %) of patients, a second operation was required for close or tumor-positive surgical margins. A second study evaluated the performance of another handheld gamma camera in 15 SNOLL procedures [49]. The authors reported that the handheld gamma camera was considered to be easy to use and does not increase operating time.

3.4.3 Breast Tumor-Seeking Radiotracers

Soluri et al. performed the first radioguided biopsies of breast lesions using a handheld gamma camera and ^{99m}Tc-sestamibi in 2003 [50]. High-resolution handheld gamma camera images were able to guide biopsy toward breast cancer in 7 out of 10 patients. Thereafter, the same group mounted the handheld gamma camera on an x-ray guided vacuum biopsy device and fused the high-resolution scintigraphic images with the stereotactic mammographic images. In five patients, a biopsy was taken from the breast tissue with the low, intermediate, and high uptake of ^{99m}Tc-Bombesin, which is taken up by the Bombesin receptors. Authors describe that the highest uptake region corresponded to the breast cancer region with the highest number of microvessels, which is the most important tumor zone to analyze [51]. Later similar conclusions were drawn by the same group in a study with ten patients [52].

Evangelista et al. evaluated in 18 patients the feasibility of a PGC for guiding surgical treatment in locally advanced breast cancer after neo-adjuvant chemotherapy [53]. PGC imaging was more accurate than conventional scintimammography for the detection of residual breast cancer (sensitivity: 50 vs. 26.6 %, respectively). Still, a clear benefit for guiding breast tumor surgery after neo-adjuvant chemotherapy is not shown. Breast surgery is always recommended in these patients, even if no clinical or radiological lesion is detected. The use of PGC does not avoid preoperative tumor localization by wire-guided or radioguided localization [54].

3.5 Experiences in Melanoma Sentinel Lymph Node Biopsy

The usefulness of PGCs and handheld gamma cameras for melanoma surgery is clearly more obvious than for breast cancer surgery secondary to the greater degree of unpredictability of the lymphatic drainage from the primary site of melanoma than from the primary breast cancer site. Vidal-Sicart et al. were the first who described the use of a PGC in five difficult melanoma cases. In this group, 4 of 5 patients had a primary lesion in the head region, and the remaining patient had a lesion on a lower limb. In total, 12 SLNs were detected using only the gamma probe, and two additional SLNs were found by the PGC [14]. Dengel et al. used a prototype large field of view PGC and compared its performance with preoperative conventional lymphoscintigraphy and intraoperative gamma probe findings in 20 melanoma patients [55]. Preoperative lymphoscintigraphy detected 29 node basins containing SLNs, while the pre-incision PGC images detected only 27 node basins. The explanation given by the authors was that this had to do with a delay of more than 20 h from injection to PGC imaging and relatively low radiotracer activity in those nodes. Intraoperative use of the gamma probe ultimately detected 46 SLNs in total, but two of them were missed on initial gamma probe screening. Thus, intraoperative imaging detected two additional nodes in 2/20 (10 %) of the patients.

In 2012, Stoffels et al. included 60 patients (38 melanoma, 22 other cutaneous malignancies) for a SLN procedure using a SFOV PGC [56]. The PGC visualized all 126 preoperatively identified SLNs by SPECT/CT. More importantly, 23 additional SLNs in 15 patients (25 %) were identified using the PGC, and intraoperative imaging extended the operating time with up to 5 min. Two of these additional nodes showed metastatic involvement preventing a false-negative procedure in two patients. Olcott and colleagues showed in 39 patients that intraoperative imaging using a handheld gamma camera successfully visualized 86 of the 92 SLNs detected by the gamma probe and detected 12 additional nodes that were missed by the gamma probe [39].

In some cases, intraoperative imaging helped determine that the signal picked up by the gamma probe was in fact produced by the radiotracer injection site.

Recently, a study has started to evaluate the above mentioned findings in 100 melanoma patients [57]. Intraoperatively, the SLN biopsy will be performed using only a gamma probe guided by the preoperative SPECT/CT images. At the end of the surgery, intraoperative imaging by a PGC will verify whether any SLNs are missed. The main endpoints of the study are: the number of additional SLNs with corresponding pathology detected using intraoperative imaging and the extended surgery time due to intraoperative imaging.

3.6 Experiences in Head and Neck Sentinel Lymph Node Biopsy

The procedure of SLN biopsy in the head and neck region is challenging because of the unpredictable lymphatic drainage and presence of several vital structures and often SLNs are located close to the primary lesion. For melanoma, the results from SLN biopsy are often less successful in this area, with higher false-negative results compared to other sites [58]. Unfortunately, the high radioactive signal of the radiotracer injection site can cause difficulty in localizing nearby SLNs. In 2005, the first head and neck cancer case was published using a PGC by Tanaka and colleagues [12]. Preoperative conventional lymphoscintigraphy visualized an increased activity near the radiotracer injection site, which was not clearly identifiable as a SLN. High-resolution images obtained with the PGC clearly visualized this node separate from the radiotracer injection site. Later, more case reports demonstrated that high-resolution imaging with a PGC is able to visualize near the injection site located SLNs missed by preoperative lymphoscintigraphy and SPECT/CT [59] or gamma probe localization [60]. Hellingman et al. showed in a phantom model that SLNs can be detected at a distance of 3 mm from the radiotracer injection site. Routine use of the PGC did prevent a false-negative procedure thanks to the detection of an additional tumor-positive SLN [61].

In 2008, Tsuchimochi et al. compared the detection of SLNs by a SFOV PGC with that of conventional lymphoscintigraphy in eight oral cancer patients [62]. The number of detected SLNs was the same for both systems, but conventional lymphoscintigraphy required a longer acquisition time to produce the same quality images. In 2010, Vermeeren et al. published the results of intraoperative imaging in 25 patients (10 oral cancer and 15 head neck melanoma cases) [63]. The PGC visualized all 70 SLNs which were preoperatively identified on SPECT/CT. SLNs at difficult sites could be localized more efficiently, and in six patients, nine additional nodes (one tumor positive) were identified by post-excision intraoperative imaging. Figure 3.5 shows an example of comparing pre- and post-excision images until all preoperatively indicated SLNs are removed.

Two other studies evaluated the use of a hybrid tracer, both fluorescent and radioactive, in head and neck procedures. Intraoperatively, a gamma probe, a PGC, and a fluorescence camera were used in order to locate the SLNs. Van den Berg and colleagues demonstrated that detection with the gamma probe was hampered due to the high background signal coming from the injection site in 4 out of 14 oral cavity cancer patients. Although the PGC was able to distinguish these SLNs from the injection site, fluorescence imaging proved to be the most accurate technology for the identification of these nodes during surgery [19]. Later the same group showed in another study ($n=25$) that the PGC detected nine additional SLNs missed by the gamma probe in 8/25 patients [64].

3.7 Experiences in Urogenital Sentinel Node Lymph Biopsy

Besides the classical applications of lymphatic mapping, experiences are gained in urogenital SLN biopsies [65]. Urogenital procedures can be divided into open (penile and vulvar cancer) and laparoscopic (prostate, testicular, kidney, cervix,

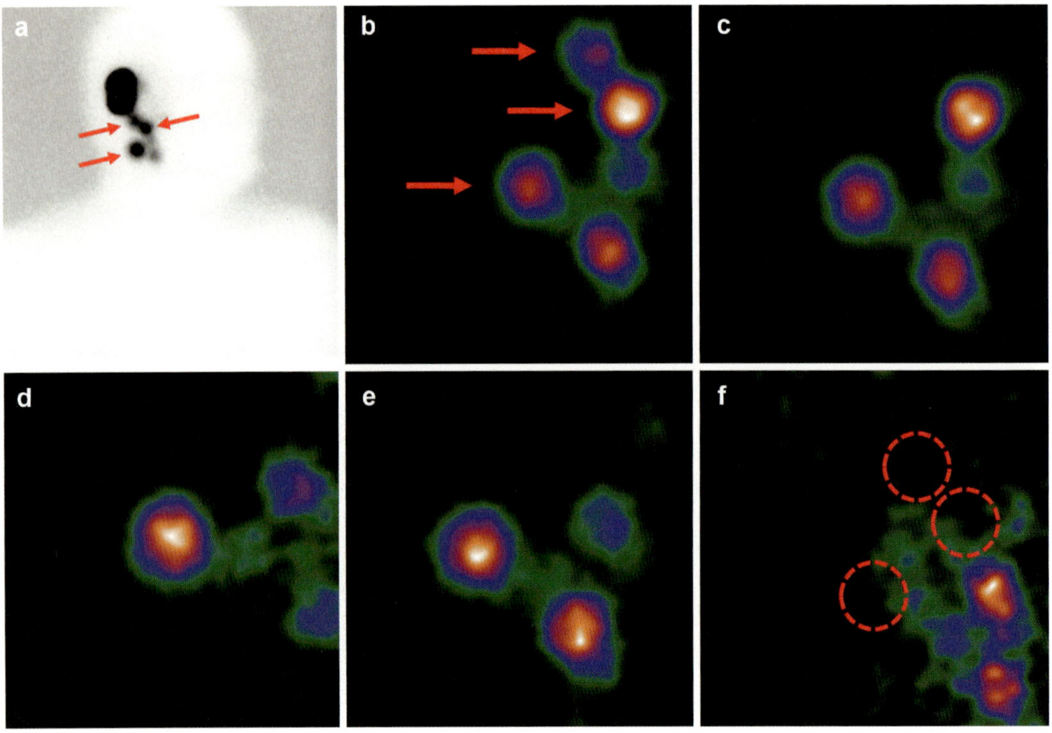

Fig. 3.5 Planar lymphoscintigraphy (**a**) after 2 h depicted the injection site and 5 radioactive hotspots corresponding three SLNs (*red arrows*) and two higher echelon nodes. A pre-incision PGC image (**b**) visualizes all five hotspots. After the excision of the first SLN, a new PGC image was obtained (**c**), which shows that the most cranial SLN was removed. The following PGC images (**d**, **e**) were taken after the removal of five other lymph nodes until all three SLNs (*red dashed circles*) were removed and only residual radioactivity was left of the higher echelon nodes (**f**)

and endometrial cancer) procedures. The first reported use of a SFOV PGC fitted with a pinhole collimator during laparoscopic urological surgery was in 2009 [13]. A total of 59 SLNs were found and the PGC enabled real-time identification in 18/20 patients (90 %). In the other two patients, SLNs could be localized with the laparoscopic gamma probe, but no identification with the PGC could be accomplished. This PGC does not allow overall visualization of the whole lymphatic drainage in wide areas such as the abdomen due to the limited field of view. Therefore, intraoperative imaging combined with preoperative conventional gamma camera imaging (and, especially in the abdomen, SPECT/CT images) is absolutely needed. The PGC is capable to detect two different signals using the dual-isotope imaging mode: the signal of ^{99m}Tc-nanocolloid for the visualization of the SLNs, plus the signal of an ^{125}I-seed which can be placed on the tip of the laparoscopic gamma probe. Location of the ^{125}I-seed can be identified as a green circle on the screen. When the green circle and the radioactive ^{99m}Tc hot spot matches on the screen, the SLN is correctly identified. The same group used this approach in 18 patients (6 renal cell carcinoma, 8 prostate, and 4 testicular cancer) with drainage to para-aortic nodes. SPECT/CT visualized SLNs in all patients, while the PGC enabled intraoperative SLN visualization in 15/18 patients. Two patients had also non-visualization on preoperative conventional lymphoscintigraphy, and one had a very weak hot spot. Authors concluded that although intraoperative imaging was of no additional value to preoperative SPECT/CT imaging, it offered the main advantage of monitoring SLN excision in the para-aortic region [66]. Once the pattern of lymph drainage is correctly identified, the use of the PGC increases the sensitivity in the SLN detection. Especially those closely located in areas of high physiologic activity, such as the liver (for para-aortic nodes) or the radiotracer injection site (e.g., parametrial nodes in cervical cancer) [14]. Furthermore, Brouwer and colleagues demonstrated in nine patients with testicular cancer that the PGC detected all 21 identified SLNs on SPECT/CT plus five additional SLNs [67]. In a larger study with 55 prostate cancer patients, the PGC was not able to detect 29/178 (16 %) SLNs detected by SPECT/CT [68]. However, intraoperative imaging was useful for localizing nodes in 15 patients (27 %), because localization with only the gamma probe was not successful. More importantly, 17 additional SLNs (two tumor-positive nodes) were detected by post-excision imaging.

Finally, a SFOV PGC was used in two other studies including 15 vulvar and 65 penile cancer patients. The main endpoint of both studies was to evaluate the use of a hybrid tracer, which was both fluorescent and radioactive. Although the PGC was used before and after SLN, its performance was not mentioned in the vulvar cancer study [69]. In the penile study, however, a remaining SLN was identified in 6/65 patients using the PGC after no residual activity was detected during initial scanning with the gamma probe. One of those additional SLNs was tumor positive and prevented a false-negative procedure [70].

3.8 Experiences in Minimally Invasive Radioguided Parathyroidectomy in Primary Hyperparathyroidism

Primary hyperparathyroidism is caused by inappropriately high secretion of parathyroid hormone (PTH) by one or more enlarged parathyroid glands. Preoperative scintigraphic identification of a solitary parathyroid adenoma characterized by clear ^{99m}Tc-sestamibi uptake is the main inclusion criterion for radioguided minimally invasive parathyroidectomy. Conventional gamma probe guidance enables the surgeon to perform a rather small incision and intraoperative parathyroid adenoma localization. Kitagawa et al. were the first who detected a parathyroid gland with a large field of view PGC in 2002 [6]. They speculated that this intraoperative imaging approach can result in smaller incisions, lower postoperative complications, and less operative time than do traditional techniques. In a following case report, the same group reported that after the excision of some tissue, intraoperative imaging revealed still an abnormal uptake in vivo. Radioguided surgery was continued and an abnormal parathyroid gland behind the right carotid artery near the right recurrent laryngeal nerve was identified [71]. This finding suggests that radioguided parathyroidectomy using intraoperative imaging is useful for localizing ectopic parathyroid tumors, which is later confirmed by case series from other groups [72–74].

Ortega and colleagues reported in their preliminary experience ($n=5$ patients) that use of the gamma probe can be avoided if a SFOV PGC is available [75]. Other studies confirmed this based on their experiences using a handheld gamma camera in 7 and 11 patients [38, 76]. The main advantage of intraoperative imaging is the morphological expression of anatomical structures and the possibility of obtaining special angle (lateral) views which provide more information than is acquired using a gamma probe. Moreover, incomplete washout of the isotope from the thyroid may produce misleading records from the gamma probe. In 2007, Ortega and colleagues speculated in the same preliminary report that it would even be possible to replace the preoperative conventional ^{99m}Tc-sestamibi scans and the intraoperative determinations of PTH, although larger studies were needed to confirm this [75]. Other groups pointed out that it would be difficult to perform minimally invasive radioguided parathyroidectomy without preoperative imaging, because it enables surgical planning and a better selection of patients suitable for minimally invasive radioguided parathyroidectomy [77]. Two years later, the hypothesis that intraoperative imaging eliminates the need for intraoperative PTH measurements was tested in 15 patients. Intraoperative imaging located all parathyroid adenomas, without the use of a gamma probe, and post-excision images

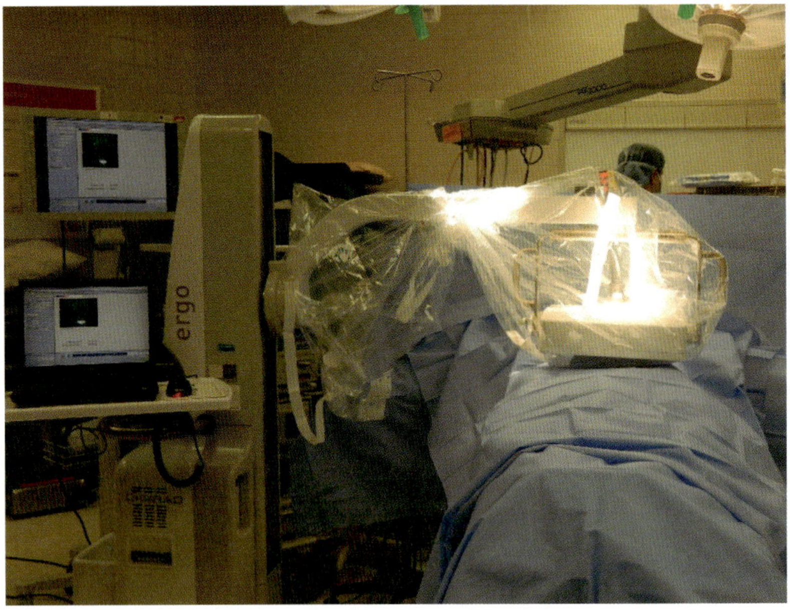

Fig. 3.6 Digital photo demonstrating the intraoperative large field of view PGC (Ergo, Digirad) setup for a pre-incision intraoperative neck image of the parathyroid adenoma (Provided courtesy of Dr. Nathan C. Hall, The Ohio State University Wexner Medical Center, Columbus, USA)

confirmed complete removal of the pathologic tissue. Again, these findings suggested that intraoperative determinations of PTH might not be needed when intraoperative imaging is used [78].

In 2012, Fujii and colleagues used a handheld gamma camera in 16 patients to proof that intraoperative PTH measurements are not needed in selected cases of single adenomas with a positive preoperative ^{99m}Tc-sestamibi scan [79]. Estrems and colleagues prospectively studied 29 patients with primary hyperparathyroidism, comparing the diagnostic effectiveness of intraoperative imaging using a PGC with the results obtained from preoperative techniques (ultrasound scan plus ^{99m}Tc-sestamibi scintigraphy). Results of this study show that the sensitivity and specificity of intraoperative PGC imaging were superior to those of the preoperative techniques. Preoperative techniques had a 79 % sensitivity and 93 % specificity for locating the pathologic parathyroid glands by side, while intraoperative PGC imaging showed sensitivity and specificity values of 90 and 96 %, respectively [80].

Recently, in 2015, Hall and colleagues evaluated the use of a large field of view PGC for radioguided parathyroid adenoma removal (Fig. 3.6). Intraoperative imaging did not show increased uptake of ^{99m}Tc-sestamibi in 13/20 patients after initial specimen excision. In the remaining 7/20 patients, residual neck activity and/or absent ex vivo specimen activity prompted excision of additional tissue, ultimately leading to complete parathyroid adenoma resection in 20/20 (100 %) patients. More interesting, the data showed that the operating time could be reduced with 22 min on average using intraoperative imaging instead of intraoperative PTH assessment [81]. Finally, in 2015, Casáns-Tormo and colleagues pointed out that intraoperative 3D imaging using freehand SPECT, providing additional information about depth, might be useful for minimally invasive radioguided parathyroidectomy as well [82].

It can be concluded that intraoperative gamma camera imaging has the potential to replace the use of conventional handheld gamma probes during radioguided parathyroid surgery, although the available evidence is limited to a small number of studies which each contain less than 30 patients. Furthermore, initial speculations of Kitagawa and colleagues that intraoperative imaging using a portable or handheld gamma camera might facilitate smaller incisions and less operative time have been proved in later studies. Nevertheless, intraoperative gamma camera imaging cannot replace preoperative gamma camera imaging, since preoperative imaging is important for establishing appropriate patient selection for radioguided parathyroid surgery.

3.9 Experiences in Radioguided Bone Lesion Localization

The principle of radioguided bone lesion localization is that after preoperative bone scintigraphy, a handheld gamma probe is used intraoperatively for tumor localization. Radioguided surgery is a good option when the bone tumor is difficult to localize, and completeness of the tumor excision can be estimated based on the gamma probe readings. Intraoperative imaging using bulky large field of view PGCs in radioguided bone lesion localization was described since 1980 [83–87]. In 2002, D'Errico and colleagues were the first who described the use of a SFOV handheld gamma camera for radioguided bone tumor biopsy in five patients [11]. These authors concluded that high-resolution intraoperative imaging over conventional gamma probe readings had the advantage that it detects bone lesions faster and more clearly than a gamma probe, especially when bone lesions are deeply located or near other radioactive sources, e.g., urine in the bladder. In 2010, Infante and colleagues mentioned that both the information of a handheld gamma camera and the use of a gamma probe are complementary to each other [88]. Intraoperative imaging provides visual confirmation of the bone lesion excision, while handheld gamma probe readings help to exactly localize the lesion. These results were later confirmed in a study with 12 patients [89].

3.10 Experiences in Other Clinical Applications

SFOV PGCs and handheld gamma cameras have been used for other applications in radioguided surgery (colon and thyroid) as well as in monitoring fusion throughout different body systems (brain, heart, and bone grafts). However, only limited experience has been gained in these particular fields. Preoperative imaging cannot be performed when an intraoperative radiotracer injection is needed. In these situations, intraoperative imaging using a portable or handheld gamma camera has even more value such as in colon SLN procedures [90].

Frontado-Morales et al. described the first radioguided surgery procedure for the treatment of locoregional lymph node recurrences in persistent differentiated papillary thyroid cancer using a SFOV PGC in 2012 [91]. Preoperatively, a radiotracer was injected directly into the lesions by ultrasound guidance. Later Bellotti and colleagues adopted this procedure using a handheld gamma camera in 22 patients. In total, 39 pathologic nodes were injected and 61 nodes were removed. Among the removed nodes, 22 (36.1 %) were additional radioactive nodes [92].

Bedside scintigraphic imaging can also be helpful to monitor blood perfusion after injecting a radiotracer in the vascular system. Therefore, the feasibility of SFOV PGCs is evaluated in: (1) cerebral perfusion scintigraphy for the diagnosis of brain death [93], (2) intraoperative assessment of bone graft vascularization [94], and (3) continuous monitoring of blood leakage in isolated limb perfusion [95].

Conclusions

Intraoperative small and large field of view gamma cameras and handheld gamma cameras have the potential to be used more widely in radioguided surgery. As advancing molecular imaging technologies will broaden clinical indications, these intraoperative cameras will probably be used and integrated with other imaging modalities (e.g., fluorescence imaging) in the near future. The feasibility and clinical safety of these systems have been proved in many publications. Preoperative lymphatic mapping with a conventional large field of view gamma camera remains the modality of choice. Intraoperative small and large field of view gamma cameras and handheld gamma cameras are mainly useful as intraoperative imaging tool in conjunction with handheld gamma detection probes. The usefulness of intraoperative real-time imaging is clear: (1) when no conventional gamma camera is available; (2) when an intraoperative radiotracer injection is needed; and (3) in difficult SLN cases such as near the injection site, deeply located SLNs, or nodes with a low radiotracer uptake. Intraoperative pre- and post-excision imaging has demonstrated that this approach is able to detect SLNs initially missed by gamma probe screening, which in rare cases prevent false-negative procedures. Unfortunately, these findings are based on single-center experiences with a limited number of patients. As for future studies, the added value of intraoperative imaging has to be proven in multicenter studies. A strict surgical protocol is critical to investigating the impact of intraoperative imaging on the detection of additional SLNs and the potential resultant finding of nodal metastases in such additional SLNs.

References

1. Vermeeren L, Klop WM, van den Brekel MW, Balm AJM, Nieweg OE, Valdés Olmos RA. Sentinel node detection in head and neck malignancies: innovations in radioguided surgery. J Oncol. 2009;2009:681746. doi:10.1155/2009/681746.
2. Soluri A, Pani R. Italian National Research Council (CNR). Miniaturized gamma camera with very high spatial resolution. Italian patent RM97A000233. 23 Apr 1997.
3. Scopinaro F, Di Luzio E, Pani R, De Vincentis G, Lamberini MP, Ballesio L, Tombolini V, De Cesare A. Sentinel node biopsy in breast cancer: use of an imaging probe. In: Limouris GS, Biersack HJ, Kouris KC, Frangos SA, Shukla SK, editors. Radionuclides for lymph nodes - current status and future aspects. Athen: Mediterra Publishers; 1999. p. 60–5.
4. Menard L, Charon Y, Solal M, Ricard M, Laniece P, Mastrippolito R, Pinot L, Valentin L. Performance characterization and first clinical evaluation of a intraoperative compact gamma imager. Proceeding 1998 IEEE Nuclear Science Symposium Conference Record. Toronto, 1999;2:1289–94.
5. Soluri A, Scafe R, Burgio N, Schiaratura A. Italian National Research Council (CNR). High spatial resolution scintigraphic device having collimator with integrated crystals. Italian patent RM2001A000279. 23 May 2001.
6. Kitagawa W, Shimizu K, Kumita SI, Akasu H, Kumazaki T, Tanaka S. Radio-guided parathyroidectomy for primary hyperparathyroidism combined with video-assisted surgery using the solid-state, multi-crystal gamma camera. J Surg Oncol. 2002;80: 173–5. doi:10.1002/jso.10120.
7. Pitre S, Ménard L, Ricard M, Solal M, Garbay JR, Charon Y. A hand-held imaging probe for radioguided surgery: physical performance and preliminary clinical experience. Eur J Nucl Med Mol Imaging. 2003;30:339–43. doi:10.1007/s00259-002-1064-2.
8. Abe A, Takahashi N, Lee J, Oka T, Shizukuishi K, Kikuchi T, Inoue T, Jimbo M, Ryuo H, Bickel C. Performance evaluation of a hand-held, semiconductor (CdZnTe)-based gamma camera. Eur J Nucl Med Mol Imaging. 2003;30:805–11. doi:10.1007/s00259-002-1067-z.
9. Tsuchimochi M, Sakahara H, Hayama K, Funaki M, Ohno R, Shirahata T, Orskaug T, Maehlum G, Yoshioka K, Nygard E. A prototype small CdTe gamma camera for radioguided surgery and other imaging applications. Eur J Nucl Med Mol Imaging. 2003;30:1605–14. doi:10.1007/s00259-003-1301-3.
10. Tsuchimochi M, Hayama K. Intraoperative gamma cameras for radioguided surgery: technical characteristics, performance parameters, and clinical applications. Phys Med. 2013;29:126–38. doi:10.1016/j.ejmp.2012.05.002.
11. D'Errico G, Rosa MA, Soluri A, Scafè R, Galli M, Chiarini S, Burgio N, Schiaratura A, Massa R, Scopinaro F. Radioguided biopsy of osteoid osteoma: usefulness of imaging probe. Tumori. 2002;88:S30–2.
12. Tanaka C, Fujii H, Shiotani A, Kitagawa Y, Nakamura K, Kubo A. Sentinel node imaging of laryngeal cancer using a portable gamma camera with CdTe semiconductor detectors. Clin Nucl Med. 2005;30:440–3.
13. Vermeeren L, Valdés Olmos RA, Meinhardt W, Bex A, van der Poel HG, Vogel WV, Sivro F, Hoefnagel CA, Horenblas S. Intraoperative radioguidance with a portable gamma camera: a novel technique for laparoscopic sentinel node localisation in urological malignancies. Eur J Nucl Med Mol Imaging. 2009;36:1029–36. doi:10.1007/s00259-009-1100-6.
14. Vidal-Sicart S, Paredes P, Zanón G, Pahisa J, Martinez-Román S, Caparrós X, Vilalta A, Rull R, Pons F. Added value of intraoperative real-time imaging in searches for difficult-to-locate sentinel nodes. J Nucl Med. 2010;51:1219–25. doi:10.2967/jnumed.110.074880.
15. Chapman J, Hugg J, Vesel J, Bai C, Blevis I, Barrett H, et al. Performance measurement of scintillation cameras. Rosslyn: National Electrical Manufacturers Association; 2007. NEMA NU 1.
16. Bhatia BS, Bugby SL, Lees JE, Perkins AC. A scheme for assessing the performance characteristics of small field-of-view gamma cameras. Phys Med. 2015;31:98–103. doi:10.1016/j.ejmp.2014.08.004.
17. Sánchez F, Benlloch JM, Escat B, Pavón N, Porras E, Kadi-Hanifi D, Ruiz JA, Mora FJ, Sebastià A. Design and tests of a portable mini gamma camera. Med Phys. 2004;31:1384–97.
18. Pouw B, van der Ploeg IM, Muller S, Valdés Olmos RA, Janssen-Pinkse LK, Oldenburg HS, Vrancken Peeters MT. Simultaneous use of an 125I-seed to guide tumour excision and 99mTc-nanocolloid for sentinel node biopsy in non-palpable breast-conserving surgery. Eur J Surg Oncol. 2015;41: 71–8.

19. van den Berg NS, Brouwer OR, Klop WMC, Karakullukcu B, Zuur CL, Tan IB, Balm AJ, van den Brekel MW, Valdés Olmos RA, van Leeuwen FW. Concomitant radio- and fluorescence-guided sentinel lymph node biopsy in squamous cell carcinoma of the oral cavity using ICG-99mTc-nanocolloid. Eur J Nucl Med Mol Imaging. 2012;39:1128–36. doi:10.1007/s00259-012-2129-5.
20. Haneishi H, Onishi Y, Shimura H, Hayashi H. Simultaneous acquisition and image synthesis of gamma cameras and optical cameras for sentinel lymph node identification during radioguided surgery. IEEE Trans Nucl Sci. 2007;54:1703–9. doi:10.1109/TNS.2007.906160.
21. Haneishi H, Shimura H, Hayashi H. Image synthesis using a mini gamma camera and stereo optical cameras. IEEE Trans Nucl Sci. 2010;57:1132–8. doi:10.1109/TNS.2010.2044805.
22. Lees JE, Bassford DJ, Blake OE, Blackshaw PE, Perkins AC. A Hybrid Camera for simultaneous imaging of gamma and optical photons. J Instrum. 2012;7:P06009. doi:10.1088/1748-0221/7/06/P06009.
23. Lees JE, Bugby SL, Bhatia BS, Jambi LK, Alqahtani MS, McKnight WR, Ng AH, Perkins AC. A small field of view camera for hybrid gamma and optical imaging. J Instrum. 2014;9:C12020. doi:10.1088/1748-0221/9/12/C12020.
24. Hellingman D, Vidal-Sicart S, de Wit-van der Veen LJ, Paredes P, Valdés Olmos RA. A new portable hybrid camera for fused optical and scintigraphic imaging: first clinical experiences. Clin Nucl Med. 2015. [Epub ahead of print].
25. Wendler T, Herrmann K, Schnelzer A, Lasser T, Traub J, Kutter O, Ehlerding A, Scheidhauer K, Schuster T, Kiechle M, Schwaiger M, Navab N, Ziegler SI, Buck AK. First demonstration of 3-D lymphatic mapping in breast cancer using freehand SPECT. Eur J Nucl Med Mol Imaging. 2010;37:1452–61. doi:10.1007/s00259-010-1430-4.
26. Freesmeyer M, Winkens T, Opfermann T, Elsner P, Runnebaum I, Darr A. Real-time ultrasound and freehand-SPECT. Experiences with sentinel lymph node mapping. Nuklearmedizin. 2014;53:259–64. doi:10.3413/Nukmed-0680-14-06.
27. Freesmeyer M, Opfermann T, Winkens T. Hybrid integration of real-time US and freehand SPECT: proof of concept in patients with thyroid diseases. Radiology. 2014;271:856–61. doi:10.1148/radiol.14132415.
28. Bricou A, Duval M-A, Charon Y, Barranger E. Mobile gamma cameras in breast cancer care – a review. Eur J Surg Oncol. 2013;39:409–16. doi:10.1016/j.ejso.2013.02.008.
29. Goto M, Okuyama C, Kubota T, Ushijima Y, Nishimura T. Assessment of the solid-state gamma camera to depict axillary sentinel lymph nodes in breast cancer patients. Ann Nucl Med. 2005;19:627–31. doi:10.1007/BF02985058.
30. Kerrou K, Pitre S, Coutant C, Rouzier R, Ancel PY, Lebeaux C, Huchet V, Montravers F, Pascal O, Duval MA, Lefebvre F, Menard L, Uzan S, Charon Y, Barranger E. The usefulness of a preoperative compact imager, a hand-held gamma-camera for breast cancer sentinel node biopsy: final results of a prospective double-blind, clinical study. J Nucl Med. 2011;52:1346–53. doi:10.2967/jnumed.111.090464.
31. Vidal-Sicart S, Vermeeren L, Solà O, Paredes P, Valdés-Olmos RA. The use of a portable gamma camera for preoperative lymphatic mapping: a comparison with a conventional gamma camera. Eur J Nucl Med Mol Imaging. 2011;38:636–41. doi:10.1007/s00259-010-1682-z.
32. Scopinaro F, Pani R, Soluri A, Pellegrini R, Scafè R, De Vincentis G, Capoccetti F, David V, Chiarini S, Stella S. Detection of sentinel node in breast cancer: pilot study with the imaging probe. Tumori. 2000; 86:329–31.
33. D'Errico G, Scafé R, Soluri A, Schiaratura A, Mangano AM, David V, Scopinaro F. One-inch field of view imaging probe for breast cancer sentinel node location. Nucl Instrum Methods Phys Res. 2003;497:105–9. doi:10.1016/S0168-9002(02)01898-3.
34. Aarsvod JN, Greene CM, Mintzer RA, Grant SF, Styblo TM, Alazraki NP, Patt BE, Caravaglia GM, Li J, Iwanczyk JS. Intraoperative gamma imaging of axillary sentinel lymph nodes in breast cancer patients. Phys Medica. 2006;21:76–9. doi:http://dx.doi.org/10.1016/S1120-1797(06)80030-X.
35. Mathelin C, Salvador S, Huss D, Guyonnet JL. Precise localization of sentinel lymph nodes and estimation of their depth using a prototype intraoperative mini gamma-camera in patients with breast cancer. J Nucl Med. 2007;48:623–9.
36. Motomura K, Noguchi A, Hashizume T, Hasegawa Y, Komoike Y, Inaji H, Saida T, Koyama H. Usefulness of a solid-state gamma camera for sentinel node identification in patients with breast cancer. J Surg Oncol. 2005;89:12–7. doi:10.1002/jso.20162.
37. Mathelin C, Salvador S, Bekaert V, Croce S, Andriamisandratsoa N, Liégeois P, Prados E, Guyonnet JL, Grucker D, Brasse D. A new intraoperative gamma camera for the sentinel lymph node procedure in breast cancer. Anticancer Res. 2008;28:2859–64.
38. Soluri A, Trotta C, Scopinaro F, Tofani A, D'Alessandria C, Pasta V, Stella S, Massari R. Radioisotope guided surgery with imaging probe, a hand-held high-resolution gamma camera. Nucl Instrum Methods Phys Res Sect A. 2007;583:366–71. doi:10.1016/j.nima.2007.09.031.
39. Olcott P, Pratx G, Johnson D, Mittra E, Niederkohr R, Levin CS. Clinical evaluation of a novel intraoperative handheld gamma camera for sentinel lymph node biopsy. Phys Med. 2014;30:340–5. doi:10.1016/j.ejmp.2013.10.005.
40. Chondrogiannis S, Ferretti A, Facci E, Marzola MC, Rampin L, Tadayyon S, Maffione AM, Reale D, Mencarelli R, Marcolongo A, Rubello D. Intraoperative hand-held imaging γ-camera for sentinel node detection in patients with breast cancer: feasibility evaluation and preliminary experience on 16 patients. Clin Nucl Med. 2013;38:e132–6. doi:10.1097/RLU.0b013e31827a278d.

41. Cardona-Arboniés J, Mucientes-Rasilla J, Moreno Elola-Olaso A, Salazar-Andía G, Prieto-Soriano A, Chicharo de Freitas J, Román-Santamaría JM, Carreras-Delgado JL. Contribution of the portable gamma camera to detect the sentinel node in breast cancer during surgery. Rev Esp Med Nucl Imagen Mol. 2012;31:130–4. doi:http://dx.doi.org/10.1016/j.remn.2011.05.007.
42. Soluri A, Massari R, Trotta C, Tofani A, Di Santo G, Di Pietro B, Di Paolo ML, Roncacci A, Amanti C, Scopinaro F. Small field of view, high-resolution, portable γ-camera for axillary sentinel node detection. Nucl Instrum Methods Phys Res Sect A. 2006;569:273–6. doi:10.1016/j.nima.2006.08.027.
43. Scopinaro F, Tofani A, di Santo G, Di Pietro B, Lombardi A, Lo Russo M, Soluri A, Massari R, Trotta C, Amanti C. High-resolution, hand-held camera for sentinel-node detection. Cancer Biother Radiopharm. 2008;23:43–52. doi:10.1089/cbr.2007.364.
44. Goñi Gironés E, Vicente García F, Serra Arbeloa P, Estébanez Estébanez C, Calvo Benito A, Rodrigo Rincón I, Camarero Salazar A, Martínez Lozano ME. Evaluation of the efficacy of sentinel node detection in breast cancer: chronological course and influence of the incorporation of an intra-operative portable gamma camera. Rev Esp Med Nucl Imagen Mol. 2013;32:343–9. doi:http://dx.doi.org/10.1016/j.remn.2013.02.008.
45. Duch J. Portable gamma cameras: the real value of an additional view in the operating theatre. Eur J Nucl Med Mol Imaging. 2011;38:633–5. doi:10.1007/s00259-011-1761-9.
46. Vidal-Sicart S, Rioja ME, Paredes P, Keshtgar MR, Valdés Olmos RA. Contribution of perioperative imaging to radioguided surgery. Q J Nucl Med Mol Imaging. 2014;58:140–60.
47. Paredes P, Vidal-Sicart S, Zanón G, Roé N, Rubí S, Lafuente S, Pavía J, Pons F. Radioguided occult lesion localisation in breast cancer using an intraoperative portable gamma camera: first results. Eur J Nucl Med Mol Imaging. 2008;35:230–5. doi:10.1007/s00259-007-0640-x.
48. Lombardi A, Nigri G, Scopinaro F, Maggi S, Mattei M, Bonifacino A, Parisella M, Soluri A, Amanti C. High-resolution, handheld camera use for occult breast lesion localization plus sentinel node biopsy (SNOLL): a single-institution experience with 186 patients. Surgeon. 2015;13:69–72. doi:10.1016/j.surge.2013.10.005.
49. Bricou A, Duval MA, Bardet L, Benbara A, Moreaux G, Lefebvre F, Menard L, Pinot L, Charon Y, Tengher Barna I, Soussan M, Sellier N, Barranger E. Is there a role for a handheld gamma camera (TReCam) in the SNOLL breast cancer procedure?. Q J Nucl Med Mol Imaging. 2015. [Epub ahead of print].
50. Soluri A, Scafè R, Capoccetti F, Burgio N, Schiaratura A, Panic R, Pellegrini R, Cinti MN, Mechella M, Amanti A, David V, Scopinaro F. Imaging probe for breast cancer localization. Nucl Instrum Methods Phys Res Sect A. 2003;497:114–21. doi:10.1016/S0168-9002(02)01900-9.
51. Soluri A, Scopinaro F, De Vincentis G, Varvarigou A, Scafé R, Massa R, Schillaci O, Spanu A, David V. 99MTC [13LEU] bombesin and a new gamma camera, the imaging probe, are able to guide mammotome breast biopsy. Anticancer Res. 2003;23:2139–42.
52. Di Santo G, Archimandritis S, Soluri A, Trotta C, Massari R, Parisella MG, Anastasia A, Mattei M, Monteleone F, Chiacchiararelli L, Varvarigou A, Scopinaro F. High-resolution scintigraphy and 99mTc Bombesin are able to guide Mammotome biopsy and to detect lymph node invasion. Nucl Instrum Methods Phys Res Sect A. 2006;569:171–4. doi:10.1016/j.nima.2006.08.013.
53. Evangelista L, Cervino AR, Sanco R, Bignotto M, Saibene T, Michieletto S, Ghiotto C, Bozza F, Paiusco M, Saladini G. Use of a portable gamma camera for guiding surgical treatment in locally advanced breast cancer in a post-neoadjuvant therapy setting. Breast Cancer Res Treat. 2014;146:331–40. doi:10.1007/s10549-014-3007-6.
54. Bricou A, Barranger E. Response to the article by Evangelista et al.: use of a portable gamma camera for guiding surgical treatment in locally advanced breast cancer in a post-neoadjuvant therapy setting. Breast Cancer Res Treat 2014. Breast Cancer Res Treat. 2014;148:231–2. doi:10.1007/s10549-014-3062-z.
55. Dengel LT, More MJ, Judy PG, Petroni GR, Smolkin ME, Rehm PK, Majewski S, Williams MB, Slingluff Jr CL. Intraoperative imaging guidance for sentinel node biopsy in melanoma using a mobile gamma camera. Ann Surg. 2011;253:774–8. doi:10.1097/SLA.0b013e3181f9b709.
56. Stoffels I, Poeppel T, Boy C, Mueller S, Wichmann F, Dissemond J, Schadendorf D, Rosenbaum-Krumme S, Klode J. Radio-guided surgery: advantages of a new portable γ-camera (Sentinella) for intraoperative real time imaging and detection of sentinel lymph nodes in cutaneous malignancies. J Eur Acad Dermatol Venereol. 2012;26:308–13. doi:10.1111/j.1468-3083.2011.04057.x.
57. ClinicalTrials.gov Website (a service of the U.S. National Institutes of Health). Available at: https://clinicaltrials.gov/ct2/show/NCT02416336?term=sentinella&rank=1. Accessed 10 Jun 2015. Clinicaltrails.gov Identifier: NCT02416336.
58. Carlson GW, Page AJ, Cohen C, Parker D, Yaar R, Li A, Hestley A, Delman KA, Murray DR. Regional recurrence after negative sentinel lymph node biopsy for melanoma. Ann Surg. 2008;248:378–86. doi:10.1097/SLA.0b013e3181855718.
59. Vidal-Sicart S, Brouwer OR, Mathéron HM, Bing Tan I, Valdés-Olmos RA. Sentinel node identification with a portable gamma camera in case without visualization on conventional lymphoscintigraphy and SPECT/CT. Rev Esp Med Nucl Imagen Mol. 2013;32:203–4. doi:10.1016/j.jmb.2005.03.040.
60. Mayoral M, Paredes P, Sieira R, Vidal-Sicart S, Marti C, Pons F. The added value of a portable gamma camera for intraoperative detection of sentinel lymph node in squamous cell carcinoma of the oral cavity: a

case report. Rev Esp Med Nucl Imagen Mol. 2014;33:237–40. doi:10.1016/j.remn.2013.12.007.
61. Hellingman D, de Wit-van der Veen LJ, Klop WMC, Valdés-Olmos RA. Detecting near-the-injection-site sentinel nodes in head and neck melanomas with a high-resolution portable gamma camera. Clin Nucl Med. 2014;40:e11–6. doi:10.1097/RLU.0000000000000370.
62. Tsuchimochi M, Hayama K, Oda T, Togashi M, Sakahara H. Evaluation of the efficacy of a small CdTe γ-camera for sentinel lymph node biopsy. J Nucl Med. 2008;49:956–62. doi:10.2967/jnumed.108.050740.
63. Vermeeren L, Valdés Olmos RA, Klop WMC, Balm AJ, van den Brekel MW. A portable gamma-camera for intraoperative detection of sentinel nodes in the head and neck region. J Nucl Med. 2010;51:700–3. doi:10.2967/jnumed.109.071407.
64. Borbón-Arce M, Brouwer OR, van den Berg NS, Mathéron H, Klop WM, Balm AJ, van Leeuwen FW, Valdés-Olmos RA. An innovative multimodality approach for sentinel node mapping and biopsy in head and neck malignancies. Rev Esp Med Nucl Imagen Mol. 2014;33:274–9. doi:10.1016/j.remn.2013.11.005.
65. Giammarile F, Vidal-Sicart S, Valdés Olmos RA. Uncommon applications of sentinel lymph node mapping: urogenital cancers. Q J Nucl Med Mol Imaging. 2014;58:161–79.
66. Vermeeren L, Meinhardt W, Bex A, van der Poel HG, Vogel WV, Hoefnagel CA, Horenblas S, Valdés Olmos RA. Paraaortic sentinel lymph nodes: toward optimal detection and intraoperative localization using SPECT/CT and intraoperative real-time imaging. J Nucl Med. 2010;51:376–82. doi:10.2967/jnumed.109.071779.
67. Brouwer OR, Valdés Olmos RA, Vermeeren L, Hoefnagel CA, Nieweg OE, Horenblas S. SPECT/CT and a portable gamma-camera for image-guided laparoscopic sentinel node biopsy in testicular cancer. J Nucl Med. 2011;52:551–4. doi:10.2967/jnumed.110.086660.
68. Vermeeren L, Valdés Olmos RA, Meinhardt W, Bex A, van der Poel HG, Vogel WV, Sivro F, Hoefnagel CA, Horenblas S. Intraoperative imaging for sentinel node identification in prostate carcinoma: its use in combination with other techniques. J Nucl Med. 2011;52:741–4. doi:10.2967/jnumed.110.085068.
69. Mathéron HM, van den Berg NS, Brouwer OR, et al. Multimodal surgical guidance towards the sentinel node in vulvar cancer. Gynecol Oncol. 2013;131:720–5. doi:10.1016/j.ygyno.2013.09.007.
70. Brouwer OR, Van Den Berg NS, Mathéron HM, Kleinjan GH, van Driel WJ, Trum JW, Vegt E, Kenter G, van Leeuwen FW, Valdés Olmos RA. A hybrid radioactive and fluorescent tracer for sentinel node biopsy in penile carcinoma as a potential replacement for blue dye. Eur Urol. 2014;65:600–9. doi:10.1016/j.eururo.2013.11.014.
71. Kitagawa W, Shimizu K, Akasu H. Radioguided parathyroidectomy for primary hyperparathyroidism using the solid-state, multi-crystal gamma camera. Med Sci Monit. 2003;9:CS53–6.
72. García-Talavera P, González-Selma ML, Ruiz M, Gamazo C, Sainz-Esteban A, Villanueva JG, Olmos R. The value of early SPECT/CT and hand-held F -camera in radio-guided surgery. Clin Nucl Med. 2014;39:1009–11.
73. Díaz-Expósito R, Casáns-Tormo I, Cassinello-Fernández N, Ortega-Serrano J, Mut-Dólera T. Contribution of intraoperative scintigraphy to the detection of intrathyroidal parathyroid adenoma. Rev Esp Med Nucl Imagen Mol 2014;33:296–8. doi: http://dx.doi.org/10.1016/j.remn.2013.09.011.
74. Gregorio S, Serena C, Melfa GI, Lo Piccolo C, Raspanti C, Richiusa P, Costa RP, Gulotta G. The intraoperative use of the mini-gamma camera (MGC) in the surgical treatment of primary hyperparathyroidism technical reports and immediate results from the initial experience. Ann Ital Chir. 2015;86:212–8.
75. Ortega J, Ferrer-Rebolleda J, Cassinello N, Lledo S. Potential role of a new hand-held miniature gamma camera in performing minimally invasive parathyroidectomy. Eur J Nucl Med Mol Imaging. 2007;34:165–9. doi:10.1007/s00259-006-0239-7.
76. Fujii T, Yamaguchi S, Yajima R, Tsutsumi S, Uchida N, Asao T, Oriuch N, Kuwano H. Use of a handheld, semiconductor (cadmium zinc telluride)-based gamma camera in navigation surgery for primary hyperparathyroidism. Am Surg. 2011;77:690–3.
77. Rubello D, Mariani G. Hand-held gamma probe or hand-held miniature gamma camera for minimally invasive parathyroidectomy: competition, evolution or synergy? Eur J Nucl Med Mol Imaging. 2007;34:162–4. doi:10.1007/s00259-006-0250-z.
78. Cassinello N, Ortega J, Lledo S. Intraoperative real-time 99mTc-sestamibi scintigraphy with miniature gamma camera allows minimally invasive parathyroidectomy without ioPTH determination in primary hyperparathyroidism. Langenbecks Arch Surg. 2009;394:869–74. doi:10.1007/s00423-009-0523-7.
79. Fujii T, Yajima R, Yamaguchi S, Tsutsumi S, Asao T, Kuwano H. Could the eZ-SCOPE AN gamma camera replace intraoperative measurement of iPTH for PHPT? Int Surg. 2012;97:99–103. doi:10.9738/CC138.1.
80. Estrems P, Guallart F, Abreu P, Sopena P, Dalmau J, Sopena R. The intraoperative mini gamma camera in primary hyperparathyroidism surgery. Acta Otorrinolaringol Esp. 2012;63:450–7. doi:10.1016/j.otorri.2012.04.009.
81. Hall NC, Plews RL, Agrawal A, Povoski SP, Wright CL, Zhang J, Martin Jr EW, Phay J. Intraoperative scintigraphy using a large field-of-view portable gamma camera for primary hyperparathyroidism: initial experience. Biomed Res Int. 2015;2015:930575. doi:10.1155/2015/930575.
82. Casáns-Tormo I, Prado-Wohlwend S, Díaz-Expósito R, Cassinello-Fernández N, Ortega-Serrano J. E. [Initial experience in intraoperative radiolocalization of the parathyroid adenoma with freehand SPECT and comparative assessment with portable gamma-camera]. Rev Esp Med Nucl Imagen Mol.

2015;34:116–9. doi:http://dx.doi.org/10.1016/j.remn.2014.11.005.
83. Rinsky LA, Goris M, Bleck EE, Halpern A, Hirshman P. Intraoperative skeletal scintigraphy for localization of osteoid-osteoma in the spine. Case report. J Bone Joint Surg Am. 1980;62:143–4.
84. Sty J, Simons G. Intraoperative 99m technetium bone imaging in the treatment of benign osteoblastic tumors. Clin Orthop Relat Res. 1982;165:223–7.
85. Meire E, Hoogmartens M, de Roo M, Mortelmans L, Nicolai D. The peroperative use of the mobile gamma camera for the localization of spinal osteoid osteoma. Acta Orthop Belg. 1983;49:384–90.
86. Ellison MJ, Issac L, Smith WI, Donofrio RJ, Turbiner EH. Intraoperative scintigraphic localization of the nidus of osteoid osteoma. Clin Nucl Med. 1984;9:640–2. doi:10.1097/00003072-198411000-00009.
87. Osebold WR, Lester EL, Hurley JH, Vincent RL. Intraoperative use of the mobile gamma camera in localizing and excising osteoid osteomas of the spine. Spine (Phila Pa 1976). 1993;18:1816–28. doi:10.1097/00007632-199310000-00018.
88. Infante JR, Rayo JI, Serrano J, Domínguez ML, García L, Durán C. Spinal osteoblastoma resection with radioguided surgery. Rev Esp Med Nucl. 2010;29:78–80. doi:10.1016/S1578-200X(10)70011-5.
89. Infante JR, Lorente R, Rayo JI, Serrano J, Domínguez ML, García L, Moreno M. [Use of radioguided surgery in the surgical treatment of osteoid osteoma]. Rev Esp Med Nucl Imagen Mol. 2015. doi:10.1016/j.remn.2015.01.003 [Epub ahead of print].
90. Bianchi PP, Petz W, Casali L. Laparoscopic lymphatic roadmapping with blue dye and radioisotope in colon cancer. Colorectal Dis. 2011;13:67–9. doi:10.1111/j.1463-1318.2011.02786.x.
91. Frontado-Morales L, Martinez-Sanchis B, Sanchez-Vaño R, Caballero-Calabuig E, Abreu-Sanchez P, Reyes-Ojeda MD. Radioguided cervical lymphadenectomy in one case of recurrence of differentiated thyroid microcarcinoma. Rev Rev Esp Med Nucl Imagen Mol. 2012;31:106–7. doi:http://dx.doi.org/10.1016/j.remnie.2011.05.002.
92. Bellotti C, Castagnola G, Tierno SM, Centanini F, Sparagna A, Vetrone I, Mezzetti G. Radioguided surgery with combined use of gamma probe and hand-held gamma camera for treatment of papillary thyroid cancer locoregional recurrences: a preliminary study. Eur Rev Med Pharmacol Sci. 2013;17:3362–6.
93. Calvo Morón C, de la Riva Pérez PA, Cambil Molina T, Alvarez Márquez E, Castro MJ. Brain perfusion image with a portable mini-gamma camera (Sentinella®) in brain death. Rev Esp Med Nucl. 2009;28:83–4. doi:10.1016/S0212-6982(09)70705-0.
94. Krohn T, Ghassemi A, Gerressen M, Verburg FA, Mottaghy FM, Behrendt FF. Bone graft scintigraphy-a new diagnostic tool to assess perfusion during surgery. Nuklearmedizin. 2012;51:201–4.
95. Orero A, Vidal-Sicart S, Roé N, Muxí A, Rubí S, Duch J, Rull R, Pavón N, Pons F, Pavía J. Monitoring system for isolated limb perfusion based on a portable gamma camera. Nuklearmedizin. 2009;48:166–72. doi:10.3413/nukmed-0223.
96. Knoll P, Mirzaei S, Schwenkenbecher K, Barthel T. Performance evaluation of a solid-state detector based handheld gamma camera system. Front Biomed Tech. 2014;1:61–7.
97. Olcott PD, Habte F, Foudray AM, Levin CS. Characterization of performance of a miniature, high sensitivity gamma ray camera. IEEE Symp Conf Rec Nucl Sci. 2004;6:1492–7. doi:10.1109/NSSMIC.2004.1466753.
98. Ferretti A, Chondrogiannis S, Marcolongo A, Rubello D. Phantom study of a new hand-held γ-imaging probe for radio-guided surgery. Nucl Med Commun. 2013;34:86–90. doi:10.1097/MNM.0b013e32835a7ccd.
99. Bugby SL, Lees JE, Bhatia BS, Perkins AC. Characterisation of a high resolution small field of view portable gamma camera. Phys Med. 2014;30:331–9. doi:10.1016/j.ejmp.2013.10.004.

Surgical Navigation: An Overview of the State-of-the-Art Clinical Applications

4

Paulo Waelkens, Matthias N. van Oosterom, Nynke S. van den Berg, Nassir Navab, and Fijs W.B. van Leeuwen

Contents

P. Waelkens • M.N. van Oosterom
Department of Surgery, Leiden University Medical Center (LUMC), Leiden, The Netherlands

Interventional Molecular Imaging Laboratory, Department of Radiology, Leiden University Medical Center (LUMC), Leiden, The Netherlands

N.S. van den Berg • F.W.B. van Leeuwen (✉)
Interventional Molecular Imaging Laboratory, Department of Radiology, Leiden University Medical Center (LUMC), Leiden, The Netherlands

Departments of Urology and Head and Neck Surgery and Oncology, Antoni van Leeuwenhoek Hospital – Netherlands Cancer Institute (AVL-NKI), Amsterdam, The Netherlands
e-mail: f.w.b.van_leeuwen@lumc.nl

N. Navab
Computer Aided Medical Procedures (CAMP), Technische Universität München, Munich, Germany

Abstract

Anatomical and/or functional imaging modalities like computed tomography (CT), magnetic resonance imaging (MRI) and ultrasound, often combined with contrast agents, and molecular imaging modalities like single-photon emission computed tomography (SPECT) and positron emission tomography (PET) have become standard tools to aid in the diagnosis, monitoring and treatment of disease or injury. Yet, translating this wealth of detailed preoperative imaging information into better surgical treatment and clinical outcome is an ongoing challenge. Patient scans usually provide a 3D map of the disease, often placed in the context of the patient's anatomy, that surgeons can use as a reference to guide them during an intervention. It would be very convenient for the surgeon to know exactly where surgical tools are on this map relative to the target location or, even better, to be provided with an optimal path from the tools towards the target.

4.1 Introduction

An analogy can be made between surgical navigation and global positioning system (GPS)-based navigation apps available on smartphones and similar devices, as illustrated in Fig. 4.1. Smartphone navigation shows a map of our

K. Herrmann et al. (eds.), *Radioguided Surgery: Current Applications and Innovative Directions in Clinical Practice*, DOI 10.1007/978-3-319-26051-8_4

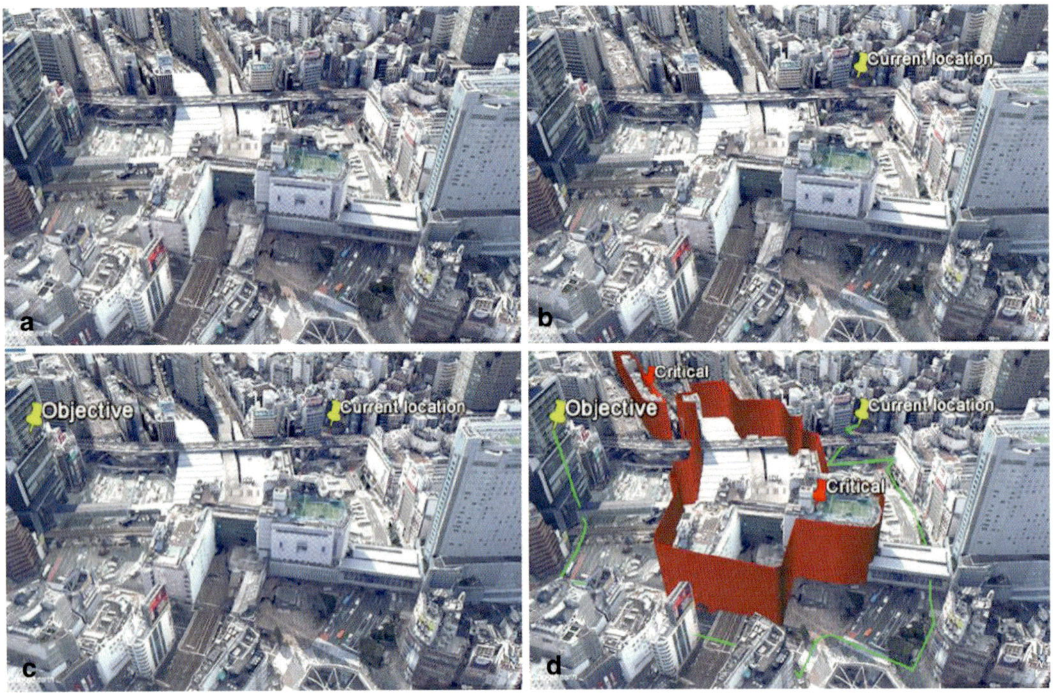

Fig. 4.1 Analogy between surgical navigation and smartphone navigation apps. (**a**): Raw 3D map of the region of interest (Depicted: Shibuya Station, Tokyo). (**b**) Current location of the surgical tools on the map, analogous to GPS localisation. (**c**): The target location for navigation, i.e. the objective, can be marked on the map. (**d**): Guidance of surgical tools to the target along optimal path (*in green*), whilst avoiding damage to nearby critical structures. Images generated with Google Earth, satellite images provided by USGS/NASA Landsat

surroundings, analogous to a patient scan (Fig. 4.1a). It shows our current location on this map (using GPS tracking), analogous to showing where surgical tools are in the image of the patient (Fig. 4.1b). The user can mark the objective on the map, analogous to marking the location of the surgical target (e.g. tumour, lymph node; Fig. 4.1c). Subsequently, the navigation app then suggests an optimal route between our current location and the objective, analogous to suggesting an optimal trajectory of the surgical tools to the target (Fig. 4.1d).

Navigation is a collective term that describes any workflow where patient scans, real-time tracking, and, occasionally, computer-aided planning are combined into real-time spatial information that provides orientation (Fig. 4.1b, c) and sometimes even guidance to reach the target location (Fig. 4.1d) during an intervention. The main benefit of this technology is the possibility to precisely indicate where structures of interest are located relative to the surgical tools in 3D. This is possible even when the structures of interest are covered by tissue and cannot be seen during surgery. Although surgical navigation technologies have not yet reached full maturity, clinical evidence already suggests it is of benefit to many clinical applications. Navigation promises to bring machine precision to clinical interventions, and will likely contribute to the emergence of more precise, less invasive and, hopefully, more effective procedures.

This chapter starts with the presentation of a typical navigation workflow and the methodologies behind this approach. Subsequently a broad overview of navigation in various clinical fields, including radioguided surgery, is provided. We close the chapter with a short discussion on the presented applications and the general developments we may expect in the upcoming years.

4.2 Navigation Workflow

The tracking systems (Fig. 4.2⑤) are an essential component in all navigation workflows as they define the intraoperative coordinate system during an intervention. They are used to estimate the position and orientation of specially marked objects (Fig. 4.2⑦, ⑧). These estimates, com-

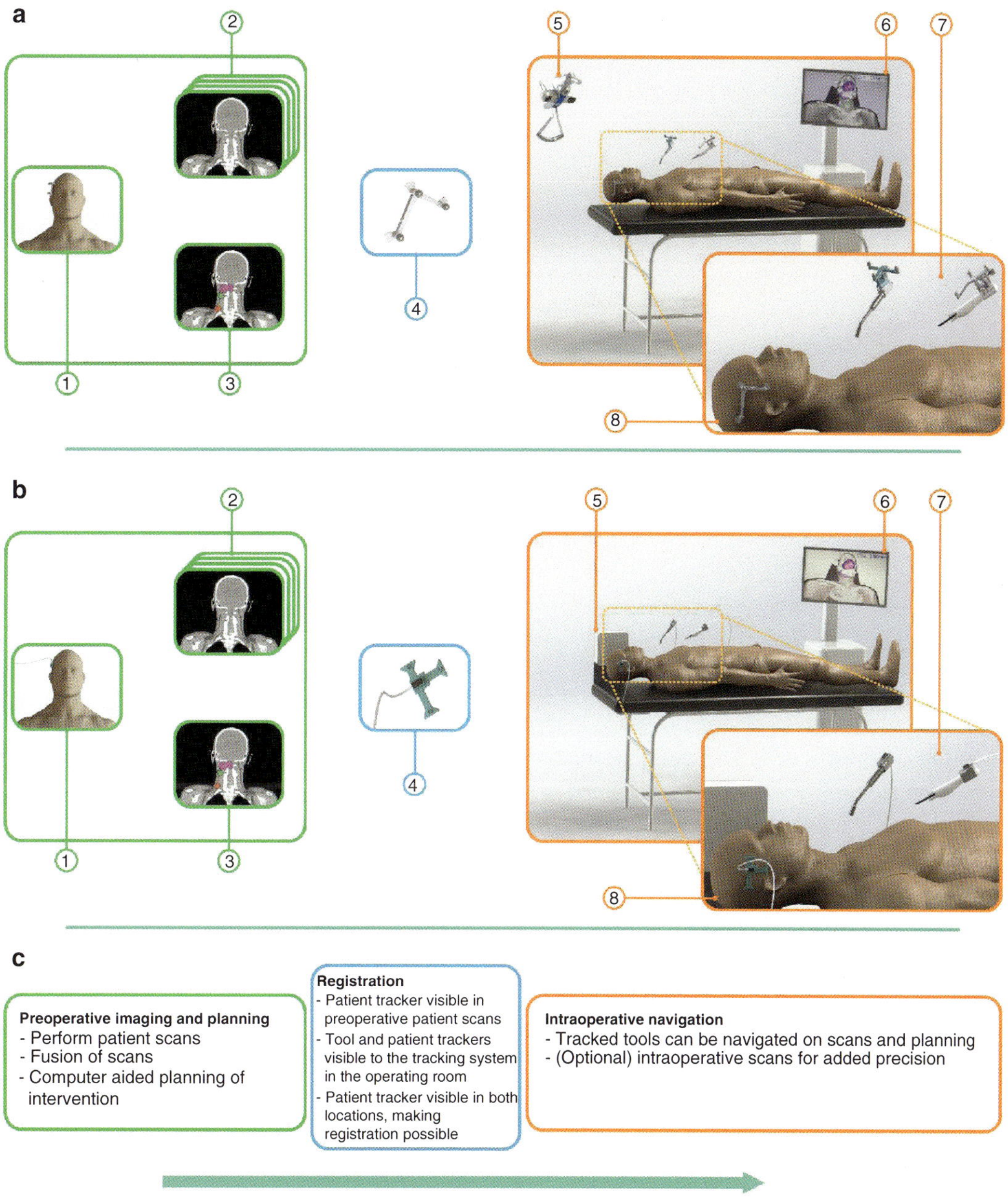

Fig. 4.2 Overview of a typical navigation workflow; (**a**) uses optical tracking and (**b**) uses electromagnetic tracking. (**c**) describes the sequence of steps in a typical workflow. ① Patient with tracker, ② multiple patient scans, ③ computer-aided planning, ④ tracker visible in preoperative and intraoperative coordinate systems, ⑤ tracking system, ⑥ navigation platform, ⑦ tracked tools, ⑧ patient with tracker on OR table. CAD models of dummy human male (by Leon Maryasin) and hospital bed (by Felipe Ospina Ochoa) found in the community library of grabcad.com

bined with registrations, enable the placement of tracked tools, patient scans and, if available, (computer-aided) planning in the same coordinate system. For object tracking, there are a number of different techniques available, e.g. near-infrared (NIR) optical tracking, electromagnetic (EM) tracking, mechanical tracking and acoustic tracking [1–4]. Of these techniques, NIR optical tracking and EM tracking are by far the most commonly used in clinical practice and will therefore be of main focus for this book chapter.

With NIR optical tracking systems (Fig. 4.2a⑤), the emission and detection of NIR light is used to determine the position of trackers in space. To obtain stereo-vision, thus depth optical perception, this NIR light has to be captured by at least two cameras in a known spatial configuration. NIR optical tracking can only work when enough fiducial markers (small objects that each approximate a point and jointly representing three noncollinear points of a tracker; see next section) are in the line of sight of these NIR cameras. Marker occlusion, e.g. by surgical staff standing between the tracking system and the fiducials, is a limitation of this tracking technique and of optical tracking in general.

EM tracking systems (Fig. 4.2b⑤), on the other hand, rely on variations in the magnetic field generated by a dedicated field generator to determine the position of sensor coils present on the tracker relative to the generator. The varying magnetic field induces current and potential in the coils. Usually, multiple coils are combined into a single tracker, and the combined readings from these coils provide enough information to estimate the position and orientation of the tracker in space. Unlike NIR tracking, EM tracking systems do not require a direct line of sight to the trackers, but they have different limitations: (1) Nearby metal objects can distort the magnetic field, leading to incorrect position and orientation estimations, and (2) the working volume of current EM tracking systems is usually smaller than that of NIR optical tracking systems.

4.2.1 Tracking

4.2.1.1 Patient Tracking

In most navigation workflows, the purpose of tracking surgical tools is to determine their position relative to the patient's anatomy and the diseased tissue therein (as in Fig. 4.1b) as such to better guide the surgeon during the procedure. The typical navigation workflow will make use of preoperative imaging, meaning that the preoperative imaging data set (Fig. 4.2①–③) has to be coupled to the interventional intraoperative coordinate system (Fig. 4.2⑤–⑧). The trick used to achieve this preoperative and intraoperative co-registration is to place a special tracker (Fig. 4.2④) at the same position on the patient during preoperative imaging and during the intervention. This tracker is, by design, both visible to the tracking system and easily segmented from the preoperative scan. Once segmented, the position of the tracker relative to the patient can be calculated, leading to a registration between the coordinates of the patient and the tracker.

To use the patient scan as a 3D map that is accurately positioned in the intraoperative coordinate system, the patient-to-tracker registration has to be coupled to the tracked position of the tracker in the intervention room. Essential requirements for precise registration are the identical placement of the tracker during preoperative imaging and during the intervention, and as little tissue deformation as possible between imaging and the intervention.

A tracker is an object that is visible to the tracking system and holds enough information for the tracking system to unambiguously establish all six degrees of freedom of the tracker in 3D space (three degrees of freedom for the position and three for the orientation). Trackers can be attached to surgical tools or to portions of the patient's anatomy, enabling their tracking (Fig. 4.2⑦, ⑧). To accomplish tracking, the position of at least three noncollinear points must be monitored, as we illustrate in Fig. 4.3. Most trackers are designed to be clearly visible to the tracking system and easy to segment from patient

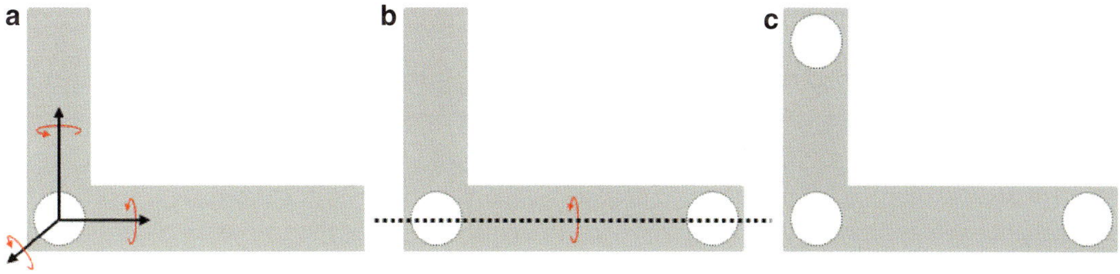

Fig. 4.3 Fiducial markers on a rigid tracker. (**a**): one fiducial, no orientation information (**b**): two fiducials, orientation around dotted line unknown (**c**): three noncollinear fiducials, unambiguous position and orientation

scans, as seen in Fig. 4.2④. Such trackers are visible both in the preoperative and in the intraoperative coordinate systems, providing the link between them and making registrations possible.

The composition of a tracker is dependent on the tracking technology that will be used during the procedure. For example, NIR optical trackers (Figs. 4.2a④ and 4.3) consist of a rigid frame holding multiple (usually three noncollinear, sometimes more) fiducial markers. A fiducial marker is small object that approximates a point. Most NIR fiducial markers are both clearly visible in preoperative scans and clearly visible to the tracking system. On the other hand, a modern EM tracker usually consists of a bundle of sensor coils inside a small case (around 0.5 cm^3) attached to a cable (wireless variants exist [5], but are uncommon) (as an example, the small black box attached to the surgical tools on Fig. 4.2b⑦ is an EM tracker). An EM tracker variant that is visible in patient scans (see Fig. 4.2b④) consists of a standard EM tracker attached to a frame that is large enough to be easily segmented in the patient scans.

The (EM and NIR optical) trackers described above provide a simple way to perform tracking and registration to the patient scans; of course, more complicated alternatives exist. For example, instead of a tracker, multiple loose fiducial markers can also be used to track the position and orientation of an object, provided at least three fiducials are noncollinear. This is equivalent to using a tracker, since both approaches provide enough measurements to cover the six degrees of freedom. Some authors report the use of fiducials which are visible in the patient scans, but not to the tracking system. For example, Krücker et al. [6] reported placing such fiducials on the patient's skin. During the intervention, the position of the fiducials then had to be marked by a tracked pointer, thus providing the connection between patient scans and tracking system.

4.2.1.2 Tracking of Surgical Tools

A similar, but simpler, approach is used to determine the position of the surgical tools in the intraoperative coordinate system. For this, a tracker is attached to the surgical tool that needs to be navigated. Here it is crucial that this tracker is placed at a predefined position on the surgical tool (see Fig. 4.2⑦), and that the tool is calibrated relative to the navigation platform. This calibration, in combination with the tracking information of the surgical tool tracker, allows tracking of the tip of the tool (or of any other part of the tool that is relevant during the intervention) thereby providing navigation from the perspective of the tip of the surgical tool. Tools like needles are routinely tracked using the methods described above. Some authors even report tracking tools to aid in implant placement [7–9]. Aside from surgical tools, it is also possible to track (handheld) imaging systems (e.g. ultrasound probes, gamma probes, portable gamma cameras and portable fluorescence imaging systems) as will be discussed later. A tracked scanning procedure performed with a handheld imaging system is referred to as "tracked freehand imaging".

4.2.1.3 Limitations and Implicit Assumptions of Tracking

Most navigation workflows make an implicit assumption about the body that is being tracked, namely, that it is a rigid body, i.e. that it has exactly the same shape any time during preoperative imaging and during surgery. If a body does not deform, it is sufficient to track the position and orientation of a tiny portion of it to know where the rest is. This is the justification for only placing a single tracker and/or a minimal amount of fiducial markers on a patient to track his or her position and orientation. Of course, the rigid body assumption may sometimes be unrealistic and can lead to mistakes. If the object being tracked is not a rigid body, the tracking approaches described in this text are, in general, inadequate. For example, a patient may change pose between preoperative imaging and the intervention without affecting the relative positions of the fiducial markers; in this case, the change in shape would not be detected by the tracking system. Surgeons must be aware of the implicit rigid body assumption of tracking systems and of the entailing limitations. In particular, it is always sensible to verify the precision of any registration between preoperative and intraoperative coordinates prior to and during an intervention, especially if a change in the shape of the patient is likely.

Current tracking systems work by tracking a relatively small number of points in 3D; in general this is not sufficient to deal with arbitrary deformations. Some authors, e.g. Krücker et al. [6] for thoracic and abdominal cavity interventions and Matziolis et al. [10] for navigated total knee arthroplasty, report the use of a redundant amount of fiducials/trackers, providing more information than necessary to obtain the six degrees of freedom of a rigid body. As a consequence, more than one rigid body could be tracked in such a workflow. This can accommodate some kinds of movement, e.g. the movement of the tibia relative to the femur. Still, these multi-rigid, landmark-based, arrangements also make implicit rigidity assumptions on the patient's shape, like the single rigid body case, and cannot accommodate arbitrary deformations particularly well. This said, redundant fiducials/trackers can be used to measure body deformation; if the spatial configuration changes during tracking, this information can be useful to correct, or at least explain, tracking errors during navigation. In addition, such findings may allow for elastic registrations which are a promising approach to handle body deformation (briefly discussed later in this chapter). Another reason for a redundant amount of fiducials, specific to optical tracking techniques, is that some fiducials may not lie in the direct line of sight of the tracking system; a large amount of fiducials reduces the chance that less than three noncollinear fiducials are visible.

On the other hand, images acquired with tracked freehand imaging are, due to tracking, automatically located in the intraoperative coordinate system; this means such images are already in the same coordinate system as the tracked surgical tools, rendering a registration between preoperative and intraoperative coordinates unnecessary. As a consequence, navigating tools in tracked freehand imaging scans is fairly straightforward. Such workflows are already reported in literature [11–13]. In the absence of specialised (and expensive) operating rooms with integrated MRI or CT scanners, tracked freehand imaging is often the only kind of 3D imaging that can be made available in the operation room. Intraoperative imaging can also be used to help verify the progress of a procedure, to cope with patient movement and sometimes even to quickly perform 3D intraoperative scans of the region of interest [11–14]. Tracked freehand ultrasound [15] is already available. An interesting novelty, especially for radioguided surgery, is tracked freehand SPECT, a SPECT generated from a tracked portable gamma camera [12, 13, 16–18].

4.2.2 Registration and Fusion

In the previous section, we explained how two coordinate systems (preoperative with patient scans and intraoperative with tracking information) can be connected via tracking of trackers, allowing objects from both coordinate systems to be shown in a single coordinate system. This connection between coordinate systems is called a

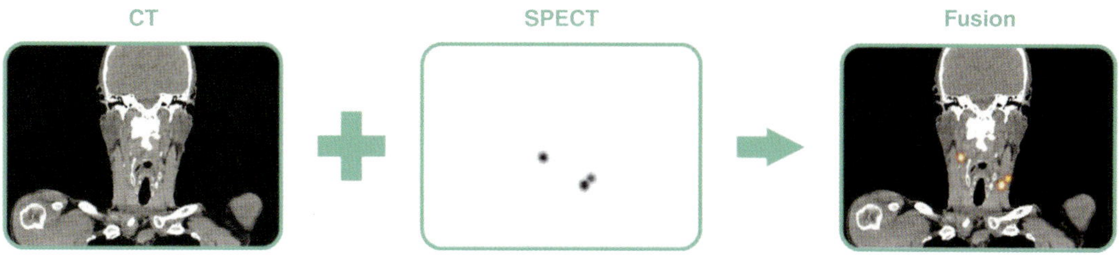

Fig. 4.4 Image fusion: CT and SPECT are registered, which enables a fused visualisation

registration. Since combining the complementary information of different patient scans allows for a more complete model of the patient, e.g. in the form of PET and MRI data, the registration concept described in the previous section should be expanded to more than two coordinate systems. This is readily possible using image registration. In fact, it is possible to register an arbitrary number of coordinate systems in a chain of registrations.

In a typical navigation workflow, all preoperative scans (Fig. 4.2②) are registered to each other. In at least one of these preoperative scans, the patient has to be outfitted with a tracker (Fig. 4.2①); this scan is then used to register the preoperative and intraoperative coordinate systems. With this registration, all other preoperative scans are also (indirectly) registered to the intraoperative coordinate system and can be navigated on. Registered patient scans are sometimes shown in composite views, where information from multiple scans is condensed into a single "fused" visualisation, as illustrated in Fig. 4.5. Note that registering multiple patient scans (i.e. performing image registrations) is often a complex and error-prone task, especially when there is deformation in the patient's anatomy between scans. For this reason image registrations should always be critically evaluated for errors and imprecisions prior to their use for navigation (or planning).

Registration methods can be separated into two types: rigid and elastic. A registration that consists exclusively of a composition of rotation and translation is called a rigid registration (see Fig. 4.5a). Rigid registrations can always be described by a transformation matrix. The vast majority of registrations currently performed in clinical practice, including most registrations using trackers or fiducials, are rigid. Rigid registrations are relatively easy to understand, fairly simple to verify, correct, and often precise enough for the intended application. But rigid registrations are, by definition, limited in the degrees of freedom that they can accommodate.

A very common example of rigid registrations is a SPECT and CT registration (see Fig. 4.4). Here a hybrid imaging device combines a measure of the distribution of a radiotracer (SPECT) with a scan of (CT) the patient's anatomy in a single imaging session; no significant patient movement is assumed during imaging, so the transformation matrix for this rigid registration is the identity matrix. Since many clinical applications only require a good alignment inside a small region of interest, rigid registrations will often be sufficient, even if a correct rigid alignment of the whole scans is not possible. In the cases where rigid registrations are not adequate to align scans as a result of extensive tissue movement, e.g. breast MRI scans [19] or preoperative to intraoperative brain scan alignment [20, 21], other types of registration are required.

Registrations that can handle arbitrary deformations, meaning random tissue movements, are called elastic or deformable registrations (see Fig. 4.5b). Elastic registrations cannot be described by a transformation matrix, due to their complexity. Instead, they are described by deformation fields. Elastic registrations are the topic of image analysis papers for decades already, but their use in clinical practice has been very limited thus far. The main reason for this is that there is a trade-off between flexibility, the ability to handle arbitrary deformations, and robustness, the ability to consistently yield reasonably precise registrations. There is not one sweet spot between

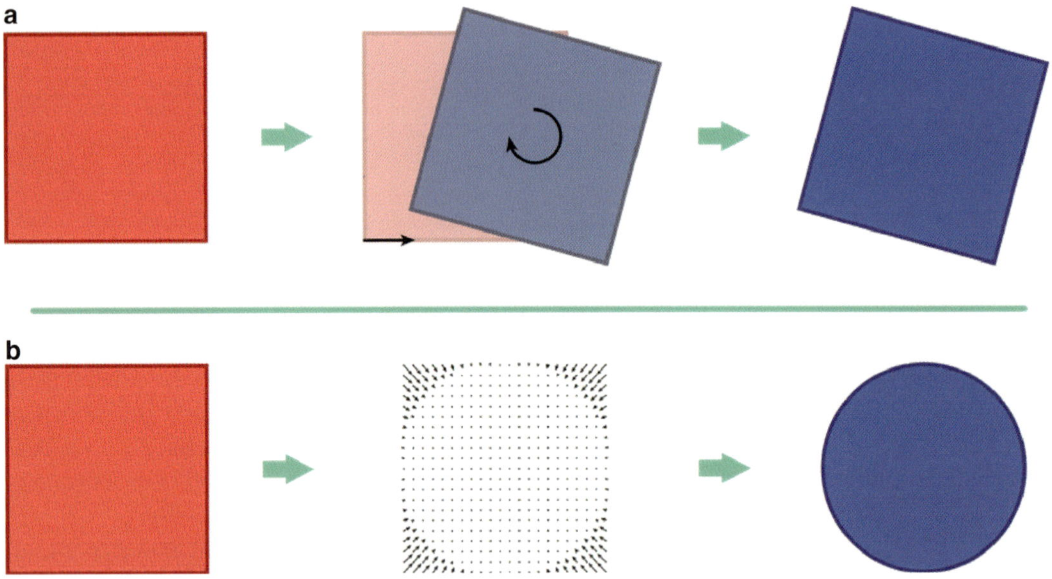

Fig. 4.5 Types of registration. (**a**): rigid registration, a composition of rotation and translation. (**b**): elastic registration, a deformation field is applied to warp the square into a circle

flexibility and robustness that works for all clinical applications, meaning an elastic registration algorithm has to be fine-tuned for each specific application. This, combined with the difficulty of finding an elastic registration method that works for the target application in the first place, greatly lowers the appeal of this technology, compared to the more generally applicable rigid registrations.

4.2.3 Computer-Aided Planning

Tracking and registration enable us to see the position of the tracked surgical tools overlaid on patient scans. The distance or the preferred route towards the target cannot be established with this information alone. Computer-aided planning software provides the navigation platform with the additional information needed to achieve both distance and route (Fig. 4.1c) estimates. To enable such planning, it is necessary to segment (i.e. define the boundaries of) the target structure in the patient scans and provide this segmentation to the navigation platform. For some surgeries, damage to critical structures must be avoided at all costs; in such cases, navigation from point A to B in a straight line does not suffice (Fig. 4.1c). Here navigation can be further improved to navigation along a path that avoids damage to nearby critical structures, as schematically shown in Fig. 4.1d. In order to provide such a "smart" route towards the target structure, it is also necessary to segment all critical structures that need to be avoided. To further clarify this approach, we illustrate how computer-aided planning fits into a navigation workflow by considering the resection of a kidney lesion (see Fig. 4.6). The starting point is the patient scan shown in Fig. 4.6a. If computer-aided planning is used, the kidney lesion and nearby critical structures are segmented (Fig. 4.6b). This segmentation can then be used to compute an optimal trajectory to the target (Fig. 4.6c). This plan is transferred to the navigation platform and can be used to position the surgical tools along the computed optimal path.

In computer-aided planning, manual and semi-automatic segmentations are currently the tools of choice in clinical practice. Manual segmentations, as their name implies, require manual drawings of the contours and interior of all structures that have to be segmented. The main advantage of manual segmentations is that the user has complete control over what label each

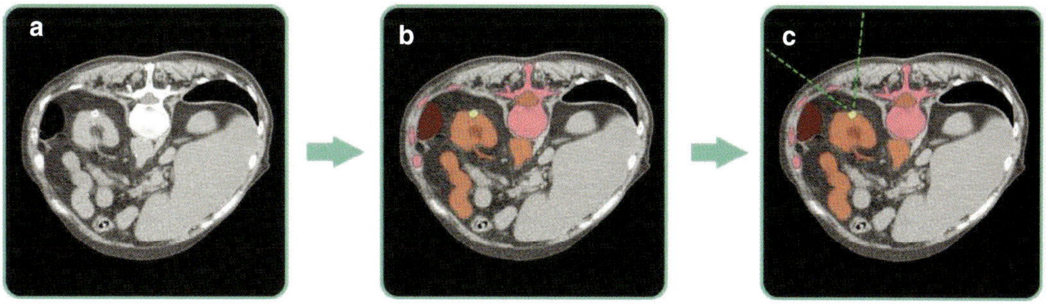

Fig. 4.6 Computer-aided planning in the treatment of a kidney lesion. (**a**): raw patient scans (**b**): segmentation of kidney lesion (*yellow*), nearby critical structures (*orange*) and nearby bones (*pink*) (**c**): optimal paths to lesion (*green dotted lines*); as short as possible whilst avoiding damage to critical structures

voxel in the 3D preoperative scan gets. However, manual segmentations can be extremely time consuming, especially for high-resolution 3D scans. Among all segmentation methods, manual segmentations, unsurprisingly, also suffer from the highest interobserver variability. A semi-automatic segmentation is a manual segmentation with some automatic assistance. For example, a drawing tool that automatically fills surrounding voxels of a similar colour, or, for example, a tool for vessel segmentation, where only the start and endpoint of the segment have to be defined manually. Semi-automatic segmentations require far less user input and can be performed significantly faster and with higher reproducibility than manual segmentations. On the other hand, the user partially surrenders the segmentation process over to the computer, thereby reducing his or her personal touch. Automatic segmentations, and in particular atlas-based segmentations [22], have improved a lot in recent years and are slowly gaining more acceptance.

A fully automatic segmentation is a segmentation that requires no user interaction. The obvious advantage of automatic segmentations is that they neither need to be performed nor supervised by a trained medical specialist. Experienced human operators, whilst usually superior to automatic methods, are subject to time constraints and susceptible to boredom, unlike machines. These time and boredom constraints are not limiting when a single segmentation of a target structure has to be performed, but can become an issue when repetitive or more extensive segmentations are required. For example, segmenting all bones in thousands of full-body scans for an anatomy experiment would certainly yield interesting insights, but very few experts would volunteer for such a tedious task. Computers do not get bored; as a consequence they can provide much more extensive segmentations than could reasonably be expected from a human expert. It goes without saying that automatic segmentations always have to be critically evaluated by an expert.

4.3 Clinical Applications of Navigation

Attempts at surgical navigation have already been reported as early as the year 1889 [23]; these involved stereotactic frames combined with generic atlases (i.e. maps) of the anatomy, used as reference during the procedure. Due to the anatomical variation found in humans, generic atlases cannot be correct for all anatomical regions of all patients; hence, they are often not reliable for precise guidance. Patient-specific approaches to navigation, where patient scans are used instead of generic atlases, only became realistic with the development of 3D imaging technologies like CT and MRI, that became commercially available in the 1970s [24] and 1980s, respectively. We focus on patient-specific navigation approaches in this chapter and do not delve further into publications from before the time of 3D imaging.

Neurosurgery is one of the pioneering fields in surgical navigation; 3D navigation experiments are reported as early as 1986 [4]. Additional neuronavigation systems and studies are reported in the 1990s, e.g. by Germano et al. [25] and Gumprecht et al. [26], among many others. The navigation workflow described in these works corresponds to the "typical" navigation workflow seen in clinical practice today, namely, navigation of the surgical tools in preoperative patient scans. The most important limitation of this approach can be seen when the intraoperative reality significantly deviates from the anatomy depicted in the preoperative scans. In this case the estimated position of the tracked tools relative to the patient's anatomy can be off by many centimetres, negating the precision benefits navigation is supposed to bring. Outside its application in neurosurgery and in external beam radiation therapy (not discussed in this chapter; see Khan et al. [27] for a review on radiation therapy), navigation is not very widespread in clinical practice thus far, even though many other clinical applications could greatly benefit from a well-thought-out navigation workflow. Mounting evidence of navigation's benefits for particular types of treatment, ideally combined with a greater awareness of what is technically feasible, should slowly change this state of affairs. To grant the reader a short overview of how navigation can be applied in various clinical fields and what the current limitations are, the remainder of this section presents selected research on needle placement, navigated resections, and navigation in orthopaedic surgeries.

4.3.1 Needle Placement

The objective of a needle placement procedure is to insert a needle into the patient so that the tip of the needle is as close as possible to the target location. Needles can be used to obtain biopsy samples, radio-frequency (RF) ablations, microwave ablations and electrode placement, among many other clinical applications. Some of these applications require a very precise needle placement, and it is expected that these will benefit most from navigation. The main challenge encountered during needle placement is that both the target location defined on imaging and, once the insertion begins, the needle tip are not visible to the physician. To compound these difficulties, the tissue (or needle) may deform during or as a result of the needle placement.

Needle navigation workflows combine patient scans with needle tracking. With tracking (and registration of the tracking system to the patient scans), the estimated (3D) position of the needle tip in the anatomy can be shown in real-time on all patient scans. In most needle navigation workflows, the target location is marked on one of the registered patient scans, as in Fig. 4.1c; this way the navigation platform can indicate the current needle trajectory or estimate the shortest route from the needle tip to the target location. A more sophisticated workflow could also incorporate the segmentation of critical structures along the possible paths of the needle, allowing for the selection of an optimal path towards the target location whilst avoiding damage to critical structures, as shown in Fig. 4.6c.

Stereotactic needle navigation is already used for decades to aid in the placement of electrodes for deep brain stimulation [28]. For more sophisticated navigation procedures, needles are usually tracked with the NIR optical or EM tracking systems. NIR optical tracking requires the tracker to be in direct line of sight of the cameras, meaning the tracker must be attached to a portion of the needle that is not inserted into the patient. Depending on the precision of the tracking system, and the distance from the tracker to the needle tip, aggravated by the possibility of needle bending, estimates of the needle tip position using NIR optical tracking may be somewhat imprecise. EM tracking does not possess the direct line of sight limitation, and trackers could be attached anywhere on or inside the needle. A particularly interesting recent development are miniaturised EM trackers with less than 1 mm in diameter, i.e. narrow enough to be placed inside needles. As a consequence, EM tracking can now be used to directly track the tip of a needle [29]. Additionally, multiple EM trackers can be used to monitor the bending of needles [30].

Müller et al. [31] investigated needle navigation for soft tissue biopsies, using NIR optical tracking. Navigated and conventional CT-guided liver needle biopsies were compared in five pigs, with a total of 20 tumours biopsied. The authors report that the navigated biopsies, on average, involved significantly fewer CT scans ($p=.01$) and lower dose length products ($p=.001$) compared to the conventional biopsies. Krücker et al. [6] describe the navigation of needles for biopsies and RF ablations, mostly targeted at liver and kidney lesions. Their trial involved 51 navigated needle placements in 40 procedures with a workflow consisting of segmenting the needle target location in preoperative CT scans, sometimes combined with PET scans. During the intervention, navigation of the (EM) tracked needle was combined with conventional ultrasound and 1–5 intraoperative CT scans, to make a correct placement more likely. Both during registration and needle placement, the patient needed to hold his or her breath, to minimise registration errors. The authors compared the precision of conventional image guidance with that of navigation for 19 targets (liver, kidney, neck and paracardiac mediastinum). The authors report a significantly ($p=.0006$) better precision using navigation: range [0.4–12.1 mm] with median 2.5 mm, against range [3.3–81.9 mm] with median 14.8 mm. Additionally one interventional radiologist assessed the utility of all 51 placements: 22 of the placements (43 %) would be very difficult or impossible to perform without navigation and an additional 24 placements (47 %) were facilitated by navigation. This study puts needle navigation in a very positive light, though the authors point out that the number of patients was relatively small and that a statistically meaningful comparison of outcomes with a control group was not performed.

Ungi et al. [11] propose a radiation-free, ultrasound-only workflow for navigated facet joint injections. The assumption is that this workflow yields the same clinical outcome as alternatives using fluoroscopy or CT imaging, whilst minimising radiation exposure of the patient and surgical crew. The suggested method would work as follows: (1) a tracked freehand ultrasound scan of the spine segment to be treated is performed prior to needle insertion; (2) after imaging, the target location is segmented in the reconstructed 3D ultrasound volume; and (3) the tracked needle is then navigated to the target. Recall that both tracked tools and images acquired with tracked freehand imaging are in the intraoperative coordinate system, so, in this case, no registration step is required prior to navigation. A particular problem in conventional ultrasound-guided needle placement is that the ideal needle path is often blocked by the transducer during insertion. Hence, separating the imaging and needle insertion steps is a sensible approach. The authors performed 100 facet joint injections in cadaveric lamb models, 50 using the conventional ultrasound-guided method and 50 with the suggested (navigated) method. This increased the insertion success rate 94 % vs. 44 % and significantly shortened insertion times.

4.3.2 Navigated Resections

The surgical removal of all, or part, of an organ, tissue or structure is often performed to treat diseases like cancer. To avoid recurrences, it is important to remove all tumorous tissue during surgery. Ideally the tumour should not be pierced during surgery, to avoid the spillage and possible spread of tumour cells. To accomplish both a thorough tumour removal and minimise spillage, surgeons usually define a safety margin surrounding the tumour and perform the resection around this margin; all tissue inside the safety margin is removed. The resected specimen is then sent to pathology to check for positive margins, i.e. the presence of tumour cells in the edges of the excised specimen. Ideally, pathology should confirm negative specimen margins in all tumour resections. Unfortunately this is not always the case; for example, Jacobs [32] cites reports of positive margin findings ranging from 20 % to as high as 70 % for partial mastectomies. Identification of the boundary between the diseased and healthy tissues can be addressed by the use of tracers, especially radionuclides, as described in detail in other chapters of this book. Imprecise surgical resection, can probably be improved by navigation. For example, navigation is widely used to resect brain tumours; some of the first navigation systems were designed for neurosurgery applications [2, 25, 26]. On the one hand, the brain is quite susceptible to damage, so surgical interventions should be as precise and minimally invasive as possible, yielding good disease treatment whilst minimising the chance of permanent neurological damage. Moreover, the brain is embedded in a rigid bone case (the neurocranium), meaning it does not deform significantly between imaging and surgery. This strong need for precision combined with the favourable rigidity of the target anatomy led to the development of clinically and commercially successful neuronavigation systems (using NIR optical tracking), which make use of preoperative CT or MRI scans. Over the years, attempts to integrate many neurosurgery specific tools, like pointer tools or even entire surgical microscopes [3, 26], have been reported.

Many resections, including brain tumour resections, involve significant tissue deformation during surgery, making traditional preoperative scan-based navigation on progressively more imprecise. To counter this, intraoperative CT and MRI systems have been suggested [33, 34]. Due to their relatively high price, complicated logistics, large volume, and relatively long acquisition times, it is questionable if these imaging systems will find widespread adoption in clinical settings. Tracked freehand imaging may prove to be a more viable intraoperative imaging solution. Unsgaard et al. [14] describe a modern neuronavigation workflow for brain tumour resections with preoperative MRI for initial planning and multiple intraoperative tracked ultrasound scans to monitor the progress of the resection and to cope with brain shift [20]. The system used by the authors simultaneously shows the position of the tracked instruments side-by-side on the preoperative MRI and on the latest ultrasound volume. Whenever significant tissue changes occurred, a new ultrasound scan was performed and the navigation procedure was adapted. In addition to more accurate navigation, the authors report that intraoperative ultrasound was very useful in detecting residual tumour after the planned resection was performed. In their subjective experience, in over half of the 91 procedures investigated, residual tumour was discovered in resections that were otherwise considered to be complete. The system described by the authors used NIR optical tracking.

Radioguided interventions are interventions that make use of tracers, especially radioactive tracers that allow for SPECT and PET imaging; fluorescent and hybrid fluorescent-radioactive tracers are also used for some applications [35–37]. Tracers mainly aid in the detection of target structures (like tumours or lymph nodes) and in more precise refinement of their borders. Tracers can be of use both preoperatively, enabling SPECT/CT (Fig. 4.5) and PET/CT scans, and intraoperatively, providing real-time acoustic or visual feedback from radiation or fluorescence readings [38–41].

SPECT, and to a lesser extent PET, scans are generally used to preoperatively identify the lesions that should be taken out during surgery using specialised imaging devices, like gamma probes (1D) or gamma/fluorescence cameras (2D) [42, 43]. A logical evolution of this is to track the intraoperative devices, allowing navigation of them on the preoperative images, possibly reducing the time needed and increasing the accuracy of the intraoperative radioactive hotspot localisation. Brouwer et al. [44] successfully navigated a tracked gamma probe in preoperative SPECT/CT images towards sentinel lymph nodes in ten patients with penile carcinoma. Here preoperative SPECT/CT-based navigation was combined with the intraoperative acoustic feedback produced by the tracked gamma probe. Tracked gamma probes can be used even more extensively in navigation workflows, for the generation of freehand SPECT [16] scans, that can be created during both the pre- and intraoperative process. Freehand SPECT scans have a smaller field of view and may have lower resolution than traditional SPECT scans, but they can be performed with cheaper and significantly less bulky devices. A particular advantage of freehand SPECT is that multiple scans can be performed during surgery if necessary, allowing the surgeon to double-check his or her work thereby decreasing the chance of incomplete resections. Rahbar et al. [45] performed navigated parathyroidectomy combining both preoperative SPECT/CT and freehand SPECT. Other authors report performing navigated sentinel lymph node biopsies on freehand SPECT scans in, for example, breast [12] and head and neck cancer [13, 46]. Recently, Engelen et al. [47] reported on the use of the freehand SPECT technology in combination with a mobile gamma camera. Compared to the gamma probe-based procedure, the use of a mobile camera could speed up the generation of the freehand SPECT, and the sensitivity of the camera might help improve lesion resolvability. All freehand SPECT works cited here used NIR optical tracking to track the gamma probes.

With the introduction of hybrid tracers, that contain both a radioactive and a fluorescent label (e.g. indocyanine green (ICG)-^{99m}Tc-nanocolloid [38, 39, 48]), the field of radioguided surgery further expanded. These tracers can extend navigation workflows based on SPECT/CT and freehand SPECT with intraoperative fluorescence image guidance. Brouwer et al. [49] presented a proof of concept via navigation of a tracked fluorescence laparoscope towards the hybrid tracer-containing sentinel lymph node seen on preoperative SPECT/CT. Here, as soon as the fluorescence laparoscope was near enough to the sentinel lymph node, fluorescence imaging could be performed to complement the navigation. A requirement for a successful hybrid workflow is that navigation leads the laparoscope to less than 1 cm from the target location, since fluorescence signal depth penetration is only around 1 cm in human soft tissue [50]. The benefit provided by the fluorescence imaging is that a real-time visual feedback of the tracer with respect to the local anatomy is provided. This real-time feedback can be used to better cope with potential inaccuracies in the SPECT/CT-based navigation, e.g. due to patient movement and tissue deformation.

4.3.3 Navigated Orthopaedic Surgeries

Orthopaedic surgeries are performed to treat fractures and congenital musculoskeletal malformations and to replace worn out joints with implants, among many other applications. Many orthopaedic surgeries, especially procedures involving implant placement, are focused on bones, making them particularly promising candidates for navigation. Bones, unlike soft tissue, usually do not deform. This rigidity should, therefore, lead to precise registrations and, as a consequence, precise navigations. The assumption is that the machine precision provided by navigation leads to a faster and more precise implant placement. This increased implant placement accuracy may lead to a better clinical outcome, e.g. increased range of motion, better joint stability, increased implant longevity and later onset of arthritis.

Rambani et al. [51] reviewed numerous applications of navigation in orthopaedic surgery, with an emphasis on navigated total knee arthroplasty (TKA) and total hip arthroplasty (THA). The authors pointed out that both for TKA and THA, correct implant alignment is essential to increase implant longevity and to achieve a good functional outcome. It was assumed that navigation may improve implant alignment compared to conventional TKA and THA. However, a recent meta-analysis involving 3423 patients (33 studies) concluded that navigated TKA brings no clear benefits in clinical outcome compared to conventional TKA, whilst at the same time, the mean duration of surgery was increased by 23 % [52]. On the other hand, a meta-analysis of three THA studies ($n=250$) concluded that navigation in THA improves the precision of acetabular cup placement [53]. Taking both these studies into account, the authors conclude that the potential benefits of navigation both for TKA and THA are not yet clearly proven or disproven and suggest multicentre randomised controlled trials with long-term follow-up for these procedures.

Larson et al. [7] described the navigated placement of pedicle screws in paediatric patients with congenital spine deformity. Their workflow consisted of an initial planning of the screw placement performed on preoperative CT scans. Then, during surgery, one or more intraoperative CT scans of the spine, with an optical tracker screwed onto the patient, were used for surgical navigation (as in Fig. 4.1b). This form of navigation allowed the authors to measure the width and depth of each screw tract, allowing screw dimensions to be custom fit to each pedicle. Results of 14 patients were presented (four cases of isolated hemivertebra and ten cases of complex spinal deformations), with a total of 142 screws placed. In this study, a 99.3 % success rate was achieved, even though the majority of screws was placed in vertebrae with congenital deformities. The authors report that comparable precision for pedicle screw placement without navigation was obtained in other studies [54], albeit for patients without congenital spine deformity.

Both Rana et al. [9] and Gander et al. [8] describe the reconstruction of unilateral orbital fractures combining the use of selective laser-melted patient-specific implants (PSIs) and navigated implant placement. Gander et al. point out that inadequate implant shape and imprecise implant placement may lead to visual disturbance and aesthetically poor results. It is assumed that PSIs have a shape that better fits to the fractured anatomy and that navigation improves the precision of the implant placement. The workflow starts with a CT scan of the patient, depicting both the fractured and the uninjured orbits, followed by a computer-aided planning step to determine the desired shape of the implant. PSIs are outfitted with ridges and landmarks, which enable navigated placement. The implants are not tracked directly; instead a tracked pointer is manually placed along the implant's ridges and landmarks during navigated insertion. Once the implant is in place, the tracked pointer can be used to verify that the implant placement is precise enough, potentially avoiding the need of additional scans to verify the implant placement after surgery. The navigation is performed on the preoperative CT scan. Both groups proceed to analyse if the proposed workflow is superior to the more traditional (manually) pre-bent titanium mesh (PBTM) implants. Based on their experiments, both groups suggest PSIs are superior to PBTM implants. Unfortunately, none of the groups directly measured the impact navigation had on the procedure or on the clinical outcome; navigation was simply used in all procedures, presumably under the assumption that this would lead to more precise (or equally precise, but faster) implant placement.

4.4 Discussion

In this chapter we described surgical navigation methods and their clinical applications over a broad range of medical fields. Navigation promises to bring machine precision to the operating room. Most authors reported a positive opinion of navigation, usually backed by experimental results from (small) clinical studies. Additionally, many authors expressed the subjective opinion that navigation was beneficial or helpful for their respective application; Krücker et al. [6] go as far as stating that "procedures were facilitated that would have otherwise been difficult or impossible to perform without this technology". These results place navigation in a good light, but there are some issues that still need to be considered.

We identified three navigation workflow variants in clinical practice. The first variant is navigation on preoperative scans alone, which is usually seen in interventions with no significant tissue deformation during surgery, for example, the navigated reconstruction of unilateral orbital fractures [8, 9]. The same type of navigation can also be used to bring surgical instruments close to the target location in (laparoscopic) surgeries, as reported by Brouwer et al. [49]. Navigation on preoperative scans is the most straightforward and probably most widely used navigation variant. In some cases, however, the navigation based on preoperative scans alone can become quite imprecise, especially in the later stages of an intervention, where significant tissue deformation and patient movement may have taken place. To date tissue deformation and patient movement between imaging and surgery present significant challenges to navigation on preoperative scans. Fortunately, many creative solutions to detect and deal with deformation are already reported in literature. Krücker et al. [6], who investigated navigation in the thoracic and abdominal cavities, mentioned breath holding and respiratory gating to minimise deformations. Using a redundant amount of fiducials, non-rigid movement could be detected. A second navigation variant combines navigation on preoperative scans with intraoperative scans. In this variant, the navigation on preoperative scans only provides rough guidance, and, whenever more precision is needed, intraoperative scans are taken. Such workflows are described in [6, 7, 14]. Navigation workflows using preoperative scans alone are unsuitable for many clinical applications. With the integration of intraoperative imaging into a workflow, such navigation can, however, be applied in a much broader range of settings. The final navigation variant is navigation on intraoperative scans alone. This variant has become practical with the recent emergence of tracked freehand imaging. Recall that both tracked tools and images from tracked freehand imaging are in the same coordinate system, meaning no registration between patient scans and surgical tools is required, thus leading to a simpler navigation workflow. This navigation variant is already reported by a few groups [11–13], and we expect this list to grow significantly with the more widespread adoption of tracked freehand imaging systems.

Regarding tracking technologies, both EM and NIR optical tracking are widely used both for freehand imaging and navigation. Both technologies work well most of the time. Tracker occlusion is the main drawback of NIR optical tracking; distortion of the magnetic field due to metallic objects and small working volume are the drawbacks of EM tracking. It is not yet clear which technology will become dominant. However, with the advent of miniaturised EM trackers, that fit inside needles and can directly track the tip [29], it seems EM tracking has an advantage, at least, in needle placement interventions.

Most navigation workflows presented in this chapter compared favourably to their conventional, non-navigated alternatives. This, however, is not sufficient evidence to make blanket statements about the usefulness of navigation in general. In fact, there also is evidence suggesting that navigation provides no tangible benefits during some types of surgery; for example, Bauwens et al. [52] pointed out that navigation seems to bring no benefits to TKA surgeries. Another important issue is the amount of evidence presented to back up the claims of the benefits of a navigation workflow. Randomised controlled trials (RCT) involving large numbers of patients, the current gold standard for clinical trials, have not been performed for any of the reported methods. An open question is how much and what kind of evidence is considered sufficient to prove the benefits (or lack thereof) of a navigation workflow. It is unclear how the alleged benefits of a particular navigation workflow compared to an equivalent non-navigated alternative should be measured. Perhaps precision should be measured directly, as reported by Krücker et al. in [6], where the needle angle insertion is measured both for the navigated and non-navigated workflows; based on these measurements, estimates of the procedures' precision can be calculated and compared. Or perhaps the clinical outcome after a number of years should be evaluated instead, as in the meta-analysis of TKA and THA clinical studies reported by Rambani et al. in [51]. Alternatively the subjective opinion of an expert [6, 14] may also provide a relevant measure. Should the experience of a surgeon also influence the measure? If so, how should one combine results from multiple surgeons with different skill sets? The lack of a consensus on how to measure the benefits of a navigation workflow surely stands in the way of large clinical trials. It is unclear when, or even if, a consensus on this measure will emerge. Even if a consensus measure emerges, one should consider if RCTs are the ideal type of trial for navigation workflows. Can clinical equipoise, i.e. the existence of a general uncertainty in the expert medical community over whether a technique is beneficial or not, be assumed for all navigation workflows? If a surgical team strongly believes a navigation workflow is superior to the alternative for a specific type of surgery, is it acceptable to perform non-navigated surgery just for the sake of a more statistically sound trial? Given all these questions, chances are RCTs will not be performed for many current and future navigation workflows. Alternative ways of gathering convincing evidence should probably be investigated. It should be pointed out that convincing evidence of the clinical benefits of a technique is a precondition for reimbursement by health insurance companies in many countries, so providing such evidence for navigated workflows is essential for them to become mainstream.

Whilst navigation is not (yet) the ultimate solution to improve surgical outcomes across the board, it does seem to be genuinely beneficial in various types of surgery. Evidence suggesting better clinical outcomes in these cases combined with ever lower barriers to its adoption leads us to believe that the use of navigation will be much more widespread in the near future, hopefully contributing to better clinical outcomes for ever more patients.

Acknowledgements This work was partially supported by a Eurostars grant (Hybrid Navigator; Grant No. E! 7555), an NWO-STW-VIDI grant (Grant No. STW BGT11272), and a European Research Council under the European Union's Seventh Framework Program (FP7/2007-2013) grant (Grant No. 2012-20120314).

References

1. Rassweiler J, et al. Surgical navigation in urology: European perspective. Curr Opin Urol. 2014;24(1): 81–97.
2. Willems P, et al. Neuronavigation and surgery of intracerebral tumours. J Neurol. 2006;253(9):1123–36.
3. Watanabe E, et al. Three-dimensional digitizer (neuronavigator): new equipment for computed tomography-guided stereotaxic surgery. Surg Neurol. 1987;27(6): 543–7.
4. Roberts DW, et al. A frameless stereotaxic integration of computerized tomographic imaging and the operating microscope. J Neurosurg. 1986;65(4):545–9.
5. Balter JM, et al. Accuracy of a wireless localization system for radiotherapy. Int J Radiat Oncol Biol Phys. 2005;61(3):933–7.
6. Krücker J, et al. Clinical utility of real-time fusion guidance for biopsy and ablation. J Vasc Interv Radiol. 2011;22(4):515–24.
7. Larson AN, et al. The accuracy of navigation and 3D image-guided placement for the placement of pedicle screws in congenital spine deformity. J Pediatr Orthop. 2012;32(6):e23–9.
8. Gander T, et al. Patient specific implants (PSI) in reconstruction of orbital floor and wall fractures. J Craniomaxillofac Surg. 2015;43(1):126–30.
9. Rana M, et al. Increasing the accuracy of orbital reconstruction with selective laser melted patient-specific implants combined with intraoperative navigation. J Oral Maxillofac Surg. 2015;73(6):1113–8.
10. Matziolis G, et al. A prospective, randomized study of computer-assisted and conventional total knee arthroplasty. J Bone Joint Surg Am. 2007;89(2):236–43.
11. Ungi T, Lasso A, Fichtinger G. Tracked ultrasound in navigated spine interventions. In: Spinal imaging and image analysis. Cham: Springer; 2015. p. 469–94.
12. Bluemel C, et al. Freehand SPECT for image-guided sentinel lymph node biopsy in breast cancer. Eur J Nucl Med Mol Imaging. 2013;40(11):1656–61.
13. Heuveling DA. Evaluation of the use of freehand SPECT for sentinel node biopsy in early stage oral carcinoma. Oral Oncol. 2015;51(3):287–90.
14. Unsgaard G, et al. Neuronavigation by intraoperative three-dimensional ultrasound: initial experience during brain tumor resection. Neurosurgery. 2002;50(4):804–12.
15. Fenster A, Downey DB, Cardinal HN. Three-dimensional ultrasound imaging. Phys Med Biol. 2001;46(5):R67.
16. Wendler T, et al. First demonstration of 3-D lymphatic mapping in breast cancer using freehand SPECT. Eur J Nucl Med Mol Imaging. 2010;37(8):1452–61.
17. Bluemel C, et al. Freehand SPECT-guided sentinel lymph node biopsy in early oral squamous cell carcinoma. Head Neck. 2014;36(11):E112–6.
18. Navab N, et al. First deployments of augmented reality in operating rooms. Computer. 2012;7:48–55.
19. Rueckert D, et al. Nonrigid registration using free-form deformations: application to breast MR images. IEEE Trans Med Imaging. 1999;18(8):712–21.
20. Roberts DW, et al. Intraoperative brain shift and deformation: a quantitative analysis of cortical displacement in 28 cases. Neurosurgery. 1998;43(4): 749–58.
21. Ferrant M, et al. Registration of 3-D intraoperative MR images of the brain using a finite-element biomechanical model. IEEE Trans Med Imaging. 2001;20(12):1384–97.
22. van Rikxoort EM, et al. Adaptive local multi-atlas segmentation: application to heart segmentation in chest CT scans. Proc. SPIE 6914, Medical Imaging 2008: Image Processing, 691407. DOI:10.1117/12.772301.
23. Kandel EI, Schavinsky YV. Stereotaxic apparatus and operations in Russia in the 19th century. J Neurosurg. 1972;37(4):407–11.
24. Beckmann E. CT scanning the early days. BJR. 2005;79(937):5–8.
25. Germano IM. The NeuroStation system for image-guided, frameless stereotaxy. Neurosurgery. 1995; 37(2):348–50.
26. Gumprecht HK, Widenka DC, Lumenta CB. BrainLab VectorVision Neuronavigation System: technology and clinical experiences in 131 cases. Neurosurgery. 1999;44(1):97–104.

27. Khan FM, Gibbons JP. Khan's the physics of radiation therapy. Philadelphia: Lippincott Williams & Wilkins; 2014.
28. Holl EM, et al. Improving targeting in image-guided frame-based deep brain stimulation. Neurosurgery. 2010;67:ons437–47.
29. Hakime A, et al. Electromagnetic-tracked biopsy under ultrasound guidance: preliminary results. Cardiovasc Intervent Radiol. 2012;35(4):898–905.
30. Lei P, et al. Real-time tracking of liver motion and deformation using a flexible needle. Int J Comput Assist Radiol Surg. 2011;6(3):435–46.
31. Müller SA, et al. Navigated liver biopsy using a novel soft tissue navigation system versus CT-guided liver biopsy in a porcine model: a prospective randomized trial. Acad Radiol. 2010;17(10):1282–7.
32. Jacobs L. Positive margins: the challenge continues for breast surgeons. Ann Surg Oncol. 2008;15(5):1271–2.
33. Maesawa S, et al. Clinical indications for high-field 1.5 T intraoperative magnetic resonance imaging and neuro-navigation for neurosurgical procedures-review of initial 100 cases. Neurol Med Chir. 2009;49(8): 340–50.
34. Grunert P, et al. Basic principles and clinical applications of neuronavigation and intraoperative computed tomography. Comput Aided Surg. 1998;3(4):166–73.
35. Mariani G, et al. A review on the clinical uses of SPECT/CT. Eur J Nucl Med Mol Imaging. 2010; 37(10):1959–85.
36. van den Berg N, et al. Hybrid tracers for sentinel node biopsy. Q J Nucl Med Mol Imaging. 2014;58: 193–206.
37. Histed SN, et al. Review of functional/anatomic imaging in oncology. Nucl Med Commun. 2012;33(4):349.
38. van den Berg NS, et al. Multimodal surgical guidance during sentinel node biopsy for melanoma: combined gamma tracing and fluorescence imaging of the sentinel node through use of the hybrid tracer indocyanine green-(99m)Tc-nanocolloid. Radiology. 2015;275(2):521–9.
39. Brouwer OR, et al. A hybrid radioactive and fluorescent tracer for sentinel node biopsy in penile carcinoma as a potential replacement for blue dye. Eur Urol. 2014;65(3):600–9.
40. KleinJan GH, et al. Optimisation of fluorescence guidance during robot-assisted laparoscopic sentinel node biopsy for prostate cancer. Eur Urol. 2014;66(6):991–8.
41. Eiber M, et al. Evaluation of hybrid 68Ga-PSMA-ligand PET/CT in 248 patients with biochemical recurrence after radical prostatectomy. J Nucl Med. 2015;56(5):668–74.
42. Povoski SP, et al. A comprehensive overview of radioguided surgery using gamma detection probe technology. World J Surg Oncol. 2009;7(1):11.
43. Heller S, Zanzonico P. Nuclear probes and intraoperative gamma cameras. Semin Nucl Med. 2011;41(3): 166–81.
44. Brouwer OR, et al. Feasibility of intraoperative navigation to the sentinel node in the groin using preoperatively acquired single photon emission computerized tomography data: transferring functional imaging to the operating room. J Urol. 2014; 192(6):1810–6.
45. Rahbar K, et al. Intraoperative 3-D mapping of parathyroid adenoma using freehand SPECT. EJNMMI Res. 2012;2(1):51.
46. Mandapathil M, et al. Freehand SPECT for sentinel lymph node detection in patients with head and neck cancer: first experiences. Acta Otolaryngol. 2014; 134(1):100–4.
47. Engelen T, et al. The next evolution in radioguided surgery: breast cancer related sentinel node localization using a freehandSPECT-mobile gamma camera combination. Am J Nucl Med Mol Imaging. 2015;5(3):233–45.
48. Brouwer OR, et al. Comparing the hybrid fluorescent–radioactive tracer indocyanine green–99mTc-nanocolloid with 99mTc-nanocolloid for sentinel node identification: a validation study using lymphoscintigraphy and SPECT/CT. J Nucl Med. 2012;53(7): 1034–40.
49. Brouwer OR, et al. Image navigation as a means to expand the boundaries of fluorescence-guided surgery. Phys Med Biol. 2012;57(10):3123.
50. Chin PT, et al. Multispectral visualization of surgical safety-margins using fluorescent marker seeds. Am J Nucl Med Mol Imaging. 2012;2(2):151.
51. Rambani R, Varghese M. Computer assisted navigation in orthopaedics and trauma surgery. Orthop Trauma. 2014;28(1):50–7.
52. Bauwens K, et al. Navigated total knee replacement. J Bone Joint Surg Am. 2007;89(2):261–9.
53. Gandhi R, et al. Computer navigation in total hip replacement: a meta-analysis. Int Orthop. 2009;33(3): 593–7.
54. Ledonio CGT, et al. Pediatric pedicle screws: comparative effectiveness and safety. J Bone Joint Surg Am. 2011;93(13):1227–34.

Tracers Applied in Radioguided Surgery

5

Anton Bunschoten, Nynke S. van den Berg, Renato A. Valdés Olmos, Jacobus A.K. Blokland, and Fijs W.B. van Leeuwen

Contents

A. Bunschoten • N.S. van den Berg
F.W.B. van Leeuwen (✉)
Interventional Molecular Imaging Laboratory, Department of Radiology, Leiden University Medical Center (LUMC), Leiden, The Netherlands
e-mail: f.w.b.van_leeuwen@lumc.nl

R.A. Valdés Olmos
Interventional Molecular Imaging Laboratory, Department of Radiology, Leiden University Medical Center (LUMC), Leiden, The Netherlands

Departments of Nuclear Medicine, Antoni van Leeuwenhoek Hospital - Netherlands Cancer Institute (AvL-NKI), Amsterdam, The Netherlands

J.A.K. Blokland
Nuclear Medicine, Department of Radiology, Leiden University Medical Center (LUMC), Leiden, The Netherlands

Abstract

Radioguided surgery (RGS) allows a surgeon to intraoperatively identify the lesions of interest. This technique relies on the accumulation of a radiotracer in the lesion(s) of interest. Such accumulation can occur via the local administration of the radiotracer, followed by local staining or passive drainage via the lymphatic system, or can occur via the systemic administration followed by retention or targeted accumulation of the radiotracer. The range of radiotracers applied in RGS varies from the radioactive isotope itself, to small molecules, peptides, antibodies, and colloids. The choice of the radionuclide depends on various factors, such as half-life, desired radiation type and energy, and (chemical) means to attach it to an active entity. An often overlooked factor is the radiation burden for the patient and the medical personnel. The introduction of optical imaging technologies, such as fluorescence and Cherenkov imaging, expands the utility of RGS.

5.1 Introduction

The concept of radioguided surgery (RGS) can provide the operating specialist with information regarding the location and margins of target lesions

K. Herrmann et al. (eds.), *Radioguided Surgery: Current Applications and Innovative Directions in Clinical Practice*, DOI 10.1007/978-3-319-26051-8_5

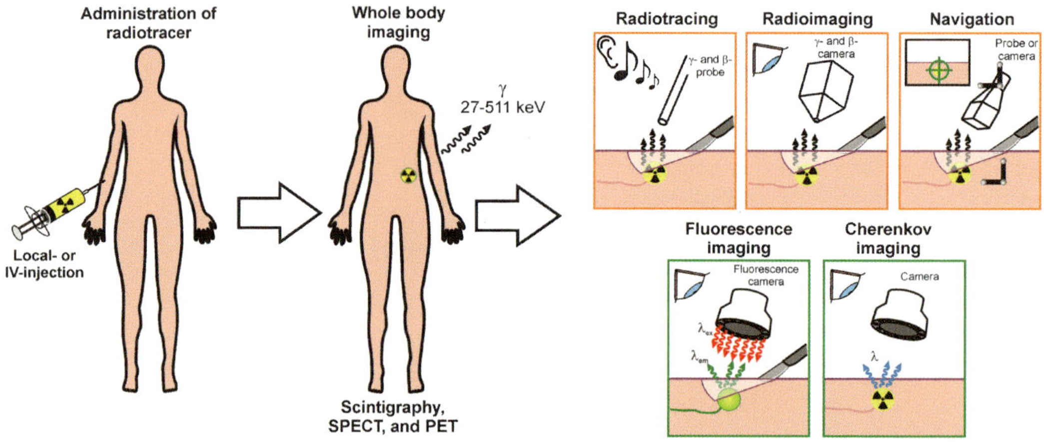

Fig. 5.1 Schematic representation of the possibilities with radio- and hybrid tracers

during surgery and as such can help improve the accuracy of the surgical procedure (Fig. 5.1). RGS requires two things: (1) the availability of a tracer emitting a nuclear signal (possibly accompanied by and optical signal) that accumulates at the site of interest and (2) (portable) detectors that can detect the tracers nuclear signal, thereby providing the surgeon with acoustic or visual feedback regarding its location. Fully integrated whole body preoperative (nuclear) imaging and intraoperative RGS using the same radiotracer (single injection) is the most superior way to perform RGS as it allows the nuclear medicine physician and surgeon to jointly generate a (virtual) roadmap regarding the location of the lesions, thereby also enabling the identification of unexpected lesions at distant locations (Fig. 5.1). During the intervention, radioguidance, possibly in combination with an optical component, can provide the surgeon with real-time information regarding the location of the lesions and helps confirm accurate lesion resection. In combination with state-of-the-art navigation equipment, the preoperative nuclear information can provide additional (virtual) intraoperative guidance to improve RGS (Fig. 5.1) [1]. The technical approach and the detectors required for RGS will be discussed in further chapters.

This chapter discusses the radio- and hybrid tracers applied in the field of RGS. Hereby we only focus on tracers that have been used in a clinical setting.

5.2 General Categories and Routes of Administration for Radiotracers

The radiotracers applied in RGS can roughly be divided into four general categories: (1) radiocolloids (Fig. 5.2), (2) small molecules (Fig. 5.3), (3) peptides (Fig. 5.4), and (4) antibodies and antibody fragments (Fig. 5.5). Radiotracers can be administered locally, e.g., when using a radiocolloid for sentinel lymph node (SLN) biopsy, or intravenously, e.g., when using targeted antibodies.

5.2.1 Local Administration

The most widespread application of RGS is the SLN biopsy procedure. For this application, radiolabeled colloid particles (Fig. 5.2) are injected into or directly surrounding the primary tumor, from which they drain via the local lymphatic pathways to the SLN(s). These lymph nodes can then be removed via RGS to be examined at pathology for the presence of metastases. Although the mechanism may differ, upon reaching the SLN(s), these radiocolloids become entrapped via interaction with macrophages and histiocytes lining the sinuses of the nodes [2]. In SLN identification applications, movement of the tracer to the SLN is a physical phenomenon driven by lymphatic flow. Hence, when the

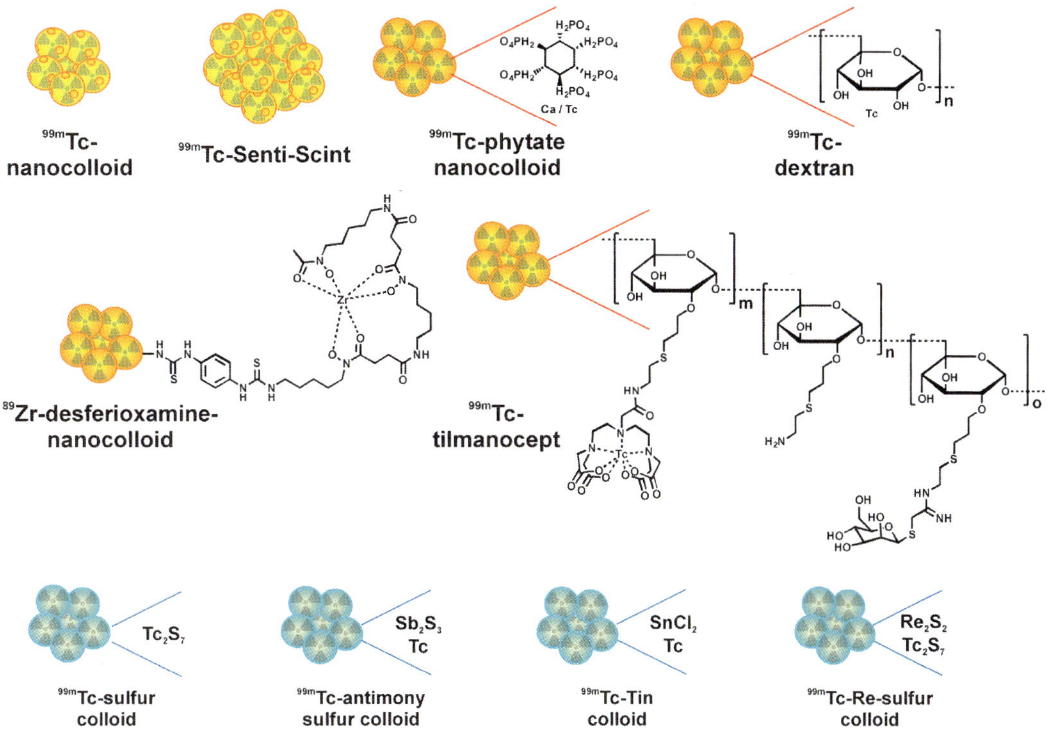

Fig. 5.2 Radiocolloids applied in RGS

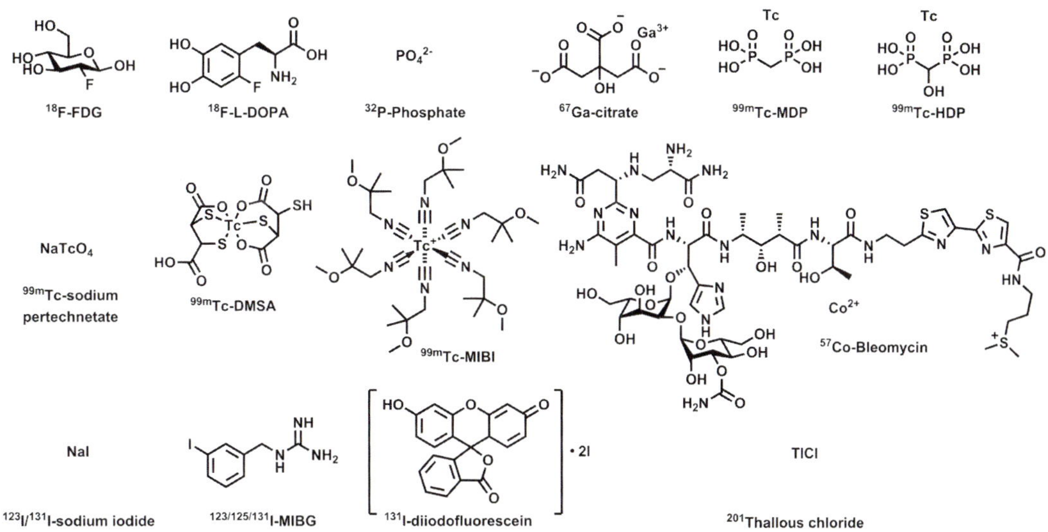

Fig. 5.3 Small-molecule radiotracers applied in RGS

lymphatic flow is abundant, e.g., following the injection of a large volume of tracer, saturation of the SLN can occur, leading to overflow into higher-echelon nodes. This effect is similar to pouring a bottle of champagne on a pyramid of champagne glasses. Initially only the first glass will fill up, but when more champagne is added, eventually all glasses will fill up. However, when

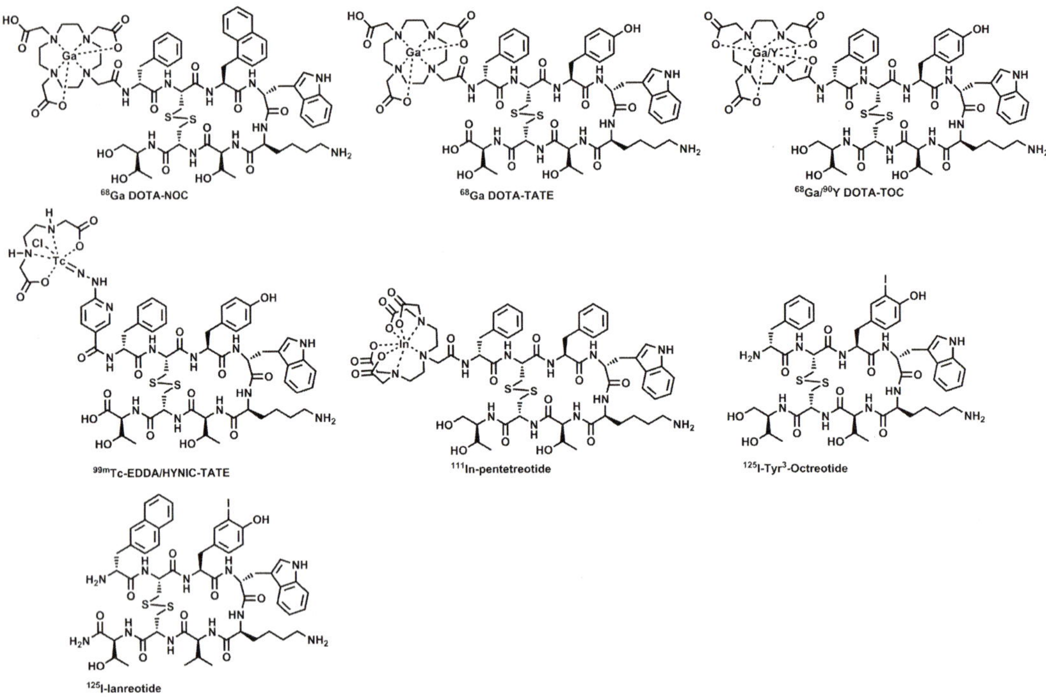

Fig. 5.4 Peptide-based radiotracers applied in RGS

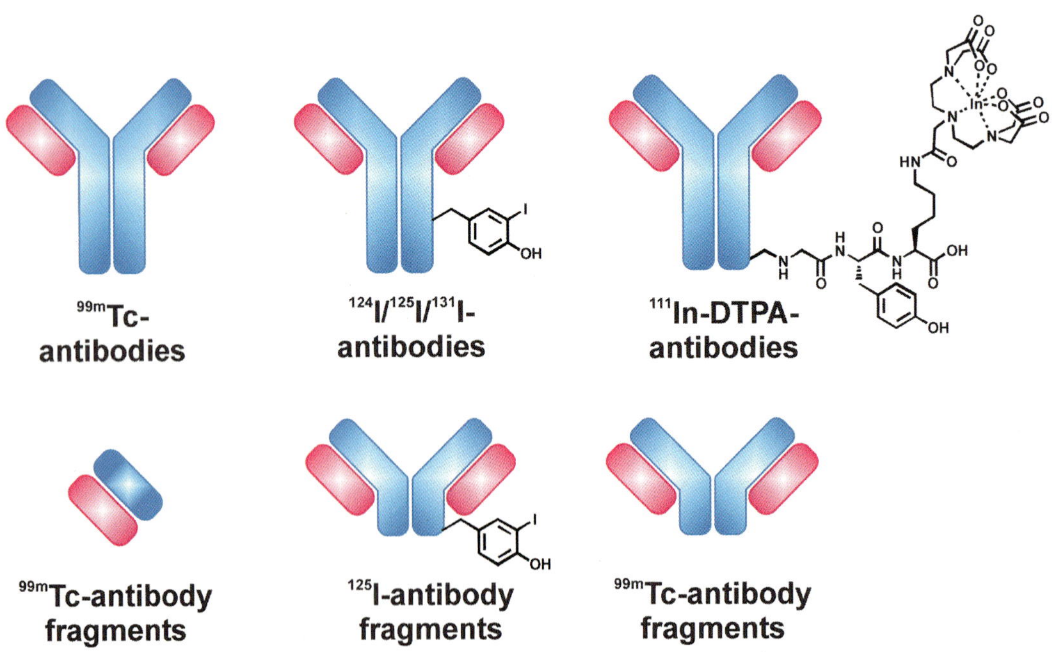

Fig. 5.5 Radiolabeled antibodies and antibody fragments applied in RIGS

the injected volume is limited and the SLN procedure is combined with dynamic imaging, retention of radiocolloid allows for accurate identification of the SLN(s).

For the radioguidance toward the sentinel lymph node in SLN biopsies in various cancer types, ^{99m}Tc-labeled radiocolloids are widely applied (Fig. 5.2). Radiocolloid labeling occurs via the complexation of ^{99m}Tc via various donor atoms in the colloids. The size of the colloidal particles is probably the most important variable and determines the tracer dynamics. Particles with a diameter above 500 nm show very limited drainage via the lymphatic system [3]. On the other side, particles between 5 and 12 nm can penetrate the capillary membranes and rapidly migrate through the lymphatic system and thus require targeting mechanisms using, e.g., mannose to be retained in the SLN [4–6]. Obviously here the chance of overflow to higher-echelon nodes is greatest. Medium-sized colloidal particles ranging between 10 and 200 nm are reported to show the best balance between drainage kinetics via the lymphatics and retention in the SLN(s) [2, 7]. An overview of the different SLN tracers and their sizes has been provided by van den Berg et al. [8].

A local injection, guided by ultrasound or X-ray imaging, with, e.g., (large) ^{99m}Tc-labeled colloidal particles, can also be used to mark nonpalpable (breast) tumors, essentially providing temporary radioactivity–based tattoos. This approach was shown a valid alternative to wire-guided localization (WGL), in which a hooked wire is placed preoperatively to locate the tumor during surgery [9]. The procedure that applies radioactive signatures of a radiocolloid to intraoperatively excise the tumors under RGS is called radioguided occult lesion localization (ROLL) [10]. A similar procedure, where a radioactive titanium seed is placed to locate the tumor, is called radioguided seed localization (RSL). If this procedure is performed with a radiolabeled colloidal particle that also drains to the SLN(s), ROLL can be combined with a SLN biopsy procedure, which has been named sentinel node and occult lesion localization (SNOLL) [10, 11].

5.2.2 Intravenous Administration

The class of small molecule-based radiotracers is the oldest and most diverse class of tracer used in medicine. It consists of radiolabeled molecules mimicking hormones, such as metaiodobenzylguanidine (MIBG) [12]; amino acids, such as 3,4-dihydroxyphenylalanine (DOPA) [13], glucose, such as fluorodeoxyglucose (FDG) [14]; and mimicking building blocks, such as bisphosphonates (Fig. 5.3) [15]. In general these tracers are widely available and/or easy to prepare locally. After distribution through the patients' venous system, these tracers show increased uptake in diseased areas based on the increased metabolism and/or increased proliferation of malignant cells in comparison to healthy tissue.

Although somewhat larger than the small molecules, the relatively small size of receptor targeting peptides (Fig. 5.4) means that they have favorable kinetics. Since they can be produced synthetically, this class of compounds is relatively cheap compared to, e.g., antibodies. Moreover, the variety in which peptide sequences can be produced, and thus the variety of receptors that can potentially be targeted using such compounds, is endless.

To introduce a radionuclide in peptide tracers, in most tracers a bifunctional linker is introduced (Fig. 5.4). Such a bifunctional linker consists of donor atoms or groups that can form a complex with the radionuclide and a reactive group to allow conjugation to the targeting peptide. The introduction of the isotope can be performed just before applying the radiotracer. Generally receptor targeted peptides are injected intravenously to allow distribution via the blood circulation and finally targeting of a disease specific receptor.

In radioimmunoguided surgery (RIGS), radiolabeled antibodies or antibody fragments (Fig. 5.5) are used to target receptor molecules expressed on the lesion(s) of interest. Such antibodies are raised against a specific biomarker that is overexpressed in certain malignancies. The advantages of using an antibody as targeting moiety are their high specificity, affinity, and avidity for the biomarker it has been raised against. Conversely, nonspecific uptake in organs such as the liver and spleen may increase the radiation burden for the patient. At the same time, long circulation times of antibodies demand a long time interval between administration and imaging and/or RIGS. This interval can vary significantly from 2 to 24 days to allow sufficient clearance of unbound antibodies [16–18]. Several options are available to deal with the circulation times: (1) use of isotopes with a long half-life such as ^{89}Zr, ^{111}In, or ^{125}I, to ensure the presence of a radioactive signal after multiple days; (2) pretargeting, which is the use of a reactive or bivalent antibody, followed after a couple of days with the (reactive) radioisotope [19, 20]; and (3) use antibody fragments that show an increased clearance rate [21]. To introduce a radionuclide in the antibodies, three options are available. Either the radionuclide is complexed by donor atoms of the antibody itself (e.g., ^{99m}Tc) via covalent conjugation to amino acids in the antibody (e.g., ^{125}I) or via the before mentioned bifunctional linkers (e.g., ^{111}In) (Fig. 5.5).

To accommodate an additional optical signal, any one of the above tracer types may be converted into hybrid entities that include dyes [22]. Alternatively, the generation of Cherenkov light by beta-emitting isotopes can also enable optical guidance [23].

5.3 Radionuclides

Numerous radionuclides are available, or can be produced, for applications in nuclear imaging, RGS, radiotherapy, or combinations hereof. The choice for the (ideal) radionuclide is based on the availability of the radionuclide and the application for which it will be used. Ideally, a balance between the clinical demands (e.g., half-life, radiation type, radiation energy) and the ability to (chemically) attach the radionuclide to the tracer is found. Table 5.1 contains the physical characteristics of the radionuclides applied in RGS to date.

Table 5.1 Characteristics of radionuclides clinically applied for RGS

Radioisotope	Half-life	Radiation	Energy	Example of use during RGS
^{18}F	110 min	β^+	634 keV	Desai et al. [14]
^{32}P	14.3 days	β^-	690 keV	Selverstone et al. [24]
^{57}Co	271.8 days	β^-	14 keV	Woolfenden et al. [25]
		γ	122, 136 keV	
^{67}Ga	3.26 days	β^-	84 keV	Schattner et al. [26]
		γ	93, 184, 300 keV	
^{68}Ga	67.7 min	β^+	1.90 MeV	Kaemmerer et al. [27]
^{89}Zr	78.4 h	β^+	389 keV	Heuveling et al. [28]
		γ	909 keV	
^{90}Y	64 h	β^-	2.3 MeV	Collamati et al.[29]
^{99m}Tc	6.0 h	γ	141 keV	Gommans et al.[30]
^{111}In	2.80 days	γ	171, 245 keV	Panareo et al.[31]
^{123}I	13.2 h	β^-	23, 127 keV	Gallowitsch et al.[32]
		γ	27, 31, 159 keV	
^{124}I	4.18 days	β^+	1.5, 2.1 MeV	Strong et al. [33]
		γ	603, 1.69 MeV	
^{125}I	60.1 days	γ	27, 35 keV	Hinkle et al. [34]
^{131}I	8.02 days	β^-	606 keV	Jager et al. [35]
		γ	364 keV	
^{201}Tl	73 h	γ	71, 167 keV	Ubhi et al. [36]

Emissions >10 keV and abundance >5 % are included

For the selection of an isotope, radiation exposure of the patient and the medical personnel is also a major factor that needs to be taken into account. Not only is it necessary that the (long-term) benefits for the patient outweigh the possible side effects of radiation exposure, the dose received by the surgical staff during the intervention may also limit the amount of procedures that they can perform on a yearly basis. Table 5.2 contains the range of radiation doses both patients and medical personnel receive upon a RGS procedure with a certain radionuclide. Although this table shows the upper limits and possibly overestimates the dose, it clearly illustrates the differences between various radionuclides.

The patient dose clearly increases upon increased gamma-radiation energy (0.94 mSv for 100 MBq ^{99m}Tc compared to 8.1 mSv for ^{111}In) or by applying β-particle emitting isotopes (7.0 mSv for 370 MBq ^{18}F and 13 Sv for 550 MBq ^{131}I). The patient dose is generally justified by the benefits the patient obtains from accurate imaging,

Table 5.2 Radiation exposure of patient, surgeon, and non-nuclear personnel

Radionuclide	Injected dose per procedure (MBq (Farmacon))	Effective dose per patient (mSv)	RGS time postinjection (h)	Effective dose personnel (μSv h^{-1} (vh postinjection))	Max. 20 mSv yearly dose (h years^{-1})	Max. 5 mSv yearly dose (h years^{-1})	Max. 1 mSv yearly dose (h years^{-1})
^{18}F	370 (FDG)	7.0	1	35.0	571	143	29
			6	5.3	3779	945	189
	700 (FDG)	13.3	1	66.3	302	75	15
			6	10.0	1998	499	100
^{32}P	–	–	–	–	–	–	–
^{57}Co	37 (cyanocobalamin)	77.7	24	2.3	8696	2174	435
^{67}Ga	150 (citrate)	15	6	3.7	5357	1339	268
^{68}Ga	180	–	2	6.3	3175	794	159
^{89}Zr	37 (mAb)	22.2	72	3.4	5897	1474	295
^{90}Y	200 (mAb)	–	12	12.3	1627	407	81
^{99m}Tc	100 (nanocolloid)	0.94	1	1.9	10,335	2584	517
			24	0.14	147,322	36,830	7366
	700 (nanocolloid)	6.6	1	13.6	1476	369	74
			24	0.95	21,046	5261	1052
^{111}In	150 (pentetreotide)	8.1	24	10.1	1973	493	99
			48	7.9	2527	632	126
^{123}I	100 (MIBG)	1.3	4	3.6	5506	1377	275
			24	1.3	15,738	3935	787
^{124}I	180 (mAb)	–	168	9.6	2094	523	105
^{125}I	7 (albumin)	1.5	48	0.2	86,039	21,510	4302
^{131}I	100 (MIBG)	14	2	6.5	3058	764	153
	550 (sodium iodide)	13.10^{3}	24	33.2	602	150	30
	4000 (sodium iodide)	96.10^{3}	120	171	117	29	6
^{201}Tl	70 (TlCl)	15.4	1	1.2	16,101	4025	805

for the calculation, an average dose based on literature procedures was used. Data for the effective dose (mSv.MBq^{-1}) and for the effective dose rate (μSv.m^{2}.(h.MBq)$^{-1}$ were obtained from literature

The physical half-life was taken into account, not the biological half-life. Personnel were estimated to be on 1 m of the patient on average, and 1 m^{2} of the personnel was exposed to the source radiation therapy (e.g., ^{131}I), and/or RGS. Nevertheless, the choice for the radionuclide should be made carefully. For instance, the choice for applying ^{89}Zr results in a considerable radiation dose (22.2 mSv for 37 MBq ^{89}Zr). Radionuclides emitting β^--particles only show a high radiation burden for the patient, because this radiation has a very limited penetration. Radionuclides emitting β^+-particles and gamma-emission also generate a radiation burden for the medical personnel.

The radiation dose received by the medical personnel, e.g., the surgeon and the OR personnel, upon RGS, also deserves careful consideration. In contrast to the justification for the patient, medical personnel has no obvious benefit from the chosen procedure or radionuclide used during the procedure except for achieving an accurate resection. Nevertheless during the, generally long, surgical procedures (multiple hours), they stand in close proximity to the patient and expose themselves to the tracer-based radiation. Based on the level of training, medical personnel is allowed to be exposed to certain levels of radiation, generally divided in maximum exposures of 20, 5, and 1 mSv per year; general surgeons and OR personnel belong to the last group. Because these values represent the upper limits of radiation exposure that is legally allowed, this may influence the amount of procedures that can be performed on a yearly basis. For example, RGS with ^{18}F (370 MBq at 1 h postinjection) results in 35 μSv. h^{-1}. This means that personnel not trained in radiation hygiene can only be present at the operation table for 29 h a year (Table 5.2). An average operation to remove malignant lesions takes 4 h, which means that this person can only perform/attend seven procedures a year. A similar procedure with ^{99m}Tc (100 MBq at 1 h postinjection) allows untrained personnel to attend 129 4-h procedures per year (Table 5.2). An important factor in these calculations is the half-life of the isotope used and the time between injection and the RGS procedure. When the accumulation of the radiotracer allows a longer time between injection and RGS, a large reduction in the radiation exposure for medical personnel can be obtained (Table 5.2). This said, often a strong signal is required during surgery to allow for RGS.

5.3.1 Gamma-Radiation

The workhorses of nuclear medicine, and in particular RGS, are radionuclides that emit γ-photons (Fig. 5.6). Gamma-emitting radionuclides allow whole body imaging using planar scintigraphy and/or single-photon emission tomography (SPECT). Especially isotopes that emit low-to-medium energy (27–245 KeV) photons, such as ^{99m}Tc, ^{111}In, and ^{125}I, have been widely used for RGS. Reasons for their popularity are: (1) availability, (2) compatibility with clinically available gamma detectors, (3) well-developed (chemical) procedures for introducing these nuclides into radiotracers, and (4) energy-dependent tissue attenuation. A high-energy γ-emitter has a higher tissue penetration, improving the accuracy of preoperative imaging, but also results in a higher chance of background signals during RGS. Furthermore, high-energy γ-emissions demand a thickly shielded detector to improve the spatial resolution. The combination of low-to-medium energy photon emission with a short-to-medium half-life of the radionuclide results in a limited radiation burden for both the patient and medical personnel.

5.3.1.1 99m-Technetium

By far the most widely applied and available radioisotope is ^{99m}Tc. ^{99m}Tc has a half-life of 6 h and emits γ-photons of 141 keV, which is in the ideal range (100–200 KeV) for γ-detection by commercially available detectors. Due to this medium energy γ-radiation, the radiation burden for both patient and medical personnel is relatively low (Table 5.2). Pertechnetate ($^{99m}TcO_4^-$) can be collected from ^{99}Mo/^{99m}Tc generators by elution with saline and there is a range of possibilities for conjugation of this isotope to generate the desired radiotracers [37, 38]. Labeling of most ^{99m}Tc-based radiotracers is

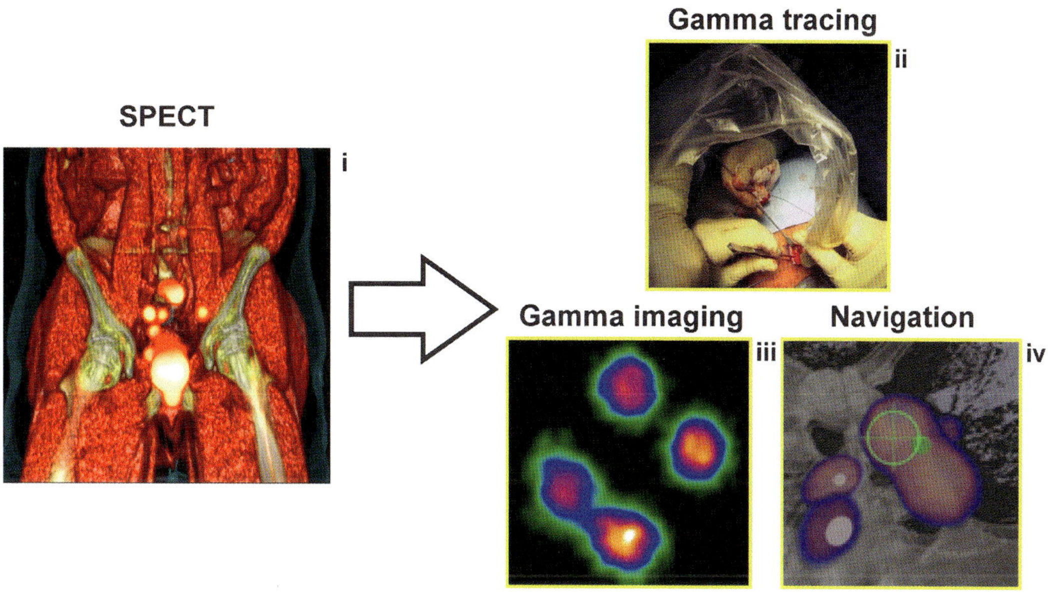

Fig. 5.6 Application of γ-emitters in RGS. (*i*) Whole body nuclear imaging by SPECT; (*ii*) intraoperative gamma tracing with acoustic gamma probe; (*iii*) intraoperative gamma imaging with gamma camera; (*iv*) virtual navigation based on preoperative SPECT imaging or intraoperative freehand γ-detection

performed by reducing the pertechnetate obtained from the generator with Sn(II)-based reducing agents in the presence of the coordinating agent of choice. Technetium can be stabilized through coordination to several donor atoms, e.g., N, O, P, S, and As [38]. Direct metal coordination can be achieved by small molecules that form the radiotracer together with ^{99m}Tc (such as hexakis-2-methoxy-2-methyl-isonitrile complex (MIBI) (Fig. 5.3)) [39], or it can be the functional part of a peptide, protein, or inorganic tracer itself (such as ^{99m}Tc-UBI$_{29–41}$ [40], ^{99m}Tc-nanocolloid, and ^{99m}Tc-sulfur colloid (Fig. 5.2) [30, 41]). Other than direct metal coordination, metal coordination can also occur through bifunctional chelates, for example, by applying hydrazinonicotinic acid (HYNIC) and diethylene triamine pentaacetic acid (DTPA) [42, 43].

Numerous materials have been applied to form radiocolloids for local injection, resulting in a large size range. Several inorganic particles are clinically applied for SLN biopsy and SNOLL applications such as ^{99m}Tc-sulfur colloid (15–5000 nm unfiltered or 15–400 nm filtered) [7, 11, 44, 45] (the United States) and ^{99m}Tc-antimony trisulfide (3–30 nm) [7, 45, 46] (Australia and Canada) (Fig. 5.7). ^{99m}Tc–tin colloids have also been applied, mainly in Japan. Their size can be controlled by the concentration of stannous chloride and ^{99m}Tc, resulting in particles of 50–1500 nm (Fig. 5.7) [45]. In some cases, like with ^{99m}Tc-rhenium sulfide (NanoCis) (20–100 nm), the stability and the formation of micro aggregates have limited use of the tracer [7, 46, 47]. Also organic-based colloid particles are applied for radioguided SLN biopsies. ^{99m}Tc-phytate particles (Fig. 5.2) are formed by the interaction of stannous phytate with Ca^{2+} present in serum. The size of these particles depends on the calcium concentration and in vitro experiments showed a size range of 150–1500 nm [45]. In Europe, ^{99m}Tc-labeled human serum albumin (HSA)-based colloids are most widely used for SLN biopsy procedures. HSA-nanocolloid (Nanocoll; mean diameter 20 nm; range 10–100 nm, Fig. 5.2) has shown to provide a superior retention in the SLN compared to radiolabeled HSA (vasculosis; mean

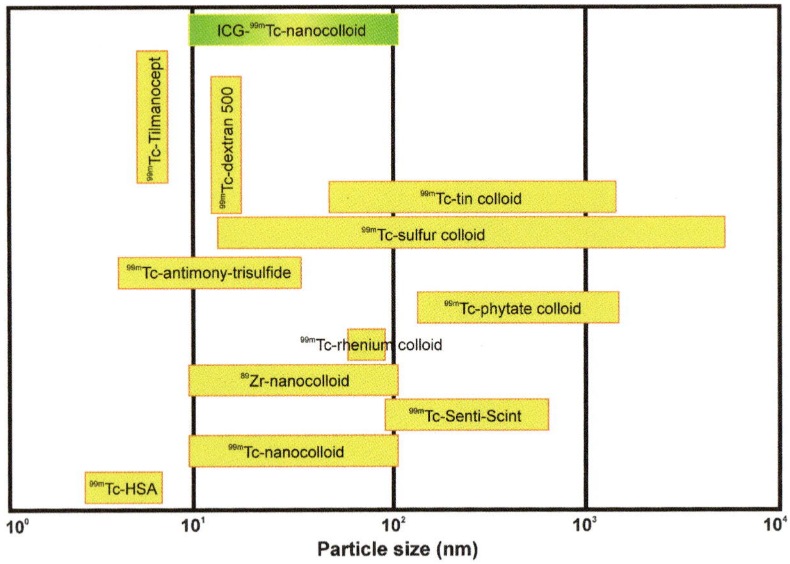

Fig. 5.7 Various size ranges of radiocolloids applied in RGS

diameter 7 nm) and is therefore widely applied [6, 30]. Next to the SLN biopsy, Nanocoll is also often used for ROLL and SNOLL procedures [48], sometimes in combination with large ^{99m}Tc-labeled albumin aggregates (e.g., ^{99m}Tc-MAA (10–90 μm) for-tumor demarcation [10]. Even the larger HSA-nanocolloid (SentiScint; mean diameter 205 nm; range 100–600 nm; Fig. 5.2) has shown promising results during SLN procedures [49, 50]. ^{99m}Tc-labeled dextran-based nanoparticles (14 nm) have been used for lymphatic mapping in, e.g., colon and breast cancer [51, 52]. A small dextran-based colloid (7 nm) with DTPA and mannose moieties conjugated to its structure has been developed for SLN mapping (Tilmanocept) (Fig. 5.2) [53–55]. This tracer is claimed to show faster clearance from the injection site and to have a stronger interaction with phagocytes [42].

Next to local administration, ^{99m}Tc-labeled compounds can also be administered intravenously. The most simple form herein is the ability of "free" ^{99m}Tc-pertechnetate to accumulate in the thyroid, due to its resemblance to iodine. Next to thyroid scintigraphy to evaluate for hot/cold nodules, pertechnetate can also be used for radioguidance during thyroidectomy [56].

Conjugated to six methoxyisobutylisonitrile ligands, ^{99m}Tc forms the hydrophobic and positively charged ^{99m}Tc-sestamibi (Fig. 5.3), which is rapidly taken up by mitochondria in (hyper)active cells. Next to its common application in cardiac imaging [57], ^{99m}Tc-sestamibi was also shown to allow the evaluation of tumor margins in patients with breast cancer showing promising results for the detection of small foci [58]. Furthermore, the normal distribution of ^{99m}Tc-sestamibi was evaluated in 5 volunteers followed by the RGS of one patient suspected of a brain tumor. ^{99m}Tc-sestamibi-based RGS resulted in the accurate detection and removal of the brain lesions diagnosed as metastases of renal cell carcinoma [59]. Due to its uptake in (hyper)active cells, ^{99m}Tc-sestamibi has also been applied in the detection of abnormalities in the (para)thyroid [60–64].

^{99m}Tc-dimercaptosuccinic acid (DMSA) (Fig. 5.3) is believed to accumulate in tumors due to their acidic environment [65]. Therefore, ^{99m}Tc-DMSA has been applied for the detection of thyroid cancer. In a study it was compared in 25 patients to ^{111}In-pentetreotide (see below) [66]. Although better results were found for ^{99m}Tc-DMSA, it is no longer commercially available [67].

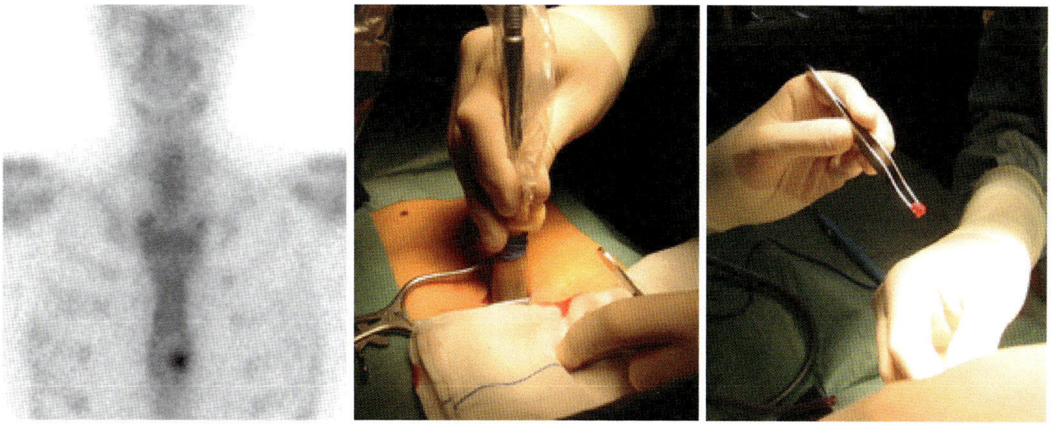

Fig. 5.8 Patient with a sternal metastasis, resected via ^{99m}Tc-MDP RGS

Bisphosphonates have a high affinity for hydroxyapatite, the mineral present in bones. Bisphosphonates especially tend to accumulate in sites of active bone formation, which occurs in bone lesions. Therefore, ^{99m}Tc-labeled bisphosphonates have been applied for radioguided biopsies and surgery of bone lesions. RGS based on ^{99m}Tc-medronic acid (MDP) and ^{99m}Tc-oxidronate (HDP) (Figs. 5.3 and 5.8) was shown to reduce the procedure time and to improve the localization of the lesions [15, 68–70].

Coordinated by HYNIC and ethylenediamine N,N'-diacetic acid (EDDA), ^{99m}Tc has also been conjugated to receptor targeting peptides such as the somatostatin analogue octreotate (Fig. 5.4). Upon intravenous administration, the peptide targets the somatostatin receptors, commonly overexpressed on neuroendocrine tumors. This radiotracer was used for RGS of four carcinoids and five pancreatic neuroendocrine tumors, resulting in accurate detection of the lesions and an increased detection of lymph node metastases [43].

^{99m}Tc has also been used to label antibodies, e.g., SM3 against polymorphic epithelial mucin and H17E2 against placental- and germ cell alkaline phosphatases; both are biomarkers that are overexpressed in ovarian cancer (Fig. 5.5). In 16 patients (1 patient for H17E2 and 15 patients for SM3), these labeled antibodies were shown to allow detection of ovarian cancer, both in vivo and in excised tissue specimens [71]. An ^{99m}Tc-labeled antibody fragment against carcinoembryonic antigen (CEA) (IMMU 4-Fab) (Fig. 5.5) was applied for RIGS in 65 patients with colorectal tumors resulting in more accurate diagnosis and in determining the extent of the lesion and possible lymph node intrusion [72]. ^{99m}Tc labeled anti-CEA antibody fragment F023C5 was unsuccessful in the detection of lesions in one lung cancer patient, but did show an increased uptake of radioactivity ex vivo [67, 73].

5.3.1.2 111-Indium

^{111}In is a γ-emitter with a half-life of 2.8 days. Similar to ^{99m}Tc, the photon energies of ^{111}In (171 and 245 keV) are in the optimum range for commercial gamma cameras. Due to the higher energy γ-radiation and the longer half-life, the radiation burden for patients and medical personnel is higher compared to ^{99m}Tc (Table 2). ^{111}In is produced by proton irradiation of ^{112}Cd and can be incorporated in radiotracers via bifunctional chelates such as DTPA and 1,4,7,10-tetraazacyclododecane-1,4,7,10-tetraacetic acid (DOTA), which can be chemically conjugated to targeting moieties such as a peptides, antibodies, and proteins.

For the RGS toward, e.g., neuroendocrine tumors, thyroid carcinomas, and meningiomas, ^{111}In-labeled somatostatin analogues are widely applied (Fig. 5.4) [31, 66, 74–78]. The mechanism of tracer uptake is based on intravenous administration of the tracer, followed by specific binding to the somatostatin receptor. Panareo et al. reported that use of ^{111}In-DTPA-D-Phe^1-octreotide (^{111}In-pentetreotide) resulted in the excision of non-palpable neuroendocrine breast tumors that were not detected by conventional imaging techniques [31]. The use of a gamma probe in ^{111}In-DTPA-D-Phe^1-octreotide RGS towards midgut carcinoid and endocrine pancreatic tumors in 21 patients allowed detection of all tumor lesions >5 mm, while SPECT failed to detect lesions <9 mm [75].

Intravenous administration of ^{111}In-labeled anti-TAG72 (a tumor-associated glycoprotein) antibodies has been used for RIGS of colorectal carcinoma (37 patients) and ovarian cancer (5 patients). This resulted in the detection of several lesions that would have been missed by standard surgical exploration [79, 80]. RIGS towards prostate-specific membrane antigen (PSMA) using the antibody ^{111}In-capromab pendetide has been reported in one patient, which resulted in the excision of a tumor positive lymph node (Fig. 5.5) [81]. RIGS with ^{111}In has also been performed via a pretargeting approach [20]; in 13 patients with thyroid carcinoma, approximately 4 days after injection of a bivalent antibody directed against CEA and DTPA, ^{111}In-di-DTPA-tyrosyl-lysine was injected [82]. 3 ± 1 days after injection of the radiotracer, patients underwent RGS. Small lesions with a diameter below 0.3 cm could be detected successfully using this approach [19].

5.3.1.3 57-Cobalt

^{57}Co is mainly a γ-emitter that emits photons of 122 and 136 keV. This radionuclide has a long half-life of 271.8 days. Due to its long half-life and the emission of low-energy β^--particles, the radiation burden for the patient is high (Table 2). This radioisotope is produced by proton irradiation of natural iron and nickel. Bleomycin, a cytostatic, was labeled with ^{57}Co via complexation of the bivalent cobalt ion by the molecule itself. 21 lung cancer patients were injected intravenously with bleomycin (Fig. 5.3), which was labeled via complexation of the divalent ^{57}cobalt ion [83]. Bleomycin itself binds and damages DNA and is therefore most active against fast dividing cells, such as in malignant tissue. ^{57}Co-labeled bleomycin was shown to allow the detection of lung tumors that would otherwise be missed [25]. However, the long half-life of ^{57}Co prevented dissemination of this technology.

5.3.1.4 67-Gallium

^{67}Ga is a γ-emitter (93, 184, and 300 keV) with a half-life of 3.26 days. Due to its medium half-life, high γ-energy emission (300 keV), and β^--emission, the use of ^{67}Ga results in a considerable radiation burden for the patient (Table 5.2). ^{67}Ga is produced by the irradiation of ^{68}Zn by charged particles, e.g., protons. After production the gallium is coordinated with citric acid to form gallium citrate (Fig. 5.3), which in itself is administered as radiotracer. ^{67}Ga-citrate is often used as radiotracer to detect inflammatory lesions, based on the transchelation of the ^{67}Ga to lactoferrin and siderophores released by leukocytes and microorganisms located at the site of infection [84, 85]. ^{67}Ga citrate has also been reported by Schattner et al. in the RGS toward extranodal lymphoma in one patient, where accumulation in the lesion was most likely caused by necrotic tissue and inflammatory responses [26].

5.3.1.5 123-Iodine

^{123}I is mainly a γ-emitter that emits photons of 27, 31, and 159 keV. Also this radionuclide emits β^--particles of 23 and 127 keV. The isotope has a half-life of 13.2 h. Due to its short half-life, the radiation burden caused by using this isotope is relatively low, although it is higher than ^{99m}Tc (Table 5.2). ^{123}I is produced by proton irradiation of ^{124}Xe, resulting in ^{123}Xe that subsequently decays to ^{123}I. Radioiodination, with all isotopes of iodine, is mainly performed by electrophilic substitution, which requires the (in situ) generation of I^+ species. These species can be obtained by the generation of mixed halogen species. Examples of applied oxidizing reagents that can generate mixed radiohalogen species are chloramine-T, iodogen, and N-chlorosuccinimide [86]. Mixed radiohalogen species (XCl) readily react with activated aryl compounds, such as phenols, resulting in mono- or disubstitution at positions ortho to the hydroxyl group. Proteins can be radioiodinated due to the presence of tyrosine residues, although also histidine, tryptophan, and cysteine are sensitive to radioiodination [86, 87]. Non-activated aryl compounds can be radioiodinated via isotopic exchange, in which a non-radioactive iodine isotope is exchanged for a radioactive isotope, or via the electrophilic substitution of a stannylated precursor [88, 89]. Finally also radioiodine-labeled prosthetic groups can be added to the targeting moiety via a selective reaction, for instance, via conjugation to amine reactive groups [86, 87].

^{123}I has been used for RGS of thyroid cancer, both as Na^{123}I and as ^{123}I-MIBG (Fig. 5.3) [32, 90]. Injection of Na^{123}I will result in the accumulation in hyperactive regions of the thyroid, while ^{123}I-MIBG will accumulate in adrenergic tissue such as thyroid tumors. Because ^{131}I (see below) is less expensive, better available, and also often used for therapy, this isotope often replaces ^{123}I in thyroid-related procedures [67]. ^{123}I-MIBG has been applied for RGS-based detection of neuroblastoma (41 procedures) [12, 91] and for the detection of neuroendocrine tumors (4 patients) [66, 92].

5.3.1.6 125-Iodine

^{125}I is a γ-emitter with a half-life of 60.1 days that emits low-energy photons (35 keV). The low-energy photon emissions makes this isotope less suitable for whole body imaging, but well suited for RGS due to its low background radiation. ^{125}I is produced by neutron irradiation of ^{124}Xe, which leads to ^{125}Xe that then decays to ^{125}I. The labeling chemistry for this isotope essentially is identical to that of ^{123}I.

For RGS using the sodium salt to detect thyroid malignancies, generally other iodine isotopes are applied. ^{125}I has been used for the labeling of MIBG (Fig. 5.3). In a direct comparison between ^{123}I-MIBG (36 cases) and ^{125}I-MIBG (30 cases) for RGS in neuroblastoma patients, ^{125}I-MIBG showed a higher specificity. This difference can be explained by the low-energy emission of ^{125}I, which resulted in a lower background signal from surrounding tissue [91, 93].

There are also examples where iodination was used in combination with targeting peptides. For example, the somatostatin analogue ^{125}I-Lanreotide was used in 13 patients with breast carcinoma resulting in accurate positive margin resection [94]. Furthermore it was applied in 2 patients with gastrinomas, which are gastrin-secreting tumors that also overexpress the somatostatin receptor [95]. A different somatostatin analogue, ^{125}I-Tyr^3-octreotide, was applied in 12 patients suspected of neuroendocrine tumors or gastrinomas showing promising results in tumor-specific accumulation and intraoperative detection (Fig. 5.4) [96].

The long half-life of ^{125}I makes it ideal for RIGS with complete antibodies (Fig. 5.5). Most clinical radioiodinated RIGS studies using ^{125}I have been performed with antibodies targeting the tumor-associated glycoprotein 72 (anti-TAG-72), e.g., primarily in colorectal cancer but also in gastric, pancreatic, ovarian, lung, prostate, and breast cancer. It started with the murine B72.3 antibody, followed by the second-generation antibodies: CC49 and the humanized HuCC49 (for an extensive review, see ref. [67]). Alternatively, A_5B_7 (52 patients) [97] and CL58 (29 patients), targeting the carcinoembryonic antigen (CEA), resulted in the detection of colorectal cancer lesions [98]. ^{125}I-labeled F(ab')$_2$ antibody fragments, containing both binding domains of a whole antibody without the Fc region, directed against CEA (F023C5) were explored for RIGS. In a small patient group, F023C5 was used to identify breast and colorectal cancer. However, due to a low tumor detection rate during RGS (40 %), the investigators advised the use of more specific antibodies [99, 100]. Antibodies against the tumor-associated antigen 17-1A (EpCAM) has been radiolabeled with ^{125}I and applied in multiple patients to assist in locating non-palpable colorectal tumors or aiding in determining the resection margins [101–103]. Wang et al. intravenously injected ^{125}I-labeled antibodies (3H11) against human gastric cancer cells in 35 patients and showed high specificity and accuracy in detecting the lesions [67, 104].

Although little chemistry is involved, a completely different application of ^{125}I can be found in ^{125}I-labeled titanium seeds [105–107]. In a procedure called radioguided seed localization (RSL), these seeds are placed under ultrasound or X-ray guidance to mark non-palpable breast tumors. It can be considered an alternative to WGL and ROLL and is of particular interest for use in a neoadjuvant setting. The systemic treatment, applied in the neoadjuvant setting to reduce the tumor volume before surgery, demands a considerable time (several weeks) between tumor localization and the actual surgery. WGL and ROLL are not ideal as they require the insertion of a twisted marker before treatment and/or the injection of ^{99m}Tc-labeled colloids just before surgery. ^{125}I-labeled seeds require only one procedure to place them and they remain detectable after >30 weeks [108]. Studies evaluating RSL showed a reduction in reoperations due to positive tumor margins and an increased patient convenience compared to the WGL [9, 109]. In comparison with ROLL, RSL showed the same surgical outcome in breast-conserving surgery [108].

5.3.1.7 131-Iodine

^{131}I emits both γ- and β$^-$-radiation of 364 and 606 keV, respectively, and has a half-life of 8 days. ^{131}I is produced by neutron irradiation of natural tellurium. The labeling chemistry for this isotope resembles that of ^{123}I. ^{131}I induces a large radiation burden for the patient, as a result of its β$^-$-emission. This, in combination with the accumulation of sodium iodide in the thyroid, has led to the therapeutic use of this isotope against thyroid malignancies. Due to the γ-emission, the isotope can be used for RGS, but caution is necessary with respect to the exposure of the medical personnel due to the large dosages (>1 GBq) used for therapeutic applications.

One of the first RGS studies reported in the literature applied ^{131}I-labeled diiodofluorescein (Fig. 5.3) to locate brain tumors [110, 111]. Fluorescein was shown to distribute throughout the body, but was slower cleared form the malignant tissue, which resulted in a detectable signal from the tumor between 3 and 8 h postinjection [112]. This observation led to the development of radioiodinated fluorescein. In 340 patients suspected of a space-occupying brain lesion, the detection of diiodofluorescein by a Geiger-Müller tube had an accuracy of 95 % [111].

^{131}I is the most used isotope to treat abnormalities of the thyroid and RGS towards, thyroid cancer [113–115]. However, after iodine-based therapy, many recurrent thyroid cancers are iodine insensitive and therefore other tracers have to be used for imaging and RGS (such as ^{99m}Tc-MIBI and ^{99m}Tc-DMSA). For the detection of neuroendocrine tumors, the use of ^{131}I-MIBG (Fig. 5.3) was shown feasible [116]. However, hepatic clearance can result in high background signals overshadowing the lesion of interest, which limits the application of all iodine-labeled MIBG tracers for the detection of neuroendocrine tumors in the area of the adrenal gland [66].

^{131}I has also been used for labeling of antibodies and antibody fragments, which resulted in the accurate detection of small lesions and allowed the evaluation of the resection margins (Fig. 5.5) [16, 35, 117, 118]. However, due to its β$^-$-emission and relatively high-energy γ-photons, ^{131}I has been replaced by other iodine isotopes, such as ^{125}I, for RIGS applications.

5.3.1.8 201-Thallium

^{201}Tl is a γ-emitter that emits photons of 71 and 167 keV. T and the isotope has a half-life of 73 h. ^{201}Tl causes a considerable radiation dose for the patient, although the exposure for the medical personnel is relatively low (Table 5.2).

The radionuclide is produced by proton irradiation of ^{203}Tl, which yields ^{201}Pb that then decays into ^{201}Tl. An intravenous injection of ^{201}Thallous chloride (TlCl; Fig. 5.3) has been used in one RGS case towards parathyroid adenoma [36]. Since ^{201}Tl showed an increased uptake in areas of high cellular density with increased regional blood flow, the authors claim it allowed removal of the tumor, which was not detected by visible inspection.

5.3.2 Positron Radiation

A prominent part of nuclear medicine, and radiochemistry, focuses on radionuclides that emit β$^+$-particles or positrons in combination with positron emission tomography (PET). The emitted positrons travel a maximum of a couple of millimeters through human tissue before they reach thermal energies and annihilate with an electron [119]. This annihilation results in the emission of two high-energy photons of 511 keV, which travel in opposite direction from the point of annihilation (180±0.25°). Compared to SPECT imaging, PET imaging has a higher sensitivity and spatial resolution in whole body imaging. Because of these advantages, and their abundant clinical use, positron emitters have also been explored for RGS (Fig. 5.9).

Unfortunately, the advantages that apply for whole body imaging cannot be directly translated to RGS. Accurate localization of high-energy photons requires extensive shielding of the detectors, which generally converts them into heavy (and relatively large) devices. An interesting alternative is the selective detection of the positrons themselves. Due to the very limited range of positrons in tissue (<2 mm), this may yield a superficial detection technique that could allow for the accurate delineation of tumor margins. The fact that it is not straightforward to detect β^+-particles over the background of high-energy photons is underlined by the fact that there are only few reports that describe the intraoperative use of a β^+-selective probe [33, 120].

5.3.2.1 18-Fluorine

The most widely used β^+-emitter is ^{18}F, which emits β^+-particles of 634 keV and has a half-life of 110 min. Although high-energy photons (511 keV) are generated by the annihilation of the β^+-particles, the effective dose for the patient is relatively low. However, the high-energy photons result in a relatively high radiation burden for the

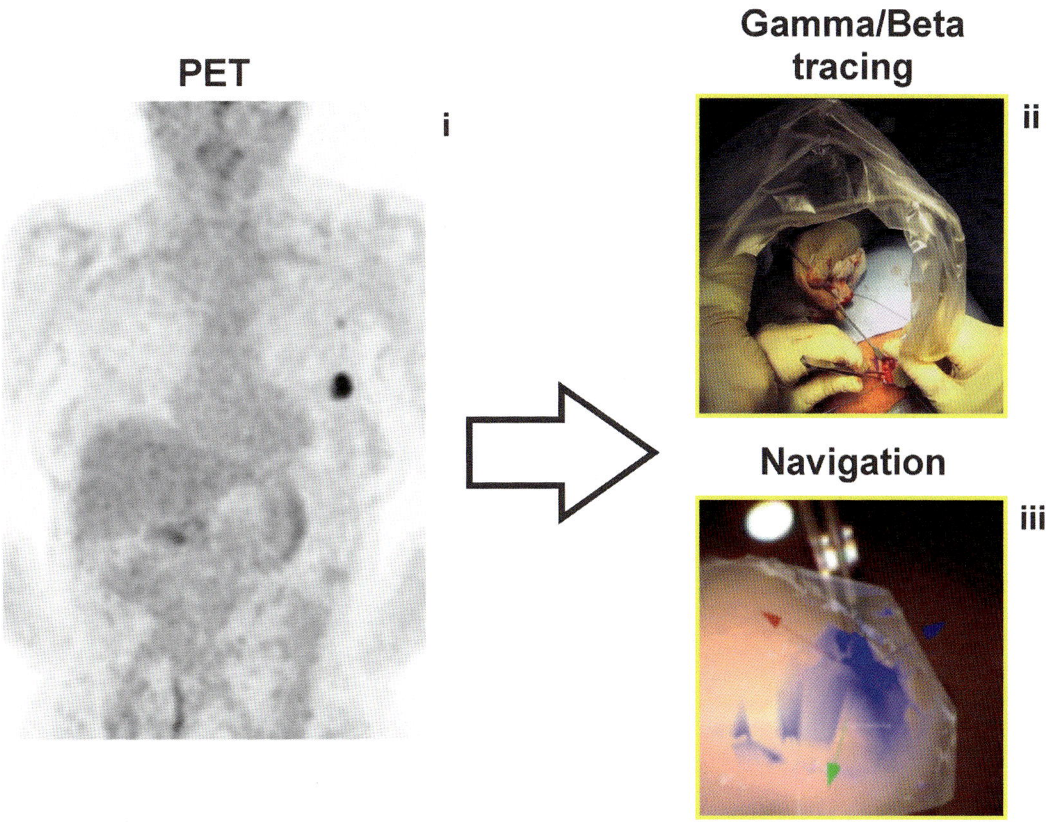

Fig. 5.9 Application of β-emitters in RGS. (*i*) Whole body nuclear imaging by PET; (*ii*) intraoperative gamma and beta tracing with acoustic probes; (*iii*) virtual navigation based on preoperative PET imaging or intraoperative freehand β-detection

medical personnel (Table 5.2). ^{18}F is generated by proton irradiation of $H_2{}^{18}O$ or $^{18}O_2$ [121] and can be covalently incorporated in radiotracers via nucleophilic or electrophilic introductions, for which multiple reagents have been developed, e.g., [^{18}F]-F^--kryptofix [121]. An alternative approach would be to incorporate ^{18}F (in the form of aluminum fluoride) in a chelate (NOTA), thereby allowing labeling of tracers by simple mixing just before administration [122].

2-Deoxy-2-(^{18}F)fluoro-D-glucose (^{18}F-FDG) (Fig. 5.3), a glucose in which the hydroxyl group at the 2-position is replaced via nucleophilic substitution by ^{18}F, is the most widely applied tracer in modern nuclear medicine and can be used to highlight areas with a high metabolic activity. ^{18}F-FDG has also been applied for RGS approaches because of its widespread use and tumor accumulating characteristics. Yet, due to its short half-life, the interval between tracer administration and surgery is limited. Furthermore certain (metabolic active) organs and tissues are known to accumulate ^{18}F-FDG, e.g., the heart, brains, and bladder, which may obscure detection of lesions in these anatomies.

Early ^{18}F-FDG RGS studies have been performed with non-optimized gamma cameras (detection windows around 124, 150, 200, and 255 KeV), resulting in low-radiation detection [14]. More optimized high-energy gamma detectors have later been used to locate, e.g., colorectal tumors and lymphoma, which resulted in the removal of non-palpable and difficult to locate lesions [120, 123–125]. Next to high-energy gamma detectors, also β-sensitive probes were applied [120]. Although the authors claim the selective detection of β-particles, the detection up to 6 cm raises some questions about the selectivity of the probe [120].

A case study has also been reported regarding RGS with ^{18}F-L-DOPA (Fig. 5.3). Increased uptake of ^{18}F-L-DOPA in tumors is caused by the upregulation of amino-acid transporters, to supply the malignancy in their demand for nutrients. The application of ^{18}F-L-DOPA in RGS with a high-energy gamma detector resulted in the successful removal of multiple neuroendocrine tumors and metastases [13].

5.3.2.2 68-Gallium

^{68}Ga is a positron emitter that emits β^+-particles of 1.9 MeV and has a half-life of 67.7 min. We were not able to find information about the effective dose for patients; a high radiation burden can be expected based on the high-energy β^+-particles and the 511 keV photons generated by positron annihilation. For the medical personnel the radiation burden is caused by the 511 keV photons and is therefore similar for most β^+-emitters (Table 5.2). ^{68}Ga can be eluted from a ^{68}Ga-generator; a stationary phase with absorbed ^{68}Ge is eluted with an acidic mobile phase, which takes the generated ^{68}Ga with it. Such a generator can be maintained at location, e.g., a nuclear facility in a medical center. For RGS applications similar advantages and disadvantages can be expected as described above for ^{18}F. From the chemical perspective, ^{68}Ga can, however, be more easily incorporated in a radiotracer via chelation by a bifunctional chelate conjugated to the targeting moiety. DOTA has been the chelate of choice in the clinically used ^{68}Ga-based radiotracers, although other and possibly better chelates are available, e.g., NOTA and TRAP [126, 127]. Due to the requirement of a chelate in combination with a short half-live, ^{68}Ga has been predominantly used in combination with peptide constructs. For RGS applications, ^{68}Ga was incorporated in the somatostatin analogues DOTA-NOC and DOTA-octreotate (DOTA-TATE) (Fig. 5.4). These radiotracers have been successfully used for RGS towards gastroenteropancreatic neuroendocrine tumors. In 9 patients, the RGS approach with a high-energy gamma detector allowed detection of 94 % of lesions (up to 5 mm tumors) compared to 69 % by preoperative PET imaging and 50 % by surgical palpation [27].

5.3.2.3 89-Zirconium

^{89}Zr has both β^+- and γ-emissions of 389 and 909 keV, respectively, and has a half-life of 78.4 h. Due to the high-energy emissions and medium half-life, ^{89}Zr causes a considerable radiation burden for the patient. Also the radiation dose for the medical personnel is slightly higher compared to other β^+-emitters due to the additional γ-emission. ^{89}Zr is produced by proton irradiation of ^{89}Y and can be incorporated in a radiotracer via the bifunctional chelate desferrioxamine.

In a pilot study with ^{89}Zr-desferioxamine-nanocolloid (Fig. 5.2) for SLN mapping by Heuveling et al., a higher resolution in the pre-operative nuclear imaging (PET vs SPECT) was observed [28]. The authors claim that, by using a β-selective probe, RGS based on ^{89}Zr-desferrioxamine-nanocolloid should provide a similar or better intraoperative detection, compared to ^{99m}Tc-nanocolloid, especially for localization of a SLN near the injection site. This was however not (yet) shown.

5.3.2.4 124-Iodine

^{124}I is a γ- and $β^+$-emitter that emits photons of 0.6 and 1.7 MeV and $β^+$-particles of 1.5 and 2.1 MeV. ^{124}I has a half-life of 4.18 days. Due to its little use in (clinical) research, we were not able to find information about the effective dose for patients. A high radiation burden can be expected based on the high-energy emissions and long half-life. The exposure for medical personnel is considerable (Table 5.2). ^{124}I is produced by proton irradiation of ^{124}Te. The conjugation chemistry for this isotope is similar to that of the other iodine isotopes reported above.

Although ^{124}I is mainly used for PET imaging, this isotope has been applied in RIGS tracing both the positrons and the high-energy photons (511 keV) originating from ^{124}I-labeled antibodies against A33 transmembrane glycoprotein (huA33) and against carbonic anhydrase IX (cG250) [33]. Detection was performed by both a high-energy gamma detector and a β-selective detector. In four patients a high correlation between γ- and $β^+$-detection was determined and the authors claim that the β-probe showed a higher tumor to background signal compared to the high-energy gamma probe.

5.3.3 Electron Radiation

$β^-$-particle or electron-emitting radionuclides have been applied for RGS for two reasons. The first reason is the clinical application of $β^-$-emitters for radiotherapy, which allows RGS toward the residual lesion based on other emissions of the radionuclide. The second reason for using a (pure) $β^-$-emitter in combination with a $β^-$-specific detector for RGS is the very limited range of $β^-$-particles in tissue. Any uptake in nearby healthy tissue or radiation of a nearby injection site is attenuated before reaching the detector. This would result in a lower background and a better delineation of the margins around the lesion of interest. Unfortunately a (pure) $β^-$-emitter does not allow preoperative whole body imaging for surgical planning and an approximate location of the lesion of interest has to be known to be able to locate it with a $β^-$-specific probe.

5.3.3.1 32-Phosphorus

^{32}P emits $β^-$-particles of 690 keV and has a half-life of 14.3 days. Due to its limited use in clinical research, we were not able to find information about the effective dose for patients or medical personnel. ^{32}P is produced by neutron irradiation of ^{32}S. One of the first studies on RGS reported on in 1949, applying a Geiger-Müller device, was performed with $^{32}P\text{-}PO_4^{2-}$ (Fig. 5.3). The accumulation and turnover of the phosphate ion were found higher in tumor tissue compared to healthy brain tissue, thereby allowing the identification of cerebral gliomas in 14 patients [24]. Due to its $β^-$-emission, ^{32}P has not been widely applied for RGS, but for research purposes, multiple methods are available to label all kind of tracers with this isotope [128, 129].

5.3.3.2 90-Yttrium

^{90}Y emits $β^-$-particles of 2.3 MeV and has a half-life of 64 h. The high-energy $β^-$emission results in a high radiation burden for the patient, and therefore, this isotope is mainly used for therapeutic purposes. However, the additional X-ray generation and the use of high therapeutic dosages cause considerable radiation exposure for the medical personnel. ^{90}Y is a decay product of ^{90}Sr, which is produced upon uranium and plutonium fission in nuclear power plants. Small-scale ^{90}Y generators based on ^{90}Sr have been developed, which can be used for the production of ^{90}Y with high specific activity [130]. These generators can be operated at the local nuclear facility of medical centers. Although ^{90}Y is almost purely a β^--emitter, SPECT imaging has been performed based on Bremsstrahlung, which originates from the loss of kinetic energy from the high-energy electrons (β^-) resulting in the emission of photons [131]. Also PET imaging is possible due to the rare (1 in 32 million transitions) β^-/β^+-pair formation, of which the β^+ can subsequently annihilate with an electron to produce two photons of 511 keV [132, 133]. ^{90}Y can be incorporated in radiotracers by binding it to the bifunctional chelate DOTA, which can be conjugated to a variety of targeting moieties.

Recently the use of a β^--specific probe in combination with the ^{90}Y-labeled somatostatin analogue DOTA-TOC (Fig. 5.4) was suggested for the detection of meningioma and high-grade glioma [29]. In this study, PET imaging was performed with ^{68}Ga-DOTA-TOC and provided quantitative information about the uptake of the tracer. Based on this information, the required dosage of ^{90}Y-DOTA-TOC was calculated to discriminate the lesion of interest from the surrounding healthy tissue with a β^--specific probe [29]. Based on this preoperative ^{68}Ga-based imaging and calculations, the authors concluded that RGS based on ^{90}Y-DOTA-TOC should be possible [29].

5.4 Hybrid Imaging and Detection Platforms (Table 5.3)

Hybrid imaging combines two imaging modalities, e.g., nuclear and luminescence imaging, in a single approach. It was already introduced in 1948 by Moore et al. who radiolabeled diiodofluorescein, resulting in a tracer that has both a nuclear and a fluorescent component. Luminescence imaging in the clinic has been performed based on fluorescence and Cherenkov luminescence (CL) and can provide high-resolution imaging in the operating theatre to aid the surgeon in detecting the lesion of interest (Fig. 5.11b). The advantage of luminescence-guided surgery over radioguided surgery lies in the limited tissue attenuation of visible light [138]; like with β^--particle or electron-emitting radionuclides, imaging of optical signals is less hindered by background signals originating from the injection site or from tracer accumulation in the vicinity of the lesion of interest. However, due to the limited tissue penetration of light (<1 cm) [138], luminescence imaging is not suitable for whole body imaging. Therefore, the application of a radio- and luminescent tracer combines the best of both worlds.

Two subclasses of hybrid tracers have been reported for clinical use, being the combination of a radionuclide and a fluorescent label on a single tracer (Fig. 5.11a) or the detection of the Cherenkov luminescence (CL) emitted by β^+/β^--emitting isotopes (Fig. 5.11b). Fluorescence imaging is based on the excitation of a fluorescent label with light, which results in the emission of light of a longer wavelength. The advantage of fluorescence imaging is that it provides real-time high-resolution information. Yet, fluorescence imaging requires the addition of a fluorescent label to the imaging tracer, the excitation light has to be blocked from reaching the camera, and background fluorescence can occur originating from endogenous fluorophores.

Cherenkov photons (Cherenkov Luminescence; CL) originate from charged particles (β+ /β−) that travel through a medium faster than the speed of light in that same medium. CL occurs in tissue when the emitted charged particles have energies higher than 0.21 MeV. The intensity of CL is around three orders of

Table 5.3 Optical characteristics of clinically applied hybrid tracers

Optical component	λ_{exc} (nm)	λ_{em} (nm)	Example of use during RGS
Diiodofluorescein	488	515	Moore et al. [134]
I-Methylene blue	670	680	Cundiff et al. [135]
ICG-nanocolloid	780	820	van der Poel et al. [136]
Cherenkov luminescence	na	>200	Spinelli et al. [137]

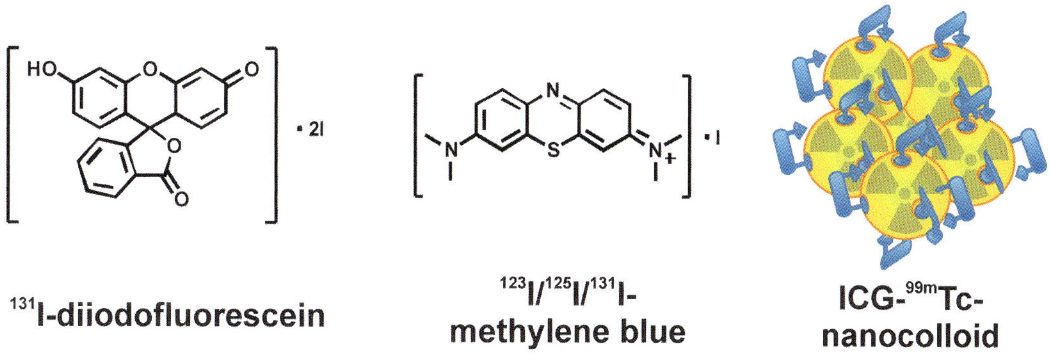

Fig. 5.10 Hybrid imaging tracers applied in RGS

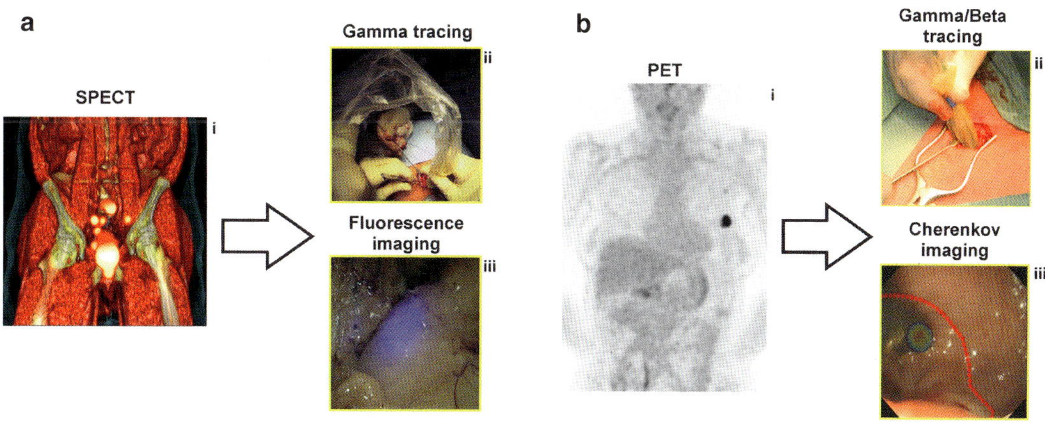

Fig. 5.11 Application of hybrid tracers in RGS. (**a**) Hybrid tracers combining nuclear imaging with fluorescence imaging: (*i*) whole body nuclear imaging; (*ii*) intraoperative tracing with acoustic probe; (*iii*) intraoperative fluorescence imaging. Real-time fluorescence overlaid with white-light image. (**b**) Hybrid imaging based on Cherenkov luminescence emitted by β^+/β^--emitting isotopes: (*i*) whole body nuclear imaging; (*ii*) intraoperative tracing with acoustic probe; (*iii*) intraoperative optical imaging. CL images overlaid with white-light photograph. *With kind permission from Springer Science and Business Media* [139]

magnitude lower than that obtained with fluorescence imaging, but during the decay of the isotope, it provides a continuous spectrum with peak emission in the UV range [140]. The advantage of CL is that no additional label is required next to the β -particle emitting radionuclide and that there is virtually no background signal because no external excitation light is required. However, since the CL intensity is tracer dose dependent, it may negatively influence the dose received by the patient and surgical staff [23]. Furthermore, low signal intensity means long acquisition times and absolute darkness are needed to generate an image and thus real-time guidance is not possible.

The earliest example of a hybrid tracer of the first subclass is ^{131}I-diiodofluorescein (Fig. 5.10), which was reported by Moore et al. in 1948. Fluorescein was already reported for the detection of malignant tissue by UV-light irradiation and visible detection of the fluorescence (λ_{em} = 520 nm) by eye [112]. By radioiodination, this fluorescent tracer could be detected using a Geiger-Müller tube [110, 111]. Both the radiosignal and the fluorescence detection could be used to localize brain lesions [134].

The radioiodinated (^{123}I, ^{125}I, and ^{131}I) derivative of methylene blue (Fig. 5.10), a blue dye commonly used for optical visualization of the lymphatic ducts, has been used for lymphatic mapping and RGS toward SLN(s), which resulted in the successful removal [135, 141–143]. Although methylene blue was shown to possess fluorescence properties [144], these were not exploited within the clinical studies.

For SLN biopsy procedures, the hybrid radioactive and fluorescent tracer indocyanine green (ICG)-^{99m}Tc-nanocolloid was introduced (Fig. 5.10). The tracer was formed via the noncovalent interaction between the near-infrared fluorescent dye ICG and the albumin components of ^{99m}Tc-nanocolloid [6, 136]. An early reproducibility study showed the behavior of the hybrid tracer being identical to its parental compound ^{99m}Tc-nanocolloid [145]. Next to preoperative SLN mapping, intraoperative radioguidance and fluorescence guidance to the SLN(s) were facilitated. The latter allowing the optical verification of the location of the SLN, which was not possible with the parental compound [146, 147]. The addition of real-time fluorescence imaging during the RGS procedure was considered especially valuable during the detection of SLNs close to the injection site of the radiocolloid [148], and enabled optical detection of SLN(s) failed to accumulated the traditionally used blue dye [146].

Cherenkov photons originate from charged particles (β^+/β^-) that travel through a medium faster than the speed of light in that same medium. CL occurs in tissue when the emitted charged particles have energies higher than 0.21 MeV. The intensity of CL is around three orders of magnitude lower than that obtained with fluorescence imaging, but during the decay of the isotope, it provides a continuous spectrum with peak emission in the UV range [140]. The advantage of CL is that no additional label is required next to the β-particle emitting radionuclide and that there is virtually no background signal because no external excitation light is required. However, since the CL intensity is tracer dose dependent, it may negatively influence the dose received by the patient and surgical staff [23]. Furthermore, low signal intensity means long acquisition times and absolute darkness are needed to generate an image and thus real-time guidance is not possible.

For CL imaging, all β^+- and β^--emitters used in clinical practice can potentially be used. This said, the amount of clinical reports on CL imaging is limited. Recently clinical studies with ^{131}I (for thyroid) and ^{18}F-FDG (for various malignancies) have been reported, showing the clinical feasibility of CL imaging [137, 139, 149]. In these studies superficial lesions were visualized through the skin. Technical camera development for CL imaging is moving toward endoscopic use and a laparoscopic camera for CL imaging was recently evaluated in four patients with colorectal cancer [139].

5.5 Future Perspectives

Although this chapter discusses radiotracers that have already been applied for RGS in patients, in principle all clinically used radiotracers can be applied for RGS. This includes also the tracers that are currently investigated for diagnostic imaging purposes, such as ^{18}F-fluorothymidine (^{18}F-FLT; visualizes cell proliferation), ^{18}F- and ^{99m}Tc-annexin V (visualizes cell apoptosis/necrosis), ^{68}Ga-prostate-specific membrane antigen ligand (^{68}Ga-PSMA; visualizes the prostate-specific membrane antigen), ^{99m}Tc-etarfolatide (visualizes epithelial tumor cells), and various antibodies labeled with ^{89}Zr [150–152]. Also in the preclinical field, several promising radio- and hybrid tracers are being developed that might be applicable in RGS and image-guided surgery [153–158]. Although the recent reemergence of image-guided surgery has boosted the preclinical activities regarding tracer development for this application, the "from molecule to man" translation of these activities remains limited.

Interesting recent developments in the choice of radionuclides for RGS are the steps toward the application of β^+- (e.g., ^{18}F and ^{89}Zr) and β^--emitters (^{90}Y) for RGS. Especially the selective detection of the β-particles can potentially improve the resolution in RGS. However, the application of these radionuclides increases the radiation dosages obtained by patients (both β^-- and β^+-emitters) and medical personnel (mainly β^+-emitters). This aspect needs to be resolved in order to implement such RGS procedures in an everyday clinical practice. One suggestion would be to improve the specificity and especially the sensitivity of the imaging modalities, both nuclear and optical, which would allow the application of lower dosages of these radiotracers.

5.6 Concluding Remarks

As can be concluded from the described applications of radioisotopes in RGS, the most used radioisotopes are ^{99m}Tc (radiocolloids and ^{99m}Tc-sestamibi), ^{111}In (^{111}In-somatostatin analogues), and ^{125}I (^{125}I-MIBG and ^{125}I-labeled antibodies). This originates mainly from their easy availability, their preferred medium to low-energy photon emission, and their ease of incorporation into radiotracers. Interesting new developments are focusing on surgical guidance toward β-emitters and the inclusion of optical guidance methods. A critical point in the development of new RGS procedures and the use of certain radionuclides is the radiation exposure of the surgical staff. Especially the need for isotopes with high-energy emissions may limit the clinical application due to restrictions in the radiation exposure of the medical personnel.

Acknowledgments This work was financially supported by a Netherlands Organisation for Scientific Research VIDI grant (NWO; STW BGT 11272).

References

1. Brouwer OR, Buckle T, Bunschoten A, Kuil J, Vahrmeijer AL, Wendler T, Valdes-Olmos RA, van der Poel HG, van Leeuwen FWB. Image navigation as a means to expand the boundaries of fluorescence-guided surgery. Phys Med Biol. 2012;57(10): 3123–36.
2. Uren RF. Lymphatic drainage of the skin. Ann Surg Oncol. 2004;11(3 Suppl):179S–85.
3. Ege GN. Internal mammary lymphoscintigraphy. The rationale, technique, interpretation and clinical application: a review based on 848 cases. Radiology. 1976;118(1):101–7.
4. Henze E, Schelbert HR, Collins JD, Najafi A, Barrio JR, Bennett LR. Lymphoscintigraphy with Tc-99m-labeled dextran. J Nucl Med. 1982;23(10):923–9.
5. Sarin H. Physiologic upper limits of pore size of different blood capillary types and another perspective on the dual pore theory of microvascular permeability. J Angiogenes Res. 2010;2:14.
6. van Leeuwen AC, Buckle T, Bendle G, Vermeeren L, Valdes Olmos R, van der Poel HG, van Leeuwen FWB. Tracer-cocktail injections for combined pre- and intraoperative multimodal imaging of lymph nodes in a spontaneous mouse prostate tumor model. J Biomed Opt. 2011;16(1):016004.
7. Mariani G, Erba P, Villa G, Gipponi M, Manca G, Boni G, Buffoni F, Castagnola F, Paganelli G, Strauss HW. Lymphoscintigraphic and intraoperative detection of the sentinel lymph node in breast cancer patients: the nuclear medicine perspective. J Surg Oncol. 2004;85(3):112–22.
8. Van den Berg NS, Buckle T, Kleinjan GI, Klop WM, Horenblas S, Van Der Poel HG, Valdes-Olmos RA, Van Leeuwen FI. Hybrid tracers for sentinel node biopsy. Q J Nucl Med Mol Imaging. 2014;58(2):193–206.
9. Pouw B, de Wit-van der Veen LJ, Stokkel MP, Loo CE, Vrancken Peeters MJ, Valdes Olmos RA. Heading toward radioactive seed localization in non-palpable breast cancer surgery? A meta-analysis. J Surg Oncol. 2015;111(2):185–91.
10. Thind CR, Tan S, Desmond S, Harris O, Ramesh HS, Chagla L, Ray A, Audisio R, SNOLL. Sentinel node and occult (impalpable) lesion localization in breast cancer. Clin Radiol. 2011;66(9):833–9.
11. Lavoue V, Nos C, Clough KB, Baghaie F, Zerbib E, Poulet B, Lefrere Belda MA, Ducellier A, Lecuru F. Simplified technique of radioguided occult lesion localization (ROLL) plus sentinel lymph node biopsy (SNOLL) in breast carcinoma. Ann Surg Oncol. 2008;15(9):2556–61.
12. Heij HA, Rutgers EJ, de Kraker J, Vos A. Intraoperative search for neuroblastoma by MIBG and radioguided surgery with the gamma detector. Med Pediatr Oncol. 1997;28(3):171–4.
13. Arbizu J, Rodriguez-Fraile M, Dominguez-Prado I, Garrastachu P, Rotellar F, Sangro B, Richter JA. Whole body 18fluoro-L-dopa PET-CT: a useful tool for location and surgical guidance in primary carcinoid tumours. Eur J Nucl Med Mol Imaging. 2008;35(8):1577.
14. Desai DC, Arnold M, Saha S, Hinkle G, Soble D, Fry J, DePalatis LR, Mantil J, Satter M, Martin Jr EW. Correlative whole-body FDG-PET and intraoperative gamma detection of FDG distribution in colorectal cancer. Clin Positron Imaging. 2000;3(5): 189–96.
15. Krag DN, Ford PV, Patel M, Schneider PD, Goodnight Jr JE. A simplified technique to resect abnormal bony radiolocalizations using a gamma counter. Surg Oncol. 1992;1(5):371–7.
16. Martin DT, Hinkle GH, Tuttle S, Olsen J, Nabi H, Houchens D, Thurston M, Martin Jr EW. Intraoperative radioimmunodetection of colorectal tumors with a hand-held radiation detector. Am J Surg. 1985;150: 672–5.
17. Agnese DM, Abdessalam SF, Burak Jr WE, Arnold MW, Soble D, Hinkle GH, Young D, Khazaeli

MB, Martin Jr EW. Pilot study using a humanized CC49 monoclonal antibody (HuCC49DeltaCH2) to localize recurrent colorectal carcinoma. Ann Surg Oncol. 2004;11(2):197–202.
18. Nieroda CA, Milenic DE, Colcher D, Schlom J. Monoclonal antibodies for use in radioimmunoguided surgery (RIGS). In: Martin Jr EW, editor. Radioimmunoguided surgery (RIGS) in the detection of colorectal cancer. Austin: R. G. Landes Company; 1994. p. 7–27.
19. de Labriolle-Vaylet C, Cattan P, Sarfati E, Wioland M, Billotey C, Brocheriou C, Rouvier E, de Roquancourt A, Rostene W, Askienazy S, Barbet J, Milhaud G, Gruaz-Guyon A. Successful surgical removal of occult metastases of medullary thyroid carcinoma recurrences with the help of immunoscintigraphy and radioimmunoguided surgery. Clin Cancer Res. 2000;6(2):363–71.
20. Sharkey RM, Chang CH, Rossi EA, McBride WJ, Goldenberg DM. Pretargeting: taking an alternate route for localizing radionuclides. Tumour Biol. 2012;33(3):591–600.
21. Nelson AL. Antibody fragments: hope and hype. MAbs. 2010;2(1):77–83.
22. van Leeuwen FWB, Hardwick JC, van Erkel AR. Luminescence-based imaging approaches in the field of interventional (molecular) imaging. Radiology. 2015;276(1):12–29.
23. Chin PTK, Welling MM, Meskers SC, Valdes Olmos RA, Tanke H, van Leeuwen FWB. Optical imaging as an expansion of nuclear medicine: Cerenkov-based luminescence vs fluorescence-based luminescence. Eur J Nucl Med Mol Imaging. 2013;40(8):1283–91.
24. Selverstone B, Sweet WH, Robinson CV. The clinical use of radioactive phosphorus in the surgery of brain tumors. Ann Surg. 1949;130(4):643–51.
25. Woolfenden JM, Nevin WS, Barber HB, Donahue DJ. Lung cancer detection using a miniature sodium iodide detector and cobalt-57 bleomycin. Chest. 1984;85(1):84–8.
26. Schattner A, Cohen A, Wolfson L, Melloul M. Unexplained systemic symptoms and Gallium-67 – guided decisions. Am J Med Sci. 2001;321(3):198–200.
27. Kaemmerer D, Prasad V, Daffner W, Haugvik SP, Senftleben S, Baum RP, Hommann M. Radioguided surgery in neuroendocrine tumors using Ga-68-labeled somatostatin analogs: a pilot study. Clin Nucl Med. 2012;37(2):142–7.
28. Heuveling DA, van Schie A, Vugts DJ, Hendrikse NH, Yaqub M, Hoekstra OS, Karagozoglu KH, Leemans CR, van Dongen GA, de Bree R. Pilot study on the feasibility of PET/CT lymphoscintigraphy with 89Zr-nanocolloidal albumin for sentinel node identification in oral cancer patients. J Nucl Med. 2013;54(4):585–9.
29. Collamati F, Pepe A, Bellini F, Bocci V, Chiodi G, Cremonesi M, De Lucia E, Ferrari ME, Frallicciardi PM, Grana CM, Marafini M, Mattei I, Morganti S, Patera V, Piersanti L, Recchia L, Russomando A, Sarti A, Sciubba A, Senzacqua M, Camillocci ES, Voena C, Pinci D, Faccini R. Toward radioguided surgery with beta(−) decays: uptake of a somatostatin analogue, DOTATOC, in meningioma and high-grade glioma. J Nucl Med. 2015;56(1):3–8.
30. Gommans GM, Gommans E, van der Zant FM, Teule GJ, van der Schors TG, de Waard JW. 99mTc Nanocoll: a radiopharmaceutical for sentinel node localisation in breast cancer – in vitro and in vivo results. Appl Radiat Isot. 2009;67(9):1550–8.
31. Panareo S, Carcoforo P, Lanzara S, Corcione S, Bagatin E, Casali M, Costanzo A, Basaglia E, Feggi LM. Radiolabelled somatostatin analogs for diagnosis and radio-guided surgery of neuroendocrine breast cancer undetectable with conventional imaging procedures. Breast. 2008;17(1):111–4.
32. Gallowitsch HJ, Fellinger J, Mikosch P, Kresnik E, Lind P. Gamma probe-guided resection of a lymph node metastasis with I-123 in papillary thyroid carcinoma. Clin Nucl Med. 1997;22(9):591–2.
33. Strong VE, Humm J, Russo P, Jungbluth A, Wong WD, Daghighian F, Old L, Fong Y, Larson SM. A novel method to localize antibody-targeted cancer deposits intraoperatively using handheld PET beta and gamma probes. Surg Endosc. 2008;22(2):386–91.
34. Hinkle GH, Laven DL. Radionuclides. In: Martin Jr EW, editor. Radioimmunoguided Surgery (RIGS) in the detection and treatment of colorectal cancer. Austin: R. G. Landes Company; 1994. p. 29–39.
35. Jager W, Feistel H, Paterok EM, Ronay G, Tulusan AH, Wolf F, Lang N. Resection guided by antibodies (REGAJ): a diagnostic procedure during second-look operation in ovarian cancer patients. Br J Cancer Suppl. 1990;10:18–20.
36. Ubhi CS, Hardy JG, Pegg CA. Mediastinal parathyroid adenoma: a new method of localization. Br J Surg. 1984;71(11):859–60.
37. Bartholoma MD, Louie AS, Valliant JF, Zubieta J. Technetium and gallium derived radiopharmaceuticals: comparing and contrasting the chemistry of two important radiometals for the molecular imaging era. Chem Rev. 2010;110(5):2903–20.
38. Dewanjee MK. The chemistry of 99mTc-labeled radiopharmaceuticals. Semin Nucl Med. 1990;20(1):5–27.
39. Hetrakul N, Civelek AC, Stagg CA, Udelsman R. In vitro accumulation of technetium-99m-sestamibi in human parathyroid mitochondria. Surgery. 2001;130(6):1011–8.
40. Nazari B, Azizmohammadi Z, Rajaei M, Karami M, Javadi H, Assadi M, Asli IN. Role of 99mTc-ubiquicidin 29–41 scintigraphy to monitor antibiotic therapy in patients with orthopedic infection: a preliminary study. Nucl Med Commun. 2011;32(8):745–51.
41. Eshima D, Eshima LA, Gotti NM, Herda SC, Algozine CA, Burris TG, Vansant JP, Alazraki NP, Taylor AT. Technetium-99m-sulfur colloid for lymphoscintigraphy: effects of preparation parameters. J Nucl Med. 1996;37(9):1575–8.

42. Vera DR, Wallace AM, Hoh CK, Mattrey RF. A synthetic macromolecule for sentinel node detection: (99m)Tc-DTPA-mannosyl-dextran. J Nucl Med. 2001;42(6):951–9.
43. Hubalewska-Dydejczyk A, Kulig J, Szybinski P, Mikolajczak R, Pach D, Sowa-Staszczak A, Fross-Baron K, Huszno B. Radio-guided surgery with the use of [99mTc-EDDA/HYNIC]octreotate in intra-operative detection of neuroendocrine tumours of the gastrointestinal tract. Eur J Nucl Med Mol Imaging. 2007;34(10):1545–55.
44. Linehan DC, Hill AD, Tran KN, Yeung H, Yeh SD, Borgen PI, Cody 3rd HS. Sentinel lymph node biopsy in breast cancer: unfiltered radioisotope is superior to filtered. J Am Coll Surg. 1999;188(4):377–81.
45. Higashi H, Natsugoe S, Uenosono Y, Ehi K, Arigami T, Nakabeppu Y, Nakajo M, Aikou T. Particle size of tin and phytate colloid in sentinel node identification. J Surg Res. 2004;121(1):1–4.
46. Tsopelas C. Particle size analysis of (99m)Tc-labeled and unlabeled antimony trisulfide and rhenium sulfide colloids intended for lymphoscintigraphic application. J Nucl Med. 2001;42(3):460–6.
47. Hodgson N, Zabel P, Mattar AG, Engel CJ, Girvan D, Holliday R. A new radiocolloid for sentinel node detection in breast cancer. Ann Surg Oncol. 2001; 8(2):133–7.
48. Lombardi A, Nigri G, Scopinaro F, Maggi S, Mattei M, Bonifacino A, Parisella M, Soluri A, Amanti C. High-resolution, handheld camera use for occult breast lesion localization plus sentinel node biopsy (SNOLL): A single-institution experience with 186 patients. Surgeon. 2015;13(2):69–72.
49. Mirzaei S, Rodrigues M, Hoffmann B, Knoll P, Riegler-Keil M, Kreuzer W, Salzer H, Kohn H, Polyak A, Janoki GA. Sentinel lymph node detection with large human serum albumin colloid particles in breast cancer. Eur J Nucl Med Mol Imaging. 2003;30(6):874–8.
50. Jeschke S, Beri A, Grull M, Ziegerhofer J, Prammer P, Leeb K, Sega W, Janetschek G. Laparoscopic radioisotope-guided sentinel lymph node dissection in staging of prostate cancer. Eur Urol. 2008;53(1):126–32.
51. Reasbeck PG, Manktelow A, McArthur AM, Packer SG, Berkeley BB. An evaluation of pelvic lymphoscintigraphy in the staging of colorectal carcinoma. Br J Surg. 1984;71(12):936–40.
52. Xavier NL, Amaral BB, Cerski CT, Fuchs SC, Spiro BL, Oliveira OL, Menke CH, Biazus JV, Cavalheiro JA, Schwartsmann G. Sentinel lymph node identification and sampling in women with early breast cancer using 99m Tc labelled dextran 500 and patent blue V dye. Nucl Med Commun. 2001;22(10):1109–17.
53. Marcinow AM, Hall N, Byrum E, Teknos TN, Old MO, Agrawal A. Use of a novel receptor-targeted (CD206) radiotracer, 99mTc-tilmanocept, and SPECT/CT for sentinel lymph node detection in oral cavity squamous cell carcinoma: initial institutional report in an ongoing phase 3 study. JAMA Otolaryngol Head Neck Surg. 2013;139(9):895–902.
54. Sondak VK, King DW, Zager JS, Schneebaum S, Kim J, Leong SP, Faries MB, Averbook BJ, Martinez SR, Puleo CA, Messina JL, Christman L, Wallace AM. Combined analysis of phase III trials evaluating [(9)(9)mTc]tilmanocept and vital blue dye for identification of sentinel lymph nodes in clinically node-negative cutaneous melanoma. Ann Surg Oncol. 2013;20(2):680–8.
55. Wallace AM, Han LK, Povoski SP, Deck K, Schneebaum S, Hall NC, Hoh CK, Limmer KK, Krontiras H, Frazier TG, Cox C, Avisar E, Faries M, King DW, Christman L, Vera DR. Comparative evaluation of [(99m)tc]tilmanocept for sentinel lymph node mapping in breast cancer patients: results of two phase 3 trials. Ann Surg Oncol. 2013;20(8):2590–9.
56. Aras G, Gultekin SS, Kucuk NO, Demirer S, Tug T. Intraoperative gamma probe guidance with 99mTc-pertechnetate in the completion thyroidectomy. Ann Nucl Med. 2009;23(5):421–6.
57. Mandalapu BP, Amato M, Stratmann HG. Technetium Tc 99m sestamibi myocardial perfusion imaging: current role for evaluation of prognosis. Chest. 1999; 115(6):1684–94.
58. Duarte GM, Cabello C, Torresan RZ, Alvarenga M, Telles GH, Bianchessi ST, Caserta N, Segala SR, de Lima MC, Etchebehere EC, Camargo EE. Radioguided Intraoperative Margins Evaluation (RIME): preliminary results of a new technique to aid breast cancer resection. Eur J Surg Oncol. 2007;33(10):1150–7.
59. Vilela Filho O, Carneiro Filho O. Gamma probe-assisted brain tumor microsurgical resection: a new technique. Arq Neuropsiquiatr. 2002;60:1042–7.
60. Martinez DA, King DR, Romshe C, Lozano RA, Morris JD, O'Dorisio MS, Martin Jr EW. Intraoperative identification of parathyroid gland pathology: a new approach. J Pediatr Surg. 1995;30(9):1306–9.
61. Placzkowski K, Christian R, Chen H. Radioguided parathyroidectomy for recurrent parathyroid cancer. Clin Nucl Med. 2007;32(5):358–60.
62. Ikeda Y, Takayama J, Takami H. Minimally invasive radioguided parathyroidectomy for hyperparathyroidism. Ann Nucl Med. 2010;24(4):233–40.
63. Garcia-Talavera P, Gonzalez-Selma ML, Ruiz M, Gamazo C, Sainz-Esteban A, Villanueva JG, Olmos R. The value of early SPECT/CT and hand-held gamma-camera in radio-guided surgery: a case of a hard-to-locate parathyroid adenoma. Clin Nucl Med. 2014;39(11):1009–11.
64. Mariani G, Gulec SA, Rubello D, Boni G, Puccini M, Pelizzo MR, Manca G, Casara D, Sotti G, Erba P, Volterrani D, Giuliano AE. Preoperative localization and radioguided parathyroid surgery. J Nucl Med. 2003;44(9):1443–58.
65. Al-Saeedi F. Role of 99mTc-(V)DMSA in detecting tumor cell proliferation. Anal Chem Insights. 2007; 2:81–3.
66. Adams S, Acker P, Lorenz M, Staib-Sebler E, Hor G. Radioisotope-guided surgery in patients with pheochromocytoma and recurrent medullary thyroid

carcinoma: a comparison of preoperative and intraoperative tumor localization with histopathologic findings. Cancer. 2001;92(2):263–70.
67. Povoski SP, Neff RL, Mojzisik CM, O'Malley DM, Hinkle GH, Hall NC, Murrey Jr DA, Knopp MV, Martin Jr EW. A comprehensive overview of radioguided surgery using gamma detection probe technology. World J Surg Oncol. 2009;7:11.
68. Robinson LA, Preksto D, Muro-Cacho C, Hubbell DS. Intraoperative gamma probe-directed biopsy of asymptomatic suspected bone metastases. Ann Thorac Surg. 1998;65(5):1426–32.
69. Axelsson CK, Nielsen BP, Graff J. Radioisotope-guided surgical biopsy of costal metastases in breast cancer patients. Scand J Surg. 2002;91(4):333–5.
70. von Meyenfeldt EM, Siebenga J, van der Pol HA, Schreurs WM, Hulsewe KW. Radionuclide-guided biopsy of bone lesions in cancer patients; a reliable, well-tolerated technique. Eur J Surg Oncol. 2014; 40(2):193–6.
71. Ind TE, Granowska M, Britton KE, Morris G, Lowe DG, Hudson CN, Shepherd JH. Peroperative radioimmunodetection of ovarian carcinoma using a hand-held gamma detection probe. Br J Cancer. 1994;70(6):1263–6.
72. Hladik P, Vizda J, Bedrna J, Simkovic D, Strnad L, Smejkal K, Voboril Z. Immunoscintigraphy and intraoperative radioimmunodetection in the treatment of colorectal carcinoma. Colorectal Dis. 2001;3(6):380–6.
73. Mansi L, Di Lieto E, Rambaldi PF, Bergaminelli C, Fallanca F, Vicidomini G, Cuccurullo V, Mancusi R. Preliminary experience with radioimmuno-guided surgery of primary neoplasms of the lung. Minerva Chir. 1998;53(5):369–72.
74. Mansi L, Rambaldi PF, Panza N, Esposito D, Esposito V, Pastore V. Diagnosis and radioguided surgery with 111In-pentetreotide in a patient with paraneoplastic Cushing's syndrome due to a bronchial carcinoid. Eur J Endocrinol. 1997;137(6):688–90.
75. Ohrvall U, Westlin JE, Nilsson S, Juhlin C, Rastad J, Lundqvist H, Akerstrom G. Intraoperative gamma detection reveals abdominal endocrine tumors more efficiently than somatostatin receptor scintigraphy. Cancer. 1997;80(12 Suppl):2490–4.
76. Adams S, Baum RP, Hertel A, Wenisch HJ, Staib-Sebler E, Herrmann G, Encke A, Hor G. Intraoperative gamma probe detection of neuroendocrine tumors. J Nucl Med. 1998;39(7):1155–60.
77. Grossrubatscher E, Vignati F, Dalino P, Possa M, Belloni PA, Vanzulli A, Bramerio M, Marocchi A, Rossetti O, Zurleni F, Loli P. Use of radioguided surgery with [111In]-pentetreotide in the management of an ACTH-secreting bronchial carcinoid causing ectopic Cushing's syndrome. J Endocrinol Invest. 2005;28(1):72–8.
78. Gay E, Vuillez JP, Palombi O, Brard PY, Bessou P, Passagia JG. Intraoperative and postoperative gamma detection of somatostatin receptors in bone-invasive en plaque meningiomas. Neurosurgery. 2005;57(1 Suppl):107–13; discussion 107–13.
79. Krag DN, Haseman MK, Ford P, Smith L, Taylor MH, Schneider P, Goodnight JE. Gamma probe location of 111indium-labeled B72.3: an extension of immunoscintigraphy. J Surg Oncol. 1992;51(4):226–30.
80. Muxi A, Pons F, Vidal-Sicart S, Setoain FJ, Herranz R, Novell F, Fernandez RM, Trias M, Setoain J. Radioimmunoguided surgery of colorectal carcinoma with an 111In-labelled anti-TAG72 monoclonal antibody. Nucl Med Commun. 1999;20(2):123–30.
81. Anderson RS, Eifert B, Tartt S, King P. Radioimmunoguided surgery using indium-111 capromab pendetide (PROSTASCINT) to diagnose supraclavicular metastasis from prostate cancer. Urology. 2000;56(4):669.
82. Le Doussal JM, Gruaz-Guyon A, Martin M, Gautherot E, Delaage M, Barbet J. Targeting of indium 111-labeled bivalent hapten to human melanoma mediated by bispecific monoclonal antibody conjugates: imaging of tumors hosted in nude mice. Cancer Res. 1990;50(11):3445–52.
83. Eckelman WC, Rzeszotarski WJ, Siegel BA, Kubota H, Chelliah M, Stevenson J, Reba RC. Chemical and biological properties of isolated radiolabeled bleomycin preparations. J Nucl Med. 1975;16(11):1033–7.
84. Lavender JP, Lowe J, Barker JR, Burn JI, Chaudhri MA. Gallium 67 citrate scanning in neoplastic and inflammatory lesions. Br J Radiol. 1971;44:361–6.
85. Weiner R. The role of transferrin and other receptors in the mechanism of 67Ga localization. Int J Rad Appl Instrum, Part B, Nucl Med Biol. 1990;17(1):141–9.
86. Wilbur DS. Radiohalogenation of proteins: an overview of radionuclides, labeling methods, and reagents for conjugate labeling. Bioconjum Chem. 1992;3(6):433–70.
87. Sugiura G, Kuhn H, Sauter M, Haberkorn U, Mier W. Radiolabeling strategies for tumor-targeting proteinaceous drugs. Molecules. 2014;19(2):2135–65.
88. Bourdoiseau M. Iodine radiochemistry and radiopharmaceutical product labeling. Int J Rad Appl Instrum B, Nucl Med Biol. 1986;13(2):83–8.
89. Rossouw DD, Macheli L. Large-scale synthesis of no-carrier-added [123I]mIBG, using two different stannylated precursors. J Label Compd Radiopharm. 2009;52:499–503.
90. Shimotake T, Tsuda T, Aoi S, Fumino S, Iwai N. Iodine 123 metaiodobenzylguanidine radio-guided navigation surgery for recurrent medullary thyroid carcinoma in a girl with multiple endocrine neoplasia type 2B. J Pediatr Surg. 2005;40(10):1643–6.
91. Martelli H, Ricard M, Larroquet M, Wioland M, Paraf F, Fabre M, Josset P, Helardot PG, Gauthier F, Terrier-Lacombe MJ, Michon J, Hartmann O, Tabone MD, Patte C, Lumbroso J, Gruner M. Intraoperative localization of neuroblastoma in children with 123I- or 125I-radiolabeled metaiodobenzylguanidine. Surgery. 1998;123(1):51–7.
92. Einspieler I, Novotny A, Okur A, Essler M, Martignoni ME. First experience with image-guided resection of paraganglioma. Clin Nucl Med. 2014; 39(8):e379–81.

93. Ricard M, Tenenbaum F, Schlumberger M, Travagli JP, Lumbroso J, Revillon Y, Parmentier C. Intraoperative detection of pheochromocytoma with iodine-125 labelled meta-iodobenzylguanidine: a feasibility study. Eur J Nucl Med. 1993; 20(5):426–30.
94. Cuntz MC, Levine EA, O'Dorisio TM, Watson JC, Wray DA, Espenan GD, McKnight C, Meier JR, Weber LJ, Mera R, O'Dorisio MS, Woltering EA. Intraoperative gamma detection of 125I-lanreotide in women with primary breast cancer. Ann Surg Oncol. 1999;6(4):367–72.
95. Woltering EA, Barrie R, O'Dorisio TM, O'Dorisio MS, Nance R, Cook DM. Detection of occult gastrinomas with iodine 125-labeled lanreotide and intraoperative gamma detection. Surgery. 1994; 116(6):1139–46; discussion 1146–37.
96. Schirmer WJ, O'Dorisio TM, Schirmer TP, Mojzisik CM, Hinkle GH, Martin Jr EW. Intraoperative localization of neuroendocrine tumors with 125I-TYR(3)-octreotide and a hand-held gamma-detecting probe. Surgery. 1993;114(4):745–51; discussion 751–42.
97. Dawson PM, Blair SD, Begent RH, Kelly AM, Boxer GM, Theodorou NA. The value of radioimmunoguided surgery in first and second look laparotomy for colorectal cancer. Dis Colon Rectum. 1991; 34(3):217–22.
98. Gu J, Zhao J, Li Z, Yang Z, Zhang J, Gao Z, Wang Y, Xu G. Clinical application of radioimmunoguided surgery in colorectal cancer using 125I-labeled carcinoembryonic antigen-specific monoclonal antibody submucosally. Dis Colon Rectum. 2003; 46(12):1659–66.
99. Percivale P, Bertoglio S, Meszaros P, Canavese G, Cafiero F, Gipponi M, Campora E, Gasco M, Badellino F. Radioimmunoguided surgery after primary treatment of locally advanced breast cancer. J Clin Oncol. 1996;14(5):1599–603.
100. Percivale P, Bertoglio S, Meszaros P, Schenone F, Gipponi M, Moresco L, Cosso M, Badellino F. Radioimmunoguided surgery with different iodine-125 radiolabeled monoclonal antibodies in recurrent colorectal cancer. Semin Surg Oncol. 1998;15(4): 231–4.
101. Martin Jr EW, Tuttle SE, Rousseau M, Mojzisik CM, O'Dwyer PJ, Hinkle GH, Miller EA, Goodwin RA, Oredipe OA, Barth RF, et al. Radioimmunoguided surgery: intraoperative use of monoclonal antibody 17-1A in colorectal cancer. Hybridoma. 1986;5 Suppl 1:S97–108.
102. Nieroda CA, Mojzisik C, Hinkle G, Thurston MO, Martin Jr EW. Radioimmunoguided surgery (RIGS) in recurrent colorectal cancer. Cancer Detect Prev. 1991;15(3):225–9.
103. O'Dwyer PJ, Mojzisik CM, Hinkle GH, Rousseau M, Olsen J, Tuttle SE, Barth RF, Thurston MO, McCabe DP, Farrar WB, et al. Intraoperative probe-directed immunodetection using a monoclonal antibody. Arch Surg. 1986;121(12):1391–4.
104. Wang C, Wang Y, Su X, Lin B, Xu X, Zhang M, Li J, Xu G. [Iodine-125 labeled monoclonal antibody 3H11: in radioimmunoguided surgery for primary gastric cancer]. Zhonghua Wai Ke Za Zhi [Chinese Journal of Surgery]. 2000;38(7):507–9.
105. Gray RJ, Giuliano R, Dauway EL, Cox CE, Reintgen DS. Radioguidance for nonpalpable primary lesions and sentinel lymph node(s). Am J Surg. 2001;182(4): 404–6.
106. van Riet YE, Maaskant AJ, Creemers GJ, van Warmerdam LJ, Jansen FH, van de Velde CJ, Rutten HJ, Nieuwenhuijzen GA. Identification of residual breast tumour localization after neo-adjuvant chemotherapy using a radioactive 125 Iodine seed. Eur J Surg Oncol. 2010;36(2):164–9.
107. Alderliesten T, Loo CE, Pengel KE, Rutgers EJ, Gilhuijs KG, Vrancken Peeters MJ. Radioactive seed localization of breast lesions: an adequate localization method without seed migration. Breast J. 2011;17(6):594–601.
108. Donker M, Drukker CA, Valdes Olmos RA, Rutgers EJ, Loo CE, Sonke GS, Wesseling J, Alderliesten T, Vrancken Peeters MJ. Guiding breast-conserving surgery in patients after neoadjuvant systemic therapy for breast cancer: a comparison of radioactive seed localization with the ROLL technique. Ann Surg Oncol. 2013;20(8):2569–75.
109. Hughes JH, Mason MC, Gray RJ, McLaughlin SA, Degnim AC, Fulmer JT, Pockaj BA, Karstaedt PJ, Roarke MC. A multi-site validation trial of radioactive seed localization as an alternative to wire localization. Breast J. 2008;14(2):153–7.
110. Moore GE. Use of radioactive diiodofluorescein in the diagnosis and localization of brain tumors. Science. 1948;107:569–71.
111. Ashkenazy M, Davis L, Martin J. An evaluation of the technic and results of the radioactive di-iodofluorescein test for the localization of intracranial lesions. J Neurosurg. 1951;8(3):300–14.
112. Moore GE. Fluorescein as an agent in the differentiation of normal and malignant tissues. Science. 1947;106(2745):130–1.
113. Morris Jr AC, Barclay TR, Tanida R, Nemcek JV. A miniaturized probe for detecting radioactivity at thyroid surgery. Phys Med Biol. 1971;16(3):397–404.
114. Scurry WC, Lamarre E, Stack B. Radioguided neck dissection in recurrent metastatic papillary thyroid carcinoma. Am J Otolaryngol. 2006;27(1):61–3.
115. Rubello D, Salvatori M, Ardito G, Mariani G, Al-Nahhas A, Gross MD, Muzzio PC, Pelizzo MR. Iodine-131 radio-guided surgery in differentiated thyroid cancer: outcome on 31 patients and review of the literature. Biomed Pharmacother. 2007;61(8):477–81.
116. Fasshauer H, Freundlieb O, Dostal G, Littmann K, Tharandt L, Strotges MW. Intraoperative localization of pheochromocytoma metastases using 131I-metabenzylguanidine. Nuklearmedizin. 1984;23(4):203–5.
117. Aitken DR, Hinkle GH, Thurston MO, Tuttle SE, Martin DT, Olsen J, Haagensen Jr DE, Houchens D, Martin Jr EW. A gamma-detecting probe for

radioimmune detection of CEA-producing tumors. Successful experimental use and clinical case report. Dis Colon Rectum. 1984;27(5):279–82.
118. Xu G, Zhang M, Liu B, Li Z, Lin B, Xu X, Jin M, Li J, Wu J, Dong Z. Radioimmunoguided surgery in gastric cancer using 131-I labeled monoclonal antibody 3H11. Semin Surg Oncol. 1994;10:88–94.
119. Sanchez-Crespo A, Andreo P, Larsson SA. Positron flight in human tissues and its influence on PET image spatial resolution. Eur J Nucl Med Mol Imaging. 2004;31(1):44–51.
120. Zervos EE, Desai DC, DePalatis LR, Soble D, Martin Jr EW. 18F-labeled fluorodeoxyglucose positron emission tomography-guided surgery for recurrent colorectal cancer: a feasibility study. J Surg Res. 2001;97(1):9–13.
121. Jacobson O, Kiesewetter DO, Chen X. Fluorine-18 radiochemistry, labeling strategies and synthetic routes. Bioconjug Chem. 2015;26(1):1–18.
122. Laverman P, McBride WJ, Sharkey RM, Eek A, Joosten L, Oyen WJ, Goldenberg DM, Boerman OC. A novel facile method of labeling octreotide with (18)F-fluorine. J Nucl Med. 2010;51(3):454–61.
123. Gulec SA, Hoenie E, Hostetter R, Schwartzentruber D. PET probe-guided surgery: applications and clinical protocol. World J Surg Oncol. 2007;5:65.
124. Vos CG, Hartemink KJ, Muller S, Oosterhuis JW, Meijer S, van den Tol MP, Comans EF. Clinical applications of FDG-probe guided surgery. Acta Chir Belg. 2012;112(6):414–8.
125. Kraeber-Bodere F, Cariou B, Curtet C, Bridji B, Rousseau C, Dravet F, Charbonnel B, Carnaille B, Le Neel JC, Mirallie E. Feasibility and benefit of fluorine 18-fluoro-2-deoxyglucose-guided surgery in the management of radioiodine-negative differentiated thyroid carcinoma metastases. Surgery. 2005;138(6):1176–82; discussion 1182.
126. Wadas TJ, Wong EH, Weisman GR, Anderson CJ. Coordinating radiometals of copper, gallium, indium, yttrium, and zirconium for PET and SPECT imaging of disease. Chem Rev. 2010;110(5):2858–902.
127. Notni J, Pohle K, Wester HJ. Comparative gallium-68 labeling of TRAP-, NOTA-, and DOTA-peptides: practical consequences for the future of gallium-68-PET. EJNMMI Res. 2012;2(1):28.
128. Clark WA, Izotova L, Philipova D, Wu W, Lin L, Pestka S. Site-specific 32P-labeling of cytokines, monoclonal antibodies, and other protein substrates for quantitative assays and therapeutic application. Bio Tech. 2002;Suppl:76–8, 80–77.
129. Randerath K, Randerath E. 32P-postlabeling methods for DNA adduct detection: overview and critical evaluation. Drug Metab Rev. 1994;26(1–2):67–85.
130. Chakravarty R, Pandey U, Manolkar RB, Dash A, Venkatesh M, Pillai MR. Development of an electrochemical 90 Sr-90 Y generator for separation of 90 Y suitable for targeted therapy. Nucl Med Biol. 2008;35(2):245–53.
131. Minarik D, Sjogreen-Gleisner K, Linden O, Wingardh K, Tennvall J, Strand SE, Ljungberg M. 90Y Bremsstrahlung imaging for absorbed-dose assessment in high-dose radioimmunotherapy. J Nucl Med. 2010;51(12):1974–8.
132. Selwyn RG, Nickles RJ, Thomadsen BR, DeWerd LA, Micka JA. A new internal pair production branching ratio of 90Y: the development of a non-destructive assay for 90Y and 90Sr. Appl Radiat Isot. 2007;65(3):318–27.
133. Lhommel R, Goffette P, Van den Eynde M, Jamar F, Pauwels S, Bilbao JI, Walrand S. Yttrium-90 TOF PET scan demonstrates high-resolution biodistribution after liver SIRT. Eur J Nucl Med Mol Imaging. 2009;36(10):1696.
134. Moore GE, Peyton WT, et al. The clinical use of sodium fluorescein and radioactive diiodofluorescein in the localization of tumors of the central nervous system. Minn Med. 1948;31(10):1073–6.
135. Cundiff JD, Wang YZ, Espenan G, Maloney T, Camp A, Lazarus L, Stolier A, Brooks R, Torrance B, Stafford S, O'Leary JP, Woltering EA. A phase I/II trial of 125I methylene blue for one-stage sentinel lymph node biopsy. Ann Surg. 2007;245(2):290–6.
136. van der Poel HG, Buckle T, Brouwer OR, Valdes Olmos RA, van Leeuwen FWB. Intraoperative laparoscopic fluorescence guidance to the sentinel lymph node in prostate cancer patients: clinical proof of concept of an integrated functional imaging approach using a multimodal tracer. Eur Urol. 2011;60:826–33.
137. Spinelli AE, Ferdeghini M, Cavedon C, Zivelonghi E, Calandrino R, Fenzi A, Sbarbati A, Boschi F. First human Cerenkography. J Biomed Opt. 2013;18(2):20502.
138. Chin PTK, Beekman CAC, Buckle T, Josephson L, van Leeuwen FWB. Multispectral visualization of surgical safety-margins using fluorescent marker seeds. Am J Nucl Med Mol Imaging. 2012;2(2):151–62.
139. Hu H, Cao X, Kang F, Wang M, Lin Y, Liu M, Li S, Yao L, Liang J, Liang J, Nie Y, Chen X, Wang J, Wu K. Feasibility study of novel endoscopic Cerenkov luminescence imaging system in detecting and quantifying gastrointestinal disease: first human results. Eur Radiol. 2015;25(6):1814–22.
140. Mitchell GS, Gill RK, Boucher DL, Li C, Cherry SR. In vivo Cerenkov luminescence imaging: a new tool for molecular imaging. Philos Trans A Math Phys Eng Sci. 2011;369(1955):4605–19.
141. Blower PJ, Kettle AG, O'Doherty MJ, Collins RE, Coakley AJ. 123I-methylene blue: an unsatisfactory parathyroid imaging agent. Nucl Med Commun. 1992;13(7):522–7.
142. Link EM, Blower PJ, Costa DC, Lane DM, Lui D, Brown RS, Ell PJ, Spittle MF. Early detection of melanoma metastases with radioiodinated methylene blue. Eur J Nucl Med. 1998;25(9):1322–9.
143. Harkrider WW, Diebold AE, Maloney T, Espenan G, Wang YZ, Stafford SJ, Camp A, Frey D, Chappuis C,

Woltering EA. An extended phase II trial of iodine-125 methylene blue for sentinel lymph node identification in women with breast cancer. J Am Coll Surg. 2013;216(4):599–605; discussion 605–596.
144. Chu M, Wan Y. Sentinel lymph node mapping using near-infrared fluorescent methylene blue. J Biosci Bioeng. 2009;107(4):455–9.
145. Brouwer OR, Buckle T, Vermeeren L, Klop WM, Balm AJ, van der Poel HG, van Rhijn BW, Horenblas S, Nieweg OE, van Leeuwen FW, Valdes Olmos RA. Comparing the hybrid fluorescent-radioactive tracer indocyanine green-99mTc-nanocolloid with 99mTc-nanocolloid for sentinel node identification: a validation study using lymphoscintigraphy and SPECT/CT. J Nucl Med. 2012;53(7):1034–40.
146. Brouwer OR, van den Berg NS, Matheron HM, van der Poel HG, van Rhijn BW, Bex A, van Tinteren H, Valdes Olmos RA, van Leeuwen FW, Horenblas S. A hybrid radioactive and fluorescent tracer for sentinel node biopsy in penile carcinoma as a potential replacement for blue dye. Eur Urol. 2014;65(3):600–9.
147. KleinJan GH, van den Berg NS, Brouwer OR, de Jong J, Acar C, Wit EM, Vegt E, van der Noort V, Valdes Olmos RA, van Leeuwen FW, van der Poel HG. Optimisation of fluorescence guidance during robot-assisted laparoscopic sentinel node biopsy for prostate cancer. Eur Urol. 2014;66(6):991–8.
148. van den Berg NS, Brouwer OR, Schaafsma BE, Matheron HM, Klop WM, Balm AJ, van Tinteren H, Nieweg OE, van Leeuwen FW, Valdes Olmos RA. Multimodal surgical guidance during sentinel node biopsy for melanoma: combined gamma tracing and fluorescence imaging of the sentinel node through use of the hybrid tracer indocyanine green-tc-nanocolloid. Radiology. 2015;275(2):521–9.
149. Thorek DL, Riedl CC, Grimm J. Clinical Cerenkov luminescence imaging of (18)F-FDG. J Nucl Med. 2014;55(1):95–8.
150. Farwell MD, Pryma DA, Mankoff DA. PET/CT imaging in cancer: current applications and future directions. Cancer. 2014;120(22):3433–45.
151. Maurer AH, Elsinga P, Fanti S, Nguyen B, Oyen WJ, Weber WA. Imaging the folate receptor on cancer cells with 99mTc-etarfolatide: properties, clinical use, and future potential of folate receptor imaging. J Nucl Med. 2014;55(5):701–4.
152. van de Watering FC, Rijpkema M, Perk L, Brinkmann U, Oyen WJ, Boerman OC. Zirconium-89 labeled antibodies: a new tool for molecular imaging in cancer patients. Biomed Res Int. 2014;2014:203601.
153. Azhdarinia A, Ghosh P, Ghosh S, Wilganowski N, Sevick-Muraca EM. Dual-labeling strategies for nuclear and fluorescence molecular imaging: a review and analysis. Mol Imaging Biol. 2012;14(3): 261–76.
154. Kuil J, Buckle T, van Leeuwen FWB. Imaging agents for the chemokine receptor 4 (CXCR4). Chem Soc Rev. 2012;41(15):5239–61.
155. Seibold U, Wangler B, Schirrmacher R, Wangler C. Bimodal imaging probes for combined PET and OI: recent developments and future directions for hybrid agent development. Biomed Res Int. 2014;2014:153741.
156. Bunschoten A, Buckle T, Visser N, Kuil J, Yuan H, Josephson L, Vahrmeijer AL, van Leeuwen FWB. Multimodal interventional molecular imaging of tumor margins and distant metastases by targeting the αvβ3 integrin. Chembiochem. 2012;13(7):1039–45.
157. Thorp-Greenwood FL, Coogan MP. Multimodal radio- (PET/SPECT) and fluorescence imaging agents based on metallo-radioisotopes: current applications and prospects for development of new agents. Dalton Trans. 2011;40(23):6129–43.
158. Kuil J, Velders AH, van Leeuwen FWB. Multimodal tumor-targeting peptides functionalized with both a radio- and a fluorescent label. Bioconjug Chem. 2010;21(10):1709–19.

6 Radiation Safety and Dosimetry

Michael Lassmann and Uta Eberlein

Contents

M. Lassmann (✉) • U. Eberlein
Department of Nuclear Medicine,
University Würzburg, Würzburg, Germany
e-mail: lassmann_m@ukw.de

Abstract

The use of radioactive substances for sentinel lymph node (SLN) biopsy needs consideration on how to optimize radiation safety issues. In this chapter an overview on basic radiation-related quantities, definitions, and on patient dosimetry is given. Values of absorbed and effective doses are provided for patients, the staff in the operation theater and in the pathology department, and for waste disposal. For radiolocalization of SLN with Tc-99m, the dose to the patients and the exposure of the staff are low; for radiopharmaceuticals with longer half-lives and/or positron emitters, individual monitoring of staff exposure and contamination should be considered for larger patient numbers.

6.1 Introduction

The use of radioactive substances for sentinel lymph node (SLN) biopsy needs the optimization of radiation safety issues for patients, for the staff in nuclear medicine departments, in the operating theater, pathology laboratories, and also the disposal of radioactive waste.

K. Herrmann et al. (eds.), *Radioguided Surgery: Current Applications and Innovative Directions in Clinical Practice*, DOI 10.1007/978-3-319-26051-8_6

6.2 Basic Quantities and Definitions

6.2.1 Absorbed Dose (*D*)

In a lot of publications in nuclear medicine, the term “dose” is used for describing the administered activity as well as the “absorbed dose.” It is, however, mandatory to distinguish between these two terms. The appropriate term for the quantity of interest in radiation protection and dosimetry, however, is “absorbed dose” (*D*), expressed in units of gray (Gy) [1].

According to ICRP103 [1], the absorbed dose is defined as the mean energy $d\varepsilon$ imparted to matter of mass dm by ionizing radiation:

$$D = \frac{d\varepsilon}{dm} \qquad (6.1)$$

The SI unit for absorbed dose is joule per kilogram (J kg^{-1}), and its special name is gray (Gy) [1]. In nuclear medicine, $d\varepsilon$ represents the number of radionuclide disintegrations in a particular volume multiplied by the energy emitted per disintegration of the radionuclide and multiplied by the fraction of emitted energy that is absorbed by a particular (target) mass.

The concept of absorbed dose is only applicable in a macroscopic scale as it is generally done in nuclear medicine dosimetry. In “macrodosimetry”, one considers mean parameters (mean doses). It should be noted that the mean absorbed dose can be calculated for a large (i.e., organ) volume or at the microscopic level, as long as the criteria applicable to macrodosimetry are met. The energy deposition, however, is a stochastic process and shows inherent statistical fluctuations. If particle flux-and energy deposition-is large enough, then the mean absorbed dose is relevant as the standard deviation due to stochastic fluctuations is small.

6.2.2 Dosimetry in Nuclear Medicine

Methods for calculating the absorbed dose from administration of a radiopharmaceutical were first standardized in the 1960s by the Medical Internal Radiation Dosimetry (MIRD) committee, with the initial aim of estimating average doses to critical organs resulting from diagnostic procedures [2]. Essentially this methodology allows the calculation of absorbed dose using the *simplified* version of the basic equation [3]:

$$\bar{D}(r_k \leftarrow r_h) = \tilde{A}_h S(r_k \leftarrow r_h) \qquad (6.2)$$

$\bar{D}(r_k \leftarrow r_h)$: the mean absorbed dose to a target region r_k from the cumulated activity in source region r_h.

$\tilde{A}_h$: the cumulated activity (i.e., the integral of the activity-time curve from zero to infinity) in a given target region r_h.

$S(r_k \leftarrow r_h)$: the radionuclide-specific *S* factor for target region r_k and source region r_h per unit cumulated activity in source region r_h.

$\tilde{A}$ denotes the total number of radioactive decays occurring within an organ in which a radiopharmaceutical accumulates (the “source organ”). The MIRD S factor accounts for the energy released from each radioactive decay and the relative geometry of the source organ and the organ for which the absorbed dose is to be calculated. Thus, the cumulated activity is dependent on biological parameters, while the *S* factor deals with the physical components of the absorbed dose.

There is no assumption made concerning the source or target, other than that the radioactive distribution is homogeneous in the source *h*: the source and target can be of any size or composition. Theoretically, if the activity in the source has a heterogeneous distribution, it is possible to subdivide the source into smaller volumes in which the activity can be considered to be homogeneous.

As the cumulated activity constitutes the sum of all radioactive emissions during the time considered, the energy deposition rate with time is not taken into account, although the absorbed dose rate (Gy s^{-1}) is known to impact on the biological consequences of the irradiation. The relevance of this is indicated by the fact that the aim of most dosimetric studies is to relate a physical parameter (i.e., energy absorbed per unit mass) to the observed biological effect: the relation between these two parameters may not be simple, and scientifically sound dosimetric protocols are simply a prerequisite for subsequent radiobiological studies.

6.2.3 Effective Dose (*E*)

For a risk assessment of medical diagnostic procedures involving ionizing radiation and radiation protection, the concept of the effective dose (*E*) has been widely adapted [1, 4]. The risk associated with the effective dose is based on assumptions such as the concept of considering the risk to the general public or to workers. This does not necessarily reflect the situation for patients in nuclear medicine as, particularly in patients with cancer, the life expectancy is likely to be different of that of the general public or of workers. Another aspect is the strong age and sex dependency of the radiation risk, which is not included in the effective dose. Therefore, the effective dose should not be used for individual risk-benefit assessments in patients; instead, the relevant quantity is the equivalent dose or the absorbed dose to irradiated organs. However, for comparing different medical procedures, effective dose is a useful quantity [1]. It is defined as

$$E = \sum_T \omega_T H_T \tag{6.3}$$

where ω_T is the tissue weighting factor for the tissue *T* and represents the radiation sensitivity for stochastic radiation damage of each tissue considered. The sum over all tissue weighting factors is 1: $\Sigma_T\ \omega_T = 1$. H_T is the organ dose (unit: Sv) caused by internal or external exposure. For nuclear medicine applications using beta and gamma emitters, the organ doses are calculated by multiplying the absorbed dose (unit: Gy) by the radiation weighting factor for photons and electrons (=1 Sv/Gy). According to ICRP103 [1], the effective dose *E* is then the arithmetic mean of the gender-specific organ doses $H^M{}_T$ (male) and $H^F{}_T$ (female):

$$E = \sum_T \omega_T \cdot \frac{H_T^M + H_T^F}{2} \tag{6.4}$$

Table 6.1 summarizes the tissue weighting factors according to ICRP103.

According to ICRP103 [1], the occupational exposure in planned exposure situations should be limited to an effective dose of 20 mSv per year, averaged over defined 5-year periods (100 mSv in 5 years), with the further provision that the effective dose should not exceed 50 mSv in any single year. For public exposure in planned exposure situations, ICRP recommends that the limit should be expressed as an effective dose of 1 mSv in a year. The annual exposure of the hands and feet should not exceed 500 mSv (organ dose) in occupational exposure; no values are provided by the ICRP for the general public.

6.2.4 External Exposure

The absorbed dose *D* imparted by the external exposure of a point source and by penetrating radiation, an activity *A* at a distance *r*, an exposure rate constant Γ (dependent on the isotope), and an exposure duration Δ*t* is described by Eq. 6.5:

$$D = \frac{\Gamma \cdot A \cdot \Delta t}{r^2} \tag{6.5}$$

An overview of the most common exposure rates, exposure durations, distances, activities to be

Table 6.1 Tissue weighting factors according to ICRP103 [1]

Tissue	ω_T	$\Sigma_T\ \omega_T$
Bone marrow (red), colon, lung, stomach, breast, remainder tissues[a]	0.12	0.72
Gonads	0.08	0.08
Bladder, esophagus, liver, thyroid	0.04	0.16
Bone surface, brain, salivary glands, skin	0.01	0.04
	Total	1.00

[a]Remainder tissues: adrenals, extrathoracic (ET) region, gall bladder, heart, kidneys, lymphatic nodes, muscle, oral mucosa, pancreas, prostate (male), small intestine, spleen, thymus, uterus/cervix (female)

Table 6.2 External exposure rates and exposures for typical SLN applications

Isotope	Tc-99m	In-111	F-18	Co-57
Exposure rate	22 μSv m²/(GBq h)	87 μSv m²/(GBq h)	37 μSv m²/(GBq h)*	15 μSv m²/(GBq h)
Typical activity	10 MBq	150 MBq	75 MBq	<1 MBq
Exposure for 2 h at a distance of 0.3 m	0.005 mSv	0.03 mSv	0.1 mSv**	<0.0003 mSv

Data taken from the radionuclide and radiation protection handbook [5]
*Similar exposure rate constants for many other PET nuclides
**4 h after administration of 300 MBq F-18-FDG

expected, and potential exposure scenarios and exposures in SLN procedures is provided in Table 6.2 (data taken from Delacroix et al. [5]). With the exception of the application of PET nuclides and In-111, the exposure scenarios do not exceed 0.06 mSv for the hands and 0.005 mSv for body exposure. For comparison, the total effective dose to individual members of the public should not exceed 1 mSv per year [1]. Concerning contamination of the hands, the dose rate after contamination with a droplet of 0.05 ml and an activity of 1 kBq leads to an exposure dose rate of 9 μSv/h, 0.06 mSv/h, and 0.8 mSv/h for Tc-99m, In-111, and F-18, respectively [5].

Reported radiation exposures for Tc-99m-based procedures were less than 0.4 mSv for the surgeon hands and 0.02 mSv for the surgeon body [6]. In procedures involving Tc-99m and in typical quality assurance procedures, therefore, the exposure by external irradiation is low. Special precaution measures, however, might need to be considered when applying SLN diagnostics after the use of PET-tracers such as F-18.

6.3 Patient Dosimetry for SLN Diagnostics with Tc-99m

6.3.1 Patients

As has been stated in the EANM-EORTC general recommendations for sentinel lymph node diagnostics in melanoma [7], lymphoscintigraphy is a procedure involving low activities. The estimated local radiation dose varies depending on the administered activity, injection site, volume of tracer, the application of multiple injections, and retention time [8]. The different radiopharmaceuticals used for SLN imaging are associated with minor differences in dosimetry. The local absorbed dose at the injection site with respect to the most common radiocolloids is less than 50 mGy/MBq [8–10].

For breast cancer, Waddington et al. estimated the mean absorbed dose to the tissue of the affected breast to be 0.72 mGy/MBq resulting in an absorbed dose of 11 mGy for a tracer administration of 15 MBq [8]. The sentinel lymph node itself will receive an absorbed dose between 0.44 and 2.5 mGy/MBq depending on the size of the lymph node, assuming 1.0 % uptake of tracer and physical half-life. Taking all other organs that are also irradiated into account, Waddington et al. estimate the effective dose for SLN diagnostics in breast cancer to 0.3 mSv for an injection of 15 MBq Tc-99m-colloids [8]. For this procedure, dosimetry data were also published by Law et al. [11]. These authors report an effective dose of 5.1 μSv/MBq, a value which is significantly lower than the 21 μSv/MBq reported by Waddington et al. [8]. Values from Waddington et al. are also systematically higher with respect to the upper limit of breast absorbed dose (720 vs 35 μGy for the injected breast). Cremonesi et al. [12] estimated a mean of 0.8 mGy/MBq at the injected breast and 0.05 mGy/MBq at the sentinel lymph node. Extensive calculations performed at the Memorial Sloan Kettering Cancer Center have confirmed the safety of the procedure for breast cancer by reporting an effective dose around 0.2 mSv [13].

Melanoma originates from skin tissue that is relatively less radiosensitive than many other tissues; the tissue weighting factor defined by the International Committee of Radiation Protection

(ICRP) for the determination of effective dose is 0.01 for skin compared to 0.05 for breast according to ICRP60 [4] or 0.12 according to ICRP103 [1]. Hence, in patients with melanoma, the local radiation dose contributes little to the effective dose. In melanoma patients, the radiolabeled colloid migrates minimally throughout the bloodstream or reticuloendothelial system (RES) or beyond the SLN and second-echelon lymph nodes. Assuming that 20 % of the administered activity has been absorbed in the RES systemically, the effective dose is calculated as 2 μSv/MBq in a "worst-case" calculation [7, 14]. This corresponds to 0.04 mSv after an injection of 20 MBq of 99mTc-labeled small colloid.

Although no dose values have been reported for other applications besides breast cancer and melanoma, it can be safely assumed that the absorbed doses and effective doses for these procedures are in the same range [15, 16].

It should be noted that adoption of SPECT/CT imaging protocols for SLN in melanoma will increase both local radiation dose and effective dose due to inclusion of the CT procedure, the dosimetry being dependent upon both the site of the melanoma and the CT acquisition parameters selected. A low-dose CT scan with a field of view limited to avoid radiosensitive tissues can help to keep the effective dose to a minimum. For a low-dose CT for attenuation correction, for patients undergoing a sentinel lymph node lymphoscintigraphy in breast cancer, an effective dose of 2.4 mSv has been reported [11]. The total exposure in such cases is the emission-generated dose plus the transmission-generated effective dose.

6.3.2 Pregnancy

Pregnant patients could be offered the SLN biopsy after careful counseling regarding the safety and efficacy of the procedure. According to international guidelines, the risk to the fetus is considered negligible for investigations exposing a fetus to <1 mSv. Gentilini et al. report in breast cancer patients that the estimated absorbed dose to the embryo/fetus per unit activity is 5 μGy/MBq [17]. As reported also for melanoma [7], the dose to the fetus from a SLN examination will generally be below the 1 mSv limit for increased stochastic risk generally applied to fetal radiation hygiene. Only in a melanoma located rather close to the fetus (over the lower abdomen or back) the theoretical risk of exceeding 1 mSv is a relevant question. In such a case, the two important modifications that may reduce fetal radiation exposure will be (1) to reduce activity injected, preferably less than 30–40 MBq, and to collect the image data twice the normal duration and (2) short time interval—always following a 1-day protocol—from injection to operation [7].

6.3.3 Lactating Women

The presence of ^{99m}Tc in breast milk has not been reported, but it has been recommended in some publications that lactation be suspended for nursing mothers for 24 h after radiopharmaceutical administration, since radiocolloid will be excreted from the breast milk during this period [18, 19].

6.4 Patient Dosimetry for Other Isotopes

In case of other isotopes (e.g., In-111 or F-18), data for the patient exposure can be taken from the corresponding ICRP tables ICRP [20–22] or from the review article of Eberlein et al. [23]. For an administered activity of 350 MBq F-18, the effective dose is 6.6 mSv, for 185 MBq In-111 10 mSv.

6.5 Staff Exposure for SLN Diagnostics with Tc-99m[1]

6.5.1 General Rules

Within the EU, national implementations of the following EU Directives apply with respect to

[1] This chapter is taken from the "EANM-EORTC general recommendations for sentinel node diagnostics in melanoma" [7] and is reprinted with kind permission of Springer Science + Business Media.

radiation protection aspects of the clinical practice of nuclear medicine. Applying the 1990 Recommendations of the ICRP [4], the Basic Safety Standards Directive (Council Directive 97/43/EURATOM 2007[2]) enforces a general radiation protection framework to ensure the safety of employees and the public. The Medical Exposures Directive (Council Directive 96/29/EURATOM 2006[3]) reinforces the need for justification, optimization, and limitation of all exposures and places additional specific requirements on stated duty holders, especially in respect to the practical aspects of a medical exposure—its referral, individual justification, and execution—including the training and competence of all staff whose actions contribute to the procedure(s) performed.

6.5.2 Staff in Nuclear Medicine Department

To comply with regulatory requirements, including those mandated by the Medical Exposures Directive within the EU and those in force elsewhere [24], radiocolloid administration and preoperative diagnosis will be performed by trained nuclear medicine personnel working in controlled environments. The administered activities in lymphoscintigraphy are low compared with those used in most other nuclear medicine procedures. Any increase in the occupational exposure of nuclear medicine staff due to a SLN procedure will be minimal as they are already categorized as radiation workers. The highest doses received by the hands of the staff have been recorded for the physician who administers the tracer [25]; however, it is far below the ICRP annual dose limits for the extremities of a radiation worker [4]. One potential cause of significant exposure exists however—if transmission imaging using a radioactive ^{57}Co flood source is performed, the source must not be held directly during image acquisition.

6.5.3 Staff in Operating Room

Radiation exposure to operating room personnel arising from the handling of radioactive specimens from SLN procedures is minimal. Studies demonstrate that the occupational doses are insignificant, the mean whole body dose received by surgical staff has been measured to be <1 μSv per operation [8, 26–28], with the maximum effective dose to the surgeons involved reported to be <2 μSv [8, 29] [30] . The radiation dose to the hands of the surgeon has been estimated to be 5–94 μSv per patient [14]. When the surgical procedure is performed 24 h after injection, the absorbed doses to the hands of the medical staff may potentially be minimized [25, 31]. The monitoring of operating room personnel for occupational exposure to radiation is unnecessary during sentinel lymph node biopsy. Additional shielding and monitoring devices are not required in the operating room.

6.5.4 Pregnant Staff in Operating Room

One circumstance requiring specific consideration is that of the pregnant female surgeon or scrub nurse regularly performing or assisting the procedure. A pregnant surgeon who participates in <100 SLN operations will stay below the limit of radiation exposure as recommended for pregnant women [28].

6.5.5 Staff in Pathology Department

The pathology staff usually spends a shorter time manipulating the radioactive tissue specimens than the does the surgeon and at a longer time interval after injection; their exposure will therefore be lower. Even personnel performing an unusually high number of procedures receive

[2]Replaced by Council Directive 2013/59/EURATOM 2013.

[3]Replaced by Council Directive 2013/59/EURATOM 2013.

radiation doses well below established limits for members of the general public [32]. Under any circumstances, radiation exposure to the pathology staff is low and should not normally require badge monitoring.

6.5.6 Radiation Safety Precautions

Labeling the pathology specimens – When transporting the specimens to the laboratory, many institutions seal them in suitable containers with outer labels indicating radioactive content [31]; however, labeling is not required if the surface dose rate is <5 μGy/h [33]. Even if an institution does not label specimens, all personnel handling them must be properly trained and authorized and the specimens should be transferred promptly.

6.5.7 Radioactive Clinical Waste

While surgical instruments and pathology slides appear to stay at background radiation levels, measurable contamination of absorptive surgical sponges and other materials used in the handling of radioactive tissues is observed, especially when they are used in the vicinity of the injection site [8, 34]. Although a negligible contamination hazard, this would constitute radioactive clinical waste. It is advisable to monitor these materials for contamination, and if contaminated, the trash should be held for decay-in-storage before disposal.

6.6 Staff Exposure for Other Isotopes

As discussed previously, the radiation exposure to personnel from low activities of Tc-99m for sentinel lymph node procedures is low. These results should not be applied to the use of other radiopharmaceuticals and considerably higher activities of Tc-99m.

For F-18-FDG, Povoski et al. [35] report on the occupational radiation exposure to intraoperative and perioperative personnel from F-18-FDG-radioguided surgical procedures after administration of around 700 MBq.[4] The authors report on a mean effective dose per case of 0.2 mSv received by the surgeon. Lower doses are reported for the anesthetist, scrub technologist, postoperative nurse, circulating nurse, and preoperative nurse. This exposure is, on a per case basis, rather low. However, for larger patient numbers, individual monitoring of exposure and contamination should be considered.

For In-111-labeled compounds, there are, unfortunately, at present no systematically collected exposure data available for SLN procedures. Therefore, one should also consider monitoring the staff in this case (see also Table 6.2).

6.7 Discussion and Conclusion

Radiolocalization of SLN with Tc-99m is associated with low levels of radiation exposure. Radiation exposure monitoring or limitation of the number of performed SLN procedures as well as additional shielding is not required for staff in the operating room and pathology department. In principle, there is no contraindication for SLN biopsies in pregnant patients; it is, however, common to reduce the activity. For radiopharmaceuticals with longer half-lives and/or positron emitters, individual monitoring of staff exposure and contamination should be considered for larger patient numbers.

References

1. ICRP. Publication 103: The 2007 recommendations of the International Commission of Radiological Protection. Ann ICRP. 2007;37(2–4).
2. Loevinger R, Budinger TF, Watson EE. MIRD Primer for absorbed dose calculations. New York: The Society of Nuclear Medicine; 1989.
3. Bolch WE, Eckerman KF, Sgouros G, Thomas SR. MIRD pamphlet No. 21: a generalized schema for radiopharmaceutical dosimetry – standardization of

[4] This activity is more typical for North America; in Europe, the administered activities are, in many countries, considerably lower and in the range of 250–350 MBq [36].

nomenclature. J Nucl Med. 2009;50(3):477–84. doi:10.2967/jnumed.108.056036.
4. ICRP. Publication 60: 1990 recommendations of the International Commission on Radiological Protection. Ann ICRP. 1991;21(1–3):1–201.
5. Delacroix D, Guerre JP, Leblanc P, Hickman C. Radionuclide and radiation protection data handbook 2nd edition (2002). Radiat Prot Dosimetry. 2002;98(1):9–168.
6. Mariani G, Giuliano AE, Strauss HW. Radioguided surgery – A comprehensive team approach. New York: Springer; 2008.
7. Chakera AH, Hesse B, Burak Z, Ballinger JR, Britten A, Caraco C, Cochran AJ, Cook MG, Drzewiecki KT, Essner R, Even-Sapir E, Eggermont AM, Stopar TG, Ingvar C, Mihm Jr MC, McCarthy SW, Mozzillo N, Nieweg OE, Scolyer RA, Starz H, Thompson JF, Trifiro G, Viale G, Vidal-Sicart S, Uren R, Waddington W, Chiti A, Spatz A, Testori A, European Association of Nuclear Medicine-European Organisation for Research. EANM-EORTC general recommendations for sentinel node diagnostics in melanoma. Eur J Nucl Med Mol Imaging. 2009;36(10):1713–42. doi:10.1007/s00259-009-1228-4.
8. Waddington WA, Keshtgar MR, Taylor I, Lakhani SR, Short MD, Ell PJ. Radiation safety of the sentinel lymph node technique in breast cancer. Eur J Nucl Med. 2000;27(4):377–91.
9. Bronskill MJ. Radiation dose estimates for interstitial radiocolloid lymphoscintigraphy. Semin Nucl Med. 1983;13(1):20–5.
10. Castronovo Jr FP, McKusick KA, Strauss HW. Dosimetric consequences of radiopharmaceutical infiltrations. Invest Radiol. 1994;29(1):59–64.
11. Law M, Ma WH, Leung R, Li S, Wong KK, Ho WY, Kwong A. Evaluation of patient effective dose from sentinel lymph node lymphoscintigraphy in breast cancer: a phantom study with SPECT/CT and ICRP-103 recommendations. Eur J Radiol. 2012;81(5):e717–20. doi:10.1016/j.ejrad.2012.01.035.
12. Cremonesi M, Ferrari M, Sacco E, Rossi A, De Cicco C, Leonardi L, Chinol M, Luini A, Galimberti V, Tosi G, Veronesi U, Paganelli G. Radiation protection in radioguided surgery of breast cancer. Nucl Med Commun. 1999;20(10):919–24.
13. Pandit-Taskar N, Dauer LT, Montgomery L, St Germain J, Zanzonico PB, Divgi CR. Organ and fetal absorbed dose estimates from 99mTc-sulfur colloid lymphoscintigraphy and sentinel node localization in breast cancer patients. J Nucl Med. 2006;47(7):1202–8.
14. Alazraki N, Glass EC, Castronovo F, Olmos RA, Podoloff D. Procedure guideline for lymphoscintigraphy and the use of intraoperative gamma probe for sentinel lymph node localization in melanoma of intermediate thickness 1.0. J Nucl Med. 2002;43(10):1414–8.
15. Alkureishi LW, Burak Z, Alvarez JA, Ballinger J, Bilde A, Britten AJ, Calabrese L, Chiesa C, Chiti A, de Bree R, Gray HW, Hunter K, Kovacs AF, Lassmann M, Leemans CR, Mamelle G, McGurk M, Mortensen J, Poli T, Shoaib T, Sloan P, Sorensen JA, Stoeckli SJ, Thomsen JB, Trifiro G, Werner J, Ross GL, European Association of Nuclear Medicine Oncology C, European Sentinel Node Biopsy Trial C. Joint practice guidelines for radionuclide lymphoscintigraphy for sentinel node localization in oral/oropharyngeal squamous cell carcinoma. Eur J Nucl Med Mol Imaging. 2009;36(11):1915–36. doi:10.1007/s00259-009-1248-0.
16. Giammarile F, Bozkurt MF, Cibula D, Pahisa J, Oyen WJ, Paredes P, Olmos RV, Sicart SV. The EANM clinical and technical guidelines for lymphoscintigraphy and sentinel node localization in gynaecological cancers. Eur J Nucl Med Mol Imaging. 2014;41(7):1463–77. doi:10.1007/s00259-014-2732-8.
17. Gentilini O, Cremonesi M, Trifiro G, Ferrari M, Baio SM, Caracciolo M, Rossi A, Smeets A, Galimberti V, Luini A, Tosi G, Paganelli G. Safety of sentinel node biopsy in pregnant patients with breast cancer. Ann Oncol. 2004;15(9):1348–51. doi:10.1093/annonc/mdh355.
18. Lloyd MS, Topping A, Allan R, Powell B. Contraindications to sentinel lymph node biopsy in cutaneous malignant melanoma. Br J Plast Surg. 2004;57(8):725–7. doi:10.1016/j.bjps.2003.12.028.
19. Giammarile F, Alazraki N, Aarsvold JN, Audisio RA, Glass E, Grant SF, Kunikowska J, Leidenius M, Moncayo VM, Uren RF, Oyen WJ, Valdes Olmos RA, Vidal Sicart S. The EANM and SNMMI practice guideline for lymphoscintigraphy and sentinel node localization in breast cancer. Eur J Nucl Med Mol Imaging. 2013;40(12):1932–47. doi:10.1007/s00259-013-2544-2.
20. ICRP. Publication 106: Radiation dose to patients from radiopharmaceuticals: addendum 3 to ICRP publication 53. Ann ICRP. 2008;38(1–2):1–197.
21. ICRP. Publication 80: Radiation dose to patients from radiopharmaceuticals: addendum 2 to ICRP publication 53. Ann ICRP. 1998;28(3):1–126.
22. ICRP. Publication 53: Radiation dose to patients from radiopharmaceuticals. Ann ICRP. 1987;18(1–4):1–377.
23. Eberlein U, Broer JH, Vandevoorde C, Santos P, Bardies M, Bacher K, Nosske D, Lassmann M. Biokinetics and dosimetry of commonly used radiopharmaceuticals in diagnostic nuclear medicine – a review. Eur J Nucl Med Mol Imaging. 2011;38(12):2269–81.
24. Michel R, Hofer C. Radiation safety precautions for sentinel lymph node procedures. Health Phys. 2004;86(2 Suppl):S35–7.
25. Nejc D, Wrzesien M, Piekarski J, Olszewski J, Pluta P, Kusmierek J, Jeziorski A. Sentinel node biopsy in skin melanoma patients – measurements of absorbed doses of radiation to the hands of medical staff. J Surg Oncol. 2006;93(5):355–61. doi:10.1002/jso.20474.
26. Sera T, Mohos G, Papos M, Osvay M, Varga J, Lazar M, Kiss E, Kapitany K, Dobozy A, Csernay L, Pavics L. Sentinel node detection in malignant melanoma patients: radiation safety considerations. Dermatol Surg. 2003;29(2):141–5. doi:29036 [pii].
27. Stratmann SL, McCarty TM, Kuhn JA. Radiation safety with breast sentinel node biopsy. Am J Surg. 1999;178(6):454–7.

28. Klausen TL, Chakera AH, Friis E, Rank F, Hesse B, Holm S. Radiation doses to staff involved in sentinel node operations for breast cancer. Clin Physiol Funct Imaging. 2005;25(4):196–202. doi:10.1111/j.1475-097X.2005.00611.x.
29. Glass EC, Essner R, Morton DL. Kinetics of three lymphoscintigraphic agents in patients with cutaneous melanoma. J Nucl Med. 1998;39(7): 1185–90.
30. Schauer AJBW, Reiser M, Possinger K. Main techniques of sentinel lymph node labeling. The sentinel lymph node concept. Berlin: Springer; 2005.
31. Strzelczyk I, Finlayson C. Sentinel node biopsy: ALARA and other considerations. Health Phys. 2004;86(2 Suppl):S31–4.
32. Glass EC, Basinski JE, Krasne DL, Giuliano AE. Radiation safety considerations for sentinel node techniques. Ann Surg Oncol. 1999;6(1):10–1.
33. IAEA. Radiation Safety Practice in Nuclear Medicine. In: Nuclear Medicine Resources Manual. 2006. IAEA, Vienna, pp 509–21.
34. Nugent N, Hill AD, Casey M, Kelly L, Dijkstra B, Collins CD, McDermott EW, O'Higgins N. Safety guidelines for radiolocalised sentinel node resection. Ir J Med Sci. 2001;170(4):236–8.
35. Povoski SP, Sarikaya I, White WC, Marsh SG, Hall NC, Hinkle GH, Martin Jr EW, Knopp MV. Comprehensive evaluation of occupational radiation exposure to intraoperative and perioperative personnel from 18F-FDG radioguided surgical procedures. Eur J Nucl Med Mol Imaging. 2008;35(11):2026–34. doi:10.1007/s00259-008-0880-4.
36. Boellaard R, O'Doherty MJ, Weber WA, Mottaghy FM, Lonsdale MN, Stroobants SG, Oyen WJ, Kotzerke J, Hoekstra OS, Pruim J, Marsden PK, Tatsch K, Hoekstra CJ, Visser EP, Arends B, Verzijlbergen FJ, Zijlstra JM, Comans EF, Lammertsma AA, Paans AM, Willemsen AT, Beyer T, Bockisch A, Schaefer-Prokop C, Delbeke D, Baum RP, Chiti A, Krause BJ. FDG PET and PET/CT: EANM procedure guidelines for tumour PET imaging: version 1.0. Eur J Nucl Med Mol Imaging. 2010;37(1):181–200. doi:10.1007/s00259-009-1297-4.

Part III

Clinical Application: Breast

7 Radioguided Sentinel Lymph Node Mapping and Biopsy in Breast Cancer

Andrea V. Barrio and Hiram S. Cody III

Contents

A.V. Barrio • H.S. Cody III (✉)
Breast Service, Department of Surgery, Memorial Sloan Kettering Cancer Center, 300 East 66th Street, New York, NY, USA
e-mail: barrioa@mskcc.org; codyh@mskcc.org

Abstract

The histologic status of the axillary lymph nodes remains one of the most important prognostic indicators in breast cancer and impacts recommendations for adjuvant therapy. Axillary lymph node dissection, once considered standard care for axillary staging in all patients with breast cancer, has been largely replaced by sentinel lymph node (SLN) biopsy in patients with a clinically negative axilla and in a select group of patients with node-positive breast cancer. The SLN can be mapped using radioisotope, blue dye, or a combination of both, utilizing a variety of injection techniques with comparable results and similar false-negative rates. In this chapter, we will review the lymphatic drainage patterns of the breast, the technique of SLN biopsy (with particular attention to the radiosurgical aspects), and the clinical implications of the results.

7.1 Introduction

The histologic status of the axillary lymph nodes remains one of the most important prognostic indicators in breast cancer and impacts recommendations for adjuvant therapy. Axillary lymph node dissection (ALND), once considered standard care for axillary staging in all patients with breast cancer, has been largely

K. Herrmann et al. (eds.), *Radioguided Surgery: Current Applications and Innovative Directions in Clinical Practice*, DOI 10.1007/978-3-319-26051-8_7

replaced by sentinel lymph node (SLN) biopsy in patients with a clinically negative axilla and in a select group of patients with node-positive breast cancer. A study-level meta-analysis of eight randomized controlled trials comparing SLN biopsy to ALND demonstrated no difference in overall survival (hazard ratio [HR] = 1.07), disease-free survival (HR = 1.00), or regional lymph node recurrence (odds ratio [OR] = 1.65) between SLN biopsy and ALND [1], rendering ALND obsolete in clinically node-negative breast cancer patients. The SLN can be mapped using radioisotope, blue dye, or a combination of both, utilizing a variety of injection techniques with comparable results and similar false-negative rates [2, 3]. In this chapter, we will review the lymphatic drainage patterns of the breast, the technique of SLN biopsy (with particular attention to the radiosurgical aspects), and the clinical implications of the results.

7.2 Lymphatic Drainage Patterns in the Era of Modern Lymphoscintigraphy

Modern techniques of lymphoscintigraphy have defined the lymphatic drainage of the breast with a new degree of precision. Estourgie et al. have reported on 691 clinically node-negative breast cancer patients in whom 700 SLN biopsy procedures were done, preceded by lymphoscintigraphy using technetium 99m-nanocolloid injected directly into the tumor. They observed axillary drainage in 95 %, internal mammary (IM) drainage in 22 % (usually in combination with axillary), isolated IM drainage in 0–5.8 %, infraclavicular drainage in 2.7 %, interpectoral drainage in 2.2 %, supraclavicular drainage in 0.5 %, and no lymphatic drainage in 3 % (Fig. 7.1) [4]. Axillary and IM drainage were observed from all quadrants of the breast, but IM drainage was more frequent and axillary drainage less frequent from the lower inner quadrant (Table 7.1) [5]. Uren et al. have reported on 217 breast cancer patients in whom isotope was injected peritumorally; 93 % had axillary drainage, but 50 % had non-axillary drainage (most of these IM), and 7 % had isolated non-axillary drainage [6]. Like Estourgie, Uren found drainage to the IM nodes from all four quadrants of the breast, suggesting that tumor location alone is not the sole determinant of non-axillary lymphatic drainage [6].

7.3 Isotope Mapping Agents

Technetium 99m—widely available, inexpensive, and with a low radiation dose—has become the isotope of choice for SLN mapping in breast cancer. A wide variety of carrier particles have been used, as reviewed by Wilhelm et al. [7]. Technetium 99m sulfur colloid (Tc 99m sulfur colloid) is the only registered radiopharmaceutical for lymphoscintigraphy in the United States and therefore is the predominant radioisotope used. Tc-99m-nanocolloidal albumin is widely used in Europe and Tc-99m-antimony trisulfide colloid in Australia; both provide accurate localization of the sentinel node, but neither agent is commercially available in the United States.

7.4 Particle Size

The large particle size of Tc 99m sulfur colloid (mean = 300 nm) raises theoretical concerns that movement of this tracer beyond the injection site into lymphatic vessels and nodes may be limited. To overcome this potential liability, many have advocated using "filtered" Tc 99m sulfur colloid that has been passed through a 220 nm filter. A multi-institutional study by Martin et al. demonstrated that the use of filtered or unfiltered technetium sulfur colloid had no impact on the number of sentinel nodes identified, indicating that passage of the unfiltered colloid into the lymphatic system was not compromised by its larger particle size [8]. Moreover, in a study of 134 breast cancer patients, Linehan et al. reported a superior sentinel node identification rate with unfiltered versus filtered isotope (88 % vs. 73 %, respectively;

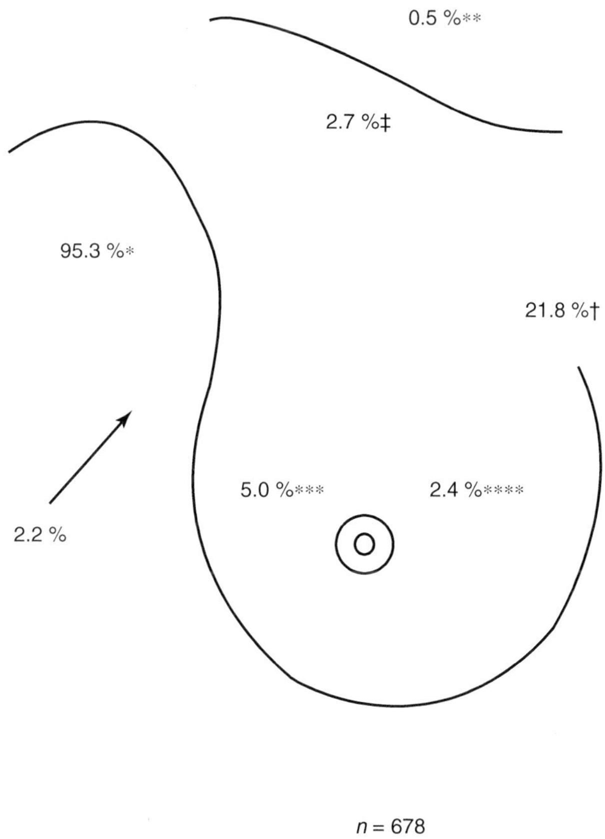

Fig. 7.1 Drainage patterns of the breast identified by scintigraphy, showing overall lymphatic drainage ($n=678$) (Adapted from Estourgie et al. [4]) *axillary; † internal mammary; ‡infraclavicular; **supraclavicular; ***lateral intramammary region; ****medial intramammary region; → interpectoral

Table 7.1 Lymphatic drainage pattern to the axilla and internal mammary nodes by tumor location in early-stage breast cancer patients ($n=678$)

Tumor location	Axillary drainage (%)	IMN drainage (%)	IMN drainage only (%)
UOQ	96	10	2
UIQ	93	32	3
LOQ	98	30	1
LIQ	88	52	6
Central	100	24	0

Adapted from Estourgie et al. [5]
IMN internal mammary node, *UOQ* upper outer quadrant, *UIQ* upper inner quadrant, *LOQ* lower outer quadrant, *LIQ* lower inner quadrant

$p=0.03$) [9]. The most frequent reason for failed localization in the filtered group was a diffusely "hot" axillary bed, not the failure to find a single "hot" node [9].

7.5 Technique of Isotope Injection

A wide variation in isotope technique has been reported in the literature with seemingly similar success and false-negative rates. Technique varies with respect to volume, timing, location (intraparenchymal, subareolar, or intradermal), and depth of injection, although early sentinel node studies reported similar outcomes despite this wide variation [2].

7.5.1 Volume of Injection

The volumes of radioisotope injection reported in the literature range from 0.05 to 16 mL, suggesting that the optimal volume for injection has not been determined [10]. Proponents of low-volume injection argue that the normal lymphatic physiology is not disrupted by the small volume, with Tanis et al. reporting an identification rate of 99 % with 0.2 mL volume of tracer [10]. Advocates of larger-volume injection report higher identification rates [11], although many have observed that the larger injection site "hot spot"/"blast zone" may interfere with both lymphoscintigraphy and with the identification of nearby SLNs at surgery. Regardless of volume, SLN identification rates in large contemporary studies are high (93–98 %), and there is no standard for volume of injection [10].

7.5.2 Timing of Injection

Blue dye travels quickly from the injection site to the SLN and is therefore injected in the OR immediately prior to surgery. Radiocolloid can be observed in lymphatics and nodes within minutes of injection, but scintigraphic images are typically taken within 30 min to 2 h of injection. Lymphatic mapping need not be done on the day of surgery. Winchester et al. reported improved sentinel node identification with day-before mapping compared to same-day mapping (97 % vs. 83 %) and a comparable number of SLNs obtained (2.8 vs. 3.8) [12]. McCarter et al. compared day-before with same-day isotope injection and found no difference in the SLN identification rate or number of SLNs obtained, but observed that *day-before injection must account for the 6-h half-life of Tc 99m*; by giving 0.5 mCi to day-before and 0.1 mCi to same-day patients, the authors observed comparable isotope counts at surgery [13].

7.5.3 Location of Injection

Location of injection varies widely among institutions, with studies reporting intradermal, subdermal, subareolar, peritumoral/intraparenchymal, and intratumoral injections. A nonrandomized study of 298 patients comparing intradermal ($n=164$) to intraparenchymal ($n=134$) isotope injection at our institution demonstrated a higher sentinel node identification rate with intradermal versus intraparenchymal injection (98 % vs. 89 %) [14]. A recent meta-analysis of 183 sentinel node articles, which included patients with a pathologically negative SLN followed by a completion ALND, compared 4 single-site injection locations (peritumoral, subareolar, intratumoral, and intradermal) and 3 multiple site injection locations (peritumoral and intradermal, peritumoral and areolar, and intradermal and areolar) and analyzed false-negative rates by injection location. No significant variation in false-negative rate was identified between these location categories ($p=0.95$) [3]. Although there was a trend toward a lower numerical false-negative rate with intratumoral (2.5 %) and intradermal (5 %) injection, there were too few cases to establish significance, and therefore no "best" location site for injection could be recommended [3]. Two randomized studies have compared localization of the SLN by injection route. Povoski et al. randomized 400 breast cancers to intradermal (ID) ($n=133$), intraparenchymal (IP) ($n=134$), or subareolar (SA) ($n=133$) injection with approximately 0.4 mCi of filtered Tc 99m sulfur colloid. SLN localization by preoperative lymphoscintigraphy was significantly higher in the ID group compared to the IP and SA group [95 % (ID) vs. 62 % (IP) vs. 72 % (SA); $p<0.001$]. Intraoperative SLN identification was also significantly higher in patients receiving ID injection (100 %) compared to IP (90 %) or SA (95 %). Mean time to first localization and time to harvest first SLN was significantly decreased with the ID injection route compared to IP and SA routes, confirming the superiority of the ID injection route for SLN biopsy in breast cancer patients [15]. The FRANSENODE trial prospectively randomized 449 early-stage (T0–T1) breast cancer patients to peritumoral injection (PT) versus periareolar (PA) injection with unfiltered Tc 99m sulfur colloid. The authors reported a higher SLN detection rate by lymphoscintigraphy with PA injection [85 % (PA) vs. 73 % (PT); $p=0.03$]; however, no significant difference in intraoperative SLN identification was noted by method of injection ($p=0.16$). It should be noted that the method of PA injection (subareolar vs. intradermal) was not specified by the authors, which limits interpretation of these results [16].

7.5.4 Superficial versus Deep Injection

Although location of injection may result in comparable false-negative rates in the axilla, the deep and superficial lymphatics of the breast may not drain to the same axillary nodes. Furthermore, lymphatic drainage of the breast is not always to the axilla, as demonstrated by Estourgie et al. and Uren et al. [5, 6]. Depth of injection affects drainage to IM nodes; intradermal or superficial isotope injections achieve high success rates in the axilla but rarely drain to IM nodes, which require a deeper intraparenchymal injection. Martin et al. imaged IM nodes in only 1.2 % of patients following intradermal injection compared to 9 % after intraparenchymal injection [14]. In comparison, Estourgie et al. documented internal mammary node drainage in 21.8 % of patients after intraparenchymal injection [5]. A recent meta-analysis of superficial versus deep injection of radioactive tracer and blue dye for SLN mapping in breast cancer patients showed no significant difference in axillary sentinel node identification rate on lymphoscintigraphy ($p=0.19$) or during surgery ($p=0.54$), but found significantly more non-axillary drainage on lymphoscintigraphy with deep injections (OR = 3.00, 95 % confidence interval [CI] 1.92–4.67, $p<0.001$) [17]. Clearly, if the goal is to map IM and other non-axillary sites, then deeper injections are required, but whether it is necessary to do so remains unclear.

7.6 Isotope Versus Blue Dye

The SLN literature to date supports the use of isotope alone, blue dye alone, or both. A meta-analysis published in 2005 which included 69 trials demonstrated a higher SLN identification rate with dual mapping (91.9 %) compared to isotope alone (89.2 %) or blue dye alone (83.1 %) ($p=0.007$). Although on univariate analysis, the false-negative rate was lower for dual mapping than for blue dye alone ($p=0.047$), the use of tracer was not an independent predictor for lowered false-negative rate on multivariate analysis [18]. A more recent study-level meta-analysis published in 2012 demonstrated the highest false-negative rate with the use of blue dye alone (8.6 %, 95 % CI 6.7–10.8 %). The largest difference in false-negative rate was between blue dye alone and blue dye + isotope ($p=0.018$); comparison of single-agent dye versus single-agent isotope did not result in a significant difference in false-negative rates ($p=0.37$) [3].

7.7 Technique of SLN Biopsy

Lymphoscintigraphy images, if taken, should be present in the OR, and the surgeon must aim to identify at least as many axillary SLNs with the handheld gamma probe as are seen by the gamma camera; even if SLNs are not seen on the lymphoscintigram, they will still be found by the handheld gamma probe in a substantial majority of cases.

Counts are typically taken of the injection site in the breast and over the axilla. After making the axillary incision and entering the clavipectoral fascia, the dissection is directed by the identification of blue lymphatics and/or blue nodes (if dye is used), and by "hot spots" as identified by the gamma probe, taking care not to pick up false counts by inadvertently "looking back" toward the injection site in the breast. All blue and/or "hot" nodes are removed and submitted as SLNs.

As defined by blue dye, the SLN is a node which is blue or contiguous with a blue lymphatic, and as defined by isotope, the SLN is a node which meets a threshold value, typically expressed as a ratio [19]. McMasters et al. have popularized the "10 % rule" in which all nodes with counts ≥ 10 % of the "hottest" node are submitted as SLNs, and Martin et al. have found that among SLN-positive patients, the "hottest" SLN is the positive node 80 % of the time [2]. Of note, it is not sufficient to remove only the "hottest" node: Martin et al. projected a false-negative rate of 13 % if only the "hottest" node had been removed ($p = 0.01$) and also observed that there was no single count ratio which identified the positive SLN in all cases [8].

Nodes which are replaced by tumor may not pick up dye or isotope, and a final element of SLN biopsy is careful palpation of the axilla, submitting any palpably suspicious nodes even if they are neither blue nor "hot"; we have observed a reduction in false-negative rate from 14 % to 4.6 % by doing so [14].

7.7.1 Extra-axillary Drainage

Although the axilla remains the primary drainage site for the breast, drainage to extra-axillary sites, particularly the IM nodes, is well recognized. Based on the experience of the 1950s and 1960s with extended radical mastectomy (which routinely removed IM nodes), IM node metastases were found in as many as 18–33 % of patients with early-stage breast cancer [20], although a randomized trial found no survival advantage for extended radical versus radical mastectomy at 30 years follow-up [21]. In recent years when IM nodes have routinely received no local treatment, they are the first site of treatment failure in <1 % of cases [20]. In six contemporary series of IM SLN biopsy (Table 7.2) [4, 22, 23, 24, 25, 26], only 1 % of patients had isolated IM node metastases (Table 7.2). IM node metastases have a prognostic importance comparable to that of axillary nodes, but in an era when the decision for adjuvant systemic therapy and node field radiotherapy is increasingly based on the characteristics of the primary tumor, IM node status would rarely change systemic and local treatment. There may be a role for IM node mapping and SLN biopsy in patients with locally recurrent breast cancer, for whom prior axillary surgery (SLN biopsy or ALND) has altered the lymphatic drainage of the breast and in whom we have performed reoperative SLN biopsy and observed a significant increase in non-axillary lymphatic drainage [27]. Of note, this is a clinical setting in which systemic adjuvant therapy would be given regardless of regional node status.

7.7.2 SLN Biopsy after Neoadjuvant Chemotherapy

Following neoadjuvant chemotherapy (NAC), the success rate of SLN biopsy is somewhat lower (~90 %) and the false-negative rate somewhat higher (~10 %) than for SLN biopsy in general [28]. Since about 40 % of node-positive patients become node negative ("ypN0") following NAC, it is logical to ask whether SLN biopsy would allow them to avoid ALND, and two recent prospective trials, ACOSOG 1071 [29] and SENTINA [30], have addressed this issue. Both confirm lower success rates (80–93 %) and higher false-negative rates (12.6–14.2 %) than for SLN biopsy in general, and both emphasize the importance of technique. The false-negative rate was minimized by the use of dual-agent (dye + isotope) versus single-agent mapping (9–11 % vs. 16–20 %) and by the removal of at least 3 SLNs (5–9 % vs. 24–31 % if only 1 SLN was removed) [29, 30].

Table 7.2 Internal mammary sentinel lymph node biopsy

Author	IMN imaged (%)	IMN found (%)	IMN positive (%)	IMN-only positive (%)
Van der Ent (2001) ($n = 256$)	25	16	4	1.2
Estourgie (2003) ($n = 691$)	22	19	3	1.3
Farrús (2004) ($n = 120$)	17	12	1.6	0
Leidenius (2006) ($n = 984$)	14	11	1.8	0.8
Madsen (2007) ($n = 506$)	22	17	4	1
Heuts (2009) ($n = 1{,}008$)	20	14	3	0.9

IMN internal mammary node

Table 7.3 Comparison of intradermal and intraparenchymal isotope injection

	Intradermal injection ($n=164$) (%)	Intraparenchymal injection ($n=134$) (%)	p value
Isotope success	93	84	0.04
Blue dye success	82	72	0.08
Total success (isotope and/or blue dye)	98	89	0.008
Isotope/dye concordance[a]	92	93	NS

Adapted from Martin et al. [14]
NS non-significant
[a]Includes cases with isotope and blue dye found in axilla (intradermal, $n=125$; intraparenchymal, $n=86$)

7.8 The Memorial Sloan Kettering Cancer Center Approach

Our current, standard technique of SLN biopsy involves a single intradermal injection of 0.1 mCi of unfiltered Tc 99m sulfur colloid in 0.05 mL of isotonic saline directly over the tumor site on the morning of surgery (or 0.5 mCi the afternoon before) [13]. In our experience, intradermal injection has resulted in a higher identification rate when compared to intraparenchymal injection (Table 7.3) [14], and we have consciously elected to maximize our success in the mapping of axillary SLN with the understanding that we will identify IM nodes less often. Static lymphoscintigraphy is performed on all patients 30 min to 2 h following isotope injection to evaluate the lymphatic drainage pattern. For early-stage breast cancer, we have found lymphoscintigraphy to be far less useful than for melanoma, where it is critical in identifying unexpected patterns of lymphatic drainage.

We continue to map SLN with blue dye and isotope, finding in our early experience that this maximized our success rate (97 %) and minimized our false-negative rate (5 %) [2, 31]. Among 255 patients with *positive SLNs*, we have shown that 11 % were found by either blue dye alone or isotope alone and would have been missed by reliance on a single modality [32]. With experience, our success in isotope mapping has increased and the marginal benefit of blue dye has declined; among our more recent patients with positive SLN, only 2 % were found by *blue dye alone* [33].

We remove a median of 2–3 SLNs per procedure. No absolute number of SLN is required, *except for node-positive patients following NAC, in which case we require the removal of at least 3*. We always aim to remove the "hottest" SLN and have found that for additional "hot" SLNs, an SLN-to-background count ratio of 4:1 optimizes the false-negative rate. Since 98 % of positive SLNs are found within the first 3 SLNs removed, and 99 % within the first 4, we rarely remove more than 3–4 [34]. At the end of the procedure, we routinely remove any palpably suspicious nodes as well.

Under this algorithm, the radiation dosage of 0.1 mCi of Tc 99m sulfur colloid is trivial—approximately 0.4 % of that given for a bone scan—and only a small fraction of this dose reaches the SLN. Accordingly, we use no special radiation precautions during surgery or in the handling of the surgical specimens [35].

Conclusion

SLN biopsy is one of the great success stories in contemporary surgical oncology, and radioisotope has played a major role. Lymphoscintigraphy has given us a detailed understanding of the lymphatic drainage patterns of the breast, demonstrating the ipsilateral axilla to be the primary drainage site but identifying non-axillary sites as well. Isotope mapping has helped to maximize the success and minimize the false-negative rates of SLN biopsy and has performed well despite wide variations in technique. For SLN biopsy done after NAC, an expanding paradigm for drug development, isotope will remain a crucial element in maintaining performance characteristics.

There are some challenges. We are entering an era in which treatment decisions for breast cancer are increasingly based on the molecular profile of the primary tumor, in which systemic therapy clearly contributes to *local and distant* control of disease, and in which locoregional relapse occurs less often than it has historically. The next generation of surgical trials will compare SLN biopsy to no axillary surgery at all, and in this setting, the role of lymph node staging will continue to decline.

References

1. Wang Z, Wu LC, Chen JQ. Sentinel lymph node biopsy compared with axillary lymph node dissection in early breast cancer: a meta-analysis. Breast Cancer Res Treat. 2011;129(3):675–89.
2. Martin RC, Fey J, Yeung H, Borgen PI, Cody 3rd HS. Highest isotope count does not predict sentinel node positivity in all breast cancer patients. Ann Surg Oncol. 2001;8(7):592–7.
3. Pesek S, Ashikaga T, Krag LE, Krag D. The false-negative rate of sentinel node biopsy in patients with breast cancer: a meta-analysis. World J Surg. 2012;36(9):2239–51.
4. Estourgie SH, Tanis PJ, Nieweg OE, Valdes Olmos RA, Rutgers EJ, Kroon BB. Should the hunt for internal mammary chain sentinel nodes begin? An evaluation of 150 breast cancer patients. Ann Surg Oncol. 2003;10(8):935–41.
5. Estourgie SH, Nieweg OE, Olmos RA, Rutgers EJ, Kroon BB. Lymphatic drainage patterns from the breast. Ann Surg. 2004;239(2):232–7.
6. Uren RF, Howman-Giles RB. The role of nuclear medicine. In: Cody HS, editor. Sentinel lymph node biopsy. London: Martin Dunitz; 2002. p. 19–44.
7. Wilhelm AJ, Mijnhout GS, Franssen EJ. Radiopharmaceuticals in sentinel lymph-node detection – an overview. Eur J Nucl Med. 1999;26(4 Suppl):S36–42.
8. Martin 2nd RC, Edwards MJ, Wong SL, Tuttle TM, Carlson DJ, Brown CM, Noyes RD, Glaser RL, Vennekotter DJ, Turk PS, Tate PS, Sardi A, Cerrito PB, McMasters KM. Practical guidelines for optimal gamma probe detection of sentinel lymph nodes in breast cancer: results of a multi-institutional study. For the University of Louisville Breast Cancer Study Group. Surgery. 2000;128(2):139–44.
9. Linehan DC, Hill AD, Tran KN, Yeung H, Yeh SD, Borgen PI, Cody 3rd HS. Sentinel lymph node biopsy in breast cancer: unfiltered radioisotope is superior to filtered. J Am Coll Surg. 1999;188(4):377–81.
10. Tanis PJ. Methodology and implications of lymphatic mapping and sentinel lymphadenectomy. Amsterdam: Print Partners Ipskamp BV; 2002.
11. Krag DN, Ashikaga T, Harlow SP, Weaver DL. Development of sentinel node targeting technique in breast cancer patients. Breast J. 1998; 4:67–74.
12. Winchester DJ, Sener SF, Winchester DP, Perlman RM, Goldschmidt RA, Motykie G, Martz CH, Rabbitt SL, Brenin D, Stull MA, Moulthrop JM. Sentinel lymphadenectomy for breast cancer: experience with 180 consecutive patients: efficacy of filtered technetium 99m sulphur colloid with overnight migration time. J Am Coll Surg. 1999;188(6):597–603.
13. McCarter MD, Yeung H, Yeh S, Fey J, Borgen PI, Cody 3rd HS. Localization of the sentinel node in breast cancer: identical results with same-day and day-before isotope injection. Ann Surg Oncol. 2001;8(8):682–6.
14. Martin RC, Derossis AM, Fey J, Yeung H, Yeh SD, Akhurst T, Heerdt AS, Petrek J, VanZee KJ, Montgomery LL, Borgen PI, Cody 3rd HS. Intradermal isotope injection is superior to intramammary in sentinel node biopsy for breast cancer. Surgery. 2001;130(3):432–8.
15. Povoski SP, Olsen JO, Young DC, Clarke J, Burak WE, Walker MJ, Carson WE, Yee LD, Agnese DM, Pozderac RV, Hall NC, Farrar WB. Prospective randomized clinical trial comparing intradermal, intraparenchymal, and subareolar injection routes for sentinel lymph node mapping and biopsy in breast cancer. Ann Surg Oncol. 2006;13(11):1412–21.
16. Rodier JF, Velten M, Wilt M, Martel P, Ferron G, Vaini-Elies V, Mignotte H, Bremond A, Classe JM, Dravet F, Routiot T, de Lara CT, Avril A, Lorimier G, Fondrinier E, Houvenaeghel G, Avigdor S. Prospective multicentric randomized study comparing periareolar and peritumoral injection of radiotracer and blue dye for the detection of sentinel lymph node in breast sparing procedures: FRANSENODE trial. J Clin Oncol. 2007;25(24):3664–9.
17. Ahmed M, Purushotham AD, Horgan K, Klaase JM, Douek M. Meta-analysis of superficial versus deep injection of radioactive tracer and blue dye for lymphatic mapping and detection of sentinel lymph nodes in breast cancer. Br J Surg. 2015;102(3):169–81.
18. Kim T, Giuliano AE, Lyman GH. Lymphatic mapping and sentinel lymph node biopsy in early-stage breast carcinoma: a metaanalysis. Cancer. 2006;106(1): 4–16.
19. McMasters KM, Reintgen DS, Ross MI, Wong SL, Gershenwald JE, Krag DN, Noyes RD, Viar V, Cerrito PB, Edwards MJ. Sentinel lymph node biopsy for melanoma: how many radioactive nodes should be removed? Ann Surg Oncol. 2001;8(3):192–7.
20. Klauber-DeMore N, Bevilacqua JL, Van Zee KJ, Borgen P, Cody 3rd HS. Comprehensive review of the management of internal mammary lymph node metastases in breast cancer. J Am Coll Surg. 2001;193(5): 547–55.
21. Veronesi U, Valagussa P. Inefficacy of internal mammary nodes dissection in breast cancer surgery. Cancer. 1981;47(1):170–5.

22. van der Ent FW, Kengen RA, van der Pol HA, Povel JA, Stroeken HJ, Hoofwijk AG. Halsted revisited: internal mammary sentinel lymph node biopsy in breast cancer. Ann Surg. 2001;234(1):79–84.
23. Farrús B, Vidal-Sicart S, Velasco M, Zanón G, Fernández PL, Muñoz M, Santamaría G, Albanell J, Biete A. Incidence of internal mammary node metastases after a sentinel lymph node technique in breast cancer and its implication in the radiotherapy plan. Int J Radiat Oncol Biol Phys. 2004;60(3):715–21.
24. Leidenius MH, Krogerus LA, Toivonen TS, Leppänen EA, von Smitten KA. The clinical value of parasternal sentinel node biopsy in breast cancer. Ann Surg Oncol. 2006;13(3):321–6.
25. Madsen E, Gobardhan P, Bongers V, Albregts M, Burgmans J, De Hooge P, Van Gorp J, van Dalen T. The impact on post-surgical treatment of sentinel lymph node biopsy of internal mammary lymph nodes in patients with breast cancer. Ann Surg Oncol. 2007;14(4):1486–92.
26. Heuts EM, van der Ent FW, von Meyenfeldt MF, Voogd AC. Internal mammary lymph drainage and sentinel node biopsy in breast cancer - A study on 1008 patients. Eur J Surg Oncol. 2009;35(3):252–7.
27. Port ER, Garcia-Etienne CA, Park J, Fey J, Borgen PI, Cody 3rd HS. Reoperative sentinel lymph node biopsy: a new frontier in the management of ipsilateral breast tumor recurrence. Ann Surg Oncol. 2007;14(8):2209–14.
28. van Deurzen CH, Vriens BE, Tjan-Heijnen VC, van der Wall E, Albregts M, van Hilligersberg R, Monninkhof EM, van Diest PJ. Accuracy of sentinel node biopsy after neoadjuvant chemotherapy in breast cancer patients: a systematic review. Eur J Cancer. 2009;45(18):3124–30.
29. Boughey JC, Suman VJ, Mittendorf EA, Ahrendt GM, Wilke LG, Taback B, Leitch AM, Kuerer HM, Bowling M, Flippo-Morton TS, Byrd DR, Ollila DW, Julian TB, McLaughlin SA, McCall L, Symmans WF, Le-Petross HT, Haffty BG, Buchholz TA, Nelson H, Hunt KK. Sentinel lymph node surgery after neoadjuvant chemotherapy in patients with node-positive breast cancer: the ACOSOG Z1071 (Alliance) clinical trial. JAMA. 2013;310(14):1455–61.
30. Kuehn T, Bauerfeind I, Fehm T, Fleige B, Hausschild M, Helms G, Lebeau A, Liedtke C, von Minckwitz G, Nekljudova V, Schmatloch S, Schrenk P, Staebler A, Untch M. Sentinel-lymph-node biopsy in patients with breast cancer before and after neoadjuvant chemotherapy (SENTINA): a prospective, multicentre cohort study. Lancet Oncol. 2013;14(7):609–18.
31. Linehan DC, Hill AD, Akhurst T, Yeung H, Yeh SD, Tran KN, Borgen PI, Cody 3rd HS. Intradermal radiocolloid and intraparenchymal blue dye injection optimize sentinel node identification in breast cancer patients. Ann Surg Oncol. 1999;6(5):450–4.
32. Cody 3rd HS, Fey J, Akhurst T, Fazzari M, Mazumdar M, Yeung H, Yeh SD, Borgen PI. Complementarity of blue dye and isotope in sentinel node localization for breast cancer: univariate and multivariate analysis of 966 procedures. Ann Surg Oncol. 2001;8(1):13–9.
33. Derossis AM, Fey J, Yeung H, Yeh SD, Heerdt AS, Petrek J, VanZee KJ, Montgomery LL, Borgen PI, Cody 3rd HS. A trend analysis of the relative value of blue dye and isotope localization in 2,000 consecutive cases of sentinel node biopsy for breast cancer. J Am Coll Surg. 2001;193(5):473–8.
34. McCarter MD, Yeung H, Fey J, Borgen PI, Cody 3rd HS. The breast cancer patient with multiple sentinel nodes: when to stop? J Am Coll Surg. 2001;192(6):692–7.
35. Cody 3rd HS, Borgen PI. State-of-the-art approaches to sentinel node biopsy for breast cancer: study design, patient selection, technique, and quality control at Memorial Sloan-Kettering Cancer Center. Surg Oncol. 1999;8(2):85–91.

Radioguided Surgery for Non-palpable Breast Lesions: I-125 Radioactive Seed Localization

8

Richard J. Gray, Charles E. Cox, and Emilia L. Dauway

Contents

Abstract

Because of several disadvantages, alternatives to wire localization (WL) for surgery of non-palpable breast lesions have been widely pursued. Radioactive seed localization (RSL) is a technique that has gained acceptance in many practices throughout the world and has been shown to be a safe, effective alternative to WL. RSL allows the localization procedure to be scheduled on a different day from the operative procedure, the operative incision to be planned with no regard for the entry point used for localization, and ongoing feedback as to the location of and distance from the lesion throughout the operation. Herein we describe the procedure, the available evidence of its effectiveness and safety, and the key issues in starting a RSL program.

R.J. Gray (✉)
Section of Surgical Oncology, Department of Surgery, Mayo Clinic, Scottsdale, AZ, USA
e-mail: gray.richard@mayo.edu

C.E. Cox
McCann Foundation Endowed Professor of Breast Surgery, Department of Surgery, University of South Florida, College of Medicine, Tampa, FL, USA

E.L. Dauway
Consultant Surgeon Senior Lecturer Department of Surgery, University of Queensland Mater Misericordiae Hospital, Queensland, QLD, Australia

K. Herrmann et al. (eds.), *Radioguided Surgery: Current Applications and Innovative Directions in Clinical Practice*, DOI 10.1007/978-3-319-26051-8_8

8.1 Introduction

Screening mammography has led to the more frequent detection of non-palpable breast lesions and non-palpable breast cancers. Therefore, radiologic localization of such lesions remains an important part of the breast surgeon's armamentarium. For decades the standard procedure for pre-excision localization has been wire localization (WL), in which a hooked wire is placed under mammography, ultrasound (US), or magnetic resonance imaging (MRI) guidance (Fig. 8.1). Unfortunately, WL has several persistent disadvantages. Localization takes place almost exclusively the same day as the operation, producing scheduling challenges in coordinating the placement of the wire and the operative procedure. In most practices this coordination eliminates the ability to perform a WL breast operation as the first case of the morning. In addition, wires can be displaced at post-localization mammography or transport [1–8] and have been transected during operative excision [1, 2, 4, 5, 7, 9–11]. The ideal entry site for localization of the lesion is often far from the location of the ideal incision for the operative excision of the lesion. This may result in a compromise at one of these sites or extensive subcutaneous dissection to retrieve the wire into the incision. Finally, the surgeon's ability to perceive the position of the lesion intraoperatively is based on the trajectory of the wire and a mental reconstruction of the available imaging. This leads to difficulty in maintaining dissection planes an appropriate distance from the lesion and in estimating the distal end of the wire. As a result, the reported rates of inadequate margins of excision for patients undergoing WL breast surgery are often greater than 30 % and as high as 73 % when the histology is unknown [12–15].

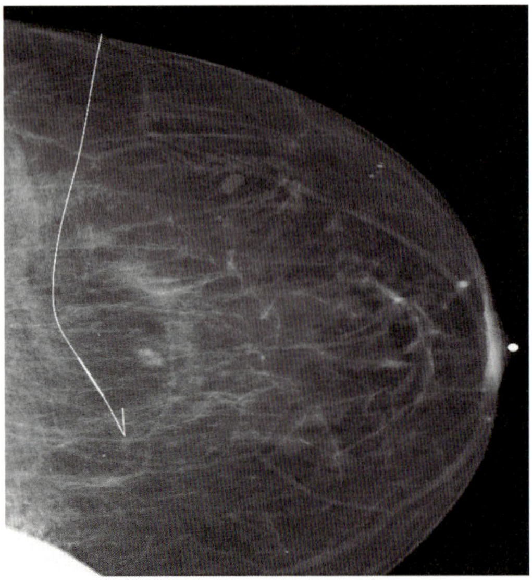

Fig. 8.1 Post-localization mammogram showing wire localization

Radioactive seed localization (RSL) is an alternative to WL that overcomes many of these disadvantages. RSL utilizes a titanium seed measuring 4.5 mm by 0.8 mm containing an I-125 dose of 0.100–0.150 mCi which is placed at the site of the non-palpable lesion by mammographic or US guidance (Figs. 8.2 and 8.3). These I-125 seeds are commonly used in prostate brachytherapy. The surgeon is able to use a gamma probe set to detect I-125 to guide the excision of the targeted lesion. This source of the low-energy gamma photon of I-125 (35 keV) can be detected as a distinct source from the Tc-99-labeled sulfur colloid (140 keV) used for sentinel lymph node (SLN) mapping and biopsy by selecting the appropriate energy range on any commercially available gamma probe [16]. Because the I-125 seed is contained within the breast, it is not subject to displacement and the localization procedure can be performed days in advance of the planned operation, thus uncoupling the schedules of the radiological localization and the operation. In some practices, RSL has even been placed prior to neoadjuvant

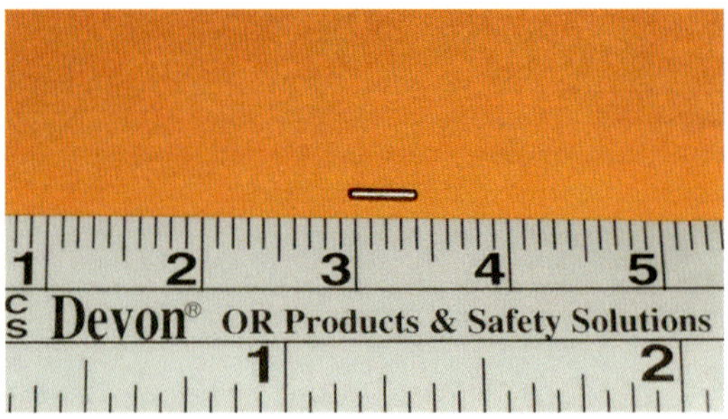

Fig. 8.2 Radioactive I-125 seed

chemotherapy with a gap of as long as several months between the localization and the operative excision [17]. The localization procedure can utilize the simplest angle of approach without consideration of the skin entry site, and the surgeon does not need to take into consideration the entry point in planning the incision as one would with WL. The gamma photon activity of the I-125 seed can be detected transcutaneously, allowing the skin incision to be more precisely placed while still allowing for a distant incision to be chosen for improved cosmesis if desired. The continuous gamma count and/or audible feedback allow constant reorientation during the procedure which may translate into better management of margins.

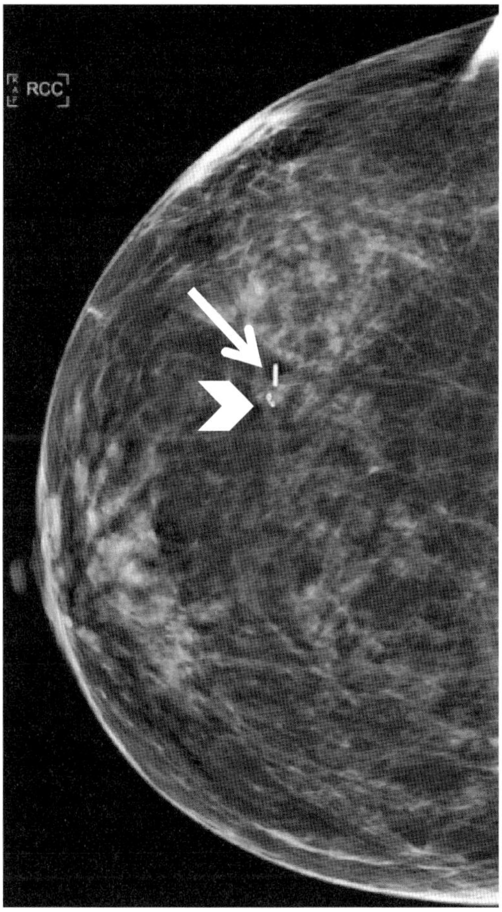

Fig. 8.3 Post-localization mammogram showing radioactive seed (*arrow*) and prior biopsy marking clip (*arrowhead*)

8.2 History of Radioactive Seed Localization

RSL was first described by two of us (CEC, ED) in a pilot study of 25 patients at the University of South Florida/H. Lee Moffitt Cancer Center [18] including establishing radiation safety and reliability of localization using these I-125 seeds [18]. This was followed by the first randomized, prospective trial which demonstrated improved margin management when compared to WL with no significant difference in operative time or excision volume [19]. Prospective validation of RSL was next reported in single-site studies from the University of South Florida/H. Lee Moffit Cancer Center and the Mayo Clinic in Arizona [20, 21]. RSL was then further validated in an expanded series including all three Mayo Clinic sites [22]. Since that time, multiple series have reported on RSL from worldwide institutions, all of which reported RSL to be preferred over WL or other techniques (Table 8.1).

8.3 Methods of Radioactive Seed Localization

8.3.1 Radiologic Localization

The RSL procedure begins with accurate placement of the seed at the site of the targeted breast lesion. The I-125 seed passes through an 18-guage needle, and early reports utilized a spinal needle with the tip occluded by bone wax for delivery of the I-125 seed to the lesion of interest. The seed is deployed by insertion of a stylette through the tip of the needle and bone wax [18–21]. Commercially available, preloaded needles are now offered for the localization procedure. Other than the different device itself, the localization procedure is performed the same as for WL and can be accomplished under US or mammographic guidance. Currently, MRI-guided deployment of an I-125 seed is not recommended due to the inability to use radiation detection equipment in these rooms, so clip placement by MRI followed by mammographically guided seed localization is utilized.

Table 8.1 Studies of radioactive seed localization versus other methods

Study (year)	*N*	Study type	Lesion retrieval rate for RSL (%)	Margins	Operative time	Localization time	Specimen volume
Gray (2001) [19]	97	Randomized vs. WL	100	Favor RSL	Not different	NR	Not different
Gray (2004)[a] [21]	199	Cohort vs. WL	100	Favor RSL	NR	NR	NR
Hughes (2008)[a] [22]	482	Cohort vs. WL	100	Favor RSL	NR	NR	NR
Mariscal Martinez (2009) [23]	134	Randomized vs. WL	100	Not different	Not different	Favor RSL	Not different
Rao (2010) [24]	88	Cohort vs. WL	100	Not different	NR	NR	NR
Lovrics (2011) [25]	305	Randomized vs. WL	100	Not different	Favor RSL	Not different	Not different
Murphy (2013) [26]	687	Cohort vs. WL	100	Not different	Favor WL	NR	Not different
Donker (2013)[b] [27]	154	Cohort vs. ROLL	100	Not different	NR	NR	NR

RSL radioactive seed localization, *WL* wire localization, *ROLL* radioguided occult lesion localization, *NR* not reported
[a]Some patients overlapped in these studies
[b]Included neoadjuvant chemotherapy patients only

After local anesthesia is administered to the chosen skin entry site, the lesion is visualized by US or mammogram and the needle containing the I-125 seed is advanced to or into the lesion. The stylette is then advanced to deploy the I-125 seed and the needle pulled back slightly to allow confirmation that the I-125 seed has separated from the needle and has not remained adherent to the occlusive material. The needle is withdrawn and mammography is used to confirm accurate deployment of the I-125 seed (Fig. 8.3). Similar to wire localization, more than one I-125 seed can be placed to bracket the area of intended excision (Fig. 8.4). Bracketing may be useful for patients with a lesion and associated microcalcifications, a broad area of microcalcifications, or a lesion with additional satellite lesion(s). It can be critical in the performance of oncoplastic excision of large volumes of breast tissue for such indications.

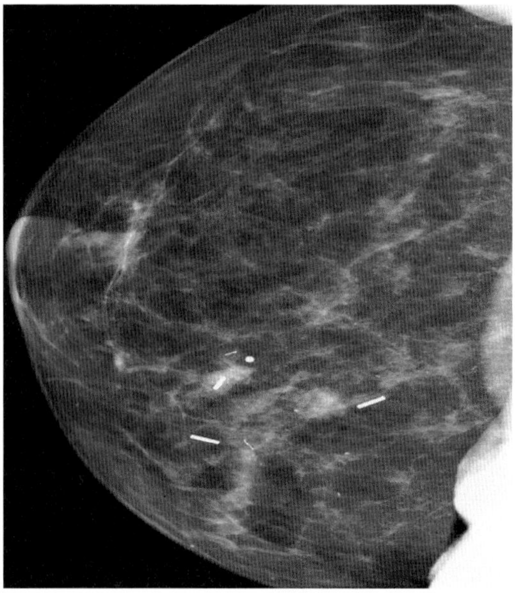

Fig. 8.4 Post-localization mammogram after bracketing radioactive seed localization

The approximately 60-day half-life of I-125 allows the localization procedure to occur well in advance of the planned operative excision [17], but in the United States, owing to the principle of the lowest possible radiation dose, the gap between these procedures is generally 5 days or fewer [16, 28]. This time frame results in a radiation dose to the residual breast tissue that is equal

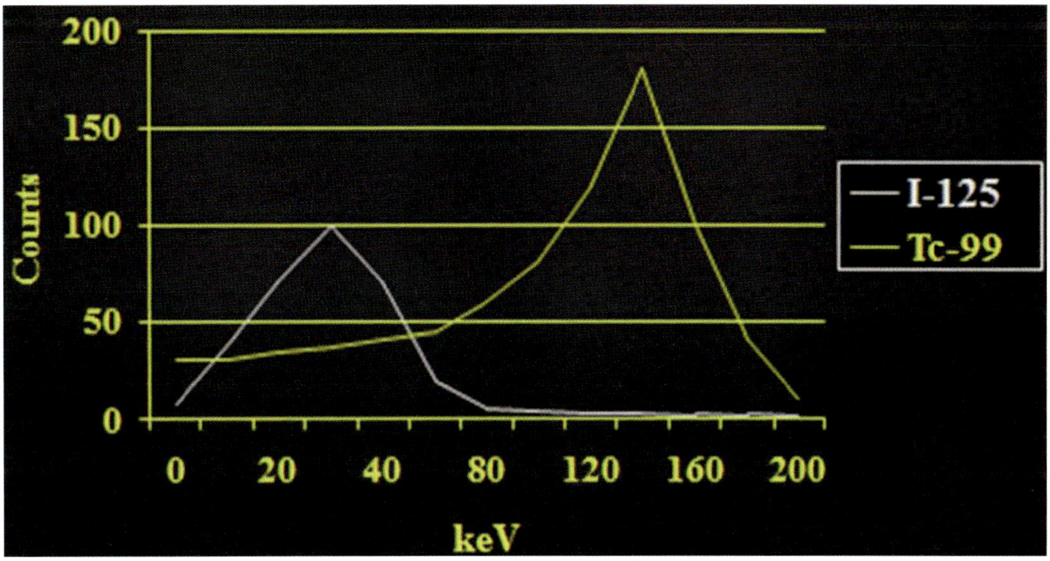

Fig. 8.5 Gamma photon energy detection for I-125 radioactive seed versus Tc-99 sulfur colloid used for sentinel lymph node biopsy

to or less than the skin dose from screening mammography [16]. The radiation doses from the I-125 seed to the patient, healthcare providers, the patients' family or friends, the general public, and even a breast-feeding infant are so low that no special precautions or labeling is necessary while the seed remains in place [16].

8.3.2 Surgical Excision

The surgical excision of a lesion after seed localization is accomplished using a standard handheld gamma probe that most surgeons use for SLN detection. These gamma probes have settings available for the detection of specific isotopes, including I-125 used for RSL and Tc-99 sulfur colloid used for SLN mapping and biopsy. Setting the probe to I-125 allows for the selective detection of the position of the radioactive seed, though some Compton scatter from a strong dose of Tc-99 (such as at the SLN injection site within the breast) will cause some gamma photon activity to be detected even at the I-125 setting (Fig. 8.5). Guided by the post-localization mammography, the gamma probe is scanned over the breast until the focus of most intense activity is detected (Fig. 8.6). This is the skin site closest to the site of the lesion which is often the best site for the incision, but any site may be used. Once an incision site is chosen and the incision is

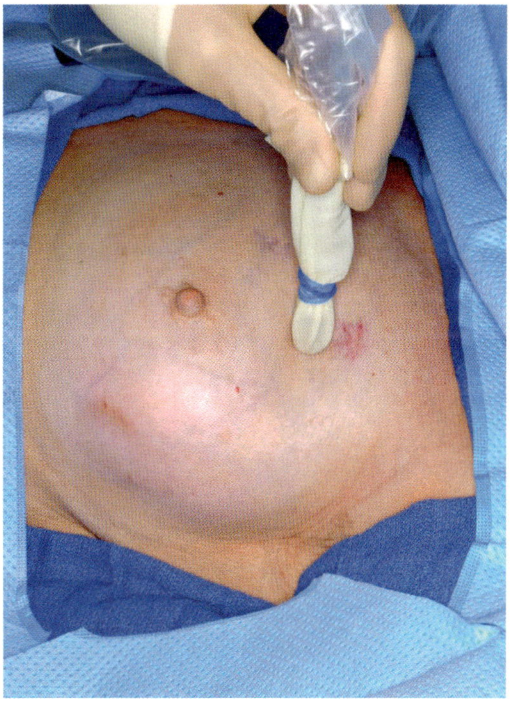

Fig. 8.6 Transcutaneous localization of I-125 seed with gamma probe

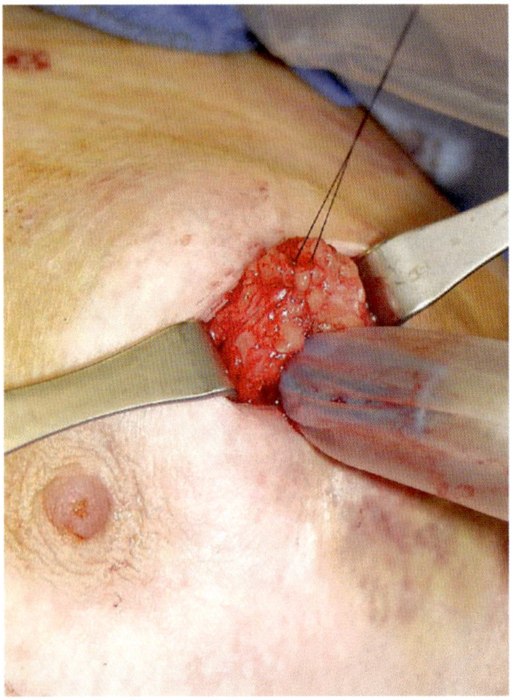

Fig. 8.7 Intraoperative assessment of depth of I-125 seed/lesion with gamma probe

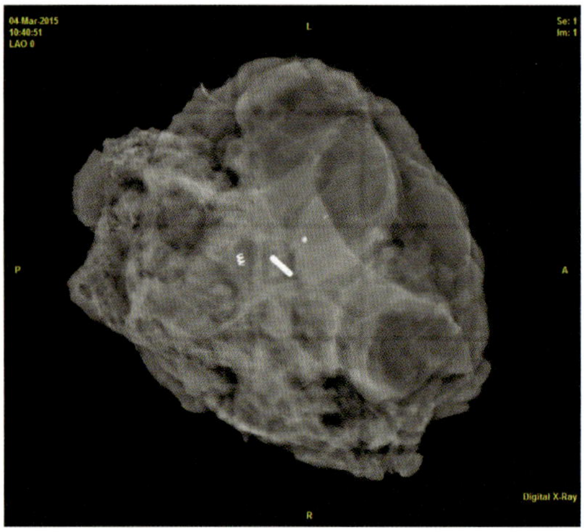

Fig. 8.8 Specimen radiograph with I-125 seed and biopsy clip

made, the gamma probe is used to guide the surgeon to the lesion. The gamma counts and/or audible feedback from the gamma probe allows a judgment as to the distance from the I-125 seed (and therefore the lesion) from any angle so that planes of dissection can be developed and maintained at an appropriate distance from the lesion without excessive normal breast tissue. The surgeon is clearly aware when he or she is deep to the seed and can safely come under the lesion based on this feedback (Fig. 8.7). The dissection through the breast tissue should be performed preferably with a scalpel or electrocautery device, rather than scissors. However, if scissors are used, then care should be taken not to cut through the titanium encasement of the I-125 seed. Since the surgeon should be aware of the location of the I-125 seed throughout the dissection with the use of the probe, this is unlikely and has yet to be reported.

The gamma probe is also used to confirm that the I-125 seed is contained within the resected specimen and that no remaining I-125 activity remains within the breast (except minor Compton scatter from Tc-99 as applicable) and to judge the adequacy of the margins of excision based on the level of gamma activity at each. The excised tissue specimen is then submitted for specimen radiography, providing additional confirmation that the targeted lesion and I-125 seed have been excised and maintaining documentation of this (Fig. 8.8). The seed-containing surgical specimen is transported for pathologic assessment with radioactive material labeling to alert the pathology providers that an I-125 seed is present and needs to be recovered for appropriate decay and disposal.

8.3.3 Pathologic Processing

The pathology staff retrieve the I-125 seed during the gross examination, sectioning, and processing of the surgical specimen [29]. Because of the low dose of radiation from the I-125 seed, there is no need for radiation protective equipment, and it is unnecessary for radiation badges to be worn by the pathology staff [16, 29]. After standard inking of margins, the specimen is serially sectioned and the I-125 seed located. Identification of the I-125 seed can be aided with the use of a gamma probe or other radiation detection device as needed [29]. If properly positioned, the location of the I-125 seed within the specimen assists the pathology personnel in identifying the breast lesion. Once identified, the I-125 seed is placed into a lead container and returned to nuclear medicine for long-term decay. Some have employed permanent containers within the pathology suite for decay, but this is not common and the required period of decay before disposal is approximately 2 years [16, 29]. If pathologic review is performed at a different institution than the institution that placed the I-125 seed, the I-125 seed can be removed prior to transporting the specimen. Otherwise, the pathology laboratory receiving the I-125 seed and specimen must be authorized to receive and handle radioactive materials including disposal of the I-125 seeds. Written protocols must be in place to ensure tracking of I-125 seeds throughout the process.

8.4 Evidence and Outcomes in Radioactive Seed Localization

RSL has been consistently shown to be an effective alternative to WL that is preferred by physicians and patients. Many studies have demonstrated other advantages, less consistently including lower rates of inadequate margins of excision, smaller specimen volumes and/or weights, shorter operative times, less pain for patients, and greater patient convenience.

8.4.1 Early Studies in the United States

The pilot study of RSL by Dauway et al. reported in 1999 found that the operative time from incision to specimen removal was 4.60 ± 0.49 min (range, 1–8 min) and specimen radiography and pathologic examination confirmed the retrieval of the I-125 seeds and lesions in all cases [18]. The first randomized, prospective trial by Gray et al. of 97 patients with non-palpable breast lesions randomized to RSL or WL demonstrated that RSL was associated with fewer patients requiring margin re-excision (26 % vs. 57 %, $p=0.02$) [19]. There were no significant differences between RSL and WL in mean times for operative excision (5.4 vs. 6.1 min, respectively) or radiographical localization (13.9 vs. 13.2 min, respectively). There were also no significant differences in the subjective ease of the procedures as rated by surgeons, radiologists, and patients [19].

In 2003, Cox and colleagues reported on 124 patients undergoing RSL breast procedures and found that it would be feasible to eliminate specimen radiography in 79 % of the cases based on intraoperative detection of gamma activity and pathologic gross identification of the targeted lesion [20]. As would be expected, avoiding specimen radiography reduced operative times. No seed migration was documented, and the I-125 seeds were again retrieved in 100 % of cases [20]. In a 2004 prospective validation of RSL in which 100 patients were compared to the immediately preceding cohort of 100 WL patients, Gray and colleagues reported that RSL was associated with lower rates of inadequate (<2 mm) margins of excision (10 % vs. 24 %, respectively, $p=0.01$) and was rated as more convenient by patients if the localization was at least 1 day prior to the operation [21]. There were no differences in the patients' ratings of pain or the SLN identification rates which were 100 % in both groups [21]. In an expanded series including all three Mayo Clinic sites, RSL was again shown to be associated with better margin management with the margins of the first specimen being >2 mm in 73 % of RSL patients versus 54 % of WL patients ($p<0.001$) and a second operation for margins being required in 8 % of RSL patients versus 25 % of WL patients ($p<0.001$). This series also found improved patient ratings of convenience with RSL but no difference in patient pain [22].

8.4.2 European Studies of Radioactive Seed Localization and Use after Neoadjuvant Therapy

The first European trial of RSL was reported from Barcelona in 2009 and was a prospective randomized study of RSL versus WL for 134 breast cancer patients undergoing breast-conserving surgery and SLN biopsy [23]. All lesions were successfully excised and the mean time needed for radiologic localization was significantly shorter for RSL ($p<0.001$). No statistical differences were found for the other parameters studied including specimen volume, rates of negative margins, and the rates of SLN identification [23]. This report was quickly followed by a report from Catharina Hospital in the Netherlands on 325 consecutive women undergoing RSL breast surgery for histologically proven malignancy [30]. Complete tumor removal was achieved in 95 % of these procedures. The same group also reported that 47 consecutive patients had successful RSL when undergoing I-125 seed placement before starting neoadjuvant chemotherapy. The operations were performed after a mean of 170 days (range, 70–220) from localization to surgery and the rate of positive margins was 6 % [17].

The Netherlands Cancer Institute compared the results of RSL after neoadjuvant chemotherapy ($n=71$) to radioguided occult lesion localization (ROLL, $n=83$) and found no differences in the rates of reoperation for inadequate margins, the median closest margin measurement, or the weight of specimens. They concluded that RSL simplified scheduling and was preferred [27]. RSL has also been utilized at the Netherlands Cancer Institute to localize lymph nodes with known metastases prior to neoadjuvant chemotherapy which they dubbed the MARI (marking the axilla with radioactive iodine seed) procedure. After neoadjuvant chemotherapy, the marked lymph nodes were removed followed by complete axillary lymph node dissection, and among the 15 patients studied, the pathologic response to chemotherapy in the RSL-marked lymph node was indicative of the overall response [31]. In a separate report, this group assessed the reliability of the positioning of I-125 seed radiologically and found that after a mean time in situ of 59 days (range 3–136 days), the mean seed migration was 0.9 mm. No differences in migration were found based on lesion type, days in situ, type of surgery, or radiologic method used to guide I-125 seed placement [32].

8.4.3 Evidence from Implementation Studies

Experiences with RSL program implementation and complications over time have also been reported [24, 26, 28]. In an initial experience with RSL in a US public healthcare system, Rao and colleagues reported no seed migration and 100 % success excising the targeted lesions [24]. They found on a matched-pair analysis that there was a 12 % lower rate of inadequate margins of excision (42 % for RSL vs. 54 % for WL), but this was not significant ($p=0.46$), perhaps due to small sample size. Importantly, this group reported on the serious consequences of misplacing an I-125 seed after it was removed from a patient; this resulted in the regulatory authorities temporarily suspending the RSL program [24].

In a retrospective review of 1000 consecutive RSL procedures performed at a single institution, 14 % of patients had more than one I-125 seed placed for a given procedure, 97 % of patients achieved negative margins at the first operation, and SLN identification was successful in 99.8 % of cases [28]. Adverse events included three I-125 seeds (0.3 %) not deployed correctly on the first attempt and 30 I-125 seed (2.6 %) displaced from the breast specimen during excision of the targeted lesion. All I-125 seeds were successfully retrieved, with no radiation safety concerns. When outcomes were analyzed by surgeon experience, there was no evidence of a learning curve [28].

In 2013 the group at Memorial Sloan Kettering Cancer Center reported their initial 6-month experience with 432 RSL procedures and compared the outcomes to the 256 WL procedures of the preceding 6-month period [26]. Positive margins were present in 7.7 % of RSL versus 5.5 % of WL patients, and an additional 16.9 % of RSL versus 19.9 % of WL had margins <1 mm ($p=0.38$). The median operative time was longer for lumpectomy and sentinel lymph node biopsy in the RSL group (55 vs. 48 min, $p<0.0001$). There was no significant difference in the volume of tissue excised between groups [26].

8.4.4 Canadian Randomized Trial of Radioactive Seed Localization

The largest prospective, randomized trial of RSL versus WL was a multi-institutional trial in Canada [25]. A total of 305 women with invasive or in situ carcinoma underwent randomization that was centralized, concealed, and stratified by surgeon. The procedures were performed at three sites, by seven surgeons. Using intention-to-treat analysis, there were no differences in positive margins rates for RSL vs. WL (10.5 % and 11.8 %, respectively, $p=0.99$) or for margins <1 mm (RSL 19 % and WL 22 %; $p=0.61$), though there was a significantly higher proportion of multifocal disease in the RSL group. Mean operative time was significantly shorter for RSL and surgeons rated RSL as significantly easier. Specimen volume, weight, reoperation rates, localization times, and radiologists' ranking of ease were similar for the two groups [25].

8.4.5 Systematic Review and Meta-Analysis of Radioactive Seed Localization

A systematic review [33] and a meta-analysis [34] of RSL studies have been published. The systematic review compared the outcomes of RSL versus standard WL in the management of non-palpable breast cancers. Eight studies were considered clinically relevant to the study. The analysis demonstrated an overall combined odds ratio (OR) of 0.51 (95 % CI, 0.36–0.72; $z=3.88$; $p=0.0001$) for involved surgical margin status, an OR of 0.47 (95 % CI, 0.33–0.69; $z=3.96$; $p<0.0001$) for reoperation rates, and mean difference (MD) of −1.32 (95 % CI, −2.32, −0.32; $z=2.58$; $p=0.01$) for operative time favoring RSL over WL. There was no significant difference found for volume of tissue excised [33]. In the meta-analysis, 4280 patients in 16 articles were considered eligible for inclusion for examination of the rates of positive margins and reoperation. After contacting the authors and exclusion of duplicate patient reports, 3168 patients were analyzed. Margins of resection, though reported differently by different institutions (0–2 mm from resection margin), were positive/inadequate in 10.3 % (range, 3–30 %) of the patients having RSL resections. This resulted in a final re-excision rate of 14.2 % (range, 4–42 %).

8.4.6 Summary of Evidence

The available individual studies, meta-analysis [34], and review articles [33, 35–37] demonstrate that RSL is clearly safe, feasible, and effective for the localization and surgical excision of non-palpable breast lesions. It is at least as effective as WL (and ROLL) in achieving negative margins of excision for malignant lesions without compromising localization times, operative times, specimen volumes, or the patient experience. In many of the studies, these factors were better for RSL and in no study was WL superior to RSL in any of these measures except operative time in one study of early experience. On the basis of this evidence, RSL should be considered at least the equal of what is widely considered the "gold standard" for the localization of breast lesions while at a minimum providing more flexible scheduling procedures for patients and providers.

8.5 Issues in Establishing a Radioactive Seed Localization Program

While having a RSL program has many advantages, starting a program involves significant effort in achieving multidisciplinary coordination and regulatory compliance. The most significant obstacles have been reported to be administrative barriers, billing and coding, not having a multidisciplinary team that is supportive of RSL, and radiation safety/regulatory issues.

8.5.1 Administrative Barriers

The identification and coordination of a multidisciplinary team to plan a RSL program, gain regulatory approval, and produce institutional changes in procedural flow and billing require considerable effort. Physicians interested in RSL have been able to drive such change but not without institutional support. Thus it is important for a breast care team to assure institutional administrative support early in RSL program planning to assure success. The ability to achieve improved scheduling flexibility and higher patient satisfaction [21, 22, 36] is important to institutional administrators and helps achieve buy-in for these efforts. RSL program institution often requires many months of planning which is best sustained through administrative support to the physician leaders of these programs.

In many practices, the place where radiologic localization occurs is different from where the operative excision occurs which may also be different from where the pathologic processing occurs. In such circumstances, the administrative leadership for each site must be willing to coordinate their efforts in achieving regulatory approval when operating under separate licenses. Some programs have required creative protocols to avoid licensure conflicts such as the surgeon inking and serially sectioning the specimen in order to retrieve the radioactive seed before submitting the specimen to another site for pathologic assessment. Such protocols, however, can only be achieved if the administrative and regulatory issues are identified appropriately, usually through strong administrator-physician partnership.

8.5.2 Billing and Coding

Billing and coding for RSL has become simplified in recent years. In the United States, the Current Procedural Terminology (CPT) codes used for the RSL radiological localization procedure and surgical excision procedure are now the same as those used for WL procedures. It is important, however, to consult with one's billing and coding personnel to assure the appropriate transition to such billing to avoid miscoding or the use of miscellaneous codes that may reimburse at lower rates. RSL programs appear to be cost-effective [38].

8.5.3 Multidisciplinary Support

RSL programs are often desired by surgeons, but the procedure requires willing partners in breast imaging, nuclear medicine, pathology, and radiation safety. Failures in attempts to establish RSL programs are often precipitated by a lack of coordinated effort from each of these disciplines. Successful efforts generally involve planning meetings of individuals from each of these disciplines with an agreement that all judge the effort in establishing a RSL program to be worthwhile. Each participant must be invested since each plays a crucial role in assuring nuclear regulatory approval, realistic and safe protocols, and the needed communication lines required if unexpected events or problems arise. Even after the RSL program begins, follow-up assessments can assure that all procedures are working properly and any safety or "near-miss" events are addressed among all the disciplines to avoid risks of nuclear regulatory noncompliance [24].

8.5.4 Radiation Safety and Nuclear Regulatory Compliance

For the clinicians involved, part of the beauty of transitioning to a RSL program is that no new skills or capital equipment are required. The team must, however, be trained in safe handling of the I-125 seeds and in procedures for identification of I-125 seeds to assure safe return. The surgeon involved may need certification from the radiation safety officer or committee on the safe handling of radioactive material. He or she also plays an important role in developing a fail-safe plan for identifying and recovering each I-125 seed.

Nuclear medicine physicians and radiation safety officers are valuable partners in developing a RSL program because of their knowledge of nuclear regulatory compliance and the facilities and protocols available for receipt, storage, and decay of radioactive materials. Similarly, a process for tracking the I-125 seeds must be established including receipt by the institution, distribution for the localization procedure, retrieval from the pathology department, and return to nuclear medicine for decay or return to the vendor. In the United States, the use of I-125 seeds for breast lesion localization is performed under the direction of the diagnostic authorized users of radioactive material.

Post-localization mammogram and specimen radiographs are strongly advised for all RSL cases to document I-125 seed placement in the patient and I-125 seed removal from the patient, respectively. That the source is no longer in the patient can also be documented by identification of the I-125 seed by the pathologist based on institutional practice [20]. One must document a proper nuclear survey if these requirements are not met. These records must be available for review to meet nuclear safety regulations. Radiation safety requirements vary by country and state. It is therefore essential that your radiation safety officer investigate the necessary steps within your country and state to gain this approval. RSL has been endorsed by the US Nuclear Regulatory Commission which has provided guidance at its website. In Europe, there are generally nuclear regulations for each country in addition to those of the European Union which must be met.

The institutional protocol should include steps to ensure safety and that no I-125 seed will be misplaced or lost. In general, it is required (and is wise regardless of regulatory requirement) to mark the specimen with a radioactive material label to assure every handler is aware of the presence of a radioactive device within the specimen. The low dose of the I-125 seed means there is no need for providers or patients to undergo any special monitoring or labeling [16]. The radiation exposure to the residual breast tissue from the I-125 seed after a typical dose, exposure time, and lumpectomy volume is similar to the peak skin dose from a standard two-view mammogram [16].

8.5.5 Lost I-125 Seed Protocol

Developing a fail-safe I-125 seed identification procedure in case of a lost I-125 seed is essential. If the plane of surgical dissection passes through the plane of the I-125 seed or a hematoma containing the I-125 seed, it can become free in the surgical field and then lost into suction devices, sponges, or elsewhere [24, 28]. The surgeon must use the gamma probe intraoperatively to assure the I-125 seed is within the excised specimen before passing the specimen off the field and must also assure no remaining I-125 activity is within the breast (other than minor background gamma activity detected from the Compton scatter of the Tc-99 used for the SLN injection). If the I-125 seed is not identified within the specimen, the gamma probe should be used to scan the lumpectomy cavity for the displaced I-125 seed. If not identified, the gamma probe should be used to scan the suction device, suction tubing, suction canister, surgical sponges, surgical drapes, and even the operating room floor to identify the I-125 seed. If the I-125 seed remains lost, a radiation safety team should survey the operating room and any other necessary location to find the missing I-125 seed. No personnel, specimens, or other items should leave the operating room until this has been accomplished. Failing to properly identify all I-125 seeds can threaten one's nuclear regulatory license [24] and result in a threat to not only maintaining a RSL program but an institutional radioactive license.

Conclusions

RSL for non-palpable breast lesions is effective, safe, and provides important flexibility in scheduling that improves the patient experience and institutional efficiency. It is at least as effective as WL in achieving negative margins of excision for malignant lesions without compromising localization times, operative times, specimen volumes, or the patient experience.

RSL does, however, require coordinated efforts from a multidisciplinary team to implement. The actual technical procedures are easy to learn and familiar to breast imagers and surgeons. Breast surgeons' familiarity with radioguided surgery makes the procedure intuitive and welcomed. RSL is a most attractive alternative to WL for non-palpable breast lesions.

References

1. Azoury F, Sayad P, Rizk A. Thoracoscopic management of a pericardial migration of a breast biopsy localization wire. Ann Thorac Surg. 2009;87(6):1937–9.
2. Banitalebi H, Skaane P. Migration of the breast biopsy localization wire to the pulmonary hilus. Acta Radiol. 2005;46(1):28–31.
3. Davis PS, Wechsler RJ, Feig SA, March DE. Migration of breast biopsy localization wire. AJR Am J Roentgenol. 1988;150(4):787–8.
4. Helvie MA, Ikeda DM, Adler DD. Localization and needle aspiration of breast lesions: complications in 370 cases. AJR Am J Roentgenol. 1991;157(4):711–4.
5. Homer MJ, Pile-Spellman ER. Needle localization of occult breast lesions with a curved-end retractable wire: technique and pitfalls. Radiology. 1986;161(2):547–8.
6. Kopans DB. Migration of breast biopsy localization wire. AJR Am J Roentgenol. 1988;151(3):614–5.
7. Rappaport W, Thompson S, Wong R, Leong S, Villar H. Complications associated with needle localization biopsy of the breast. Surg Gynecol Obstet. 1991; 172(4):303–6.
8. Wales LR. Prevention of migration of breast biopsy localization wire. AJR Am J Roentgenol. 1988; 151(2):413.
9. Bristol JB, Jones PA. Transgression of localizing wire into the pleural cavity prior to mammography. Br J Radiol. 1981;54(638):139–40.
10. Bronstein AD, Kilcoyne RF, Moe RE. Complications of needle localization of foreign bodies and nonpalpable breast lesions. Arch Surg. 1988;123(6):775–9.
11. Homer MJ. Transection of the localization hooked wire during breast biopsy. AJR Am J Roentgenol. 1983;141(5):929–30.
12. McLaughlin SA, Ochoa-Frongia LM, Patil SM, Cody 3rd HS, Sclafani LM. Influence of frozen-section analysis of sentinel lymph node and lumpectomy margin status on reoperation rates in patients undergoing breast-conservation therapy. J Am Coll Surg. 2008; 206(1):76–82.
13. O'Sullivan MJ, Li T, Freedman G, Morrow M. The effect of multiple reexcisions on the risk of local recurrence after breast conserving surgery. Ann Surg Oncol. 2007;14(11):3133–40.
14. Thompson M, Henry-Tillman R, Margulies A, Thostenson J, Bryant-Smith G, Fincher R, Korourian S, Klimberg VS. Hematoma-directed ultrasound-guided (HUG) breast lumpectomy. Ann Surg Oncol. 2007; 14(1):148–56.
15. Velanovich V, Lewis Jr FR, Nathanson SD, Strand VF, Talpos GB, Bhandarkar S, Elkus R, Szymanski W, Ferrara JJ. Comparison of mammographically guided breast biopsy techniques. Ann Surg. 1999;229(5):625–30; discussion 630–3.
16. Pavlicek W, Walton HA, Karstaedt PJ, Gray RJ. Radiation safety with use of I-125 seeds for localization of nonpalpable breast lesions. Acad Radiol. 2006;13(7):909–15.
17. van Riet YE, Maaskant AJ, Creemers GJ, van Warmerdam LJ, Jansen FH, van de Velde CJ, Rutten HJ, Nieuwenhuijzen GA. Identification of residual breast tumour localization after neo-adjuvant chemotherapy using a radioactive 125 Iodine seed. Eur J Surg Oncol J Eur Soc Surg Oncol Br Assoc Surg Oncol. 2010;36(2):164–9.
18. EL Dauway SR, Friedland J, Berman C, Ku NN, Reintgen DS, Yeatman T, Falcone R, Crawford S, Cox CE. Innovative diagnostics for breast cancer: new frontiers for the new millennium using radioactive seed localization. Surg Forum. 1999;50:348–9.
19. Gray RJ, Salud C, Nguyen K, Dauway E, Friedland J, Berman C, Peltz E, Whitehead G, Cox CE. Randomized prospective evaluation of a novel technique for biopsy or lumpectomy of nonpalpable breast lesions: radioactive seed versus wire localization. Ann Surg Oncol. 2001;8(9):711–5.
20. Cox CE, Furman B, Stowell N, Ebert M, Clark J, Dupont E, Shons A, Berman C, Beauchamp J, Gardner M, Hersch M, Venugopal P, Szabunio M, Cressman J, Diaz N, Vrcel V, Fairclough R. Radioactive seed localization breast biopsy and lumpectomy: can specimen radiographs be eliminated? Ann Surg Oncol. 2003; 10(9):1039–47.
21. Gray RJ, Pockaj BA, Karstaedt PJ, Roarke MC. Radioactive seed localization of nonpalpable breast lesions is better than wire localization. Am J Surg. 2004;188(4):377–80.
22. Hughes JH, Mason MC, Gray RJ, McLaughlin SA, Degnim AC, Fulmer JT, Pockaj BA, Karstaedt PJ, Roarke MC. A multi-site validation trial of radioactive seed localization as an alternative to wire localization. Breast J. 2008;14(2):153–7.
23. Mariscal Martinez A, Sola M, de Tudela AP, Julian JF, Fraile M, Vizcaya S, Fernandez J. Radioguided localization of nonpalpable breast cancer lesions: randomized comparison with wire localization in patients undergoing conservative surgery and sentinel node biopsy. AJR Am J Roentgenol. 2009;193(4):1001–9.
24. Rao R, Moldrem A, Sarode V, White J, Amen M, Rao M, Andrews V, Euhus D, Radford L, Ulissey M. Experience with seed localization for nonpalpable breast lesions in a public health care system. Ann Surg Oncol. 2010;17(12):3241–6.
25. Lovrics PJ, Goldsmith CH, Hodgson N, McCready D, Gohla G, Boylan C, Cornacchi S, Reedijk M. A multicentered, randomized, controlled trial comparing radioguided seed localization to standard wire localization for nonpalpable, invasive and in situ breast carcinomas. Ann Surg Oncol. 2011;18(12):3407–14.
26. Murphy JO, Moo TA, King TA, Van Zee KJ, Villegas KA, Stempel M, Eaton A, St Germain JM, Morris E, Morrow M. Radioactive seed localization compared to wire localization in breast-conserving surgery: initial 6-month experience. Ann Surg Oncol. 2013; 20(13):4121–7.
27. Donker M, Drukker CA, Valdes Olmos RA, Rutgers EJ, Loo CE, Sonke GS, Wesseling J, Alderliesten T, Vrancken Peeters MJ. Guiding breast-conserving

surgery in patients after neoadjuvant systemic therapy for breast cancer: a comparison of radioactive seed localization with the ROLL technique. Ann Surg Oncol. 2013;20(8):2569–75.
28. McGhan LJ, McKeever SC, Pockaj BA, Wasif N, Giurescu ME, Walton HA, Gray RJ. Radioactive seed localization for nonpalpable breast lesions: review of 1,000 consecutive procedures at a single institution. Ann Surg Oncol. 2011;18(11):3096–101.
29. Graham RP, Jakub JW, Brunette JJ, Reynolds C. Handling of radioactive seed localization breast specimens in the pathology laboratory. Am J Surg Pathol. 2012;36(11):1718–23.
30. van Riet YE, Jansen FH, van Beek M, van de Velde CJ, Rutten HJ, Nieuwenhuijzen GA. Localization of non-palpable breast cancer using a radiolabelled titanium seed. Br J Surg. 2010;97(8):1240–5.
31. Straver ME, Loo CE, Alderliesten T, Rutgers EJ, Vrancken Peeters MT. Marking the axilla with radioactive iodine seeds (MARI procedure) may reduce the need for axillary dissection after neoadjuvant chemotherapy for breast cancer. Br J Surg. 2010;97(8):1226–31.
32. Alderliesten T, Loo CE, Pengel KE, Rutgers EJ, Gilhuijs KG, Vrancken Peeters MJ. Radioactive seed localization of breast lesions: an adequate localization method without seed migration. Breast J. 2011; 17(6):594–601.
33. Ahmed M, Douek M. Radioactive seed localisation (RSL) in the treatment of non-palpable breast cancers: systematic review and meta-analysis. Breast. 2013; 22(4):383–8.
34. Pouw B, de Wit-van der Veen LJ, Stokkel MP, Loo CE, Vrancken Peeters MJ, Valdes Olmos RA. Heading toward radioactive seed localization in non-palpable breast cancer surgery? A meta-analysis. J Surg Oncol. 2015;111(2):185–91.
35. Barentsz MW, van den Bosch MA, Veldhuis WB, van Diest PJ, Pijnappel RM, Witkamp AJ, Verkooijen HM. Radioactive seed localization for non-palpable breast cancer. Br J Surg. 2013;100(5):582–8.
36. Jakub JW, Gray RJ, Degnim AC, Boughey JC, Gardner M, Cox CE. Current status of radioactive seed for localization of non palpable breast lesions. Am J Surg. 2010;199(4):522–8.
37. Dua SM, Gray RJ, Keshtgar M. Strategies for localisation of impalpable breast lesions. Breast. 2011; 20(3):246–53.
38. Loving VA, Edwards DB, Roche KT, Steele JR, Sapareto SA, Byrum SC, Schomer DF. Monte Carlo simulation to analyze the cost-benefit of radioactive seed localization versus wire localization for breast-conserving surgery in fee-for-service health care systems compared with accountable care organizations. AJR Am J Roentgenol. 2014;202(6):1383–8.

Radioguided Surgery of Non-palpable Breast Lesions: Radio Occult Lesion Localization (ROLL)

9

Bas Pouw, Marie-Jeanne T.F.D. Vrancken Peeters, and Renato A. Valdés Olmos

Contents

B. Pouw, MSc (✉)
Departement of nuclear medicine, The Netherlands Cancer Institute, Amsterdam, The Netherlands
e-mail: b.pouw@nki.nl

M.-J.T.F.D. Vrancken Peeters, MD, PhD
Departement of surgical oncology, The Netherlands Cancer Institute, Amsterdam, The Netherlands

R.A. Valdés Olmos, MD, PhD
Departement of nuclear medicine, The Netherlands Cancer Institute, Amsterdam, The Netherlands

Leiden University Medical Centre, Leiden, The Netherlands

Abstract

The incidence of non-palpable breast cancer is rising since national screening programs were introduced. More than 25 % of the radiological suspicious breast lesions are considered clinically occult or non-palpable. Surgical removal of non-palpable breast tumors requires a specific approach. The main challenge of resecting non-palpable lesions is to ensure clear margins while minimizing the resection of healthy tissue and cosmetic damage. Radioguided occult lesion localization (ROLL) using a radioactive tracer (e.g., technetium 99m; half-life of approximately 6 hours) was developed in 1996 and is nowadays used in several institutes as a reliable alternative for wire-guided localization. The commonly used radiotracer is technetium 99m (Tc 99m) macroaggregate albumin (MAA) with a particle size of 10–150 μm, which can be detected by the surgeon using a gamma probe. The tracer is administered by an intratumoral injection, and accordingly, this site is surgically excised at the operating room while using a gamma probe. At the moment more than 29 peer-reviewed articles have emerged about ROLL. The general consensus is that ROLL, using Tc 99m, is preferable over wire-guided localization with the main advantages: the patient comfort, positive margins, and localization time. Furthermore, the procedure can be combined with a sentinel lymph node biopsy.

K. Herrmann et al. (eds.), *Radioguided Surgery: Current Applications and Innovative Directions in Clinical Practice*, DOI 10.1007/978-3-319-26051-8_9

9.1 Background and Clinical Application

9.1.1 General Background

The incidence of non-palpable breast cancer is rising since national screening programs were introduced. Breast cancer screening has changed the type and stage of detected breast cancer lesions. More than 25 % of the radiological suspicious breast lesions are considered clinically occult or non-palpable [1]. This includes small invasive lesions, ductal carcinoma in situ (DCIS), or smaller clusters of microcalcifications. The surgical removal of non-palpable breast tumors requires a specific approach. The main challenge of resecting non-palpable lesions is to ensure clear margins while minimizing the resection of healthy tissue and cosmetic damage [2]. For this purpose, mostly three different techniques are used for intraoperative tumor localization: wire-, ultrasound (US)-, and radioguided localization (i.e., guided by a radioactive tracer or radioactive marker). At present, wire-guided localization (WGL) is still the most commonly used technique for non-palpable breast cancer (75 %) [1, 3]. Nonetheless, wire placement is a cumbersome technique for both the surgeon and the patient. The limitations of WGL include (1) technical complications such as wire dislodging [4, 5], migration [6, 7], kinking or fracture; (2) logistic challenges as the wire is to be placed a maximum of one day in advance of surgery; (3) higher patient discomfort as opposed to alternative techniques [8, 9]; and (4) poor cosmetic outcome [10, 11]. Dislodging and poor localization are causes for relatively high irradicality rates for WGL ranging from 10 to 50 % [1, 5, 12–17]. Radioguided occult lesion localization (ROLL) using a radioactive tracer (e.g., technetium 99m) was developed in 1996 and is nowadays used in several institutes as a reliable alternative for WGL [1, 16, 18–22]. A relatively newer and still less frequently used localization technique is the ROLL technique using a radioactive marker (e.g., iodine 125 (^{125}I) marker), named radioactive seed localization (RSL) [23, 24]. One study describes the use of ROLL as an addition to WGL [25]. In this setting, the tumor localization was guided by the Tc 99m and the wire was used to guide intratumoral blue dye injection. Afterward the results of the WGL + ROLL were compared with WGL only.

9.1.2 Tracer Administration

The principle of the ROLL technique using a radioactive tracer consists of an image-guided intratumoral injection of this radioactive tracer. The most frequently used techniques to visualize the tumor are ultrasound and/or stereotaxis. The radiotracer that is commonly used is technetium 99m (Tc 99m) macroaggregate albumin (MAA) with a particle size of 10–150 μm, which is retained within the tumor without any significant migration to lymph nodes and can be detected by the surgeon using a gamma probe. The dosage of radiolabeled MAA varies from 1 MBq to 123 MBq in literature [26–28].

Both the ultrasound-guided and the stereotactic-guided administration routes enable real-time feedback about the needle tip position and the tumor location. By real-time validation of this location, a secure intratumoral injection is facilitated (Fig. 9.1). The injected suspension consists of 0.5 μg MAA radiolabeled with Tc 99m in a volume of 0.2 ml. When the lesion can be accurately visualized with both stereotaxis and ultrasound, the preferred injection method is the ultrasound-guided technique because of better needle tracking [29]. For both stereotaxis and ultrasound, a spinal needle (22 gauge) is recommended in order to facilitate the connection of the syringe with the radioactive tracer. Usually the radiologist introduces the needle into the tumor under continuous monitoring by ultrasound. Subsequently, the nuclear physician connects the syringe containing the radiotracer to the needle. A 1 ml tuberculin syringe with Luer-Lok connection is strongly recommended in order to prevent leakage of the tracer during injection. A 0.1 ml air bubble, positioned behind the radioactivity volume, in the syringe may help to flush the tracer rest from the needle. Figure 9.2 illustrates stepwise the procedure. Pitfalls during the tracer administration are spill on the skin (contamination), missed localization, and spillage to the liver by puncturing a blood vessel.

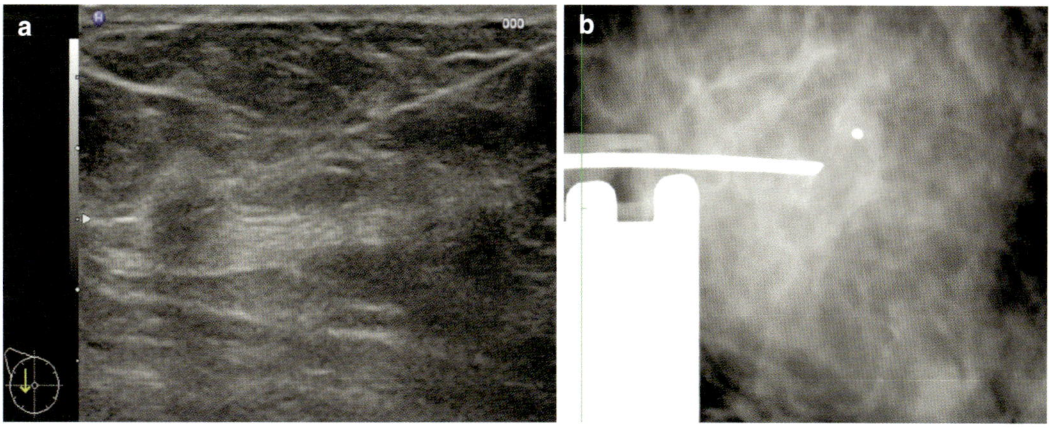

Fig. 9.1 Injection techniques. (**a**) Ultrasound-guided tracer injection. The needle is positioned in the lesion. (**b**) Stereotactic-guided tracer injection. The tip of the needle is positioned at the site of the tumor marker

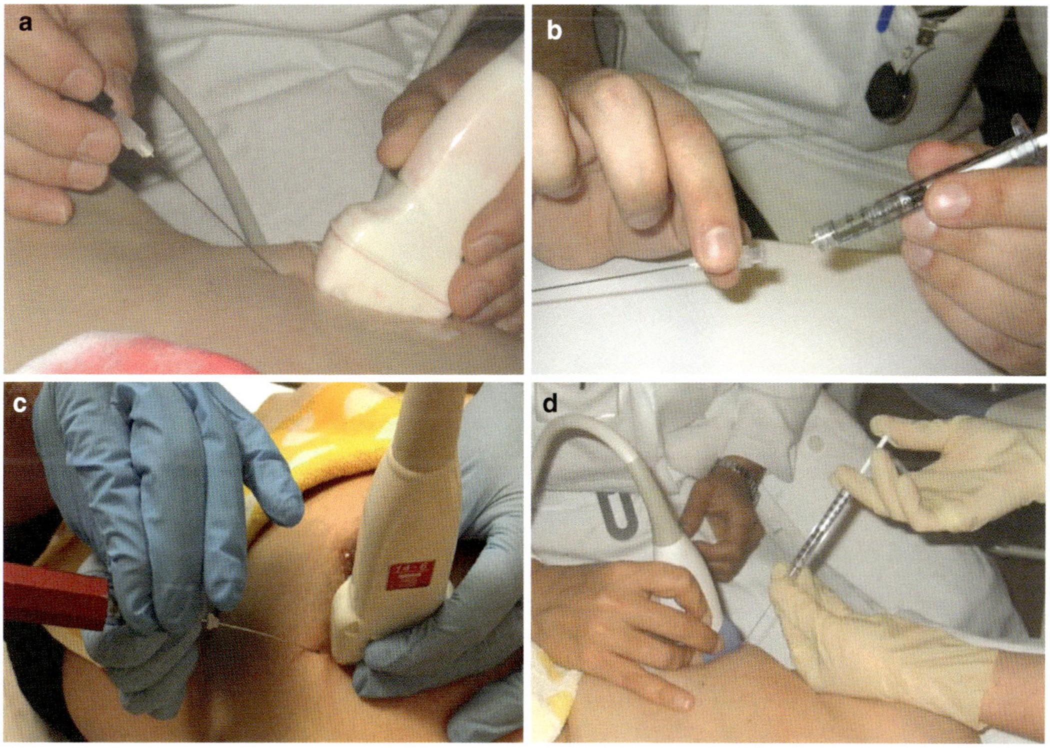

Fig. 9.2 Tracer administration procedure. (**a**) Ultrasound-guided needle tip position in the lesion. (**b**) A 1 ml tuberculin syringe with Luer-Lok connection in order to prevent leakage. (**c**) The syringe with an attached lead cover for radiation protection. (**d**) US-guided Tc 99m injection. A 0.1 ml air bubble, positioned behind the radioactivity volume, in the syringe may help to flush the tracer rest from the needle

9.1.3 Combining ROLL with SLNB

To combine ROLL with a sentinel lymph node biopsy (SLNB), two different approaches have been described in literature. For the first approach, Tc 99m MAA is injected intratumorally and Tc 99m albumin nanocolloid for the SLNB is injected subdermally at the level of the lesion [30, 31]. The

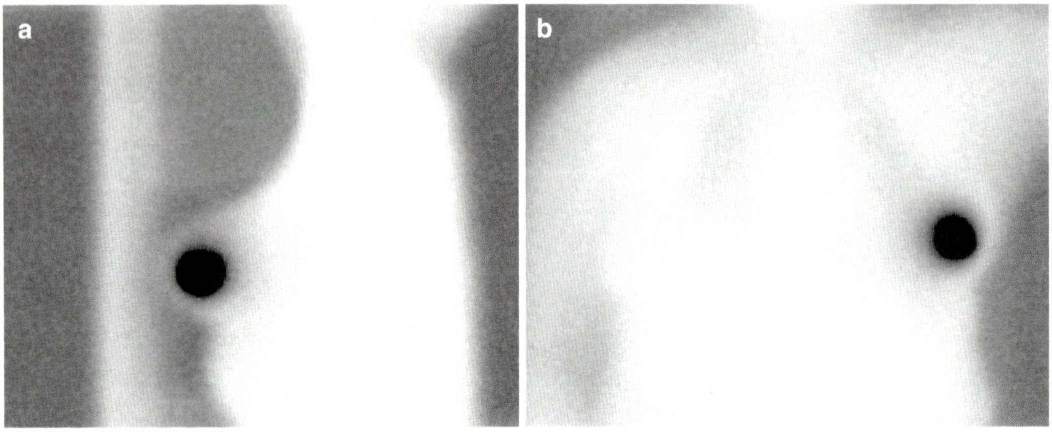

Fig. 9.3 Nuclear imaging. (**a**) A lateral and (**b**) an anterior view of the tracer deposit in the tumor

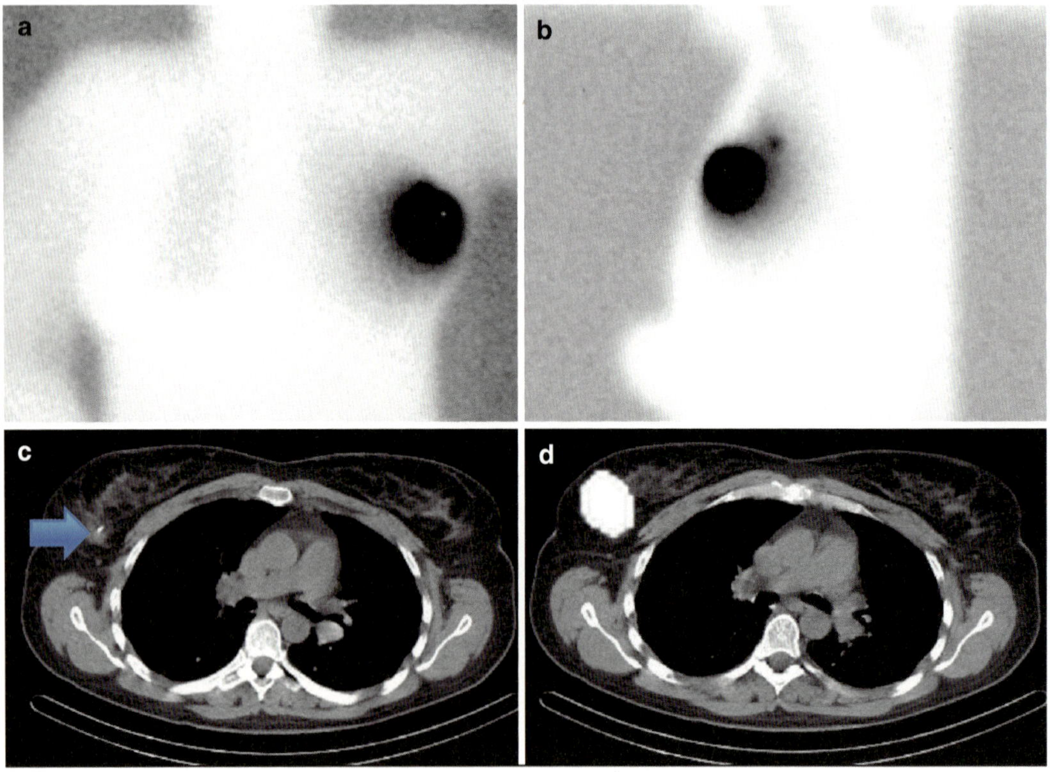

Fig. 9.4 Sentinel node+radioguided occult lesion localization (SNOLL). (**a**) anterior image with the injection site. (**b**) Lateral image with an SN. (**c**) Axial CT scan with the tumor maker indicated with the *arrow*. (**d**) Axial SPECT/CT scan with the radioactivity deposit at the site of the tumor marker

second approach combines the two procedures in one injection using Tc 99m albumin nanocolloid into the tumor. This tracer has a particle size of 5–80 nm, and a small fraction of the radioactivity migrates from the tumor to the lymph nodes which enables the use of the tracer for combined ROLL and SLNB in one session; the procedure is also called SNOLL procedure (SN+ROLL) [2,

19, 32–35] (Figs. 9.3 and 9.4). The advantage of using Tc 99m MAA is that it acts more as a point source compared to the Tc 99m albumin nanocolloid, which partially diverges into the lymphatics. The advantage of using only one tracer for both procedures is a more simplistic procedure with only one injection.

9.1.4 Imaging

Gamma camera imaging for a ROLL procedure may be performed to ensure that the radioactive tracer stays locally in the breast lesion and does not disperse though the breast parenchyma or small vessels; it is also helpful to depict contaminations, for example, on the skin. Static scintigraphic imaging 10–15 min after administration is sufficient to assess this. If contamination has occurred, skin decontamination is recommended to avoid spurious intraoperative findings [2]. When wide spread of the radiotracer through the breast parenchyma is observed, another localization technique (e.g., wire guided) should be considered; this happened in 4 out of 959 patients in a large study [2]. The necessity of gamma camera imaging after secure injection of the fluid for ROLL is according to some authors not required or recommended [26]. In case of a SNOLL procedure, imaging can be accomplished according to standard SLNB gamma camera imaging. In our institute, we obtain planar static images 15 min and 3 h after tracer injection followed by additional SPECT/CT imaging in case of inconclusive static images or aberrant drainage patterns for SLNB procedures [36] (Figs. 9.3 and 9.4). When planar images are obtained, the patient contour can be visualized by means of a flood source positioned underneath the patient during the acquisition (Fig. 9.4).

9.1.5 Surgical Localization

The radioactive tracer can be detected during operation with a gamma probe. There are many types of gamma probes available for intraoperative localization [37]. Important properties are the sensitivity, side shielding, thickness of the gamma probe, and visualization possibilities (i.e., acoustic noise and numerical display). The first three properties, which are mentioned, are all dependable on each other, and the end user should decide what parameters do best suit their needs. For example, a more focused beam, thanks to more side shielding, will result in a lower sensitivity. The surgical excision of the lesion is performed at the operating theatre. The highest Tc 99m counts detected transcutaneous with the gamma probe give insight in the location and guide the placement of the incision. During the procedure, the probe guides the location of the tumor by measuring a count drop at the border of the marked tissue and the surrounding tissue. After excision, the rest of the cavity is searched for further radioactivity exceeding the background signal (Fig. 9.5). If there remains signal in the cavity exceeding the background signal, the excision should be enlarged.

9.1.5.1 Innovative Techniques

Another approach is to use a portable gamma camera to localize the lesion and secure complete removal of the lesion. The portable gamma camera is used in conjunction with the conventional gamma probe. Paredes et al. proposed this method in 2008 (Fig. 9.6a). In this study, it was demonstrated on 43 patients that a pinhole portable gamma camera was capable of imaging the surgical bed and the specimen. There was 60 % congruence between the images in terms of appropriate excision and centricity of the radioactivity compared to histopathology [38, 39]. Freehand SPECT is another technique, which can be used to localize the radioactive lesion. This method consists of hovering an optically tracked gamma probe over the area of interest, and by measuring the radioactivity from multiple directions, a radioactivity map is reconstructed. In this way, nearly real-time localization of radioactivity is facilitated, and at the same time, navigation with depth measurements is possible [40] (Fig. 9.6b).

9.1.6 Histopathology

Frozen section analysis of imprint cytology can be performed during the procedure for confirmation of

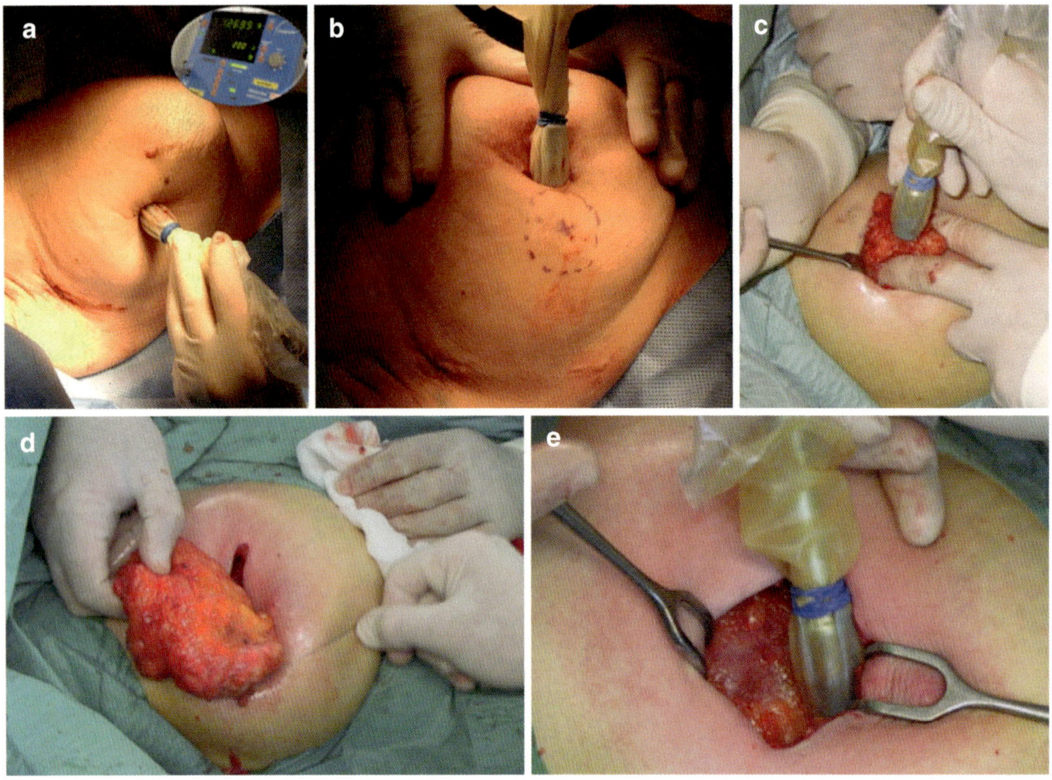

Fig. 9.5 Surgical localization. (**a**) The maximum signal of Tc 99m is measured on the skin and marked. (**b**) The surgeon decides the best approach and accordingly places the incision. (**c**) Measurement after skin incision. (**d**) Wide excision of a large tumor. (**e**) Control for residual activity after excision

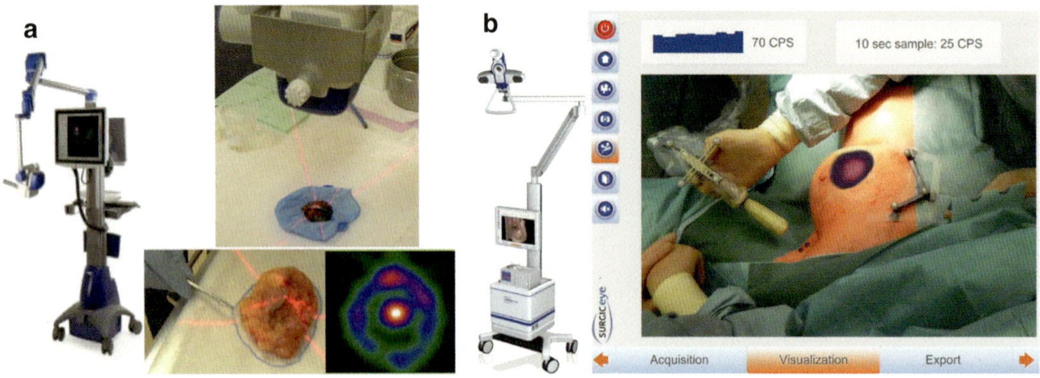

Fig. 9.6 Innovative techniques. (**a**) ROLL procedure with a portable gamma camera (Paredes et al. [38]). The radioactivity is imaged in a very short time interval. (**b**) Freehand SPECT navigation with declipse SPECT (SurgicEye GmbH, Munich, Germany) for a ROLL procedure. The location of the radioactivity is superimposed over the breast of the patient

appropriate excision. These rapid intraoperative methods of assessing the excised tissues during the operative procedure can reduce the need for a subsequent second surgical procedure [41, 42]. Alternatively, standard postoperative permanent section analysis can be performed for assessing the final status of the surgical resection margins, as well as for standard comprehensive evaluation of the primary tumor and lymph nodes. At the moment, there is no general consensus on how to manage minimally involved surgical resection margins. Adjuvant radiation and chemotherapy might be equally good compared to secondary surgery [43, 44].

9.2 Overall Results of ROLL

The first ROLL procedures are described in 1998 by Luini et al. [45], and, since then, ROLL rapidly increased in use. The rapid introduction was caused by the increased need for a proper localization method for the increasing number of non-palpable lesions and the good first results. At the moment, more than 29 peer-reviewed articles have emerged about ROLL, including multiple series of a thousand patients or more.

9.3 Results Compared to Other Techniques

9.3.1 ROLL-WGL

The largest meta-analysis comparing ROLL with WGL is the meta-analysis from Sajid et al. This study included four randomized controlled trials (RTCs) with a total of 449 patients randomized to either one of the procedures [1, 5, 18, 46]. The meta-analysis demonstrated a significant favorable outcome considering positive margins and localization time for the ROLL procedure. The localization rate, reoperation rate, complication rate, duration, specimen weight, and specimen volume were all comparable for both techniques.

The same meta-analysis describes results from other non-RCTs. Seven of these studies describe similar results as the 4 RCTs on ROLL [5, 12, 26, 46–49]. Further the results on the similarity of the excised volume and weight of the specimen concur with other publications [5, 18, 46]. Some retrospective studies do not concur with the results about the specimen volume and weight [49, 50]. Furthermore, the meta-analysis mentions studies with a reduced degree of positive margins, with 75 to 100 % margin clearance [2, 19, 34, 47, 48, 51].

9.3.2 ROLL-Ultrasound

Another localization method for non-palpable breast lesions is intraoperative ultrasound guidance [52, 53]. Ultrasound guidance seems to have strong advantages compared to surgery by palpation only. However, in contrast to invasive breast cancer, DCIS lesions are usually not visible at ultrasound, and therefore, this method is not always applicable. This could be resolved by placing a nonradioactive marker that is visible on US, but this would be a cumbersome method. A study from Krekel et al. compared WGL, ROLL, and ultrasound-guided localization [13]. This study included non-palpable lesions but excluded in situ carcinomas and neoadjuvant treated tumors, and, for this selection, it demonstrated significant favorable results for US-guided procedures based on margin status not taking unexpected DCIS component into account. When taking the unexpected DCIS component into account, there was no significant difference in margin status between the three groups. Altogether, intraoperative ultrasound use can be useful for tumor excision in certain groups, although an ultrasound-trained surgeon is required and this technique is only applicable for carcinomas visible on ultrasound.

9.3.3 ROLL (Tc-99m)-RSL (I-125-Seed)

Ahmed et al. described the comparison between ROLL and RSL, and regarding the original study comparing the techniques from Donker et al. [54, 55]. This study demonstrated comparable results between the ROLL-Tc99m technique and I-125 seed localization when used to perform breast-conserving surgery after neoadjuvant systemic treatment, although the preference was I-125 seed localization because this does not require additional radiological localization shortly before surgery, and therefore, it simplifies surgery scheduling. The largest study comparing ROLL with RSL is from Noordaa et al. [56]. In this study, 403 patient with either unifocal non-palpable DCIS or invasive carcinoma were retrospectively analyzed, 128 patients underwent RSL and 275 patients ROLL. Margin status and re-excision rates were comparable for RSL and ROLL in patients with non-palpable breast lesions. A significant lower weight of the resected specimen using RSL in the DCIS group was found. Because of the feasibility of position verification of the I-125 seed and more convenient logistics, RSL was favored over ROLL for breast-conserving therapy.

9.4 Discussion

The general consensus is that the main advantages of ROLL, using Tc 99m, over WGL are the patient comfort, positive margins, and localization time. The wire localization technique has disadvantages such as wire dislodging, worsened cosmetics, and wire migration which are all negated by the ROLL technique. The 6-hour half-life of Tc 99m allows some flexibility, up to 24 h, in planning the surgical procedure after the radiotracer injection. A possible limitation of injection of a liquid radiotracer, like Tc 99m, is the potential for dispersion of the radiotracer throughout the breast tissue. Therefore, the more recent development of RSL, using a I-125 seed, represents a very promising alternative form of radioguided surgery for non-palpable breast lesions, and for which we expect the popularity of RSL to quickly grow [57].

Working with radioactivity (tracers or markers) requires strict regulations at the nuclear medicine department and a close collaboration with the radiology department. The radiation dose for patients and involved staff is limited and comparable to SLN procedures, which are performed on a regular basis in most institutes. The radiation dose for patient and staff was analyzed by Rampaul et al. and Cremonesi et al. The dose for patients was 0.45 mGy and after 100 surgical procedures for surgeons 0.45 mGy. The mean effective dose was 0.09 mSv. These numbers did not exceed the limits established by the commission on radiological protection [58, 59].

Conclusive

ROLL, using Tc 99m, is useful for localization of non-palpable lesions in the breast; this includes invasive cancers, DCIS, or areas of microcalcifications. The general consensus is that ROLL is preferable over WGL. There are however some drawbacks considering the radiotracer distribution and decay, although in general the patient comfort, cosmetic outcome, and the localization results outweigh the drawbacks. In the future, we expect an increase in the use of RSL using I-125 seeds that act more as a point source, allow position verification by mammography, and allow more flexibility in the logistics between radiology and the surgical department.

References

1. Sajid MS, Parampalli U, Haider Z, Bonomi R. Comparison of radioguided occult lesion localization (ROLL) and wire localization for non-palpable breast cancers: a meta-analysis. J Surg Oncol. 2012;105:852–8.
2. Monti S, Galimberti V, Trifiro G, Cicco C, Peradze N, Brenelli F, et al. Occult Breast Lesion Localization plus Sentinel Node Biopsy (SNOLL): experience with 959 patients at the European Institute of Oncology. Ann Surg Oncol. 2007;14:2928–31.
3. DICA jaarrapportage 2012. http://clinicalaudit.nl/jaarrapportage. 2014. p. 1–87.
4. Ocal K, Dag A, Turkmenoglu O, Gunay EC, Yucel E, Duce MN. Radioguided occult lesion localization versus wire-guided localization for non-palpable breast lesions: randomized controlled trial. Clinics. 2011;66:1003–7.
5. Medina-Franco H, Abarca-Pérez L, García-Alvarez MN, Ulloa-Gómez JL, Romero-Trejo C, Sepúlveda-Méndez J. Radioguided occult lesion localization (ROLL) versus wire-guided lumpectomy for non-palpable breast lesions: a randomized prospective evaluation. J Surg Oncol. 2008;97:108–11.
6. Kopans DB. Migration of breast biopsy localization wire. Am J Roentgenol. 1988;151:614–5.
7. Kilcoyne RF, Moe RE, Bronstein AD. Complications of needle localization of foreign bodies and nonpalpable breast lesions. Arch Surg. 1988;123:775–9.
8. Kelly P, Winslow EH. Needle wire localization for nonpalpable breast lesions: sensations, anxiety levels, and informational needs. Oncol Nurs Forum. 1996;23:639–45.
9. Rovera F, Frattini F, Marelli M, Corben AD, Vanoli C, Dionigi G, et al. Radio-guided occult lesion localiza-

tion versus wire-guided localization in non-palpable breast lesions. Int J Surg. 2008;6 Suppl 1:S101–3.
10. Ahmed M, Hemelrijck M, Douek M. Systematic review of radioguided versus wire-guided localization in the treatment of non-palpable breast cancers. Breast Cancer Res Treat. 2013;140:241–52.
11. Dua SM, Gray RJ, Keshtgar M. Strategies for localisation of impalpable breast lesions. Breast. 2011;20: 246–53.
12. Moreno M, Wiltgen JE, Bodanese B, Schmitt RL, Gutfilen B, da Fonseca LMB. Radioguided breast surgery for occult lesion localization – correlation between two methods. J Exp Clin Cancer Res. 2008; 27:29.
13. Krekel NMA, Zonderhuis BM, Stockmann HBAC, Schreurs WH, van der Veen H, de Lange de Klerk ESM, et al. A comparison of three methods for nonpalpable breast cancer excision. Eur J Surg Oncol. 2011;37:109–15.
14. Postma EL, Witkamp AJ, van den Bosch MA, Verkooijen HM, van Hillegersberg R. Localization of nonpalpable breast lesions. Expert Rev Anticancer Ther. 2011;11:1295–302.
15. Postma EL, Verkooijen HM, Van Esser S, Hobbelink MG, van der Schelling GP, Koelemij R, et al. Efficacy of 'radioguided occult lesion localisation' (ROLL) versus "wire-guided localisation" (WGL) in breast conserving surgery for non-palpable breast cancer: a randomised controlled multicentre trial. Breast Cancer Res Treat. 2012;136:469–78.
16. Giacalone PL, Bourdon A, Trinh PD, Taourel P, Rathat G, Sainmont M, et al. Radioguided occult lesion localization plus sentinel node biopsy (SNOLL) versus wire-guided localization plus sentinel node detection: a case control study of 129 unifocal pure invasive non-palpable breast cancers. Eur J Surg Oncol. 2012;38:222–9.
17. Bishop CV, Neerhut P, Mann GB, Rose A, Collins JP. Carbon localisation of impalpable breast lesions. Breast. 2003;12:264–9.
18. Rampaul RS, Bagnall M, Burrell H, Pinder SE, Evans AJ, Macmillan RD. Randomized clinical trial comparing radioisotope occult lesion localization and wire-guided excision for biopsy of occult breast lesions. Br J Surg. 2004;91:1575–7.
19. Lavoué V, Nos C, Clough KB, Baghaie F, Zerbib E, Poulet B, et al. Simplified Technique of Radioguided Occult Lesion Localization (ROLL) Plus Sentinel Lymph Node Biopsy (SNOLL) in breast carcinoma. Ann Surg Oncol. 2008;15:2556–61.
20. Aydogan F, Ozben V, Yilmaz MH, Celik V, Uras C, Ferahman M, et al. Simultaneous excision of ipsilateral nonpalpable multiple breast lesions using radioguided occult lesion localization. Breast. 2011; 20:241–5.
21. van Esser S, Hobbelink MG, Peeters PH, Buskens E, van der Ploeg IM, Mali WP, et al. The efficacy of 'Radio guided Occult Lesion Localization' (ROLL) versus "Wire-guided Localization" (WGL) in breast conserving surgery for non-palpable breast cancer: A randomized clinical trial – ROLL study. BMC Surg. 2008;8:9.
22. Lovrics PJ, Cornacchi SD, Vora R, Goldsmith CH, Kahnamoui K. Systematic review of radioguided surgery for non-palpable breast cancer. Eur J Surg Oncol. 2011;37:388–97.
23. Murphy JO, Moo T-A, King TA, Van Zee KJ, Villegas KA, Stempel M, et al. Radioactive seed localization compared to wire localization in breast-conserving surgery: initial 6-month experience. Ann Surg Oncol. 2013;20:4121–7.
24. Alderliesten T, Loo CE, Pengel KE, Rutgers EJT, Gilhuijs KGA, Vrancken Peeters M-JTFD. Radioactive seed localization of breast lesions: an adequate localization method without seed migration. Breast J. 2011;17:594–601.
25. Gallegos Hernandez JF, Tanis PJ, Deurloo EE, Nieweg OE, Th Rutgers EJ, Kroon BBR, et al. Radioguided surgery improves outcome of therapeutic excision in non-palpable invasive breast cancer. Nucl Med Commun. 2004;25:227–32.
26. Audisio RA, Nadeem R, Harris O, Desmond S, Thind R, Chagla LS. Radioguided occult lesion localisation (ROLL) is available in the UK for impalpable breast lesions. Ann R Coll Surg Engl. 2005;87:92–5.
27. Kim J, Chung D, Spillane A. Combined radioguided occult lesion and sentinel node localization for breast cancer. ANZ J Surg. 2004;74:550–3.
28. van Rijk MC, Tanis PJ, Nieweg OE, Loo CE, Valdés Olmos RA, Oldenburg HSA, et al. Sentinel node biopsy and concomitant probe-guided tumor excision of nonpalpable breast cancer. Ann Surg Oncol. 2007; 14:627–32.
29. De Cicco C, Pizzamiglio M, Trifirò G, Luini A, Ferrari M, Prisco G, et al. Radioguided occult lesion localisation (ROLL) and surgical biopsy in breast cancer. Technical aspects. Q J Nucl Med. 2002;46:145–51.
30. De Cicco C, Trifirò G, Intra M, Marotta G, Ciprian A, Frasson A, et al. Optimised nuclear medicine method for tumour marking and sentinel node detection in occult primary breast lesions. Eur J Nucl Med Mol Imaging. 2003;31:349–54.
31. Sarlos D, Frey LD, Haueisen H, Landmann G, Kots LA, Schaer G. Radioguided occult lesion localization (ROLL) for treatment and diagnosis of malignant and premalignant breast lesions combined with sentinel node biopsy: a prospective clinical trial with 100 patients. Eur J Surg Oncol. 2009;35:403–8.
32. Kroon BB, Rutgers EJ, Nieweg OE, Deurloo EE, Besnard AP, Olmos RAV, et al. Single intralesional tracer dose for radio-guided excision of clinically occult breast cancer and sentinel node. Ann Surg Oncol. 2001;8:850–5.
33. Jackson L, Bourke AG, Abdul Aziz F, Taylor D. Radioactive seed localisation to guide removal of impalpable lymph nodes (radioguided occult lesion localisation using iodine-125 seeds, "ROLLIS"). BMJ Case Rep. 2014;2014.

34. Feggi L, Basaglia E, Corcione S, Querzoli P, Soliani G, Ascanelli S, et al. An original approach in the diagnosis of early breast cancer: use of the same radiopharmaceutical for both non-palpable lesions and sentinel node localisation. Eur J Nucl Med. 2001;28:1589–96.
35. Ahmed M, Douek M. Sentinel node and occult lesion localization (SNOLL): a systematic review. Breast. 2013;22:1034–40.
36. van der Ploeg IMC, Nieweg OE, Kroon BBR, Rutgers EJT, Baas-Vrancken Peeters M-JTFD, Vogel WV, et al. The yield of SPECT/CT for anatomical lymphatic mapping in patients with breast cancer. Eur J Nucl Med Mol Imaging. 2009;36:903–9.
37. Haigh PI, Glass EC, Essner R. Accuracy of gamma probes in localizing radioactivity: in-vitro assessment and clinical implications. Cancer Biother Radiopharm. 2000;15:561–9.
38. Paredes P, Vidal-Sicart S, Zanon G, Roé N, Rubí S, Lafuente S, et al. Radioguided occult lesion localisation in breast cancer using an intraoperative portable gamma camera: first results. Eur J Nucl Med Mol Imaging. 2008;35:230–5.
39. Vidal-Sicart S, Rioja ME, Paredes P, Keshtgar MR, Valdes Olmos RA. Contribution of perioperative imaging to radioguided surgery. Q J Nucl Med Mol Imaging. 2014;58:140–60.
40. Pouw B, de Wit-van der Veen BJ, van der Hage JA, Vrancken Peeters M-JTFD, Wesseling J, Stokkel MPM, et al. Radio-guided seed localization for breast cancer excision: an ex-vivo specimen-based study to establish the accuracy of a freehand-SPECT device in predicting resection margins. Nucl Med Commun. 2014;35:961–6.
41. Esbona K, Li Z, Wilke LG. Intraoperative imprint cytology and frozen section pathology for margin assessment in breast conservation surgery: a systematic review. Ann Surg Oncol. 2012;19:3236–45.
42. Thill M, Baumann K, Barinoff J. Intraoperative assessment of margins in breast conservative surgery-still in use? J Surg Oncol. 2014;110:15–20.
43. Silverstein MJ, Lagios MD. Should all patients undergoing breast conserving therapy for DCIS receive radiation therapy? No. One size does not fit all: an argument against the routine use of radiation therapy for all patients with ductal carcinoma in situ of the breast who elect breast conservation. J Surg Oncol. 2007;95:605–9.
44. Bijker N, van Tienhoven G. Local and systemic outcomes in DCIS based on tumor and patient characteristics: the radiation oncologist's perspective. J Natl Cancer Inst Monogr. 2010;2010:178–80.
45. Luini A, Zurrida S, Galimberti V, Paganelli G. Radioguided surgery of occult breast lesions. Eur J Cancer. 1998;34:204–5.
46. Mariscal Martínez A, Solà M, de Tudela AP, Julián JF, Fraile M, Vizcaya S, et al. Radioguided localization of nonpalpable breast cancer lesions: randomized comparison with wire localization in patients undergoing conservative surgery and sentinel node biopsy. AJR Am J Roentgenol. 2009;193:1001–9.
47. Thind CR, Desmond S, Harris O, Nadeem R, Chagla LS, Audisio RA. Radio-guided localization of clinically occult breast lesions (ROLL): a DGH experience. Clin Radiol. 2005;60:681–6.
48. Nadeem R, Chagla LS, Harris O, Desmond S, Thind R, Titterrell C, et al. Occult breast lesions: a comparison between radioguided occult lesion localisation (ROLL) vs. wire-guided lumpectomy (WGL). Breast. 2005;14:283–9.
49. Chu TYC, Lui CY, Hung WK, Kei SK, Choi CLY, Lam HS. Localisation of occult breast lesion: a comparative analysis of hookwire and radioguided procedures. Hong Kong Med J. 2010;16:367–72.
50. Zgajnar J, Hocevar M, Frkovic-Grazio S, Hertl K, Schweiger E, Besic N. Radioguided occult lesion localization (ROLL) of the nonpalpable breast lesions. Neoplasma. 2004;51:385–9.
51. Rönkä R, Krogerus L, Leppänen E, von Smitten K, Leidenius M. Radio-guided occult lesion localization in patients undergoing breast-conserving surgery and sentinel node biopsy. Am J Surg. 2004;187: 491–6.
52. Krekel NM, Haloua MH, Lopes Cardozo AM, de Wit RH, Bosch AM, de Widt-Levert LM, et al. Intraoperative ultrasound guidance for palpable breast cancer excision (COBALT trial): a multicentre, randomised controlled trial. Lancet Oncol. 2013;14:48–54.
53. Haid A, Knauer M, Dunzinger S, Jasarevic Z, Köberle-Wührer R, Schuster A, et al. Intra-operative sonography: a valuable aid during breast-conserving surgery for occult breast cancer. Ann Surg Oncol. 2007;14:3090–101.
54. Ahmed M, Douek M. ROLL versus RSL: toss of a coin? Breast Cancer Res Treat. 2013;140:213–7.
55. Donker M, Drukker CA, Valdés Olmos RA, Rutgers EJT, Loo CE, Sonke GS, et al. Guiding breast-conserving surgery in patients after neoadjuvant systemic therapy for breast cancer: a comparison of radioactive seed localization with the ROLL technique. Ann Surg Oncol. 2013;20:2569–75.
56. van der Noordaa MEM, Pengel KE, Groen E, van Werkhoven E, Rutgers EJT, Loo CE, et al. The use of radioactive Iodine-125 seed localization in patients with non-palpable breast cancer a comparison with the radioguided occult lesion localization with 99m Technetium. Eur J Surg Oncol. 2015.
57. Pouw B, de Wit-van der Veen LJ, Stokkel MPM, Loo CE, Vrancken Peeters M-JTFD, Valdés Olmos RA. Heading toward radioactive seed localization in non-palpable breast cancer surgery? A meta-analysis. J Surg Oncol. 2015;111:185–91.
58. Rampaul RS, Dudley NJ, Thompson JZ, Burrell H, Evans AJ, Wilson ARM, et al. Radioisotope for occult lesion localisation (ROLL) of the breast does not require extra radiation protection procedures. Breast. 2003;12:150–2.
59. Cremonesi M, Ferrari M, Sacco E, Rossi A, De Cicco C, Leonardi L, et al. Radiation protection in radioguided surgery of breast cancer. Nucl Med Commun. 1999;20:919–24.

Part IV

Clinical Application: Skin

Radioguided Sentinel Lymph Node Mapping and Biopsy in Cutaneous Melanoma

10

Omgo E. Nieweg, Roger F. Uren, and John F. Thompson

Contents

O.E. Nieweg, MD, PhD, FRACS (✉) • J.F. Thompson, MD, FRACS, FACS
Sydney Medical School, The University of Sydney, Sydney, NSW, Australia

Melanoma Institute Australia, 40 Rocklands Road, North Sydney, NSW 2060, Australia

The Mater Hospital, North Sydney, NSW, Australia

Royal Prince Alfred Hospital, Camperdown, NSW, Australia
e-mail: omgo.nieweg@melanoma.org.au

R.F. Uren, MD, FRACP, DDU
Sydney Medical School, The University of Sydney, Nuclear Medicine and Diagnostic Ultrasound, Suite 206, RPAH Medical Centre, 100 Carillon Ave., Newtown, NSW, Australia

Abstract

Sentinel lymph node biopsy has developed into a routine procedure to stage patients with a clinically localized melanoma. The node can be found in almost every patient. The status of the lymph nodes is the most powerful prognostic factor. Although high false-negative rates are still being published, sentinel lymph node biopsy is reliable when performed by an experienced multidisciplinary team using a meticulous technique. The Multicenter Selective Lymphadenectomy Trial I has shown that the procedure leads to improved survival when combined with completion lymph node dissection in lymph node-positive patients with an intermediate Breslow thickness melanoma. The technique of sentinel lymph node biopsy continues to evolve and its importance will expand even further when adequate adjuvant systemic therapies become available.

K. Herrmann et al. (eds.), *Radioguided Surgery: Current Applications and Innovative Directions in Clinical Practice*, DOI 10.1007/978-3-319-26051-8_10

10.1 Introduction

Approximately 1 in 50 individuals in Europe and the United States develops melanoma and 1 in 18 in Australia [1]. Every year 4 % more people are diagnosed with the disease, making melanoma the cancer with the greatest increase in incidence [2]. At the time of diagnosis, there is usually no evidence of dissemination to other sites, but one in five patients who present with a primary melanoma more than 1 mm in Breslow thickness has occult involvement of their regional lymph nodes. These nodal metastases are too small to palpate, and usually they are not detectable by ultrasound screening at this stage. If left undisturbed, such metastases later become evident. At that time, they may have generated metastases at distant sites, and these imply a dismal prognosis.

In melanoma patients, prophylactic regional node dissection had been the standard management of the regional lymph nodes for many years until randomized studies revealed that there was no overall survival benefit from this procedure [3–6]. However, improved survival compared to patients with palpable nodal disease was shown when prophylactic dissection of clinically negative lymph node fields did reveal metastases, and this was confirmed in other studies [7–11]. This survival advantage is particularly evident in patients with melanomas of intermediate Breslow thickness. These lesions have a substantial risk of lymph node involvement, while the risk of fatal blood-borne metastases to vital organs is still limited. Sentinel lymph node (SLN) biopsy was developed as a diagnostic technique to detect lymph node metastases at this early stage so that regional node dissection could be selectively carried out to gain this potential survival benefit [12].

The SLN concept of orderly progression of lymphatic metastases is logical and exciting. When first introduced, it was therefore attractive to surgeons, and it quickly developed a momentum that caused some to get carried away by their enthusiasm. The procedure was immediately embraced widely, and, like many other new surgical procedures in the past, it quickly became standard management in patients with melanoma without much scientific evidence to support it. Since then, however, much research has been undertaken. Donald Morton, who introduced the modern SLN biopsy procedure, initiated two randomized trials to assess the procedure in a scientific fashion. The final outcome of the first of these two studies, the first Multicenter Selective Lymphadenectomy Trial (MSLT-I), demonstrated its value in various respects.

The purpose of this chapter is to present a balanced summary of the current status of lymphatic mapping in melanoma and to speculate about its future, with special reference to the role of radioguided surgery. The discussion will be based largely on the data gathered at our institutions.

10.2 Definition of a Sentinel Lymph Node

The SLN procedure is based on the concept that lymphatic fluid draining from a primary tumor carries detached malignant cells through an afferent lymph vessel to a particular lymph node, where they are trapped. Such a metastasis may then generate further nodal metastases downstream through the efferent lymph vessel or may disseminate to distant sites via the bloodstream [12]. Therefore, a SLN was initially defined as "the initial lymph node to which the primary tumor drains" [12]. In the beginning, the SLN was pursued by visualization of the afferent lymph vessel using the blue dye technique, i.e., by tracing the blue-stained lymphatics to the lymph node after intradermal injection of blue dye at the primary melanoma site.

When lymphoscintigraphy was introduced, the phasing of "*the initial lymph node to which the primary tumor drains*" led to confusion because it can be interpreted in different ways. For instance, the primary tumor may drain through two separate lymph ducts to two different lymph nodes that may not necessarily be visualized simultaneously, although both are directly at risk of receiving tumor cells. When the dynamic process is observed during lymphoscintigraphy, it became clear that a more general definition was needed to include all eventualities. In 1994, our group described the SLN as "any lymph node receiving direct lymphatic drainage from the primary tumor site" [13]. This includes all possibilities including an obvious metastatic node in the draining node field that was not seen on the lymphoscintigrams and was not staining blue. In the following years, many other definitions were put forward (Table 10.1) [14–17]. Most of these new definitions are based on the techniques used to find the SLN, and they appeal because they are easier than having to scrutinize dynamic lymphoscintigrams from various angles or to carefully dissect a delicate blue lymphatic vessel to determine to which lymph node that vessel takes the tumor cells [17–21]. However, the new definitions missed the pathophysiological foundation of the SLN concept. For instance, the definition of a SLN being a blue-stained node may lead to the removal of too many lymph nodes, because the blue dye is not retained in a lymph node and will also stain nodes downstream that are not directly at risk of harboring tumor cells (so-called "second-tier" nodes). The definition of the SLN being the most radioactive node may lead to the removal of too few lymph nodes because separate lymphatic vessels originating in a tumor may drain to two lymph nodes, and one is likely to contain more of the tracer than the other.

Our original definition reflects the physiology of lymphatic drainage and the concept of stepwise spread of cancer through the lymphatic system, and this is the definition most experts now adhere to and that we advocate. This definition requires the nuclear medicine physician to perform dynamic imaging to visualize the afferent lymph vessel or vessels. The surgeon needs to have the skill and experience to find and dissect the fragile blue lymph duct through a small incision in a confined space in a lymph node basin that may be quite deep. Finding the correct node requires close cooperation from the nuclear medicine physician and the surgeon. Adherence to these principles appears to yield the best results [22].

Table 10.1 Alternative definitions of a sentinel lymph node [17]

Node closest to the primary lesion
First node depicted on the lymphoscintigraphy images
Node with the highest count rate
Any radioactive lymph node
Node with a count rate that is a certain factor higher than the background or compared to a non-sentinel lymph node
Node with a count rate that exceeds a certain fraction of the hottest lymph node
Any blue lymph node

The recommended definition is "any lymph node receiving direct lymphatic drainage from the melanoma site"

10.3 Imaging Technique

The technique of lymphatic mapping for SLN biopsy was proposed by Donald Morton (surgeon) and Ed Glass (nuclear medicine physician) in the early 1990s, and the technique was subsequently refined by others, including ourselves, over the course of many thousands of procedures. Various radiopharmaceuticals containing the radionuclide technetium-99m can be used for lymphatic mapping. The radionuclide is attached to a colloidal particle of a size that can enter the initial lymphatic capillary lumen. This occurs via the gap between the endothelial cells that line the wall of such initial lymphatics. This gap is 20 nm wide but can be wider when massage is applied to the injection site. The colloid particles can be of variable size and range from five to hundreds of nanometers. Smaller particles enter the lymphatic capillaries more readily than the larger ones. After intradermal administration, the flow rate of the tracers is about 1.5 cm/min in the head and neck, 2.5 cm/min on the trunk, 3 cm/min in the upper limb, and 10 cm/min on the lower limb [23]. However, there are multiple factors that influence the flow rate, including time of day, ambient temperature, medication, state of hydration, and exercise. There are sound reasons to assume that the lymphatic flow rate will be slower than usual during a surgical procedure. The retention of these colloidal particles in lymph nodes is not a simple mechanical filtration process. The particles are phagocytosed by macrophages and tissue histiocytes that line the subcapsular sinuses of lymph nodes, after they have been recognized as foreign to the patient.

The percentage of the injected dose that is retained in the SLN varies with the radiopharmaceutical used with smaller particles reaching the SLN more easily than larger particles. The aim of lymphatic mapping is to identify only the true SLNs (receiving tracer directly from the lesion site), and therefore it is important to have enough particles in the collecting vessel so that it can be traced directly to the lymph node in question. Sometimes second-tier lymph nodes will be seen but these should not be removed. In patients with melanoma, an average of 0.82 % of the injected dose for nanocolloid (range 0.0013–6.8 %) is accumulated [24].

The procedure is best done before wide local excision, as the risk of crossing a lymphatic watershed increases with increasing distance from the original melanoma site, and we know from experience that a different pattern of lymphatic drainage may result after wide local excision. A dose of 30–100 MBq of the radiopharmaceutical is generally used in a volume of 0.1–0.2 ml/injection. Lignocaine may be added so that the injection volume becomes 0.2–0.4 ml. The dose may be adjusted to the interval between administration and operation, keeping in mind the 6-h physical half-life of the radionuclide. The tracer is injected immediately around the melanoma or the center of the excisional biopsy site. Since the tracer is intended to delineate the drainage pathway from a tumor located in the dermal layer of the skin, the tracer is injected intradermally.

Dynamic imaging is commenced immediately. The nuclear medicine physician observes the passage of tracer through lymphatic collecting vessels and identifies the SLNs as those nodes to which a lymphatic vessel drains. The number and location of SLNs are then recorded. SLNs (interval nodes) are found outside the established nodal regions in 7 % of patients [25]. These early images visualize the lymphatic collecting vessels and can distinguish SLNs from second-tier lymph nodes. Late anterior, posterior, and lateral images are obtained 1–2 h later, and other images are acquired when required.

Single-photon emission tomography combined with computerized radiographic tomography (SPECT/CT) has proved to be a major advance and has become part of the routine SLN imaging protocol in most major melanoma treatment centers [26, 27]. This hybrid technology provides tomographic slices in every desired direction and enables visualization of nodes containing tracer from any angle. The correction for attenuation and scatter results in improved SLN identification. SPECT/CT shows SLNs that may go unnoticed with conventional imaging and provides important anatomic information about the location of nodes. Surgeons want to see the anatomy. Now they see the SLN in its anatomic habitat, which is very helpful in difficult cases. An initial study of SPECT/CT was performed in patients with conventional lymphoscintigrams that were difficult to interpret. SPECT/CT showed additional SLNs in 8 % of the patients [28]. SPECT/CT had an added value in 35 % of the study population, resulting in modification of the planned surgical procedure in terms of a longer or shorter incision, an incision at a different location, or an extra incision. The results were even better in a subsequent group of unselected melanoma patients undergoing routine SLN biopsy, with SPECT/CT providing additional useful information in 46 % of them and resulting in adjustment of the surgical approach in 29 % [29].

The nuclear medicine physician can mark the location of a SLN on the overlying skin with the patient in the position used for surgery, providing valuable orientation for the surgeon. Now that its site is known, the SLN can be examined with ultrasound. Ultrasound occasionally suggests involvement with melanoma that can be confirmed by fine needle aspiration cytology, obviating the need for the actual biopsy. The location of a lymph node can also be marked with a small permanent dermal tattoo. In some patients a biopsy is not performed because of an excessive number of SLNs, the expected complexity of the procedure, or the age or poor general health of the patient. In such patients, these lymph nodes can be followed using repeat ultrasound examination every 3 or 4 months. The dermal tattoo spots facilitate their identification among other lymph nodes.

10.4 Surgical Technique

There is a definite learning curve for this procedure, but one cannot reliably establish how many cases this requires [30]. Once the technique has been mastered, the operation is usually simple to carry out [31]. A single-day admission is customary, and the operation is typically done using general anesthesia, although it can be performed using local anesthesia. The two established techniques to find the SLN are the blue dye technique and the gamma ray detection technique. Most experts combine the two methods as they find this the easiest, quickest, and most reliable approach. We recommend that surgeons embarking upon lymphatic mapping acquire proficiency in both techniques. The probe technique is easier to learn and has a higher success rate. When lymphoscintigraphy leaves no doubt as to the number of SLNs, either technique is usually adequate. When multiple nodes light up and lymphoscintigraphy is not decisive, the blue dye can discern between a SLN on a direct drainage pathway and a second-tier node. This cannot be accomplished with the probe, since the probe does not identify lymphatic channels.

When using blue dye, the margin for the wide local re-excision of the primary melanoma biopsy site is outlined with a marker pen before injection of the blue dye, since the dye may obscure a small biopsy scar. One milliliter of vital dye (isosulfan blue, patent blue) is injected intradermally as close as possible to the melanoma site in the same manner as the radiopharmaceutical was administered. The dye is immediately taken up by the lymphatic system and stains the lymphatic channel within a few minutes. Vigorous massage of the injection site and the skin in the direction of the node field for a few minutes stimulates the lymph flow. The skin mark made by the nuclear medicine physician preoperatively and localization of the "hot" lymph node with a gamma ray detection probe through the intact skin guide the placement of the incision. When making the incision, the surgeon must bear in mind that formal regional lymph node dissection with excision of the SLN biopsy site may need to be performed at a later stage. An incision length of 2–4 cm is usually sufficient. The subcutaneous tissue is gently explored in search of a blue-stained afferent lymphatic channel underneath Scarpa's fascia or the blue-stained lymph node itself. If tracing a blue-stained lymphatic, it should be followed until it enters a blue-stained first-echelon lymph node. Lymphatic channels are fragile, requiring a subtle surgical technique. Once the SLN is identified, it is excised from the surrounding tissue while afferent and efferent lymph and blood vessels are ligated and divided. The biopsy cavity is obliterated with absorbable sutures to prevent seroma as part of the wound closure process.

The technique using a gamma detection probe exploits the presence of radiopharmaceutical that persists in the SLN after the preceding lymphoscintigraphy. The radioactivity content of a SLN exceeds that of the surrounding tissues by a factor of 600 on average. The location of the lymph node can be determined through the intact skin using the gamma detection probe. The probe guides the direction of the dissection. The features that we appreciate on a probe are a sound pitch that varies with the radioactive count rate and that has different ranges to accommodate for the great variability of count rates that may be faced. A collimator blocks gamma rays from the side and provides directionality. For some probes this can be removed during the operation to increase sensitivity when pursuing a minimally radioactive SLN in an area with a low background count rate.

10.5 Identification of Sentinel Lymph Nodes, Staging Information, and Morbidity

Using the above approaches, the SLN can be found in close to 100 % of cases and usually within 10 min [32]. SLN biopsy is a staging procedure. Staging provides prognostic information and is needed to choose the appropriate therapy for each patient. The tumor status of the SLN has been found to be the most important prognostic factor in melanoma patients with clinically negative regional lymph nodes [33, 34]. Based on these findings, the American

Joint Committee on Cancer and the Union Internationale Contre le Cancer (AJCC-UICC) included the tumor status of the SLN in the staging classification [35].

The obvious advantages of the procedure need to be weighed against its disadvantages. A 1-day admission and general anesthesia are usual. The radiopharmaceutical results in minor exposure to ionizing radiation. The morbidity of SLN biopsy is generally described as limited. A recent audit at Melanoma Institute Australia revealed a complication rate of only 1.8 %. Postoperative complications are generally minor, like seroma or infection, and tend to resolve completely. There was an initial suggestion that SLN biopsy could lead to an increase in the incidence of in transit metastases, but several subsequent studies have refuted this notion [36–38].

10.6 False-Negative Rate

The capability of lymphatic mapping to detect nodal metastases is generally believed to be good, but often the rate of false-negative procedures is calculated based on the entire group of patients or based on the group of SLN negative patients [39]. This is not correct because one cannot miss a nodal metastasis in a patient who does not have any metastases [40]. The sensitivity and the false-negative rate of a diagnostic test to detect disease should be examined in a population of patients in whom this disease is present. In other words the false-negative rate should be calculated in relation to the total number of patients who are actually lymph node positive. Also, many studies have had a follow-up interval that was too short for many nodal recurrences to become apparent. The mean interval before a missed lymph node metastasis becomes manifest is 28 months (range 4.6–106 months) in a study with a mean follow-up duration of 54 months [22]. In the Multicenter Selective Lymphadenectomy Trial (MSLT-I) that was carried out by 17 melanoma centers worldwide, all patients were followed for 10 years and the false-negative rate was 20.3 % [32]. Early studies from reputable institutions and cooperative groups around the world revealed false-negative rates ranging from 16 to 38 %, when recalculated in the appropriate fashion [39]. Even a recent study with a median follow-up period of 65 months resulted in a false-negative rate of 38 % [41]. This means that the correct SLN was not removed in almost two of every five patients. These numbers are considerably worse than the reported false-negative rates in breast cancer. A systematic literature review and meta-analysis of published studies in that disease yielded false-negative results between 0 and 3 % with a weighed combined sensitivity of 100 % [42]. At The Netherlands Cancer Institute, the poor results in melanoma were analyzed. The investigators adhered to the correct definition of a SLN and meticulously used the combined detection technique. One of two melanoma surgeons performed all the operations and once a week all procedures were evaluated in a multidisciplinary meeting. The results of 708 consecutive patients with a median follow-up of 54 months were analyzed starting with the very first patient. The false-negative rate was 5.7 %. In the first year after the SLN biopsy was introduced, this was 29.4 %. In subsequent years, it dropped to 3.0 %. False-negative SLN biopsy procedures can be attributed to the nuclear medicine physician, the surgeon, or the pathologist, but in 25–50 % of cases no cause can be established [22, 43].

10.7 Survival

After its early and rapid embracement as a routine procedure, unanswered questions soon became evident and SLN biopsy became the subject of a fierce debate [44–46]. Opposing opinions were vigorously debated, particularly concerning its impact on survival. Survival is indeed a fundamental issue. Although unusual for a diagnostic technique, it was felt that a randomized study was warranted because of the clinical importance of the subject, because of the radioactivity involved, the expensive equipment that is needed, and also because the procedure was a minimally invasive diagnostic test. A randomized trial, MSLT-I, was initiated in 1994 and was the largest and longest-running surgical melanoma trial ever. In total 2001 patients with a melanoma at least 1 mm Breslow thickness or with Clark level IV invasion were randomized to either SLN biopsy with subsequent completion lymph node dissection if the lymph node proved to be involved or to observation with lymph node dissection when a nodal metastasis became evident during follow-up. The last patient was enrolled in 2002. All patients were followed for 10 years.

The final results of MSLT-I have been published and show that the two arms of the study were well balanced for the usual prognostic factors Breslow thickness, Clark level, ulceration, primary lesion site, age, and gender [32]. SLNs were found in 99.4 % of the individuals who underwent the procedure. Lymph node metastases were present in 21 % of the entire study population. The incidence of nodal involvement was similar in the two arms of the study. The trial confirmed that the tumor status of the SLN is the strongest predictor of survival.

The patients were divided into three prespecified groups, those with a thin melanoma, defined in the trial as less than 1.2 mm Breslow thickness, those with a melanoma of intermediate Breslow thickness of 1.2–3.5 mm, and those with thicker lesions. The patients with thin melanomas were not sufficiently numerous to allow for a meaningful analysis and their results were not reported. Ten-year disease-free survival in the patients with a melanoma with a Breslow thickness of 1.2–3.5 mm was 71 % in the patients who underwent SLN biopsy compared to 65 % in the observation group ($p=0.01$). These percentages were 51 % versus 41 % in patients with thick melanomas ($p=0.03$). Most of this improvement reflected fewer regional nodal recurrences in patients who underwent immediate lymphadenectomy for tumor-positive SLNs. So, these patients were spared a nodal recurrence. A recurrence often necessitates a more extensive operation, carries more morbidity, is associated with a longer hospital stay, results in a reduced quality of life, and may involve adjuvant radiotherapy [47, 48]. Also, the published risks of recurrence in a regional nodal basin range from 2 to 10 % when lymph node dissection is performed because of a positive SLN but increases to 20 to 50 % when the procedure is done for palpable disease [49–52].

The most important results of MSLT-I concern the 1270 patients with a melanoma of intermediate Breslow thickness, and these will be discussed here in more detail. An interesting question is whether the watch-and-wait observation period during which an occult nodal metastasis grows to palpable size permits metastatic spread to other nodes within the lymph node basin. The answer is yes, as the mean total number of involved lymph nodes in patients with a tumor-positive SLN in whom early lymph node dissection was performed was 1.4, yet this number increased to 3.3 by the time lymph nodes became palpable ($p=0.0001$). The number of involved lymph nodes is a powerful prognostic factor in the AJCC-UICC staging classification, and this is clearly apparent when survival in the two lymph node-positive arms is compared [35]. Ten-year melanoma-specific survival rose from 41.5 % when nodal clearance was performed for palpable nodal disease to 62.1 % when early dissection was carried out because of an involved SLN ($p=0.006$). This represents a very substantial improvement in 10-year survival in patients who were found to be SLN positive and had an immediate completion, lymph node dissection. There was no survival difference for lymph node-positive patients with thicker melanomas, nor between the two randomized groups when the lymph node-negative patients were included.

Contemplating these outcomes, many melanomologists are excited about the exceptional 20.6 % absolute improvement in 10-year survival (from 41.5 to 62.1 %), but not everybody shares this enthusiasm. Opponents emphasize the fact that the survival benefit concerns a subgroup and point out that there is no statistically significant melanoma-specific survival difference between the entire SLN (81.4 %) and observation (78.3 %) arms in the patients with intermediate thickness melanoma, which was the primary aim of the trial [44].

One obvious reason for the lack of such a difference is that the survival gain in the node-positive 21 % target population was diluted by the other 79 % of patients without metastases who could not benefit from the procedure. Also, the number of deaths was smaller than predicted, which reduced the power of the study. The 20.3 % false-negative procedures had a similar effect. However, one should keep in mind that SLN biopsy is a staging test and that its purpose is not to improve survival per se. Its purpose is to identify patients with nodal involvement so that these patients subsequently can undergo a therapeutic procedure that should improve their chances to survive. And this is exactly what was found to be true. Other objections have been raised but the investigators have refuted these [46, 53–56]. Most of the objections appear to be based on little appreciation of the essence of the trial, which was to examine the impact on survival of the combination of SLN biopsy and lymph node dissection. In hindsight, it is clear that much of the confusion might have been prevented if melanoma-specific survival in the node-positive patients had been the designated primary aim of the trial.

10.8 New Developments

10.8.1 Need for Completion Node Dissection in Patients with a Metastatic Sentinel Lymph Node

Now that the MSLT-I has validated the role of SLN biopsy, the next important question is whether SLN-positive patients require further surgery. Completion lymph node dissection yields more nodal metastases in 12–20 % of patients. However, half of these patients harbor occult distant disease that leads to their demise, and a third of the remaining patients can still be cured when the lymph node dissection is carried out at the time that the lymph nodes become palpable [57]. Also, it is not certain that every SLN metastasis inevitably progresses to clinically relevant disease. Some observational studies indicate the need for completion lymph node dissection in all patients found to be SLN positive while others suggest that this is not always required [58, 59]. The question is particularly pertinent in patients with minimal involvement of the SLN [60]. The observational prospective Minitub study (European Organisation for Research and Treatment of Cancer) and the randomized MSLT-II study are currently addressing this question.

10.8.2 New Tracers

New tracers have been developed that are discussed in detail elsewhere in this book. The tracer Lymphoseek, which is a mannosyl diethylenetriamine-pentaacetate dextran and targets the CD206 receptor that is present in the reticuloendothelial system including lymph nodes, has been approved by the US Food and Drug Administration. It has been suggested that it is more quickly resorbed from the injection site as the size of the molecule is about 7 nm and that it is better retained in the SLN, but its superiority over traditional radiopharmaceuticals remains to be established [61].

Fluorescent tracers exploit a different type of radiation. They require a source of near-infrared light and a camera to detect the reemitted near-infrared light. The new generation of cameras combines the fluorescence image with the standard video image so that the lymph node is visualized in the surrounding tissue. The specific feature of the approach is the fact that the near-infrared light can be discerned through a layer of tissue. In our experience, this layer is very thin and better tracers need to be developed for this approach to be useful in patients with melanoma. A hybrid tracer that is both radioactive and fluorescent has also been developed and explored in clinical studies [62, 63]. This tracer allows preoperative lymphoscintigraphy and probe detection and adds the option of intraoperative fluorescence imaging. This approach appears to be useful in difficult cases [64, 65]. Such fluorescent tracers would appear to offer greatest potential in cancers of visceral organs where injection of the usual radiocolloids preoperatively is technically difficult and dynamic imaging not possible to identify the SLN receiving the lymphatic collector. Considerable effort is currently underway to apply this approach using fluorophores in patients with lung cancer and gastrointestinal cancers.

10.8.3 Innovative Imaging Technology

In addition to the near-infrared light camera, other new intraoperative imaging technologies have recently been introduced. A portable gamma camera for use in the operating theater can visualize radioactive hot spots directly in the operative field [66]. Freehand SPECT is another innovative intraoperative imaging technique [67]. This technique synchronizes information on position, orientation, and readings of the gamma ray detection probe. Intraoperatively, a three-dimensional nearly real-time image is constructed that guides the surgeon to the SLN [68].

10.8.4 Clinical Need for New Technologies

There is usually excellent drainage of the injected radiopharmaceutical from the skin, and the associated nodal basins are typically on the outside of the body. Using the conventional techniques described earlier in this chapter, the SLN can be found in close to 100 % of cases and usually within 10 min. Therefore, we feel there is little need for more advanced technology in most melanoma patients. That being said, these new technologies may be useful in difficult cases. SLN biopsy in the neck may be challenging [66]. SLN outside the usual nodal basin also come to mind. However, the main potential of these innovative diagnostic approaches as we see them is that they may facilitate SLN biopsy in other cancer types, cancers deeper inside the body, cancers with a more intricate anatomy, and cancer types with more complex lymphatic drainage than melanoma [69].

10.8.5 New Drugs for Melanoma Patients with Inoperable Metastases

Various new drugs have been introduced and have been shown to improve survival in patients with inoperable regional and visceral melanoma metastases. It is only logical that the value of these drugs is now being examined in earlier stages of the disease, for example, as adjuvant therapies in patients with operable lymph node metastases. SLN biopsy appears preeminently suitable to identify these patients. Preliminary results of a trial of adjuvant immunotherapy with ipilimumab were presented in 2014 [70]. An improved recurrence-free survival was found in patients with lymph node metastases exceeding 1 mm, but overall survival data were not available at the time of writing. The associated morbidity was considerable and five patients (1.1 %) died from the treatment. However, other adjuvant studies are in progress evaluating newer, less toxic drugs that have been more effective than ipilimumab in treating established visceral melanoma metastases.

10.9 Current Clinical Practice

Based on the currently available evidence, patients with melanomas with a Breslow thickness of 1.2–3.5 mm that is clinically localized are candidates for SLN biopsy. Primarily, it provides accurate staging and a useful guide to prognosis but the procedure also reduces their risk of nodal recurrence, and lymph node-positive patients have a 20.6 % absolute improvement in their 10-year survival. SLN biopsy can also be considered in patients outside the intermediate thickness range for staging, for providing prognostic information, and for regional disease control. The number of patients with a melanoma thinner than 1.2 mm in MSLT-I was too small to allow proper analysis, and no survival benefit was found if the melanoma was thicker than 3.5 mm. Only about 5 % of the patients with a thin melanoma have lymph node metastases. Routine SLN biopsy in these patients would have a low yield, but there are many such patients and it appears reasonable to assume that early lymph node dissection would improve their prognosis because the risk of occult distant metastases is so small. The lack of evidence is keenly felt. At Melanoma Institute Australia, SLN biopsy is considered in patients with a thin melanoma in the presence of unfavorable features such as young age, ulceration, high mitotic rate, microsatellite metastases, or lymphovascular invasion. In such patients, if the ultrasound examination of the mapped SLNs is normal, this means that the metastasis if present is less than 2 mm in diameter, and it is likely that a proportion of these patients will survive if the involved SLN is removed at the time of wide excision of the primary melanoma.

Patients with thick melanomas often have occult metastases to visceral organs and generally have a poor prognosis. Early treatment of their lymph node metastases does not improve their survival rate but does improve regional disease control.

Until further evidence becomes available, the practice at Melanoma Institute Australia is to recommend regional lymph node dissection to all patients with SLN metastases [71]. The preliminary results of adjuvant systemic therapy with ipilimumab do not warrant routine treatment with this agent for SLN-positive patients, but the results of trials of adjuvant therapy with other agents are awaited eagerly.

Conclusions

SLN biopsy is an accurate procedure to stage melanoma patients when performed by an experienced multidisciplinary team using a meticulous technique. The status of the lymph nodes is the most powerful prognostic factor. It is now clear that radioguided surgery really improves the survival rate, as MSLT-I has provided evidence that sentinel lymph node biopsy can identify lymph node-positive patients whose chance of survival at 10 years improves from 41.5 to 62.1 % with an immediate regional lymph node dissection. The technique of SLN biopsy continues to evolve and its importance will expand even further when adequate adjuvant systemic therapies become available.

References

1. Cancer Council New South Wales. http://www.cancercouncil.com.au/melanoma/2015.
2. Hollestein LM, van den Akker SA, Nijsten T, Karim-Kos HE, Coebergh JW, de Vries E. Trends of cutaneous melanoma in the Netherlands: increasing incidence rates among all Breslow thickness categories and rising mortality rates since 1989. Ann Oncol. 2012;23:524–30.
3. Veronesi U, Adamus J, Bandiera DC, Brennhovd IO, Caceres E, Cascinelli N, et al. Delayed regional lymph node dissection in stage I melanoma of the skin of the lower extremities. Cancer. 1982;49:2420–30.
4. Sim FH, Taylor WF, Pritchard DJ, Soule EH. Lymphadenectomy in the management of stage I malignant melanoma: a prospective randomized study. Mayo Clin Proc. 1986;61:697–705.
5. Balch CM, Soong SJ, Bartolucci AA, Urist MM, Karakousis CP, Smith TJ, et al. Efficacy of an elective regional lymph node dissection of 1 to 4 mm thick melanomas for patients 60 years of age and younger. Ann Surg. 1996;224:255–66.
6. Cascinelli N, Morabito A, Santinami M, Mackie RM, Belli F. Immediate or delayed dissection of regional nodes in patients with melanoma of the trunk: a randomized trial. WHO melanoma programme. Lancet. 1998;351:793–6.
7. Balch CM, Soong SJ, Gershenwald JE, Thompson JF, Reintgen DS, Cascinelli N, et al. Prognostic factors analysis of 17,600 melanoma patients: validation of the American Joint Committee on Cancer melanoma staging system. J Clin Oncol. 2001;19:3622–34.
8. Morton DL, Hoon DS, Cochran AJ, Turner RR, Essner R, Takeuchi H, et al. Lymphatic mapping and sentinel lymphadenectomy for early-stage melanoma: therapeutic utility and implications of nodal microanatomy and molecular staging for improving the accuracy of detection of nodal micrometastases. Ann Surg. 2003;238:538–49.
9. Kretschmer L, Hilgers R, Mohrle M, Balda BR, Breuninger H, Konz B, et al. Patients with lymphatic metastasis of cutaneous malignant melanoma benefit from sentinel lymphonodectomy and early excision of their nodal disease. Eur J Cancer. 2004;40:212–8.
10. Starz H, Siedlecki K, Balda BR. Sentinel lymphonodectomy and s-classification: a successful strategy for better prediction and improvement of outcome of melanoma. Ann Surg Oncol. 2004;11(3 Suppl):162S–8.
11. Nowecki ZI, Rutkowski P, Michej W. The survival benefit to patients with positive sentinel node melanoma after completion lymph node dissection may be

limited to the subgroup with a primary lesion Breslow thickness greater than 1.0 and less than or equal to 4 mm (pT2-pT3). Ann Surg Oncol. 2008;15: 2223–34.
12. Morton DL, Wen DR, Wong JH, Economou JS, Cagle LA, Storm FK, et al. Technical details of intraoperative lymphatic mapping for early stage melanoma. Arch Surg. 1992;127:392–9.
13. Uren RF, Howman-Giles R, Thompson JF, Shaw HM, Quinn MJ, O'Brien CJ, et al. Lymphoscintigraphy to identify sentinel lymph nodes in patients with melanoma. Melanoma Res. 1994;4:395–9.
14. Morton DL, Bostick PJ. Will the true sentinel node please stand? Ann Surg Oncol. 1999;6:12–4.
15. Balch CM, Ross MI. Sentinel lymphadenectomy for melanoma – is it a substitute for elective lymphadenectomy? Ann Surg Oncol. 1999;6:416–7.
16. Thompson JF, Uren RF. What is a 'sentinel' lymph node? Eur J Surg Oncol. 2000;26:103–4.
17. Nieweg OE, Tanis PJ, Kroon BBR. The definition of a sentinel node. Ann Surg Oncol. 2001;9:538–41.
18. Veronesi U, Paganelli G, Galimberti V, Viale G, Zurrida S, Bedoni M, et al. Sentinel-node biopsy to avoid axillary dissection in breast cancer with clinically negative lymph-nodes. Lancet. 1997;349:1864–7.
19. De Cicco C, Sideri M, Bartolomei M, Maggioni A, Colombo N, Bocciolone L, et al. Sentinel node detection by lymphoscintigraphy and gamma detecting probe in patients with vulvar cancer. J Nucl Med. 1997;38:33P.
20. Gershenwald JE, Tseng CH, Thompson W, Mansfield PF, Lee JE, Bouvet M, et al. Improved sentinel lymph node localization in patients with primary melanoma with the use of radiolabeled colloid. Surgery. 1998;124:203–10.
21. Boxen I, McCready D, Ballinger JR. Sentinel node detection and definition may depend on the imaging agent and timing. Clin Nucl Med. 1999;24:390–4.
22. Veenstra HJ, Wouters MJWM, Kroon BBR, Valdés Olmos RA, Nieweg OE. Less false-negative sentinel node procedures in melanoma patients with experience and proper collaboration. J Surg Oncol. 2011;104:454–7.
23. Uren RF, Hawman-Giles R, Thompson JF. Variation in cutaneous lymphatic flow rates. Ann Surg Oncol. 1997;4:279–81.
24. Jansen L. Sentinel node biopsy: evolving from melanoma to breast cancer. PhD thesis. University of Amsterdam; 2000.
25. Uren RF, Howman-Giles R, Thompson JF, McCarthy WH, Quinn MJ, Roberts JM, et al. Interval nodes: the forgotten sentinel nodes in patients with melanoma. Arch Surg. 2000;135:1168–72.
26. Valdés Olmos RA, Rietbergen DD, Vidal-Sicart S, Manca G, Giammarile F, Mariani G. Contribution of SPECT/CT imaging to radioguided sentinel lymph node biopsy in breast cancer, melanoma, and other solid cancers: from "open and see" to "see and open". Q J Nucl Medi Mol Imaging Off Publ Ital Assoc Nucl Med. 2014;58:127–39.
27. Uren RF. SPECT/CT Lymphoscintigraphy to locate the sentinel lymph node in patients with melanoma. Ann Surg Oncol. 2009;16:1459–60.
28. Van der Ploeg IM, Valdés Olmos RA, Kroon BBR, Wouters MW, van den Brekel MW, Vogel WV, et al. The yield of SPECT/CT for anatomical lymphatic mapping in patients with melanoma. Ann Surg Oncol. 2009;16:1537–42.
29. Veenstra HJ, Vermeeren L, Valdés Olmos RA, Nieweg OE. The additional value of lymphatic mapping with routine SPECT/CT in unselected patients with clinically localized melanoma. Ann Surg Oncol. 2012;19:1018–23.
30. Tanis PJ, Hart AAM, Nieweg OE, Kroon BBR. The illusion of a learning phase for lymphatic mapping. Ann Surg Oncol. 2002;9:142–7.
31. Nieweg OE, Jansen L, Kroon BBR. Technique of lymphatic mapping and sentinel node biopsy for melanoma. Eur J Surg Oncol. 1998;24:520–4.
32. Morton DL, Thompson JF, Cochran AJ, Mozzillo N, Nieweg OE, Roses DF, et al. Final trial report of sentinel-node biopsy versus nodal observation in melanoma. N Engl J Med. 2014;370:599–609.
33. Gershenwald JE, Thompson W, Mansfield PF, Lee JE, Colome MI, Tseng CH, et al. Multi-institutional melanoma lymphatic mapping experience: the prognostic value of sentinel lymph node status in 612 stage I or II melanoma patients. J Clin Oncol. 1999;17:976–83.
34. Jansen L, Nieweg OE, Peterse JL, Hoefnagel CA, Valdés Olmos RA, Kroon BBR. Reliability of sentinel lymph node biopsy for staging melanoma. Br J Surg. 2000;87:484–9.
35. Balch CA, Gershenwald JE, Soong SJ, Thompson JF, Atkins MB, Byrd DR, et al. Final version of 2009 AJCC melanoma staging and classification. J Clin Oncol. 2009;27:6199–206.
36. Estourgie SH, Nieweg OE, Kroon BBR. High incidence of in-transit metastases after sentinel node biopsy in patients with melanoma. Br J Surg. 2004;91:1370–1.
37. Veenstra HJ, Van der Ploeg IMC, Wouters MWJM, Kroon BBR, Nieweg OE. Reevaluation of the locoregional recurrence rate in melanoma patients with a positive sentinel node compared to patients with palpable nodal involvement. Ann Surg Oncol. 2010; 17:521–6.
38. Van Poll D, Thompson JF, Colman MH, McKinnon JG, Saw RP, Stretch JR, et al. A sentinel node biopsy does not increase the incidence of in-transit metastasis in patients with primary cutaneous melanoma. Ann Surg Oncol. 2005;12:597–608.
39. Nieweg OE, Tanis PJ, De Vries JDH, Kroon BBR. Sensitivity of sentinel node biopsy in melanoma. J Surg Oncol. 2001;78:223–4.
40. Nieweg OE. False-negative sentinel node biopsy. Ann Surg Oncol. 2009;16:2089–91.
41. Sakowska MM, Smith N, Coutts RJ. Twelve years' experience of sentinel lymph node biopsy for melanoma at a rural New Zealand hospital. N Z Med J. 2014;127:12–22.

42. Van der Ploeg IMC, Nieweg OE, Van Rijk MC, Valdés Olmos RA, Kroon BBR. Axillary recurrence after a tumour-negative sentinel node biopsy in breast cancer patients: a systematic review and meta-analysis of the literature. Eur J Surg Oncol. 2008;34:1277–84.
43. Karim RZ, Scolyer RA, Li W, Yee VSK, McKinnon JG, Li LXL, et al. False negative sentinel lymph node biopsies in melanoma may result from deficiencies in nuclear medicine, surgery, or pathology. Ann Surg. 2008;247:1003–10.
44. Rosenberg SA. Why perform sentinel-lymph-node biopsy in patients with melanoma? Nat Clin Pract Oncol. 2008;5:1.
45. Thomas JM. Prognostic false-positivity of the sentinel node in melanoma. Nat Clin Pract Oncol. 2008;5: 18–23.
46. Morton DL, Cochran AJ, Thompson JF. The rationale for sentinel-node biopsy in primary melanoma. Nat Clin Pract Oncol. 2008;5:510–1.
47. Garreau JR, Faries MB, Ye X, Morton DL. Mood state and melanoma outcome in the Multicenter Selective Lymphadenectomy Trial. J Clin Oncol. 2009;27:15S, abstract 9603.
48. Faries MB, Thompson JF, Cochran A, Elashoff R, Glass EC, Mozzillo N, et al. The impact on morbidity and length of stay of early versus delayed complete lymphadenectomy in melanoma: results of the Multicenter Selective Lymphadenectomy Trial (I). Ann Surg Oncol. 2010;17:3324–9.
49. Gershenwald JE, Berman RS, Porter G, Mansfield PF, Lee JE, Ross MI. Regional nodal basin control is not compromised by previous sentinel lymph node biopsy in patients with melanoma. Ann Surg Oncol. 2000;7:226–31.
50. Chao C, Wong SL, Ross MI, Reintgen DS, Noyes RD, Cerrito PB, et al. Patterns of early recurrence after sentinel lymph node biopsy for melanoma. Am J Surg. 2002;184:520–4.
51. Lee RJ, Gibbs JF, Proulx GM, Kollmorgen DR, Jia C, Kraybill WG. Nodal basin recurrence following lymph node dissection for melanoma: implications for adjuvant radiotherapy. Int J Radiat Oncol Biol Phys. 2000;46:467–74.
52. Gershenwald JE, Ross MI. Sentinel-lymph-node biopsy for cutaneous melanoma. N Engl J Med. 2011;364:1738–45.
53. Morton DL, Cochran AJ, Thompson JF. Authors' response to a letter to the editor re: sentinel node biopsy for early-stage melanoma. Ann Surg. 2007;245:828–9.
54. Morton DL, Elashoff R. Sentinel node biopsy: facts to clear the alleged clouds. Arch Dermatol. 2008; 144:685–6.
55. Sanki A, Uren RF, Moncrieff M, Tran KL, Scolyer RA, Lin HY, et al. Targeted high-resolution ultrasound is not an effective substitute for sentinel lymph node biopsy in patients with primary cutaneous melanoma. J Clin Oncol. 2009;27:5614–9.
56. Thompson JF, Cochran AJ, Faries MB. Sentinel-node biopsy in melanoma. N Engl J Med. 2014;370:2149–50.
57. Estourgie SH, Nieweg OE, Valdés Olmos RA, Hoefnagel CA, Kroon BBR. Review and evaluation of sentinel node procedures in 250 melanoma patients with a median follow-up of 6 years. Ann Surg Oncol. 2003;10:681–8.
58. Wong SL, Morton DL, Thompson JF, Gershenwald JE, Leong SP, Reintgen DS, et al. Melanoma patients with positive sentinel nodes who did not undergo completion lymphadenectomy: a multi-institutional study. Ann Surg Oncol. 2006;13:809–16.
59. Scheri RP, Essner R, Turner RR, Ye X, Wanek L, Morton DL. Do isolated tumor cells in the sentinel node in melanoma affect long-term prognosis? Ann Surg Oncol. 2007;14 Suppl:11.
60. Veenstra HJ, Brouwer OR, van der Ploeg IM, Kroon BBR, Nieweg OE. Five-year follow-up of 16 melanoma patients with a Starz I-involved sentinel node in whom completion lymph node dissection was omitted. Melanoma Res. 2012;22:436–9.
61. Vera DR, Wallace AM, Hoh CK. [(99m)Tc]MAG(3)-mannosyl-dextran: a receptor-binding radiopharmaceutical for sentinel node detection. Nucl Med Biol. 2001;28:493–8.
62. Buckle T, van Leeuwen AC, Chin PT, Janssen H, Muller SH, Jonkers J, et al. A self-assembled multimodal complex for combined pre- and intraoperative imaging of the sentinel lymph node. Nanotechnology. 2010;21:355101.
63. Brouwer OR, Buckle T, Vermeeren L, Klop WM, Balm AJ, van der Poel HG, et al. Comparing the hybrid fluorescent-radioactive tracer indocyanine green-99mTc-nanocolloid with 99mTc-nanocolloid for sentinel node identification: a validation study using lymphoscintigraphy and SPECT/CT. J Nucl Med. 2012;53:1034–40.
64. Van den Berg NS, Brouwer OR, Schaafsma BE, Matheron HM, Klop WM, Balm AJ, et al. Multimodal surgical guidance during sentinel node biopsy for melanoma: combined gamma tracing and fluorescence imaging of the sentinel node through use of the hybrid tracer indocyanine green-(99m)Tc-Nanocolloid. Radiology. 2015;275:521–9.
65. Brouwer OR, Klop WM, Buckle T, Vermeeren L, van den Brekel MW, Balm AJ, et al. Feasibility of sentinel node biopsy in head and neck melanoma using a hybrid radioactive and fluorescent tracer. Ann Surg Oncol. 2012;19:1988–94.
66. Vermeeren L, Valdés Olmos RA, Klop WM, van der Ploeg IM, Nieweg OE, Balm AJ, et al. SPECT/CT for sentinel lymph node mapping in head and neck melanoma. Head Neck. 2011;33:1–6.
67. Wendler T, Herrmann K, Schnelzer A, Lasser T, Traub J, Kutter O, et al. First demonstration of 3-D lymphatic mapping in breast cancer using freehand SPECT. Eur J Nucl Med Mol Imaging. 2010; 37:1452–61.
68. Mihaljevic AL, Rieger A, Belloni B, Hein R, Okur A, Scheidhauer K, et al. Transferring innovative freehand SPECT to the operating room: first experiences

with sentinel lymph node biopsy in malignant melanoma. Eur J Surg Oncol. 2014;40:42–8.
69. Nieweg OE. Current status of sentinel lymph node biopsy in patients with melanoma. Rozhl Chir Mesicnik Cesk Chir Spol. 2014;93:485–90.
70. Eggermont AMM, Chiarion-Sileni V, Grob JJ, Dummer R, Wolchok JD, Schmidt H. Ipilimumab versus placebo after complete resection of stage III melanoma: initial efficacy and safety results from the EORTC 18071 phase III trial. J Clin Oncol. 2014;32:LBA9008.
71. Scolyer RA, Murali R, Satzger I, Thompson JF. The detection and significance of melanoma micrometastases in sentinel nodes. Surg Oncol. 2008;17:165–74.

Part V

Clinical Application: Head and Neck

11 Radioguided Sentinel Lymph Node Mapping and Biopsy in Oral Cancer

Remco de Bree and Christina Bluemel

Contents

Abstract

Oral cancer is one of the most common head and neck malignancies. As lymph node metastases are one of the most important prognostic factors, an elective neck dissection (END) has been widely performed for accurate staging of the cervical lymph nodes. However, up to 75 % of patients are overtreated and may suffer from side effects of END. In 2001, the first results and advantages of sentinel lymph node biopsy (SLNB) as an alternative for neck staging in clinically node negative patients with oral cancer were firstly discussed in an international conference. The high detection rate, sensitivity, and low false-negative rate of SLNB was demonstrated in multicenter studies. However, due to the complex lymphatic drainage and close vicinity of the injection site, SLNB in head and neck is challenging. The development of new tracers and technologies might facilitate the intraoperative detection of SLNs and improve results of SLNB.

R. de Bree, MD, PhD (✉)
Department of Head and Neck Surgical Oncology, UMC Utrecht Cancer Center, UMCU Utrecht, Heidelberglaan 1000, Utrecht 3584 CX, The Netherlands
e-mail: r.debree@umcutrecht.nl

C. Bluemel, MD
Department of Nuclear Medicine, University Hospital of Würzburg, Würzburg, Germany

11.1 Introduction

Oral cancer is one of the most common head and neck cancers. A total of 30,260 new cases of oral cancer are estimated in the United States in 2015, and the incidence is rising [1, 2]. Squamous cell carcinoma is the most frequent tumor type in the

K. Herrmann et al. (eds.), *Radioguided Surgery: Current Applications and Innovative Directions in Clinical Practice*, DOI 10.1007/978-3-319-26051-8_11

oral cavity and has a high propensity to metastasize through lymphatics to regional lymph nodes rather than to spread hematogenously. Moreover, regional metastasis at time of diagnosis is one of the most important prognostic factors. The presence of cervical lymph node metastasis roughly reduces survival by half [3]. Patients with multiple contralateral or bilateral metastases in the neck have even a more markedly reduced survival. It is generally accepted that the neck has to be treated by surgery (i.e., neck dissection) and/or radiotherapy with or without chemotherapy when lymph node metastases are present.

Unfortunately, there is no single noninvasive imaging technique, which could detect occult (clinically undetectable) lymph node metastasis reliably enough [4, 5]. Recently a meta-analysis comparing computed tomography (CT), magnetic resonance imaging (MRI), positron emission tomography (PET), and ultrasound (US) for the detection of cervical lymph node metastasis in head and neck cancer patients with a clinically negative (cN0) neck was performed by Liao et al. [6]. The pooled estimates for sensitivity on a per-neck basis were 52 % (95 % confidence interval (CI): 39–65), 65 % (CI: 34–87), 66 % (CI: 47–80), and 66 % (CI: 45–77) for CT, MRI, PET, and US, respectively. The pooled estimates for specificity were 93 % (CI: 87–97), 81 % (CI: 64–91), 87 % (CI: 77–93), and 78 % (CI: 71–83) for CT, MRI, PET, and US, respectively. In this study, US-guided fine-needle aspiration cytology (USgFNAC) was not included, because of several methodological reasons [6]. The reported sensitivity of USgFNAC in cN0 neck was between 42 and 73 % [5, 7].

Consequently, the management of the cN0 neck is still a controversial issue. There is general agreement that elective treatment of the neck is indicated when there is a high likelihood of occult, i.e., clinically and radiologically undetectable, lymph node metastases. A neck dissection is generally performed when the neck needs to be entered to resect the primary tumor or to reconstruct the surgical defect. When the feasibility of regular follow-up is questionable, the neck will be generally treated [4, 5]. The dilemma to treat the cN0 neck applies to most early-stage (T1-T2cN0) oral squamous cell carcinomas (OSCC).

The rationale for elective (prophylactic) treatment is based on the following assumptions. First, occult metastases will inevitably develop into clinically manifest disease. Second, even with watchful waiting, some patients will develop extensive or even inoperable disease in the neck with a wait-and-see policy. Third, if left untreated, disease in the neck may be associated with a higher incidence of distant metastases developing while the undetected lymph node metastasis is growing to a clinically detectable size. The arguments against elective treatment of the neck are as follows. First a large proportion of patients are subjected to the morbidity (e.g., shoulder dysfunction [8]) and costs of unnecessary treatment. Second, such treatment may remove or destroy a barrier to cancer spread and a route of cancer spread in case of local recurrence or second primary tumor.

11.2 Sentinel Lymph Node Procedure

The standard sentinel lymph node (SLN) procedure in OSCC consists of lymphoscintigraphy, biopsy, and histopathological examination of the SLN. In a 2-day protocol 40–100 MBq and in a same-day protocol 25–40 MBq of technetium-99m (^{99m}Tc)-labelled colloidal albumin divided over 4 aliquots of 0.1–0.2 mL each is generally peritumorally submucosally injected (Fig. 11.1). In general, directly after injections, dynamic and static

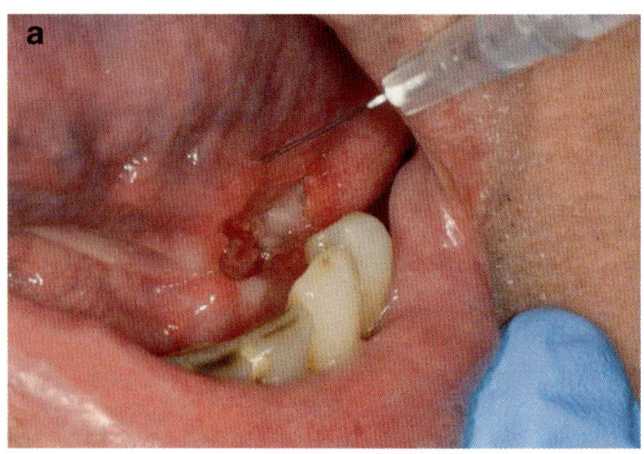

Fig. 11.1 Case of a patient with a paramedian cT1N0 floor of mouth carcinoma on the left side. (**a**) Peritumoral injection of ^{99m}Tc-labelled nanocolloid. (**b**) Dynamic scintigrams. (**c**) Planar late scintigrams. (**d**) Peritumoral injection of *patent blue*. (**e**) Gamma-probe-guided sentinel lymph node biopsy. (**f**) *Blue* coloration of sentinel lymph node. (**g**) Confirmation of hot sentinel lymph node by activity counting

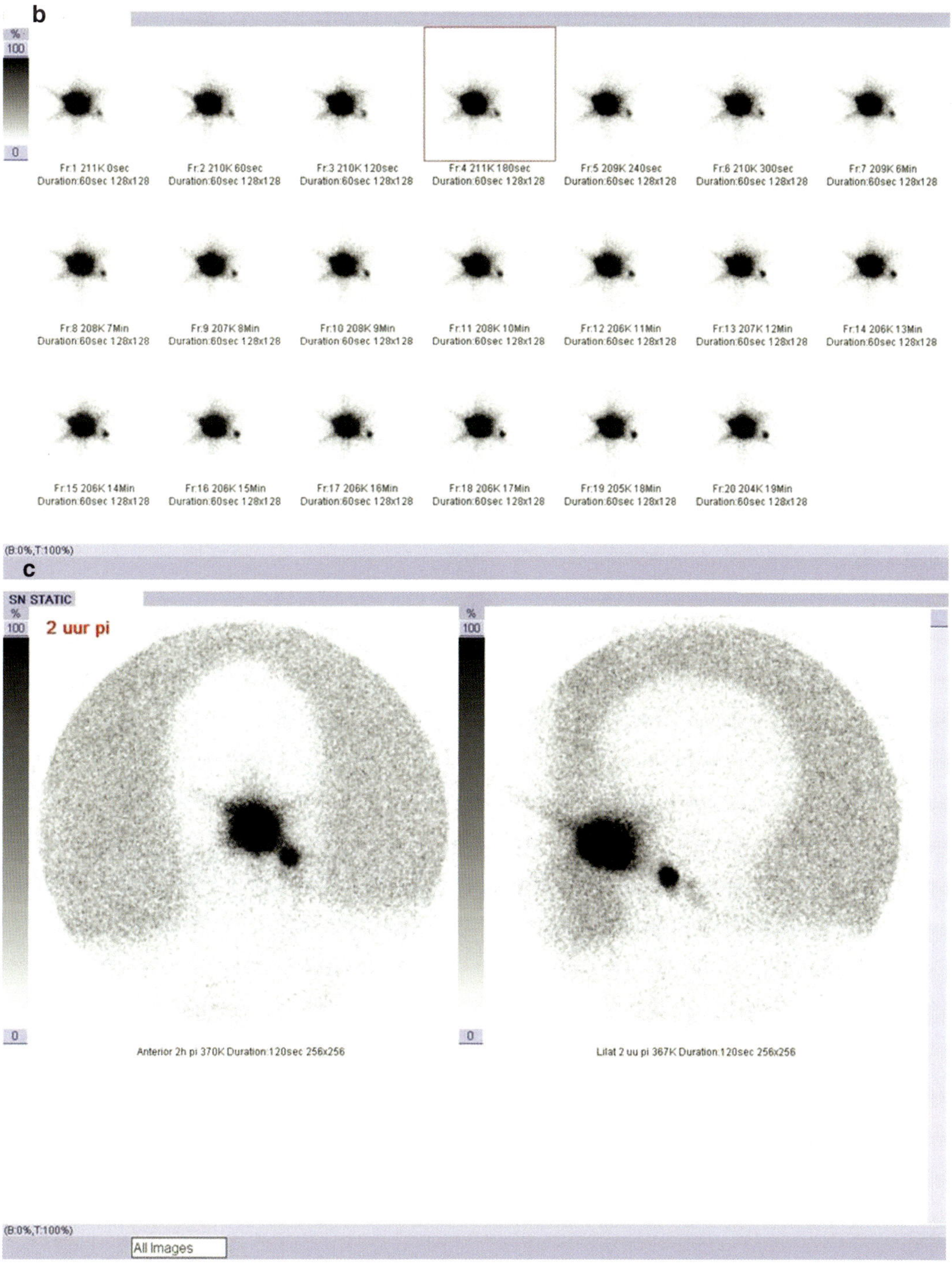

Fig. 11.1 (continued)

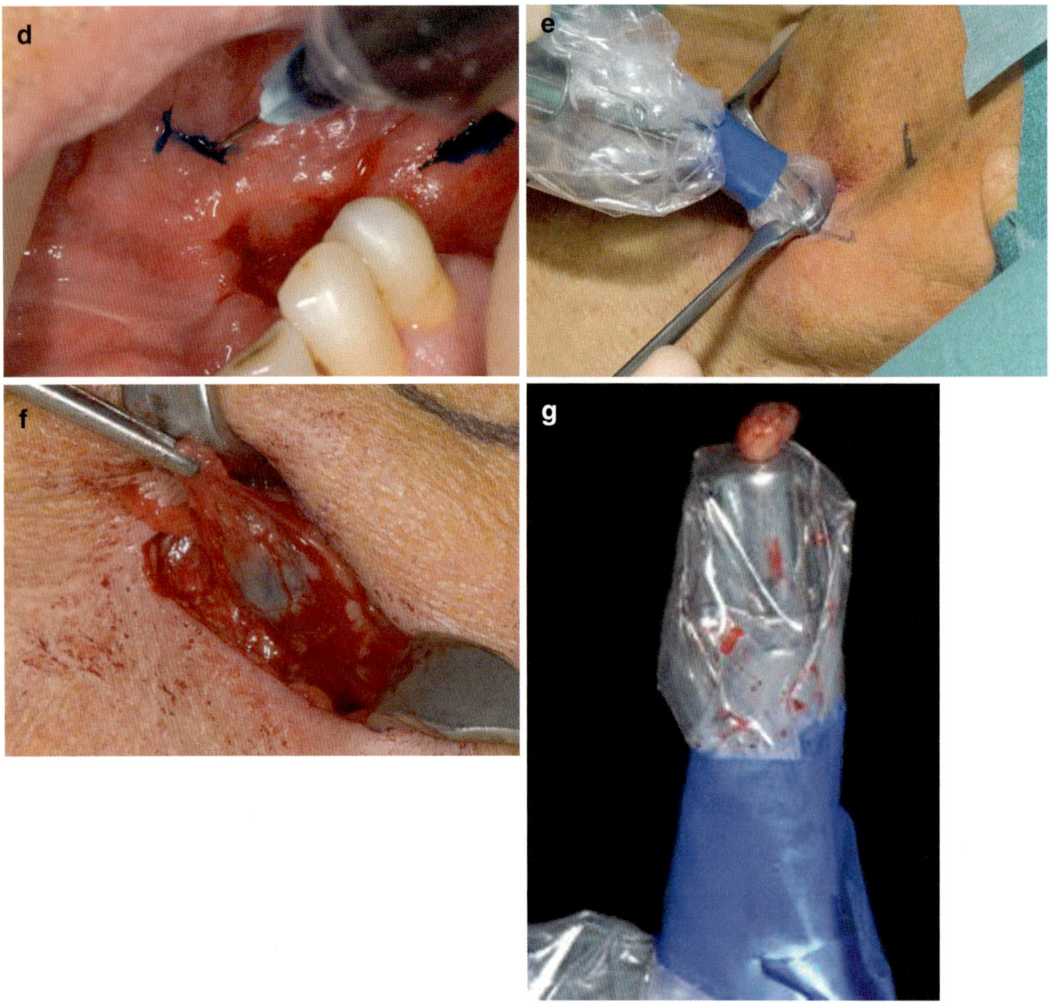

Fig. 11.1 (continued)

planar lymphoscintigraphy followed by single-photon emission tomography/computed tomography (SPECT-CT) imaging is performed [9]. Late imaging (2–4 h after injections) is generally only needed in patients with midline tumors and tumors in the oral cavity other than mobile tongue or lateral flour of mouth [10], or if no clear, SLN could be visualized in early imaging [9]. Based on the preoperative lymphoscintigraphy results, the position of the SLN is marked on the skin [9].

The main radiopharmaceutical used in Europe is ^{99m}Tc-labelled nanocolloidal albumin with a mean particle size of 8–30 nm, whereas in the United States, this tracer is not approved, and ^{99m}Tc-rhenium sulfide colloid (mean particle size 23–25 nm) and ^{99m}Tc-sulfide colloid (particle size <100–200 nm) are used. Since these radiopharmaceuticals are registered for breast cancer and melanoma, all these tracers have to be used off-label. ^{99m}Tc-labelled-tilmanocept (^{99m}Tc-diethylenetriamine pentaacetic acid-mannosyl-dextran) [11–13], a novel receptor-targeted radiopharmaceutical, recently received approval from the Food and Drug Administration (FDA) and positive statement of the European Medicines Agency (EMA) for use in SLNB for melanoma, breast cancer, and head and neck cancer. It is nonparticulate radiotracer that contains multiple mannose moieties with high affinity for the CD206 receptor found on macrophages and dendritic cells, enhancing targeting to these cells within the sentinel lymph node. In breast cancer and melanoma, it may have improved clearance from the injection site and enhanced retention within the SLN [11, 12, 14]. This tracer has only recently been tested in early oral squamous cell cancer (OSCC) [15] and head and neck cancers [13]. There have yet to be any head-to-head studies comparing ^{99m}Tc-labelled-tilmanocept to ^{99m}Tc-labelled colloids [9].

Sentinel lymph node biopsy (SLNB) is performed under general anesthesia, and intraoperative detection of the SLN is possible by a combination of peritumorally injected blue dye (coloration) and a portable, handheld gamma probe (radionuclide detection). One or more blue and/or radioactive ('hot') SLNs are identified and excised. Since the use of blue dye appeared to be of limited additional values, some surgeons do not use this dye anymore in head and neck cancers [16]. This was recently confirmed by a sensitivity of only 40 % found in 15 patients who received only intraoperative peritumorally injections of 1 % isosulfan dye [17].

After surgical removal, the SLN is investigated by meticulous histopathological examination using stepped serial sectioning and immunohistochemistry. Current best practice guidelines for the provision of SNB in early OSCC patients have been outlined, which provide a framework for the currently evolving recommendations for its use [9].

11.3 Diagnostic Value of Sentinel Lymph Node Procedure

The feasibility of the SLN concept in OSCC was first reported by Alex and Krag in 1996 [18] and has been validated in several studies in which all patients underwent an elective neck dissection (END) after SLNB [19]. The histopathological examination of the neck dissection specimen was used as reference (gold) standard. Although several studies have validated the SLNB concept in OSCC, the American College of Surgeons Oncology Group (ACOSOG) performed a validation study (Z0360) with 140 patients in 25 institutions and found a sensitivity of 90 % and a negative predictive value of 96 %, and these figures were even better for experienced surgeons [20]. A recent meta-analysis of these validation studies with 631 OSCC patients showed a pooled sensitivity and negative predictive value of 94 % and 96 %, respectively [21]. A more recent meta-analysis of 35 studies in which all 1211 patients underwent a neck dissection revealed pooled sensitivity and negative predictive value of 93 % and 97 %, respectively. [22]. Because routine histopathological examination (and not step-serial sectioning and immunohistochemistry) of the neck dissection specimen was used as the reference standard, occult micrometastases might have been missed [23], potentially contributing to higher figures for sensitivity and negative predicting value. Therefore, to investigate the accuracy and utility of SLNB only (without subsequent neck dissection in all patients), follow-up should be used as reference standard [24]. However, when new tracers or instruments are tested, the validation concept using END as reference standard should be considered.

After initial studies to validate the SLN concept in early OSCC patients, several prospective observational studies have been reported. In these studies, a neck dissection was performed only when the SLN contained a metastasis, while a watchful waiting strategy was followed when the SLN did not contain metastasis. In a European multicenter study of 134 cT1/2N0 OSCC patients, 55 patients underwent SLNB followed by END, while 79 patients underwent SLNB as the sole staging tool [25]. In 125 (93 %) patients, the SLN was successfully harvested. For the two groups together, using a reference standard of 5 years follow-up after SLNB staging, a sensitivity of 91 % and a negative predictive value of 95 % were found. In a large single center study ($n = 103$ patients), no false-negative ipsilateral findings were found. Lymphoscintigraphy revealed a hot spot in 98 %, the detection rate was 96 %, and a mean of 2.65 SLNs were harvested per patient [26]. In another single center study of 79 cT1/2N0 patients with oral and oropharyngeal SCC, lymphoscintigraphy showed a hot spot in 95 %, the perioperative detection rate was 99 %, and a mean of 2.7 SLNs were harvested for a sensitivity of 91 % and a negative predictive value of 90 % [27]. A recent meta-analysis including 847 patients from 21 studies showed a pooled sensitivity of 93 % (CI: 90–95 %) in oral cancer patients [28]. With neck dissection as reference standard, the sensitivity was 94 % (CI: 90–97 %), while when follow-up was the reference standard, a sensitivity of 91 % (CI: 84–95 %) was found. The vast majority of the studies included were performed in patients with early OSCC. The negative predictive values ranged from 88 to 100 % [28]. More recently, a retrospective study of 90 previously untreated early OSCC patients with a clinically N0 neck who underwent SLNB (only neck dissection after positive SLNB) was reported: a lymphoscintigraphic identification rate of 98 %, surgical detection rate of 99 %, and upstaging rate of 30 % were found. Using a median follow-up of 10 months, the sensitivity was 93 % and the negative predictive value was 97 % [29].

In a meta-analysis, Liao et al. [30] reported that the best negative predictive rate was the combination of CT or MRI followed by SLNB, when compared to CT or MRI in combination with US, USgFNAC, or PET. Unfortunately, the combination of USgFNAC and SLNB (only when USgFNAC is negative) was not investigated, although USgFNAC was the second best diagnostic technique after SLNB in this meta-analysis. Since SLNB is a more complex and invasive procedure, it can be anticipated that the combination of USgFNAC and SLNB is the most sensitive combination for the detection of occult lymph node metastases with less burden to the patients compared to SLNB only. This combination may be valuable also because gross lymphatic involvement potentially blocks and may alter the lymphatic drainage and reduce the accuracy of SLNB [31].

11.4 Advantages of Sentinel Lymph Node Biopsy

Occult metastases can be missed by routine histopathological techniques in up to 15.2 % [21]. In SLNB, the lymph node with the highest risk is examined by step-serial sectioning and immunohistochemistry. Since the neck contains up to about 100–150 lymph nodes per side, it is practically impossible in daily clinical practice to examine all lymph nodes from a neck dissection specimen so rigorously. Therefore, it can be expected that SLNB or SLNB assisted neck dissection stage the neck more reliable than neck dissection without SLNB [32].

The levels dissected during END depend on the expected drainage pattern of the primary tumor site. However, Civantos et al. [20] found in 14 of the 103 (13.6 %) oral cavity carcinomas and head and neck cutaneous malignancies lymph node drainage patterns outside the expected lymph node basins. These unexpected SLN localizations include not only level IV and V and the contralateral neck but also in 4 of the 43 oral cancer patients facial SLNs. Kovacs et al. [26] reported on the SLN distribution pattern in 103 patients with T1/2N0 oral and oropharyngeal cancer. Besides SLNs in level IV (18/273) and level V (5/273), also SLNs in level VI (5/273) were found. In the ACOSOG Z0360 study, 40 of the 136 patients had drainage to lymph nodes in level IV and V, of whom 5 had drainage to level IV without level I–III. Twenty-seven patients had bilateral drainage on lymphoscintigraphy [33]. Flach et al. [34] found in pretreated necks unexpected lymphatic drainage in 67 %. These findings underline the strength of SLNB in assessing individual drainage patterns.

Recently, a report of a European multicenter study on 109 oral squamous cell carcinoma patients with positive SLNB showed additional (non-SLN) metastases in 34.4 % of the neck dissection specimens. The risk of non-SLN metastases outside the adjacent basins of the positive SLN was low (7.1 %), suggesting that in the vast majority of the patients with a positive SNB, a (super)selective neck dissection may be sufficient [35]. It can be anticipated that using information obtained from the SLNB procedure, neck dissections can be tailored to the individual patient.

SLNB is less invasive than an END. Murer et al. [36] compared shoulder morbidity and postoperative complications between 33 SLNB only and 29 END OSCC patients using questionnaires and objective measures of active shoulder function. SLNB was associated with a shorter incision, significant less (no) complications, and significant better (almost normal) shoulder function. Although all the complications were minor, they all occurred in patients after END [36]. Schiefke et al. [37] also found a significant minor disturbance of shoulder function in 24 HNSCC patients receiving SNB only compared to 25 head and neck SCC (HNSCC) patients who underwent elective neck dissection assessed by patient symptom scores and objective measurements. SNB was also associated with significant less cervical skin numbness and less disturbance of protopathic (pain) sensitivity compared to END [37]. Hernando et al. [38] compared shoulder function, length of the surgical scar, degree of cervical lymphedema, neck hematoma and the presence of orocutaneous fistula in 32 SLNB patients and 41 elective selective (levels I-III) patients with early oral cancer and found statistically significant differences in shoulder function and average scar length. Neck hematomas and oro-cervical communications occurred only in the END group [38]. From these studies, it can be concluded that SNB presents less postoperative morbidity than END.

Apart from reducing neck dissection numbers, SLNB may reduce treatment costs. Using a treatment model derived from the European Sentinel Node Trial (SENT) information, O'Conner et al. [39] produced estimates for relative treatment costs between patients managed through a traditional END or SLNB pathway and found that the SLNB approach is cheaper relative to the traditional surgical approach in the centers from Spain, the United Kingdom, and the Netherlands. Kosuda et al. [40] showed that SLNB was also cost-effective (compared to END) using costs referred to billed costs based on the Japanese national insurance reimbursement system. A recent cost-effectiveness study in which five different strategies for management of the clinically N0 neck (defined as N0 after imaging and ultrasound-guided fine-needle aspiration cytology) in OSCC patients were compared predicted that the SLNB followed by neck dissection (if positive) or watchful waiting (if negative) is more cost-effective than END, watchful waiting, and gene expression proofing (GEP) followed by neck dissection (if high risk) and GEP and SN (in case of high risk GEP) followed by neck dissection (if SNB positive) or watchful waiting [41].

11.5 Limitations of Current Sentinel Lymph Node Procedure

From these data, it can be concluded that the introduction of SLNB in early oral cancer has been successful. This was recognized by the National Comprehensive Cancer Network (NCCN) and resulted in incorporation in the NCCN Clinical Practice Guidelines in Oncology of Head and Neck Cancers (version 2.2014): "Sentinel lymph node biopsy is an alternative to elective neck dissection for the identification of occult cervical metastasis in patients with early (T1 or T2) oral cavity carcinoma in centers where experience for this procedure is available. Its advantages include decreased morbidity and improved cosmetic outcome." [42] However, in some subsites of the oral cavity, e.g., floor of mouth (FOM), these results are significantly worse. With respect to FOM tumors, detection of the SLN appeared to be more difficult: SLN successfully harvested in 88 % vs. 96 % and a significantly lower sensitivity for FOM tumors compared to other sites (80 % vs. 97 %) [25]. This is probably due to the close spatial relation between the primary tumor and the first draining lymph nodes (SLNs). The injection site (around the primary tumor) produces a large hotspot on lymphoscintigraphy possibly hiding SLN(s) in the close proximity of the primary tumor ("shine through"). It is therefore of utmost importance and challenging to improve SLNB in patients with early OSCC at these subsites. Technical improvements are needed to bring SNB for carcinoma of all subsites in the oral cavity to the same high level. More precise information on the localization of the SLN may reduce operating time and the risk of damaging vulnerable structures such as nerves and vessels in the neck improving the safety during surgery. Less extensive exploration will result in less fibrosis hampering an eventual subsequent neck dissection, resulting at the end in a reduction of complications and not-intended sacrificed structures in the neck.

11.6 Improvements in Sentinel Lymph Node Procedure

Due to the anatomical complexity of the head and neck region, hybrid single-photon emission computed tomography with integrated computed tomography (SPECT-CT) might be useful in the localization of SLNs and planning of surgery in patients with OSCC (Fig. 11.2). Although SPECT-CT has the potential to detect *preoperatively* more SLNs as compared to planar lymphoscintigraphy, it still has some difficulties in visualization of SLNs in close spatial relation to the injection site [43]. Other advantages of SPECT-CT might be reduction of the misinterpretation rate (e.g., skin contamination, injection site) and better anatomical localization. SPECT-CT can improve visualization of the relation of SLNs to several vital vascular and neural structures in order to be able to easily (reducing operating time) and more safely remove these nodes [44].

Recently, a PET-tracer, zirconium-89 (^{89}Zr)-nanocolloidal albumin, dedicated to lymphatic mapping and SLN detection using high-resolution PET-CT was developed. Compared to gamma-based techniques, improved detection and more precise localization of SLNs could be achieved on PET-CT in a recently performed clinical feasibility studies. PET-CT was able to identify SLNs close to the injection site and lymphatic vessels, which were not visualized on SPECT-CT [45].

Due to its particular nature and non-standardized variation in preparation, SLNB agents, i.e., radiolabelled colloids (100–1000 nm particle diameter) are retained for prolonged periods within the injection site, which in turn contributes to the phenomenon of the shine through effect. Recently, a receptor-targeted non-particulate tracer, ^{99m}Tc-tilmanocept, was introduced, with smaller size and specific targeting the CD206 mannose receptors located on reticuloendothelial cells within lymph nodes permitting rapid clearance from the injection site and stable retention in SLNs. These characteristics may enable identification of SLNs close to the injection site and limit the visualization of second echelon lymph nodes [13, 15].

Also, intraoperative detection of SLNs close to the primary tumor is often found to be difficult, due to the high amount of radioactivity present at the injection site (i.e., primary tumor). Gamma probe detection may fail in reliable differentiation between SLN and injection site. Blue dye particles follow lymphatic vessels and accumulate in the draining lymph nodes giving them a blue staining. Real-time detection of this blue staining is only possible if there is no overlying tissue. Moreover, blue dye consists of small particles with a very poor retention in the SLN and is therefore restraint to a short period of time. This is probably due to the fast lymphatic drainage in the head and neck area. As a consequence, the use of blue dye appeared to be of limited added value in the head and neck area [32].

Technical innovations to improve intraoperative SLN localization include intraoperative real-time imaging with portable gamma cameras or handheld SPECT and fluorescence imaging. Intraoperative real-time imaging with the portable gamma camera provides an overview of all radioactive spots and can show SLNs near the injection site by adjusting its position. Another advantage may be the certainty it can provide about the completeness and accuracy of SLN excision by showing the remaining activity. This portable gamma camera was able to visualize SNs at difficult sites more efficiently and identifies 9 additional SNs in 6 of the 25 head and neck melanoma or OSCC patients [46]. Handheld SPECT is designed to determine the position of the detector relative to the patient through which 3D images are generated [47]. This provides the surgeon information about the direction and depth of the SLN in relation to the probe. The possibility of generating images in the operating room could be used again after the procedure but before closing the wounds, in order to confirm harvesting of all hot spots. In this way remaining

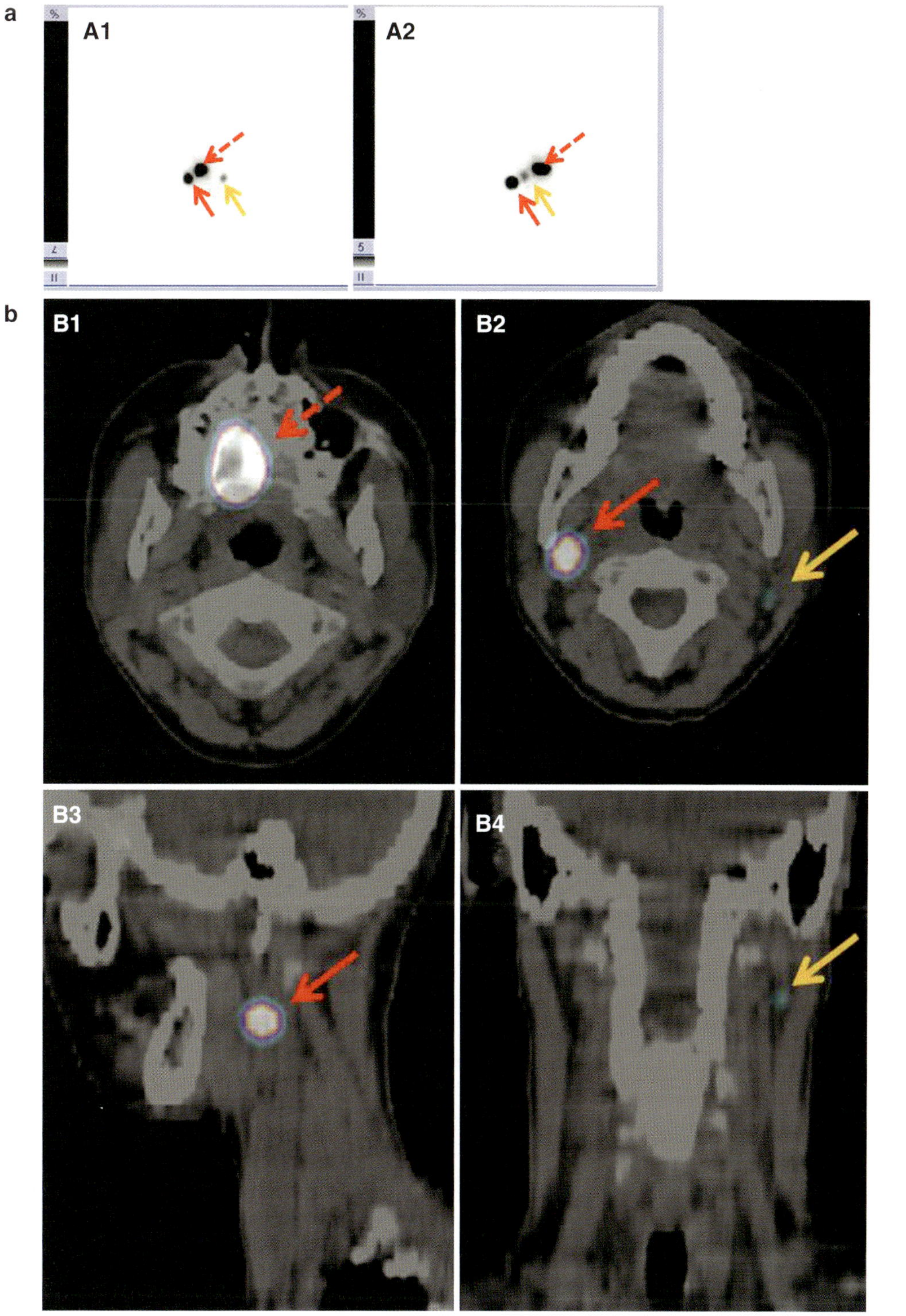

Fig. 11.2 Patient with T1 squamous cell carcinoma of the hard palate. (**a**) Static imaging from ventral (*A1*) and lateral view (*right* lateral view, *A2*) showing the injection site (*dotted arrow*) and one hot spot (SLN) on the left and right cervical region (*arrow*). (**b**) SPECT/CT for better anatomical localization showing the injection site (*dotted arrow*, *B1*) and a cluster of sentinel lymph nodes (*arrow*) in level II right (*B2* (axial view), *B3* (sagittal view)) and a single sentinel lymph node in level II left (*B2*, *B4* (coronal view))

hot spots can be excluded. Promising results in OSCC patients have been reported [48–50].

In head and neck cancer, initial studies described the feasibility of this technique. In 23 patients with T1-T2cN0 OSCC, handheld SPECT was able to detect intraoperatively all but one of the SLNs detected by preoperative imaging successfully (detection rate 98 %), including those in six patients with a tumor in the FOM. Using END as reference standard, a sensitivity of 100 % was found [51]. A study in 66 early oral OSCC patients confirmed that the use of the freehand SPECT system is feasible in the intraoperative detection of SLNs in early-stage oral cancer. Moreover, handheld SPECT provides helpful information facilitating the SLN biopsy procedure in a quarter of cases. However, freehand SPECT could not detect all SLNs, which are located in the vicinity of the injection site [52]. A further development of freehand SPECT technology is the fusion of the 3D images of freehand SPECT with ultrasound. Freehand SPECT-US was able to guide fine-needle aspiration cytology of SLNs in early-stage head and neck cancer [53].

Near-infrared (NIR) fluorescence imaging is also a very attractive option to facilitate intraoperative detection. NIR dyes have the advantage to exhibit reasonable tissue penetration of excited and emitted light with negligible autofluorescence, resulting in higher target-to-background contrast. NIR fluorescence imaging provides high-resolution images which can be obtained in real time during the surgical procedure, even if the structure of interest is covered by some tissue (in contrast to blue dye). Another advantage of NIR fluorescence imaging is that it is much better suited for detection of SLNs close to the primary, because there is negligible influence of fluorescence signal coming from the injection site.

Nowadays, the only FDA-approved NIR-fluorescent compound that has been extensively evaluated for SLN detection is indocyanine green (ICG). Because ICG alone has a poor retention in SLN, it is combined with nanocolloidal albumin. The feasibility of near NIR fluorescence-guided SLN detection has been demonstrated in HNSCC where fluorescence imaging of ICG was used as fluorescent tracer. Using ICG-^{99m}Tc-nanocolloidal albumin, in 4 of the 14 OSCC patients where the SLN was located close to the primary injection site, the SN could only be localized by fluorescence imaging [54]. The combination of ICG and a radiopharmaceutical enables the identification of SLNs more easily and rapidly than by using a radiopharmaceutical alone [55]. Other tracers with improved optical properties have been tested in HNSCC in preclinical settings [55]. Radiolabelled tracers other than colloidal albumin with other characteristics, e.g., ^{99m}Tc-tilmanocept, may improve intraoperative differentiation between SLN and injection site [13, 15]. A very recent multicenter validation study using ^{99m}Tc-tilmanocept for SLNB in head and neck squamous cell carcinoma of the skin and (mainly) oral cavity showed an SN identification rate of 97.6 %, a false-negative rate of 2.56 % and a negative predictive value of 97.8 %. At note, these high figures were also obtained in FOM cancers [13].

11.7 Conclusion and Outlook

SLNB is a reliable diagnostic staging technique of the clinically negative neck in early oral carcinoma and allows for personalized management of the neck. Using SLNB, early-stage OSCC patients can avoid from unnecessarily END, which may reduce morbidity and costs and improve quality of life. However, there is room for improvement for tumor sites with close spatial relation of the potential SLNs as in FOM tumors. New tracers for gamma imaging, PET, and fluorescence imaging, e.g. ^{89}Zr-, ICG-, and IRDye800CW-nanocolloidal albumin and ^{99m}Tc-tilmanocept, have been developed and are currently being tested in early oral cancer patients as single or hybrid tracers. These improvements may increase the sensitivity of SLNB further and limit the exploration needed to harvest SLNs, reducing the risk of complications and operating time.

Conflict of Interest The authors declare no conflict of interest.

References

1. Siegel RL, Miller KD, Jemal A. Cancer statistics, 2015. CA Cancer J Clin. 2015;65(1):5–29.
2. Braakhuis BJ, Leemans CR, Visser O. Incidence and survival trends of head and neck squamous cell carcinoma in the Netherlands between 1989 and 2011. Oral Oncol. 2014;50(7):670–5.
3. Stoeckli SJ, Alkureishi LW, Ross GL. Sentinel node biopsy for early oral and oropharyngeal squamous cell carcinoma. Eur Arch Otorhinolaryngol. 2009; 266(6):787–93.
4. Leusink FK, van Es RJ, de Bree R, Baatenburg de Jong RJ, van Hooff SR, Holstege FC, et al. Novel diagnostic modalities for assessment of the clinically node-negative neck in oral squamous-cell carcinoma. Lancet Oncol. 2012;13(12):e554–61.
5. de Bree R, Takes RP, Castelijns JA, Medina JE, Stoeckli SJ, Mancuso AA, et al. Advances in diagnostic modalities to detect occult lymph node metastases in head and neck squamous cell carcinoma. Head Neck. 2015;37:1829–39.
6. Liao LJ, Lo WC, Hsu WL, Wang CT, Lai MS. Detection of cervical lymph node metastasis in head and neck cancer patients with clinically N0 neck-a meta-analysis comparing different imaging modalities. BMC Cancer. 2012;12:236.
7. de Bondt RB, Nelemans PJ, Hofman PA, Casselman JW, Kremer B, van Engelshoven JM, et al. Detection of lymph node metastases in head and neck cancer: a meta-analysis comparing US, USgFNAC, CT and MR imaging. Eur J Radiol. 2007;64(2):266–72.
8. van Wouwe M, de Bree R, Kuik DJ, de Goede CJ, Verdonck-de Leeuw IM, Doornaert P, et al. Shoulder morbidity after non-surgical treatment of the neck. Radiother Oncol. 2009;90(2):196–201.
9. Alkureishi LW, Burak Z, Alvarez JA, Ballinger J, Bilde A, Britten AJ, et al. Joint practice guidelines for radionuclide lymphoscintigraphy for sentinel node localization in oral/oropharyngeal squamous cell carcinoma. Eur J Nucl Med Mol Imaging. 2009;36(11):1915–36.
10. Heuveling DA, Flach GB, van Schie A, van Weert S, Karagozoglu KH, Bloemena E, et al. Visualization of the sentinel node in early-stage oral cancer: limited value of late static lymphoscintigraphy. Nucl Med Commun. 2012;33(10):1065–9.
11. Wallace AM, Han LK, Povoski SP, Deck K, Schneebaum S, Hall NC, et al. Comparative evaluation of [(99m)tc]tilmanocept for sentinel lymph node mapping in breast cancer patients: results of two phase 3 trials. Ann Surg Oncol. 2013;20(8):2590–9.
12. Sondak VK, King DW, Zager JS, Schneebaum S, Kim J, Leong SP, et al. Combined analysis of phase III trials evaluating [(9)(9)mTc]tilmanocept and vital blue dye for identification of sentinel lymph nodes in clinically node-negative cutaneous melanoma. Ann Surg Oncol. 2013;20(2):680–8.
13. Marcinow AM, Hall N, Byrum E, Teknos TN, Old MO, Agrawal A. Use of a novel receptor-targeted (CD206) radiotracer, 99mTc-tilmanocept, and SPECT/CT for sentinel lymph node detection in oral cavity squamous cell carcinoma: initial institutional report in an ongoing phase 3 study. Otolaryngol Head Neck Surg. 2013;139(9):895–902.
14. Leong SP, Kim J, Ross M, Faries M, Scoggins CR, Metz WL, et al. A phase 2 study of (99m) Tc-tilmanocept in the detection of sentinel lymph nodes in melanoma and breast cancer. Ann Surg Oncol. 2011;18(4):961–9.
15. Agrawal A, Civantos FJ, Brumund KT, Chepeha DB, Hall NC, Carroll WR, et al. [Tc]tilmanocept accurately detects sentinel lymph nodes and predicts node pathology status in patients with oral squamous cell carcinoma of the head and neck: results of a phase III multi-institutional trial. Ann Surg Oncol. 2015;22(11):3708–15.
16. Ross G, Shoaib T, Soutar DS, Camilleri IG, Gray HW, Bessent RG, et al. The use of sentinel node biopsy to upstage the clinically N0 neck in head and neck cancer. Arch Otolaryngol Head Neck Surg. 2002;128(11): 1287–91.
17. Sangwan P, Nilakantan A, Patnaik U, Mishra A, Sethi A. Sentinel lymph node localization using 1 % isosulfan blue dye in cases of early oral cavity and oropharyngeal squamous cell carcinoma. Indian J Otolaryngol Head Neck Surg. 2015;67 Suppl 1:56–61.
18. Alex JC, Krag DN. The gamma-probe-guided resection of radiolabeled primary lymph nodes. Surg Oncol Clin N Am. 1996;5(1):33–41.
19. Paleri V, Rees G, Arullendran P, Shoaib T, Krishman S. Sentinel node biopsy in squamous cell cancer of the oral cavity and oral pharynx: a diagnostic meta-analysis. Head Neck. 2005;27(9):739–47.
20. Civantos FJ, Zitsch RP, Schuller DE, Agrawal A, Smith RB, Nason R, et al. Sentinel lymph node biopsy accurately stages the regional lymph nodes for T1-T2 oral squamous cell carcinomas: results of a prospective multi-institutional trial. J Clin Oncol. 2010;28(8):1395–400.
21. Thompson CF, St John MA, Lawson G, Grogan T, Elashoff D, Mendelsohn AH. Diagnostic value of sentinel lymph node biopsy in head and neck cancer: a meta-analysis. Eur Arch Otorhinolaryngol. 2013;270(7):2115–22.
22. Hassan O, Taha M, El Mehairy H. Sentinel lymph node biopsy versus elective neck dissection in evaluation of cN0 neck in patients with oral and oropharyngeal squamous cell carcinoma. Systemic review and meta-analysis study. Egypt J Ear Nose Throat Allied Sci. 2015;16:25–34.
23. Rinaldo A, Devaney KO, Ferlito A. Immunohistochemical studies in the identification of lymph node micrometastases in patients with squamous cell carcinoma of the head and neck. ORL J Otorhinolaryngol Relat Spec. 2004;66(1):38–41.
24. de Bree R. How to analyze the diagnostic value of sentinel node biopsy in head and neck cancer. Eur Arch Otorhinolaryngol. 2013;270(3):789–91.
25. Alkureishi LW, Ross GL, Shoaib T, Soutar DS, Robertson AG, Thompson R, et al. Sentinel node

biopsy in head and neck squamous cell cancer: 5-year follow-up of a European multicenter trial. Ann Surg Oncol. 2010;17(9):2459–64.
26. Kovacs AF, Stefenelli U, Seitz O, Middendorp M, Diener J, Sader R, et al. Positive sentinel lymph nodes are a negative prognostic factor for survival in T1-2 oral/oropharyngeal cancer-a long-term study on 103 patients. Ann Surg Oncol. 2009;16(2):233–9.
27. Broglie MA, Haile SR, Stoeckli SJ. Long-term experience in sentinel node biopsy for early oral and oropharyngeal squamous cell carcinoma. Ann Surg Oncol. 2011;18(10):2732–8.
28. Den Toom IJ, Heuveling DA, Flach GB, van Weert S, Karagozoglu KH, van Schie A, et al. Sentinel node biopsy for early-stage oral cavity cancer: the VU University Medical Center experience. Head Neck. 2015;37(4):573–8.
29. Govers TM, Hannink G, Merkx MA, Takes RP, Rovers MM. Sentinel node biopsy for squamous cell carcinoma of the oral cavity and oropharynx: a diagnostic meta-analysis. Oral Oncol. 2013;49(8):726–32.
30. Liao L, Hsu W, Wang C, Lo W, Lai M. Analysis of sentinel node biopsy combined with other diagnostic tools in staging cN0 head and neck cancer: a diagnostic meta-analysis. Head Neck. 2014. Epub a head of Print.
31. Hornstra MT, Alkureishi LW, Ross GL, Shoaib T, Soutar DS. Predictive factors for failure to identify sentinel nodes in head and neck squamous cell carcinoma. Head Neck. 2008;30(7):858–62.
32. Ross GL, Shoaib T, Soutar DS, MacDonald DG, Camilleri IG, Bessent RG, et al. The first international conference on sentinel node biopsy in mucosal head and neck cancer and adoption of a multicenter trial protocol. Ann Surg Oncol. 2002;9(4):406–10.
33. Farmer RW, McCall L, Civantos FJ, Myers JN, Yarbrough WG, Murphy B, et al. Lymphatic drainage patterns in oral squamous cell carcinoma: findings of the ACOSOG Z0360 (Alliance) study. Otolaryngol Head Neck Surg. 2015;152(4):673–7.
34. Flach GB, Broglie MA, van Schie A, Bloemena E, Leemans CR, de Bree R, et al. Sentinel node biopsy for oral and oropharyngeal squamous cell carcinoma in the previously treated neck. Oral Oncol. 2012;48(1):85–9.
35. Gurney BA, Schilling C, Putcha V, Alkureishi LW, Alvarez AJ, Bakholdt V, et al. Implications of a positive sentinel node in oral squamous cell carcinoma. Head Neck. 2012;34(11):1580–5.
36. Murer K, Huber GF, Haile SR, Stoeckli SJ. Comparison of morbidity between sentinel node biopsy and elective neck dissection for treatment of the n0 neck in patients with oral squamous cell carcinoma. Head Neck. 2011;33(9):1260–4.
37. Schiefke F, Akdemir M, Weber A, Akdemir D, Singer S, Frerich B. Function, postoperative morbidity, and quality of life after cervical sentinel node biopsy and after selective neck dissection. Head Neck. 2009;31(4):503–12.
38. Hernando J, Villarreal P, Alvarez-Marcos F, Gallego L, Garcia-Consuegra L, Junquera L. Comparison of related complications: sentinel node biopsy versus elective neck dissection. Int J Oral Maxillofac Surg. 2014;43(11):1307–12.
39. O'Connor R, Pezier T, Schilling C, McGurk M. The relative cost of sentinel lymph node biopsy in early oral cancer. J Craniomaxillofac Surg. 2013;41(8):721–7.
40. Kosuda S, Kusano S, Kohno N, Ohno Y, Tanabe T, Kitahara S, et al. Feasibility and cost-effectiveness of sentinel lymph node radiolocalization in stage N0 head and neck cancer. Arch Otolaryngol Head Neck Surg. 2003;129(10):1105–9.
41. Govers TM, Takes RP, Baris Karakullukcu M, Hannink G, Merkx MA, Grutters JP, et al. Management of the N0 neck in early stage oral squamous cell cancer: a modeling study of the cost-effectiveness. Oral Oncol. 2013;49(8):771–7.
42. Head and Neck Cancers. NCCN-guidelines 022014 [Internet]. 2014. http:/www.ncn.org/professionals/physician-gls/f-guidelines.asp.
43. Haerle SK, Hany TF, Strobel K, Sidler D, Stoeckli SJ. Is there an additional value of SPECT/CT over planar lymphoscintigraphy for sentinel node mapping in oral/oropharyngeal squamous cell carcinoma? Ann Surg Oncol. 2009;16(11):3118–24.
44. Wagner T, Buscombe J, Gnanasegaran G, Navalkissoor S. SPECT/CT in sentinel node imaging. Nucl Med Commun. 2013;34(3):191–202.
45. Heuveling DA, van Schie A, Vugts DJ, Hendrikse NH, Yaqub M, Hoekstra OS, et al. Pilot study on the feasibility of PET/CT lymphoscintigraphy with 89Zr-nanocolloidal albumin for sentinel node identification in oral cancer patients. J Nucl Med. 2013;54(4):585–9.
46. Vermeeren L, Valdes Olmos RA, Klop WM, Balm AJ, van den Brekel MW. A portable gamma-camera for intraoperative detection of sentinel nodes in the head and neck region. J Nucl Med. 2010;51(5):700–3.
47. Wendler T, Herrmann K, Schnelzer A, Lasser T, Traub J, Kutter O, et al. First demonstration of 3-D lymphatic mapping in breast cancer using freehand SPECT. Eur J Nucl Med Mol Imaging. 2010; 37(8):1452–61.
48. Heuveling DA, Karagozoglu KH, van Schie A, van Weert S, van Lingen A, de Bree R. Sentinel node biopsy using 3D lymphatic mapping by freehand SPECT in early stage oral cancer: a new technique. Clin Otolaryngol. 2012;37(1):89–90.
49. Mandapathil M, Teymoortash A, Heinis J, Wiegand S, Guldner C, Hoch S, et al. Freehand SPECT for sentinel lymph node detection in patients with head and neck cancer: first experiences. Acta Otolaryngol. 2014;134(1):100–4.
50. Bluemel C, Herrmann K, Muller-Richter U, Lapa C, Higuchi T, Wild V, et al. Freehand SPECT-guided sentinel lymph node biopsy in early oral squamous cell carcinoma. Head Neck. 2014;36(11):E112–6.
51. Bluemel C, Herrmann K, Kubler A, Buck AK, Geissinger E, Wild V, et al. Intraoperative 3-D imaging improves sentinel lymph node biopsy in oral cancer. Eur J Nucl Med Mol Imaging. 2014;41(12): 2257–64.

52. Heuveling DA, van Weert S, Karagozoglu KH, de Bree R. Evaluation of the use of freehand SPECT for sentinel node biopsy in early stage oral carcinoma. Oral Oncol. 2015;51(3):287–90.
53. De Bree R, Pouw B, Heuveling DA, Castelijns JA. Fusion of freehand SPECT and ultrasound to perform ultrasound guided fine-needle aspiration cytology of sentinel nodes in head and neck cancer. AJNR Am J Neuroradiol. 2015. Epub a head of Print.
54. van den Berg NS, Brouwer OR, Klop WM, Karakullukcu B, Zuur CL, Tan IB, et al. Concomitant radio- and fluorescence-guided sentinel lymph node biopsy in squamous cell carcinoma of the oral cavity using ICG-(99m)Tc-nanocolloid. Eur J Nucl Med Mol Imaging. 2012;39(7):1128–36.
55. Nakamura T, Kogashiwa Y, Nagafuji H, Yamauchi K, Kohno N. Validity of sentinel lymph node biopsy by ICG fluorescence for early head and neck cancer. Anticancer Res. 2015;35(3):1669–74.

Part VI

Clinical Application: Thyroid and Parathyroid

Radioguided Sentinel Lymph Node Mapping and Biopsy in Thyroid Cancer

12

Isabella Merante Boschin, Domenico Rubello, Christina Bluemel, Ken Herrmann, and Maria Rosa Pelizzo

Contents

I.M. Boschin • M.R. Pelizzo
Department of Surgery, University of Padova, Padova, Italy

D. Rubello, MD (✉)
Department of Nuclear Medicine, PET/CT Center, Santa Maria della Misericordia Hospital, Via Tre Martiri 140, Rovigo 45100, Italy
e-mail: domenico.rubello@libero.it

C. Bluemel • K. Herrmann
Department of Nuclear Medicine, Würzburg University, Würzburg, Gernany

Abstract

This chapter evaluates the "state-of-the-art" application of sentinel lymph node (SLN) procedure in patients with thyroid carcinoma. All PubMed/Medline listed papers including the key words "sentinel lymph node biopsy" and "thyroid carcinoma" published until January 2015 are taken into consideration. Both vital blue dye and radioisotope techniques are used in thyroid cancer patients and are discussed in this chapter. The SLN identification rates ranged from 0 to 100 % for blue dye, 64 to 100 % for radioisotopes, and 98 to 100 % for the combination of both techniques, respectively.

In conclusion, there is sufficient evidence to propagate the increasing use of the SLN technique in thyroid cancer. If the SLN is shown to consistently and accurately predict regional lymph node metastasis, a controlled randomized multicenter trial evaluating the effectiveness of this technique in patients with suspected or proven PTC is warranted.

K. Herrmann et al. (eds.), *Radioguided Surgery: Current Applications and Innovative Directions in Clinical Practice*, DOI 10.1007/978-3-319-26051-8_12

12.1 Rationale for Sentinel Node in Thyroid Cancer

12.1.1 The Concept of Sentinel Lymph Node (SLN) in Thyroid Cancer

Thyroid cancer is rare, but the most common endocrine malignancy [1, 2]. Differentiated thyroid cancer (DTC) accounts for over 90 % of thyroid malignancies and arises from thyroid follicular epithelial cells. DTC includes papillary thyroid carcinoma (PTC) and follicular thyroid carcinoma (FTC) with PTC representing more than 80 % of DTC [3]. Approximately 15 to 50% of patients with PTC have clinical evidence of cervical lymph node metastases at presentation, with up to 80% having micrometastatic disease. FTC represents about 20 % of DTC, and lymph node metastases are rare and metastatic disease mainly located in the liver and lungs; moreover, the metastatic spread happens usually by blood in FTC. FTC is typically diagnosed histopathologically, and not at cytology as for PTC.

Locoregional lymph node metastases of PTC are described to be associated with a worse prognosis, and extensive resection can improve the outcome of these patients. Therefore, correct identification of SLN involvement in PTS is crucial and impacts patient treatment and survival.

The SLN concept in DTC has been developed as an alternative to elective lymph node dissection in patients with clinically node-negative disease and was considered as an accurate technique for obtaining information about cervical lymph node involvement in patients undergoing thyroidectomy [4–6]. One of the complicating aspects in neck surgery and specifically in thyroid surgery is that the lymphatic drainage pathways are quite intricate [7]. The lymphatic vessels usually accompany blood vessels and nerves in directions that are not always predictable. The intrathyroid capillaries drain the lymphatic fluid to the lymphatic vessels associated with the capsule, potentially cross-communicating with the isthmus and the opposite lobe. Usually the superior lymphatic vessels drain the isthmus and the medial superior portion of the thyroid lobes, ascending in front of the larynx and terminating in the subdigastric lymph nodes of the internal jugular chain. The media inferior lymphatic vessels descend with the inferior vein to the pretracheal nodes. The lateral collecting vessels drain superiorly to the anterior and superior nodes of the internal jugular vein. Numerous classifications have been proposed to describe the location and the anatomic boundaries of lymph node groups in the neck. The most commonly used classifications are the ones of the American Joint Committee on Cancer (AJCC) and the American Society of Head and Neck Surgery (AHNS) [8, 9].

12.1.2 Lymph Node Metastases in Papillary Thyroid Carcinoma (PTC)

Patients with PTC frequently have lymph node metastases at the time of initial diagnosis and less frequently during successive follow-up. Incidence of metastasis is reported to range between 15 and 50 %, but microscopic metastases have been found in even up to 80 % of patients with PTC [10]. The thyroid gland has an extensive network of draining lymphatic vessels, both intraglandular and extraglandular [5, 9, 10]. Not surprisingly, the central neck compartment (level VI) is involved in approximately 90 % of patients with metastatic PTC [10, 11]; however, lateral and mediastinal compartment disease is also common [8, 9].

The involvement of lateral lymph nodes varies between 51 and 100 % in different series, with the caudal compartments involved more frequently than the cranial compartments [12]. Supraclavicular lymph nodes are the third site involved in terms of frequency, with a reported rate ranging from 10 to 52 % [11, 13]. Contralateral lymph node involvement is not rare with an incidence of up to 18 % for PTC [13, 14]. Mediastinal lymph node involvement, mostly the anterosuperior mediastinal lymph nodes, is less frequent at 1.9–15 % [11–13].

The distribution of locoregional lymph node involvement is poorly correlated to the site of the primary thyroid tumour. Even when the tumour is located in the upper third of the thyroid lobes, the subdigastric lymph nodes are often involved. Tumours located in the isthmus may cause bilateral cervical metastases with major risk of nodal recurrence on the contralateral neck side. The size of the primary tumour seems to have some importance: lymph node metastases in PTC <10 mm are usually found in the paratracheal area and rarely in the jugular nodes [8, 9]. It is important to mention that the reported incidence of regional lymphatic metastases identified in PTC patients varies according to the extent of nodal dissection performed [5, 15].

12.1.3 Prognostic Significance of Lymph Node Metastases in PTC

Surgical treatment is considered as the most effective therapy for patients with PTC. It remains controversial whether a prophylactic lymph node dissection improves the prognosis of PTC patients and whether the lymph node status predicts patient survival in PTC [4, 7, 10–13, 15]. Locoregional lymph node metastases of PTC are characterized by a worse prognosis, and extensive resection can improve the outcome of these patients. Some authors reported that nodal involvement has little influence on long-term survival of PTC patients, which is in contrast with other reports that found the presence of cervical lymph node metastases related to a worse prognosis due to an increased prevalence of locoregional recurrences; moreover, the finding of extracapsular invasion of lymph node metastases has been reported to be an indicator for the development of distant metastases and poor outcome [16, 17].

12.1.4 Surgical Techniques for Staging Neck in PTC

Currently, the extent of lymph node dissection is based predominantly on the histological type, stage of the primary tumour and the preoperative knowledge of lymph node involvement [18, 19]. In the presence of gross lymph node involvement, there is no debate about the need and prognostic benefit of a neck dissection in addition to total thyroidectomy. On the other hand, the management of a clinical N0 status node is generally much more conservative [4–7, 15].

In the absence of evidence favoring of routine prophylactic neck dissection, some surgeons perform "node picking"; while others perform lymphadenectomy of the ipsilateral central compartments. A more aggressive approach of routine prophylactic neck dissection has been suggested by some surgeons for PTC clinically lymph node negative patients secondary to the known high rate of occult micrometastatic disease in up to 80% of such PTC patients and the higher rate of locoregional recurrence of such patients who did not previously undergo routine prophylactic neck dissection [4–7, 15]. However, a general dissection of the central compartment may cause complications such as a damaged recurrent laryngeal nerve or higher hypoparathyroidism rates [7] and leads to overtreatment in patients with negative lymph nodes. The SLN procedure can avoid unnecessary lymph node dissection and reduce morbidity [7], identifying PTC patients with positive lymph nodes even if non-palpable or with a negative ultrasound (US) from true negative patients.

12.2 Methods of Sentinel Lymph Node Biopsy in PTC

12.2.1 Vital Blue Dye Technique

Early attempts of thyroid cromo-lymphoscintigraphy employed chlorophyll and Lipiodol UF in DTC, demonstrating the feasibility of the "sentinel lymph node concept" by showing coloured nodes to harbour metastasis [7]. Several studies have evaluated the vital blue dye technique for identification of the SLN in PTC [20–45] (Table 12.1).

At the time of surgery, the vital blue dye is injected intratumorally or around the tumour using a tuberculin syringe (Fig. 12.1). It is important not to mobilize the thyroid gland before blue dye injection to secure intact lymphatic drainage. The blue dye can usually be seen within seconds, sometimes only after 1–2 min, passing through lymphatic vessels towards the SLN (Fig. 12.2). Blue-stained lymph nodes are then resected with extreme caution to avoid accidental removal of parathyroid glands that can also be blue coloured. After removal, the SLNs are submitted to histopathology for frozen section analysis.

Table 12.1 Twenty-six studies considering the vital blue dye technique of SLN in thyroid surgery.

Reference	*n*. patients	p.o. diagnosis	PTCs	Vital blue dye	Volume (ml)	Timing of injection	Injection site IT or PT	*n*. patients with SLN (%)	SLN + metastasis (%)
Kelemen (1998) [20]	17	Suspicious/PTC	11	1 % isosulphan blue	0.1–0.8	After strap muscle retraction	IT	11 (100)	5 (45)
Dixon (2000) [21]	40	Suspicious/PTC	14	Isosulphan blue	0.1–0.7	After strap muscle retraction	IT	10 (71)	6 (60)
Arch-Ferrer (2001) [22]	22	PTC	22	1 % isosulphan blue	0.5	After mobilization	IT	20 (91)	17 (85)
Fukui (2001) [23]	22	PTC	22	2 % methylene blue	0.1	After mobilization	PT	21 (95)	7 (33)
Tsugawa (2002) [24]	38	PTC	38	1 % patent blue V	0.2–0.5	NA	PT	27 (71)	16 (59)
Takami (2003) [25]	68	PTC	68	1 % isosulphan blue	0.3	After strap muscle retraction	PT	63 (93)	35 (55)
Chow (2004) [26]	15	PTC	15	2.5 % patent blue V	0.1–0.5	After strap muscle retraction	IT	10 (67)	7 (70)
Dzodic (2006) [27]	40	DTC	34	1 % methylene blue	0.2	After strap muscle retraction	PT	37 (92)	7 (19)
Falvo (2006) [28]	18	PTC	18	methylene blue	0.4	After mobilization	IT	18 (100)	12 (48)
Peparini (2006) [29]	9	PTC	8	2.5 % patent blue V	0.1–1.2	NA	PT/IT	0 (0)	–
Abdalla (2006) [30]	30	Benign nodules only	0	1 % isosulphan blue	0.5–0.1	After strap muscle retraction	IT	0	0
Rubello (2006) [31]	153	PTC	153	0.5 % patent blue V	0.25	After strap muscle retraction	IT	107 (70)	36 (34)
Wang (2008) [44]	25	PTC	25	2 % methylene blue	1–2	NA	PT	22 (88)	19 (86)
Roh (2008) [32]	50	PTC	50	2 % methylene blue	0.2	After strap muscle retraction	PT	46 (92)	14 (30)
Bae (2009) [33]	11	PTC	11	2 % methylene blue	0.5	After strap muscle retraction	IT	9 (82)	5 (55)

Lee (2009) [34]	54	DTC	54	2 % methylene blue	0.1–0.5	Before mobilization	PT	50 (93)	19 (38)
Takeyama (2009) [35]	37	Suspicious/DTC	8	1 % sulphan blue	0.1	Before mobilization	PT	7 (88)	3 (43)
Anand (2009) [36]	97	Suspicious/PTC	70	1 % methylene blue	0.2–0.3	Before mobilization	PT	55 (79)	14 (25)
Cunningham (2010) [37]	211	PTC	211	1 % isosulphan blue	0.5–0.2	After mobilization	IT	192 (91)	71 (37)
Huang (2011) [38]	45	PTC	45	Methylene blue 1 %	1	After mobilization	IT	39 (87)	21 (54)
Ji (2012) [39]	114	PTC	114	Methylene blue 1 %	0.2	After strap muscle retraction	PT	84 (74)	24 (29)
Li (2012) [40]	132	PTC	NA	Methylene blue 1 %	1	24 h p.o. (US)	PT	NA	NA
Larrad (2012) [41]	23	PTC	23	Methylene blue 2 %	0.3–0.5	Not defined	PT	21 (91)	7 (33)
Hao (2012) [42]	100	PTC	100	Methylene blue 2 %	0.1–0.5	After strap muscle retraction	PT	79 (79)	48 (61)
Kaczka (2013) [45]	23	Suspected/PTC	13	Patent blue dye 1 %	0.1–1	After strap muscle retraction	IT	20 (87)	5 (25)
Jozaghi (2013) [43]	300	DTC	134	Methylene blue 1 %	0.2	After strap muscle retraction	PT	300 (100)	43 (14)

P.o. preoperative, *DTC* differentiated thyroid carcinoma, *PTC* papillary thyroid carcinoma, *NA* data non available, *IT* intratumoral, *PT* peritumoral

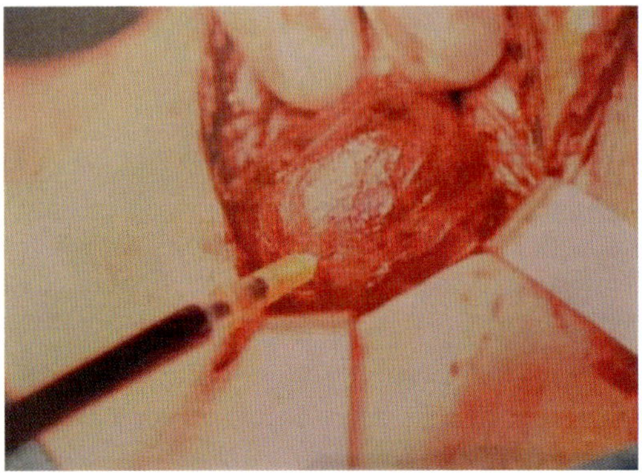

Fig. 12.1 The intranodular injection of vital blue dye at surgery

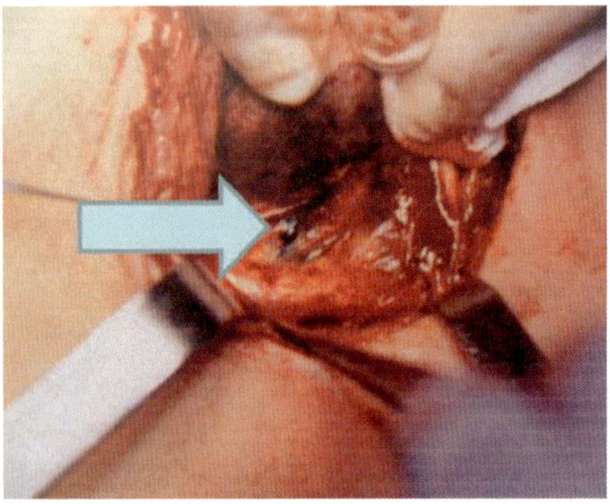

Fig. 12.2 The evidence of the lymphatic drainage by the vital blue dye at surgery

Disadvantages of the vital blue dye technique include the following: (1) risk of disruption and interruption of the lymphatic channels from the nodule, (2) difficulties in identifying SLN lying outside the central compartment; (3) need to identify the parathyroid glands prior to injection as they also take up the blue dye and (4) the technique is sometimes difficult and requires experience.

12.2.2 Lymphoscintigraphy and Intraoperative Gamma Probe Technique

To overcome some of these drawbacks, the use of preoperative lymphoscintigraphy with radiocolloids and intraoperative gamma probe detection was introduced (Table 12.2). Lymphoscintigraphy is an excellent method to visualize the lymphatic pathways and the SLN. It offers numerous important advantages compared to the vital blue dye technique: (1) preoperative injection of radiopharmaceutical eliminates risk of lymphatic disruption during operation, (2) it allows identification of SLN located outside the central compartment and (3) there is no physiological uptake in the parathyroid glands.

Current techniques use intranodular injection of 15–37 MBq ^{99m}Tc nanocolloid particles (particle size 20–80 nm) in a volume of 0.1–0.5 ml of saline. US-guided injection of the radionuclide is useful in small nodules located deep in the thyroid lobe (Fig. 12.3). Peritumoral injection should be avoided because of the high density of blood vessels in the thyroid gland with the risk of radiocolloid spillage outside the gland. Lymphatic drainage from the thyroid gland is visualized by dynamic images (1 frame per 15s, 64 × 64 matrix) in the anteroposterior projection for up to 10 min after injection. Longer acquisition times have been proposed (Fig. 12.4). Additional 5-min static images in anterior, lateral, and oblique views are usually obtained (256 × 256 matrix) for up to 1–3 h post injection or until adequate accumulation of the radiocolloid in the SLN is obtained. Surface localization of the SLN is marked with a water-resistant dye.

After a variable time interval (2–24 h), the patient is taken to the operating room for a total or near-total thyroidectomy. Following the removal of the thyroid tissue, a handheld collimated gamma probe is used to scan the central compartments (through the incision) and the lateral compartments (through skin surface) for "radioactive" lymph nodes (Fig. 12.5). SLN detection has been reported to be feasible up to 24 h post injection. A lesion-to-background ratio of 2:1 or greater is significant for SLN identification, although a smaller threshold level of 10 or 20 % is acceptable in breast cancer and melanoma.

The SLN(s) is (are) selectively excised, and the activity of the lymphatic bed is monitored

Table 12.2 Twelve studies evaluating the role of the radioisotope technique of SLN in thyroid surgery

Reference	*n.* Patients	p.o. diagnosis	PTCs	Radioisotope	Volume injected (ml)	Technique	Injection site IT or PT	*n.* patients with SLN (%)	SLN + metastasis (%)
Rettenbacher (2000) [46]	9	Suspicious/DTC	4	^{99m}Tc-labelled nanocolloid	0.5	NA	IT	4 (100)	2 (50)
Stoeckli (2003) [47]	10	Suspicious/DTC	1	^{99m}Tc-labelled sulphur colloid	0.2	US-g	PT	1 (100)	1 (100)
Pelizzo (2006) [48]	41	Suspicious/DTC	40	^{99m}Tc-labelled nanocolloid	0.1–0.2	Us-g	IT	40 (100)	21 (53)
Pelizzo (2007) [49]	25	PTC	25	^{99m}Tc-labelled nanocolloid	0.1–0.2	US-g	IT	25 (100)	12 (48)
Carcoforo (2007) [50]	64	Suspicious/PTC	59	^{99m}Tc-labelled nanocolloid	0.3	US-g	PT	57 (97)	14 (25)
Boschin (2008) [15]	65	PTC	65	^{99m}Tc-labelled nanocolloid	0.1–0.2	US-g	IT	65 (100)	34 (52)
Lee (2011) [51]	94	PTC	94	^{99m}Tc tin colloid	0.1–0.2	US-g	IT	60 (64)	19 (32)
Hao (2012) [42]	100	PTC	100	Carbon nanoparticles	0.1–0.5	NA	PT	91 (91)	45 (45)
Lee (2013) [52]	39	PTC	39	^{99m}Tc phytate (lymphoscintigraphy + SPECT/CT)	20 MBq	NA	IT	38 (97)	NA
Garcia Burillo (2013) [53]	24	PTC	24	^{99m}Tc nanocolloid	0.1–0.2	24 h p.o.	IT	23 (96)	10 (43)
Cabrera (2015) [54]	23	PTC	23	^{99m}Tc phytate (lymphoscintigraphy+SPECT/CT)	7.4 MBq 0.1	NA	PT	21 (91)	7 (30)
Carcoforo (2014) [55]	374	Suspicious/PTC	345	^{99m}Tc nanocolloidal albumin	74 MBq	24 h p.o. US	PT	372 (99.7)	55 (16)
Boni (2014) [56]	1	MTC	0	^{99m}Tc nanocolloidal albumin		US-g	IT	1 (100)	1 (100)
Puccini (2014) [57]	4	MTC	0	^{99m}Tc macrocolloid albumin	0.1–0.2	5 h p.o. US	IT	4 (100)	3 (75)

P.o. preoperative, *DTC* differentiated thyroid carcinoma, *PTC* papillary thyroid carcinoma, *NA* data non available, *US-g* ultrasound guidance, *IT* intratumoral, *PT* peritumoral

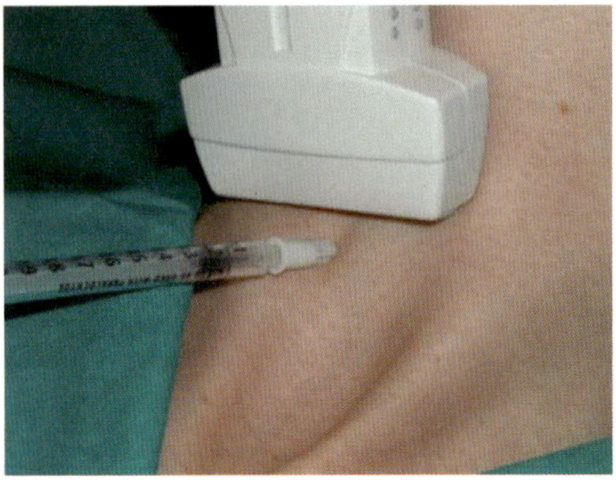

Fig. 12.3 The ultrasound-guided intranodular injection of ^{99m}Tc nanocolloid before surgery

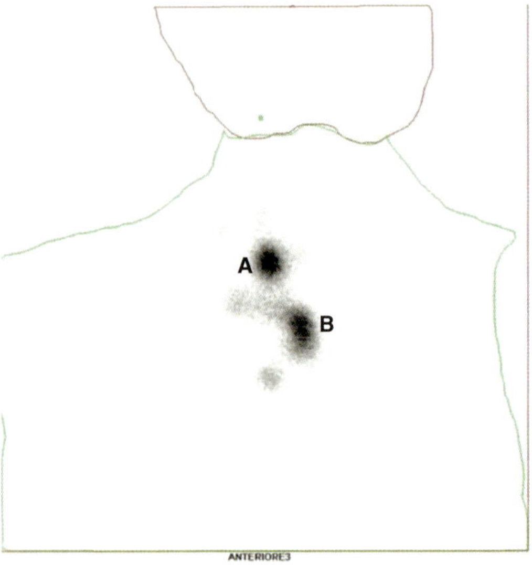

Fig. 12.4 An image at lymphoscintigraphy. *A*: the injection site, *B*: the SLN

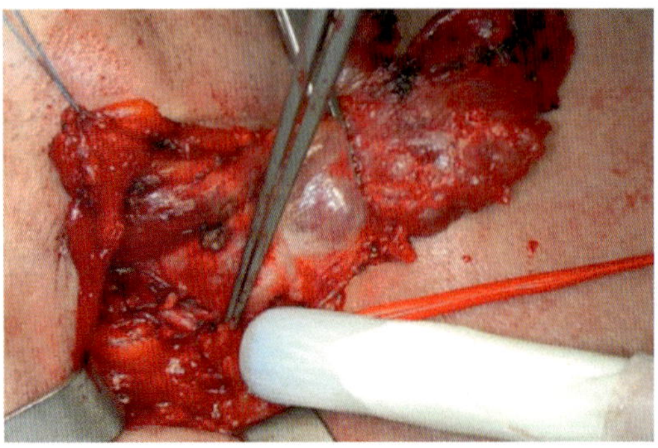

Fig. 12.5 The localization of the SLN at surgery

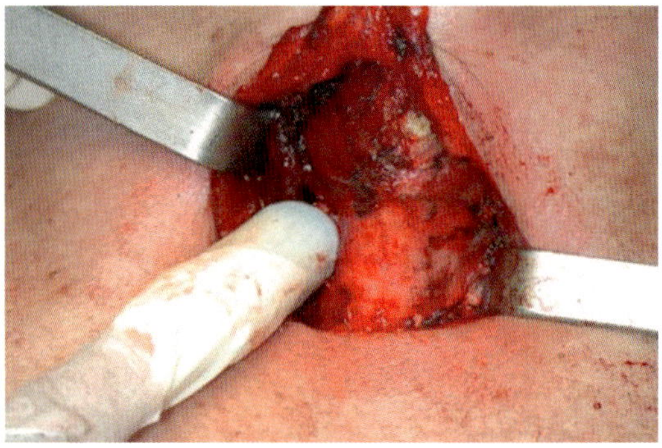

Fig. 12.6 After the SLN is excised, the activity of the lymphatic bed is monitored with the probe to verify completeness of surgical extirpation

with the handheld gamma probe to verify completeness of surgical removal (Fig. 12.6). It is important to emphasize that the thyroidectomy must precede SLN detection to avoid interference from radioactivity in the primary tumour. Finally, the SLN(s) is (are) sent for histopathology to screen for occult metastasis.

12.2.3 Combination of Vital Blue Dye and Lymphoscintigraphy and Intraoperative Gamma Probe Techniques

The combination of vital blue dye, lymphoscintigraphy, and intraoperative gamma probe techniques was described first in 2001 by Catarci et al. in 6 PTC patients (Table 12.3) [58]. They performed an intratumoral injection of 0.1 ml ^{99m}Tc-labelled colloidal albumin to visualize the SLN 2 h prior to surgery. At surgery, 0.1 ml per cm tumour diameter of Blue Patent V (2.5 %) was injected directly into the tumour, identified without dividing any structure in order to preserve the lymphatic drainage.

The SLN was identified by the flow and accumulation of the blue dye and the handheld gamma detection probe. SLN(s) was (were) correctly identified in all cases, suggesting that these techniques have a complementary role.

Table 12.3 Three studies evaluating the combination of vital blue dye technique and radioisotope technique of SLN in thyroid surgery

Reference	*n*. patients	p.o. diagnosis	PTCs	Vital blue dye Radioisotope	Volume (ml)	Timing of injection	Injection site IT or PT	*n*. patients with SLN (%)	SLN + metastasis (%)
Catarci (2001) [58]	6	PTC	6	Blue Patent V 2.5 % ^{99m}Tc-labelled colloid albumin	–0.2–0.4 –0.1	Before mobilization US-g	IT	6 (100)	4 (67)
Lee (2009) [34]	43	DTC	43	Methylene blue 2 % ^{99m}Tc-labelled tin colloid	–0.1–0.5 –0.1–0.2	Before mobilization US-g	PT IT	42 (98)	21 (50)
Huang (2011) [38]	45			Methylene blue ^{99m}Tc sulphur colloid	–1 –0.5	Before mobilization US-g	IT	45 (100)	24 (53)

P.o. preoperative, *DTC* differentiated thyroid carcinoma, *PTC* papillary thyroid carcinoma, *NA* data non available, *US-g* ultrasound guidance, *IT* intratumoral, *PT* peritumoral

12.3 Summary of Available Studies

12.3.1 Data Collection

A PUBMED search was performed on 20 January 2015 for the MeSH headings "sentinel lymph node biopsy" and "thyroid carcinoma". All original articles (retrospective and prospective) that examined the SLN techniques in human thyroid carcinoma were reviewed. The full text versions of the studies were obtained for further detailed evaluation.

Articles were subdivided depending on the technique used for SLN detection: group 1 included articles describing the vital blue dye technique, group 2 consisted of articles evaluating lymphoscintigraphy with radioisotopes and group 3 contained manuscripts involving both techniques for SLN detection. Extracted data included number of patients; preoperative diagnosis; postoperative diagnosis; SLN technique, in particular use of vital blue dye, isotope or both; volume and concentration; site of injection; time of injection; SLN detection rate; and metastatic SLN rate.

Reviews and letters were excluded [7, 59–63]. To avoid duplication of patient data in this chapter, multiple articles from the same authors and institutions were evaluated carefully for possible duplication. If this was thought likely, only the most recent article was included. Moreover, we excluded the studies of Saliba et al. and Maniakas et al. [64, 65] as they did not report the SLN technique.

Saliba et al. performed a retrospective chart review of 96 low-risk PTC patients who underwent a total thyroidectomy including SLN procedure. Patients with a negative SLN had a significantly lower postoperative thyroglobulin (Tg) level [64]. Maniakas et al. included 311 patients undergoing a total thyroidectomy and SLN biopsy for well-differentiated thyroid carcinoma in their retrospective chart review. Younger age (<45 years) and higher T category were found to be associated with a higher rate of positive SLNs [65].

12.3.2 Results of Studies

A total of 41 articles about SLN detection in thyroid carcinoma provided valuable information. Twenty-six studies reported on vital blue dye, 12 on SLN detection with radioisotopes and 3 on a combination of both techniques. The corresponding studies are summarized in Tables 12.1, 12.2, and 12.3 accordingly.

12.3.2.1 Vital Blue Dye Technique

In the 26 studies [20–45] evaluating vital dye for SLN detection, the patient number ranged between 9 [29] and 300 [43]. Further information including the preoperatively suspected diagnosis, the type of vital blue dye employed, the injected volume and injection technique are displayed in Table 12.1. The SLN was successfully visualized in a range between 0 % [29] and 100 % [20]. The SLN was positive for metastases in a range between 14 % [43] and 86 % [44].

12.3.2.2 Lymphoscintigraphy and Intraoperative Gamma Probe Technique

Table 12.2 summarizes the studies employing radioisotope-guided SLN technique [15, 42, 46–57] displaying in more detail the number of patients studied, the preoperative diagnosis and injection techniques. The SLN was successfully detected in a range of 64 % [51] to 100 % [15, 46–49, 56, 57] with corresponding detection rates of 64–100 % for intratumoral injection and 91–100 % for peritumoral injection, respectively. The identified SLN was positive for tumour cells in a range of 16 % [55] to 100 % [47].

12.3.2.3 Combination of Vital Blue Dye and Lymphoscintigraphy/Intraoperative Gamma Probe Techniques

Only three studies were reported on the combined use of vital blue dye and lymphoscintigraphy/intraoperative gamma probe techniques for SLN detection in thyroid carcinoma [34, 38, 58]. Corresponding patient numbers, preoperative diagnosis, the type of vital blue dye employed as well as injection technique and volumes are summarized in Table 12.3. In all three studies, the detection rate of the SLN was very high with 98 % [34] and 100 % [38, 58], respectively. Percentage of tumour-positive SLNs ranged between 50 % [34] and 67 % [58].

12.4 Current Status of Sentinel Lymph Node in Thyroid Cancer

The SLN technique is well standardized in melanoma and breast cancer, providing important information for patient treatment [7, 59]. The application of the SLN technique in DTC was first proposed 17 years ago by Kelemen et al. [20]. Since then the value of SLN in thyroid cancer including indications, benefits and limitations has been controversially discussed [59, 60]. Identification of the SLN is of particular value in PTC, as this tumour predominantly metastasizes lymphogenous, in contrast to the predominantly hematogeneous dissemination of FTC. Identification and resection of the SLN allow for the detection of microscopic metastatic disease, thus potentially reducing patient morbidity by avoiding unnecessary complete nodal dissection [59–63]. A topic of controversy is the prognostic significance of lymph node involvement in PTC and therefore whether accurate SLN detection is worthwhile and also questioning the indication of prophylactic lymphadenectomy of the central neck compartment [60–62].

SLN detection can be performed using vital blue dye, radioisotope-based lymphoscintigraphy and gamma probe detection as well as by the combined use of both techniques. Various studies reported in the literature have shown the isotopic procedure to be more precise (95–100 %) for SLN localization compared to vital blue dye (80–90 %); however, the isotopic procedure also has detractors [59–62]. In respect to feasibility and accuracy, preoperative lymphoscintigraphy and intraoperative gamma probe offer important advantages over the vital blue dye technique: (i) the injection of the radiopharmaceutical is done preoperatively, therefore eliminating disruption of the lymphatic vessels during the initial dissection; (ii) the use of the radiolabelled material permits to disclose the SLN that lies outside the central compartment; and (iii) there is no false-positive staining of the parathyroid glands. After identification, SLNs are selectively excised, and the activity of the lymphatic bed is assessed with the handheld gamma probe to verify background activity only within the resection bed after completion of the SLN biopsy procedure. Some authors have suggested that a combination of both procedures provides an even better yield [34, 38, 58].

Non-visualization of the lymphatics and of the SLN has been described for both techniques [59–63]. Potential explanations include lymphatic disruption during resection of the thyroid nodule, blockage of lymphatics by tumour or lymphatics, leading to a non-accessible site such as a retro-oesophageal or retrothyroid location. SLNs may occasionally be located in areas that are relatively inaccessible via a collar incision; this has been reported for both the radioisotope and the blue dye techniques [34, 38, 58]. Specific for the radioisotope technique is the requirement to remove the thyroid gland before identification of the SLN, because of the so-called "shine-through" effect. This is due to the close proximity of the central neck compartment lymph nodes to the thyroid nodes to the thyroid nodule where the radioisotope is injected.

The "shine-through" effect is especially problematic in the central neck compartment where the lymph nodes are located in close proximity to the thyroid. The "shine-through" phenomenon is also well known from SLN biopsy in oral cancers with reduced identification rates in floor of the mouth tumours due to the location of the SLNs in close vicinity of the injection site [66, 67]. Therefore, hybrid tracers [68], more specific radioactive tracers [69], intraoperative gamma cameras [70], and intraoperative 3D imaging [71] have been investigated and a multimodality approach, including preoperative hybrid imaging (SPECT/CT), has been proposed [72]. No corresponding studies are so far available for DTC, but these new approaches may also solve the "shine-through" problem in thyroid cancer. A limitation of the radioactive technique is the fact that in the majority of countries, the intraoperative use of radioactivity requires the existence of a Nuclear Medicine Unit and/or the presence of a nuclear medicine physician at surgery.

This chapter demonstrates that there is sufficient preliminary evidence to suggest the more rigorous use of the SLN technique in thyroid cancer. The utilization of SLN biopsy for PTC patients allows one to identify lymph node metastases more readily than based upon preoperative clinical exam [59–63]. Therefore, a controlled, randomized clinical trial evaluating the efficacy of SLN biopsy for identifying lymph node metastases in PTC patients and its resultant impact on management and long-term patient outcome seems warranted.

Conflict of Interest Statement The authors declare no conflict of interest with the present chapter.

References

1. Torre LA, Bray F, Siegel RL, Ferlay J, Lortet-Tieulent J, Jemal A. Global cancer statistics, 2012. CA Cancer J Clin. 2015;65(2):87–108.
2. Pellegriti G, Frasca F, Regalbuto C, Squatrito S, Vigneri R. Worldwide increasing incidence of thyroid cancer: update on epidemiology and risk factors. J Cancer Epidemiol. 2013;2013:965212.
3. Cooper DS, Doherty GM, Haugen BR, Kloos RT, Lee SL, Mandel SJ, et al. Revised American Thyroid Association management guidelines for patients with thyroid nodules and differentiated thyroid cancer. Thyroid. 2009;19(11):1167–214.
4. Pasieka JL. Sentinel lymph node biopsy in the management of thyroid disease. Br J Surg. 2001; 88(3):321–2.
5. Wiseman SM, Hicks Jr WL, Chu QD, Rigual NR. Sentinel lymph node biopsy in staging of differentiated thyroid cancer: a critical review. Surg Oncol. 2002;11(3):137–42.
6. Delbridge L. Sentinel lymph node biopsy for thyroid cancer: why bother? ANZ J Surg. 2004;74(1–2):2.
7. Rubello D, Pelizzo MR, Al-Nahhas A, Salvatori M, O'Doherty MJ, Giuliano AE, et al. The role of sentinel lymph node biopsy in patients with differentiated thyroid carcinoma. Eur J Surg Oncol. 2006; 32(9):917–21.
8. Robbins KT. Classification of neck dissection: current concepts and future considerations. Otolaryngol Clin North Am. 1998;31(4):639–55.
9. Robbins KT, Medina JE, Wolfe GT, Levine PA, Sessions RB, Pruet CW. Standardizing neck dissection terminology. Official report of the Academy's Committee for Head and Neck Surgery and Oncology. Arch Otolaryngol Head Neck Surg. 1991; 117(6):601–5.
10. Shaha AR. Management of the neck in thyroid cancer. Otolaryngol Clin North Am. 1998;31(5):823–31.
11. Mirallie E, Visset J, Sagan C, Hamy A, Le Bodic MF, Paineau J. Localization of cervical node metastasis of papillary thyroid carcinoma. World J Surg. 1999;23(9):970–3; discussion 3–4.
12. Machens A, Hinze R, Thomusch O, Dralle H. Pattern of nodal metastasis for primary and reoperative thyroid cancer. World J Surg. 2002;26(1):22–8.
13. Frankenthaler RA, Sellin RV, Cangir A, Goepfert H. Lymph node metastasis from papillary-follicular thyroid carcinoma in young patients. Am J Surg. 1990;160(4):341–3.
14. Noguchi M, Kumaki T, Taniya T, Miyazaki I. Bilateral cervical lymph node metastases in well-differentiated thyroid cancer. Arch Surg. 1990;125(6):804–6.
15. Boschin IM, Toniato A, Piotto A, Ide EC, Casara D, Guolo A, et al. 99Tc Nanocolloid sentinel node procedure in thyroid carcinoma. Langenbecks Arch Surg. 2008;393(5):705–8.
16. Yamashita H, Noguchi S, Murakami N, Kawamoto H, Watanabe S. Extracapsular invasion of lymph node metastasis is an indicator of distant metastasis and poor prognosis in patients with thyroid papillary carcinoma. Cancer. 1997;80(12):2268–72.
17. Mazzaferri EL, Kloos RT. Clinical review 128: current approaches to primary therapy for papillary and follicular thyroid cancer. J Clin Endocrinol Metab. 2001;86(4):1447–63.
18. Mazzaferri EL, Massoll N. Management of papillary and follicular (differentiated) thyroid cancer: new paradigms using recombinant human thyrotropin. Endocr Relat Cancer. 2002;9(4):227–47.
19. Watkinson JC. The British Thyroid Association guidelines for the management of thyroid cancer in adults. Nucl Med Commun. 2004;25(9):897–900.
20. Kelemen PR, Van Herle AJ, Giuliano AE. Sentinel lymphadenectomy in thyroid malignant neoplasms. Arch Surg. 1998;133(3):288–92.
21. Dixon E, McKinnon JG, Pasieka JL. Feasibility of sentinel lymph node biopsy and lymphatic mapping in nodular thyroid neoplasms. World J Surg. 2000; 24(11):1396–401.
22. Arch-Ferrer J, Velazquez D, Fajardo R, Gamboa-Dominguez A, Herrera MF. Accuracy of sentinel lymph node in papillary thyroid carcinoma. Surgery. 2001;130(6):907–13.
23. Fukui Y, Yamakawa T, Taniki T, Numoto S, Miki H, Monden Y. Sentinel lymph node biopsy in patients with papillary thyroid carcinoma. Cancer. 2001; 92(11):2868–74.

24. Tsugawa K, Ohnishi I, Nakamura M, Miwa K, Yokoyama K, Michigishi T, et al. Intraoperative lymphatic mapping and sentinel lymph node biopsy in patients with papillary carcinoma of the thyroid gland. Biomed Pharmacother. 2002;56 Suppl 1:100s–3s.
25. Takami H, Sasaki K, Ikeda Y, Tajima G, Kameyama K. Detection of sentinel lymph nodes in patients with papillary thyroid cancer. Asian J Surg. 2003; 26(3):145–8.
26. Chow TL, Lim BH, Kwok SP. Sentinel lymph node dissection in papillary thyroid carcinoma. ANZ J Surg. 2004;74(1–2):10–2.
27. Dzodic R, Markovic I, Inic M, Jokic N, Djurisic I, Zegarac M, et al. Sentinel lymph node biopsy may be used to support the decision to perform modified radical neck dissection in differentiated thyroid carcinoma. World J Surg. 2006;30(5):841–6.
28. Falvo L, Marzullo A, Palermo S, Biancafarina A, De Stefano M, Vanni B, et al. The sentinel lymph node in papillary cancer of the thyroid including histological subtype. Ann Ital Chir. 2006;77(1):13–8; discussion 8.
29. Peparini N, Maturo A, Di Matteo FM, Tartaglia F, Marchesi M, Campana EP. Blue-dye sentinel node mapping in thyroid carcinoma: debatable results of feasibility. Acta Chir Belg. 2006;106(5):523–7.
30. Abdalla HM. Feasibility of sentinel lymph node detection in nodular thyroid disease. J Egypt Natl Canc Inst. 2006;18(1):35–40.
31. Rubello D, Nanni C, Merante Boschin I, Toniato A, Piotto A, Rampin L, et al. Sentinel lymph node (SLN) procedure with patent V blue dye in 153 patients with papillary thyroid carcinoma (PTC): is it an accurate staging method? J Exp Clin Cancer Res. 2006; 25(4):483–6.
32. Roh JL, Park CI. Sentinel lymph node biopsy as guidance for central neck dissection in patients with papillary thyroid carcinoma. Cancer. 2008;113(7): 1527–31.
33. Bae JS, Park WC, Song BJ, Jung SS, Kim JS. Endoscopic thyroidectomy and sentinel lymph node biopsy via an anterior chest approach for papillary thyroid cancer. Surg Today. 2009;39(2):178–81.
34. Lee SK, Choi JH, Lim HI, Kim WW, Kim SM, Choe JH, et al. Sentinel lymph node biopsy in papillary thyroid cancer: comparison study of blue dye method and combined radioisotope and blue dye method in papillary thyroid cancer. Eur J Surg Oncol. 2009;35(9): 974–9.
35. Takeyama H, Tabei I, Uchida K, Morikawa T. Sentinel node biopsy for follicular tumours of the thyroid gland. Br J Surg. 2009;96(5):490–5.
36. Anand SM, Gologan O, Rochon L, Tamilia M, How J, Hier MP, et al. The role of sentinel lymph node biopsy in differentiated thyroid carcinoma. Arch Otolaryngol Head Neck Surg. 2009;135(12):1199–204.
37. Cunningham DK, Yao KA, Turner RR, Singer FR, Van Herle AR, Giuliano AE. Sentinel lymph node biopsy for papillary thyroid cancer: 12 years of experience at a single institution. Ann Surg Oncol. 2010;17(11):2970–5.
38. Huang O, Wu W, Wang O, You J, Li Q, Huang D, et al. Sentinel lymph node biopsy is unsuitable for routine practice in younger female patients with unilateral low-risk papillary thyroid carcinoma. BMC Cancer. 2011;11:386.
39. Ji YB, Lee KJ, Park YS, Hong SM, Paik SS, Tae K. Clinical efficacy of sentinel lymph node biopsy using methylene blue dye in clinically node-negative papillary thyroid carcinoma. Ann Surg Oncol. 2012;19(6):1868–73.
40. Li X, Ma H, Tian X, Jin X. Elective neck dissection in papillary thyroid carcinoma patients. Acta Chir Belg. 2012;112(1):44–50.
41. Larrad Jimenez A, de Quadros Borrajo P, Martin Duce A. Evaluation of the sentinel lymph node in T1-T2 papillary thyroid cancer: a preliminary study. Cir Esp. 2012;90(7):440–5. Valoracion del ganglio centinela en el cancer papilar de tiroides T1-T2. Estudio preliminar.
42. Hao RT, Chen J, Zhao LH, Liu C, Wang OC, Huang GL, et al. Sentinel lymph node biopsy using carbon nanoparticles for Chinese patients with papillary thyroid microcarcinoma. Eur J Surg Oncol. 2012; 38(8):718–24.
43. Jozaghi Y, Richardson K, Anand S, Mlynarek A, Hier MP, Forest VI, et al. Frozen section analysis and sentinel lymph node biopsy in well differentiated thyroid cancer. J Otolaryngol Head Neck Surg. 2013;42:48.
44. Wang JD, Deng XC, Jin XJ, Zhang C, Zhou JQ, Zhou QY, et al. [Surgical exploration of the sentinel lymph nodes in the papillary thyroid carcinoma]. Rev Laryngol Otol Rhinol (Bord). 2008;129(4–5):285–7. Exploration chirurgicale des ganglions sentinelles dans le cancer papillaire de la thyroide.
45. Kaczka K, Luks B, Jasion J, Pomorski L. Sentinel lymph node in thyroid tumors – own experience. Contemp Oncol (Pozn). 2013;17(2):184–9.
46. Rettenbacher L, Sungler P, Gmeiner D, Kassmann H, Galvan G. Detecting the sentinel lymph node in patients with differentiated thyroid carcinoma. Eur J Nucl Med. 2000;27(9):1399–401.
47. Stoeckli SJ, Pfaltz M, Steinert H, Schmid S. Sentinel lymph node biopsy in thyroid tumors: a pilot study. Eur Arch Otorhinolaryngol. 2003;260(7):364–8.
48. Pelizzo MR, Merante Boschin I, Toniato A, Piotto A, Bernante P, Paggetta C, et al. Sentinel node mapping and biopsy in thyroid cancer: a surgical perspective. Biomed Pharmacother. 2006;60(8):405–8.
49. Pelizzo MR, Rubello D, Boschin IM, Piotto A, Paggetta C, Toniato A, et al. Contribution of SLN investigation with 99mTc-nanocolloid in clinical staging of thyroid cancer: technical feasibility. Eur J Nucl Med Mol Imaging. 2007;34(6):934–8.
50. Carcoforo P, Feggi L, Trasforini G, Lanzara S, Sortini D, Zulian V, et al. Use of preoperative lymphoscintigraphy and intraoperative gamma-probe detection for identification of the sentinel lymph node in patients with papillary thyroid carcinoma. Eur J Surg Oncol. 2007;33(9):1075–80.

51. Lee SK, Kim SH, Hur SM, Choe JH, Kim JH, Kim JS. The efficacy of lateral neck sentinel lymph node biopsy in papillary thyroid carcinoma. World J Surg. 2011;35(12):2675–82.
52. Lee J, Na KY, Lee SJ, An YS, Yoon JK, Soh EY. The usefulness and accuracy of sentinel lymph node biopsy using single photon emission computed tomography/computed tomography with 99mTc phytate to detect locoregional lymph node metastases in patients with papillary thyroid carcinoma. J Korean Surg Soc. 2013;84(4):195–201.
53. Garcia-Burillo A, Roca Bielsa I, Gonzalez O, Zafon C, Sabate M, Castellvi J, et al. SPECT/CT sentinel lymph node identification in papillary thyroid cancer: lymphatic staging and surgical management improvement. Eur J Nucl Med Mol Imaging. 2013; 40(11):1645–55.
54. Cabrera RN, Chone CT, Zantut-Wittmann D, Matos P, Ferreira DM, Pereira PS, et al. Value of sentinel lymph node biopsy in papillary thyroid cancer: initial results of a prospective trial. Eur Arch Otorhinolaryngol. 2015;272(4):971–9.
55. Carcoforo P, Portinari M, Feggi L, Panareo S, De Troia A, Zatelli MC, et al. Radio-guided selective compartment neck dissection improves staging in papillary thyroid carcinoma: a prospective study on 345 patients with a 3-year follow-up. Surgery. 2014;156(1):147–57.
56. Boni G, Mazzarri S, Grosso M, Manca G, Biricotti M, Ambrosini CE, et al. Sentinel node radioguided biopsy in surgical management of the medullary thyroid carcinoma A case report. Ann Ital Chir. 2014;21:85(ePub).
57. Puccini M, Manca G, Ugolini C, Candalise V, Passaretti A, Bernardini J, et al. Interest of sentinel node biopsy in apparently intrathyroidal medullary thyroid cancer: a pilot study. J Endocrinol Invest. 2014;37(9):829–34.
58. Catarci M, Zaraca F, Angeloni R, Mancini B, de Filippo MG, Massa R, et al. Preoperative lymphoscintigraphy and sentinel lymph node biopsy in papillary thyroid cancer. A pilot study. J Surg Oncol. 2001;77(1):21–4; discussion 5.
59. Balasubramanian SP, Brignall J, Lin HY, Stephenson TJ, Wadsley J, Harrison BJ, et al. Sentinel node biopsy in papillary thyroid cancer--what is the potential? Langenbecks Arch Surg. 2014;399(2):245–51.
60. Gonzalez O, Zafon C, Roca I. Selective sentinel lymph node biopsy in papillary thyroid carcinoma. Endocrinol Nutr. 2013;60(3):111–4.
61. Barczynski M. Systematic review and meta-analysis of sentinel node biopsy in thyroid cancer (Br J Surg 2010; 98: 334–344). Br J Surg. 2011;98(3):344–5.
62. Raijmakers PG, Paul MA, Lips P. Sentinel node detection in patients with thyroid carcinoma: a meta-analysis. World J Surg. 2008;32(9):1961–7.
63. Doherty GM. Sentinel lymph node biopsy for papillary thyroid cancer: commentary on the Efficacy of lateral neck sentinel lymph node biopsy in papillary thyroid carcinoma by Se Kyung Lee et al. World J Surg. 2011;35(12):2683.
64. Saliba J, Payne RJ, Varshney R, Sela E, Maniakas A, Rahme E, et al. Sentinel lymph node biopsy status correlates with postoperative stimulated thyroglobulin levels in low-risk papillary thyroid cancer patients. Endocr Pract. 2014;20(5):399–404.
65. Maniakas A, Forest VI, Jozaghi Y, Saliba J, Hier MP, Mlynarek A, et al. Tumor classification in well-differentiated thyroid carcinoma and sentinel lymph node biopsy outcomes: a direct correlation. Thyroid. 2014;24(4):671–4.
66. Civantos FJ, Zitsch RP, Schuller DE, Agrawal A, Smith RB, Nason R, et al. Sentinel lymph node biopsy accurately stages the regional lymph nodes for T1-T2 oral squamous cell carcinomas: results of a prospective multi-institutional trial. J Clin Oncol. 2010; 28(8):1395–400.
67. Alkureishi LW, Ross GL, Shoaib T, Soutar DS, Robertson AG, Thompson R, et al. Sentinel node biopsy in head and neck squamous cell cancer: 5-year follow-up of a European multicenter trial. Ann Surg Oncol. 2010;17(9):2459–64.
68. van den Berg NS, Brouwer OR, Klop WM, Karakullukcu B, Zuur CL, Tan IB, et al. Concomitant radio- and fluorescence-guided sentinel lymph node biopsy in squamous cell carcinoma of the oral cavity using ICG-(99m)Tc-nanocolloid. Eur J Nucl Med Mol Imaging. 2012;39(7):1128–36.
69. Agrawal A, Civantos FJ, Brumund KT, Chepeha DB, Hall NC, Carroll WR, et al. [Tc]tilmanocept accurately detects sentinel lymph nodes and predicts node pathology status in patients with oral squamous cell carcinoma of the head and neck: results of a phase III multi-institutional trial. Ann Surg Oncol. 2015;22(11):3708–15.
70. Vermeeren L, Valdes Olmos RA, Klop WM, Balm AJ, van den Brekel MW. A portable gamma-camera for intraoperative detection of sentinel nodes in the head and neck region. J Nucl Med. 2010;51(5):700–3.
71. Heuveling DA, van Weert S, Karagozoglu KH, de Bree R. Evaluation of the use of freehand SPECT for sentinel node biopsy in early stage oral carcinoma. Oral Oncol. 2015;51(3):287–90.
72. Valdes Olmos RA, Vidal-Sicart S, Giammarile F, Zaknun JJ, Van Leeuwen FW, Mariani G. The GOSTT concept and hybrid mixed/virtual/augmented reality environment radioguided surgery. Q J Nucl Med Mol Imaging. 2014;58(2):207–15.

Radioguided Parathyroid Surgery 13

Irene Lou, Rebecca S. Sippel, and Herbert Chen

Contents

I. Lou, MD • R.S. Sippel, MD
Department of Surgery, University of Wisconsin, 600 Highland Ave., K3/705 CSC, Madison, WI 53792, USA

H. Chen, MD (✉)
Chairman, Department of Surgery, University of Alabama at Birmingham, 1808 7th Avenue South, Suite 502, Birmingham, AL 35233, USA
e-mail: herbchen@uab.edu

Abstract

Radioguided parathyroidectomy is a helpful tool in the armamentarium of parathyroid surgeons and is applicable to nearly all patients. This chapter outlines the clinical utility of this method and provides an outline for appropriate patient selection. We also highlight many of the potential advantages of a radioguided approach, paying special attention to pediatric and geriatric patients as well as focusing on challenges particular to parathyroid surgery including ectopically located glands, a history of previous neck exploration, and parathyroid carcinoma. Focused detail is provided on the technical aspects of employing a radioguided approach, and we share practical pearls as well as discuss pre- and postoperative care for these patients. Lastly, we provide three clinical case examples in which a radioguided approach to parathyroidectomy was beneficial.

K. Herrmann et al. (eds.), *Radioguided Surgery: Current Applications and Innovative Directions in Clinical Practice*, DOI 10.1007/978-3-319-26051-8_13

13.1 Introduction

The surgical management of primary hyperparathyroidism (PHPT) is shifting to a focused, more minimally invasive approach from routine bilateral neck dissection [1]. As such, multiple tools have been developed to aid this focused approach both preoperatively and intraoperatively. These tools include improved imaging techniques to identify and localize parathyroid adenomas prior to surgery, rapid intraoperative parathyroid hormone (ioPTH) measurements to indicate adequate removal of hyper-functioning parathyroid tissue, and the detection of technetium 99m sestamibi within the pathologic parathyroid gland(s) [2, 3]. These adjuncts have become particularly useful in the parathyroid surgeon's armamentarium and are often used for both directed and four-gland explorations. Radioguided parathyroid surgery is when technetium 99m sestamibi is used on the day of surgery for parathyroid gland detection.

Technetium 99m sestamibi was initially used in cardiac imaging due to its ability to concentrate in mitochondrial-rich tissues [4]. During the initial years of use, findings of "hot spots" in the neck were described. These patients were noted to have PHPT, with adenomas located in the areas corresponding to the areas of increased activity. Recently, it has been confirmed the mechanism of sestamibi uptake in enlarged human parathyroid tissue is indeed associated with mitochondria function [5]. Coakley first described the use of technetium 99m sestamibi for preoperative localizing imaging in parathyroid surgery in 1989 [6]. The first report of using a gamma probe to aid in intraoperative detection of parathyroid tissue was by Ubhi in 1984 [7], who employed the use of thallium chloride-201. Currently, technetium 99m is the most popular choice for intraoperative parathyroid localization. The first use of technetium 99m alone for intraoperative parathyroid localization using a gamma probe was reported in a small case series by Martinez in 1995 [8]. Over the next decade, this isotope was further adapted for intraoperative use, to employ gamma rays to guide dissection and confirm the etiology of resected tissue [9–11], and this technique continues to be used today [12]. A selected overview of the current literature on radioguided parathyroidectomy is shown in Table 13.1. Several early studies on the use of radioguided techniques included only PHPT patients who were successfully localized preoperatively. With increasing familiarity with

Table 13.1 Selected overview of the current literature on radioguided parathyroidectomy

Group (year)	Inclusion criteria	Patient number	Dose of Tc 99m	Additional adjuncts	Success rate[a]	Findings
Flynn [13] (2000)	1HPT, untreated, recurrent, or persistent	39	20 mCi	Methylene blue, ioPTH	89 %	MIRP decreases operative time, hospital LOS, and cost Inability to localize abnormal gland with probe in patients with inconclusive or negative preoperative localization scans
Goldstein [14] (2000)	1HPT, positive delayed scans prior to surgery	20	20 mCi	Frozen section	20/20 (100 %)	MIRP decreases operative time, hospital LOS, and cost
McGreal [15] (2001)	1HPT	75	20 mCi	–	73/75 (98 %)	MIRP is a feasible alternative to bilateral dissection, allowing guided dissection and rapid confirmation

Table 13.1 (continued)

Group (year)	Inclusion criteria	Patient number	Dose of Tc 99m	Additional adjuncts	Success rate[a]	Findings
Shabtai [16] (2003)	1HPT, excluded suspected MGD	140	15 mCi	Frozen section, ioPTH	137/140 (98 %)	Success of MIRP for single-adenoma patients comparable to bilateral exploration
Takeyama [17] (2004)	1HPT and 2HPT	27	5.4 mCi	Frozen Section	1HPT: 9/10 (90 %) 2HPT: 13/17 (76.5 %)	Intraoperative probe effective for 1HPT and 2HPT and facilitate surgery for 2HPT
Rubello [18] (2005)	1HPT, solitary adenoma found on preoperative imaging	277	1–3 mCi	ioPTH	268/277 (96.8 %)	Low-dose Tc 99m is safe and effective in MIRP Use of ioPTH can facilitate intraoperative detection of multigland parathyroid disease
Caudle [19] (2006)	1HPT, localized on preoperative imaging	140	10 mCi	Frozen Section	135/140 (96.5 %)	MIRP obviates ioPTH in well-localized patients, but beneficial to non-localized patients
H. Chen [20] (2009)	1HPT	769	10 mCi	ioPTH	757/769 (98 %)	Radioguided technique equally effective in patients with negative preoperative localization Probe helps detect ectopically located parathyroid glands
Norman [21] (2009)	1HPT, excludes MEN patients	5,000	20–25 mCi	–	4960/5000 (99.2 %)	Probe allows accurate and very rapid feedback of parathyroid physiology prior and/or after resection
Pitt [22] (2009)	1HPT, 2HPT, 3HPT with prior neck surgery	110	10 mCi	ioPTH	106/110 (96 %)	Radioguided technique is safe and effective in the reoperative neck with similar cure rates as seen with initial parathyroidectomy
J. Chen [23] (2014)	2HPT	25	20 mCi	–	24/25 (96 %)	Radioguided localization improves success rate of patients undergoing parathyroidectomy for 2HPT
Somnay [24] (2015)	3HPT, no previous neck surgery	80	10 mCi	ioPTH	80/80 (100 %)	Probe reliably localizes abnormal parathyroid tissue, including ectopically located glands

1HPT primary hyperparathyroidism, *Tc 99m* technetium 99m, *mCi* millicurie, *ioPTH* intraoperative parathyroid hormone, *MIRP* minimally invasive radioguided parathyroidectomy, *LOS* length of stay, *MGD* multiglandular disease, *2HPT* secondary hyperparathyroidism, *3HPT* tertiary hyperparathyroidism

[a]Success rate = ability of radioguided technique to identify gland(s) of interest

this technique, a radioguided approach has been expanded to include all patients with hyperparathyroidism regardless of preoperative localization status.

13.2 Patient Selection

Before proceeding with radioguided parathyroid surgery, one must consider the additional cost of the isotope injection as well as the significant coordination and cooperation required between various hospital departments. Patients arrive to the preoperative holding area on the day of surgery; however, injections usually take place in nuclear medicine, optimally around 60–90 min prior to surgery [25]. Communication between preoperative holding, nuclear medicine, and the surgical team is paramount to ensure timeliness of travel between departments and the isotope administration. If the patient is taken to the operating room too soon after injection, there may not be enough of a differential within the tissues to direct dissection. If you wait too long after injection, counts may become too weak to provide useful information. We have found that by routinely employing the radioguided technique, the teams involved develop familiarity with the workflow which helps to facilitate the process.

13.2.1 Primary Hyperparathyroidism

The vast majority of patients undergoing radioguided parathyroidectomy have a diagnosis of primary hyperparathyroidism (PHPT). Regardless of preoperative sestamibi results or suspicion for a single-gland versus multigland disease, the use of technetium 99m on the day of surgery can provide helpful guidance in the operating room [9, 20] Table 13.1. When performing a parathyroidectomy, the gamma probe provides the surgeon with immediate feedback that the excised tissue is parathyroid in origin, rather than lymph node, fat, thymus, or thyroid nodule [11]. This avoids the need to obtain a frozen section and hence can decrease total operative time.

13.2.2 Secondary and Tertiary Hyperparathyroidism

Patients diagnosed with secondary or tertiary hyperparathyroidism generally have diffuse parathyroid gland hyperplasia due to longstanding renal disease or other disorders of calcium metabolism. While the underlying etiology of hyperplasia differs between these patients and those with PHPT, the concentration of sestamibi within the glands is equivalent. For patients with secondary and tertiary hyperparathyroidism, the operative procedure of choice is bilateral neck exploration with either a subtotal or total parathyroidectomy. As both sides of the neck are to be explored, these patients often do not undergo preoperative imaging localization. These patients however often have supernumerary glands, and the probe is useful to ensure additional areas of increased activity are identified and removed [24, 26] (Table 13.1).

13.2.3 Contraindications to a Radioguided Approach

There are few contraindications to radioguided parathyroidectomy. Pregnancy at the time of parathyroidectomy is rare, and though not by itself a contraindication, the International Atomic Energy Association advocates for a strong justification and exploration of alternative techniques prior to use of nuclear medicine techniques in this population [27]. As with any medication, patients who suffer an allergic reaction as a result of isotope injection should also not have this approach. Though the exact dose limitation for technetium 99m is unknown, patients felt to have large amounts of previous exposure based on annual radiation exposure limitations set forth by the United States Nuclear Regulatory Commission [28] should not undergo the procedure. Relative contraindications include recent diagnostic imaging with technetium 99m, as it may take over 3 days to completely clear the isotope from circulation and reinjection will lead to equivocal results.

13.3 Advantages of the Radioguided Approach

There are several advantages to radioguided parathyroidectomy. The method is equally effective in patients with negative preoperative localization [20] and allows a more focused skin incision. The dosing protocols for radioguided parathyroidectomy are safe for both patients and the operative team [29, 30] (Table 13.2). Extremely high-volume centers may elect to cover the patient with a lead blanket to minimize the cumulative exposure to the operating room staff [21]. The radioguided approach is also especially helpful in the clinical situations described below.

13.3.1 Pediatric and Geriatric Patients

Radioguided parathyroidectomy has been studied at both extremes of age [31, 32], as potentially decreasing the extent of resection is advantageous in these populations. The dose of technetium 99m sestamibi administered must be adjusted for pediatric patients, and lower dose protocols have been investigated for patients of all ages [33]. Regardless of technique, age should not be a deterrent of surgical management for PHPT. In the hands of an experienced, high-volume surgeon, excellent outcomes can be achieved at all ages [34–40].

Table 13.2 Radiation exposure to surgeon and staff during radioguided parathyroidectomy, reported monitoring threshold dose limit in accordance with the US Nuclear Regulatory Commission [28]

OR team member	Exposure per case (mrem) [29]	Number of cases to reach monitoring threshold (adult)[a]	Number of cases to reach monitoring threshold (minor or pregnancy)[b]
Surgeon or first assistant	0.80	625	125
Anesthesia team	0.11	4545	909
Scrub nurse or medical student	0.46	1087	217

OR operating room, *mrem* millirem
[a]Annual monitoring threshold for an adult = 500 mrem/year
[b]Annual monitoring threshold for minors and pregnant women (throughout duration of pregnancy) = 100 mrem/year

13.3.2 Ectopic Glands

When a missing gland is encountered during a four-gland exploration, or a supernumerary gland is suspected, in vivo counts with the gamma probe can detect glands in ectopic locations such as the retroesophageal groove and carotid sheath [41, 42].

When a patient is noted to have a mediastinal gland on preoperative imaging, there is a laparoscopic gamma probe that provides excellent guidance for dissection of the mediastinum during video-assisted thoracoscopy (VATS) [43, 44]. VATS is a minimally invasive alternative to open midline sternotomy and the probe additionally can provide measurements ex vivo which can immediately confirm a parathyroid adenoma within the excised specimen.

13.3.3 Obesity

Obesity is an operative challenge to all surgeons, and the neck is no exception. Excessive amounts of subcutaneous fat and tissue may limit the quality of preoperative imaging, although several studies have shown equivalent performance of ultrasound and sestamibi when the studies are of high quality [45–47]. The large amount of soft tissue in the neck also obscures visualization and may necessitate a larger incision for adequate exposure [47]. In this difficult population, a radioguided approach can improve gland detection within a limited field and discern parathyroid tissue from surrounding neck structures. Lastly, the weight of a large amount of soft tissue may raise concerns of perioperative airway safety and management [45, 47]. Radioguidance by potentially minimizing the total operative and thus anesthesia time can aid in mitigating these concerns.

13.3.4 Reoperative Neck

Patients with persistent/recurrent disease or extensive previous cervical operations are challenging due to dense scarring and disrupted tissue planes. In addition parathyroid adenomas may be displaced from the typical locations as a result of previous exploration [22, 48]. For these reasons, precise localization is needed for optimal success [49]. This can perhaps be achieved via preoperative imaging. However, intraoperative detection with the gamma probe can limit the field of dissection minimizing the amount of exploration through scar tissue helping to keep critical structures of the neck safe.

13.3.5 Forearm Grafts

Extensive parathyroid resection via subtotal or total parathyroidectomy is indicated in familial causes of primary hyperparathyroidism, secondary hyperparathyroidism, and occasionally tertiary hyperparathyroidism. These patients have an ongoing physiologic stimulus to the remnant parathyroid tissue or a genetic alteration leading to persistent proliferation and residual tissue can become hyperplastic over time. Many of these patients have forearm grafts, not only to differentiate recurrent disease in the neck from graft hyperplasia but also to allow ease of access during reoperation. If the graft locations are not clearly marked by clips or permanent suture at the time of graft placement, finding these grafts within the forearm musculature can be difficult [26]. Several groups have described the success of using radioguidance to aid in the resection and debulking of forearm grafts [50–52].

13.3.6 Parathyroid Carcinoma

Though rare, parathyroid carcinoma commonly invades adjacent structures [53]. When parathyroid carcinoma is suspected or recognized, en bloc resection without disruption of the tumor capsule is critical in decreasing the incidence of local seeding. These deposits often vary in size and location at reoperation, and the gamma probe can help direct the surgeon to these residual areas and limit the degree of dissection through scar tissue [54].

13.4 Performing a Radioguided Parathyroidectomy

13.4.1 Preoperative Preparation

On the day of surgery, the patient will undergo injection of technetium 99m through a peripherally placed intravenous catheter. Dosing protocols vary greatly ranging from 1 millicurie (mCi) to 25 mCi [9, 21, 31, 33]. Lower dosing protocols require a shorter time interval between injection and operation, while higher doses allow for both diagnostic imaging and a longer time frame before surgery [21, 33]. We favor a mid-range dose of 10 mCi for adult patients to be injected approximately 60 min prior to surgery with no nuclear imaging the day of surgery [9]. Again, coordination within your healthcare system is of utmost important to ensure timeliness between injection and surgery. Routine use of this technique creates familiarity, therefore making delays and disruptions less likely.

The same probe that is used for sentinel lymph node biopsies in breast and melanoma cases can be programmed to be used in radioguided parathyroidectomy surgeries. Care should be taken to coordinate with the operating room to ensure there is enough equipment for all.

13.4.2 Operative Technique

The patient is positioned on the operating room table in a supine, modified beach chair position with a shoulder roll placed to allow moderate hyperextension of the neck. The amount of radiation emitting from the patient is low and rapidly deteriorates with distance; therefore, no particular safety precautions are necessary for the operating room staff [29, 30]. This procedure may be safely performed under local anesthesia, local anesthesia with monitored anesthesia laryngeal mask, or general anesthesia with an endotracheal tube based on patient, surgeon, and anesthesia preferences [21, 55]. If within your practice, an ultrasound for confirmation of localization and incision planning can be performed at this time.

As previously mentioned, the same probe used for sentinel lymph node biopsies in breast and melanoma can be used in radioguided parathyroidectomy. We use a wireless collimated 12 mm neoprobe Gamma Detection System with Bluetooth (Devicor Medical Products, Inc, Cincinnati, OH). The gamma probe is fitted with a sterile covering for use within the operative field. After the patient is appropriated prepped and draped, the probe is held over the thyroid isthmus to obtain measurements of background emissions for the thyroid (Fig. 13.1). In patients without clear localization prior to surgery, measurements can quickly be obtained in the bilateral upper and lower neck. Areas of increased counts correspond to the likely location of enlarged glands and can guide the initial incision [11].

After incision, the probe may be inserted into the wound as needed to confirm the direction and depth necessary for dissection to identify the enlarged gland(s). This is especially important when looking for ectopic glands. Tissue suspicious for parathyroid adenomas have counts measured in vivo prior to resection [56]. After excision, ex vivo counts are obtained as a percentage of the initial background value obtained (Figs. 13.2 and 13.3). The excised tissue is placed directly on the tip of the probe and importantly also held away from the patient to minimize any patient background emissions. Tissue with counts of at least 20 % of the initial background measurement is consistent with parathyroid tissue, while adipose, lymph nodes, scar, and thyroid nodules will emit counts in the single digits [11, 57].

We strongly encourage patients undergoing a directed or focused parathyroidectomy to have additional confirmation to ensure resection of all hyper-functioning tissue and to minimize the risk of persistent disease [21, 56, 58]. We therefore draw a baseline ioPTH prior to gland excision. Surgeons who routinely perform bilateral exploration with radioguidance however may choose to omit the use of any additional adjuncts [59]. Once the offending glands have been excised, it is in our practice to obtain 5, 10, and 15 min postexcision measurements of ioPTH. Our benchmark for cure is based on the Miami criterion in which we dem-

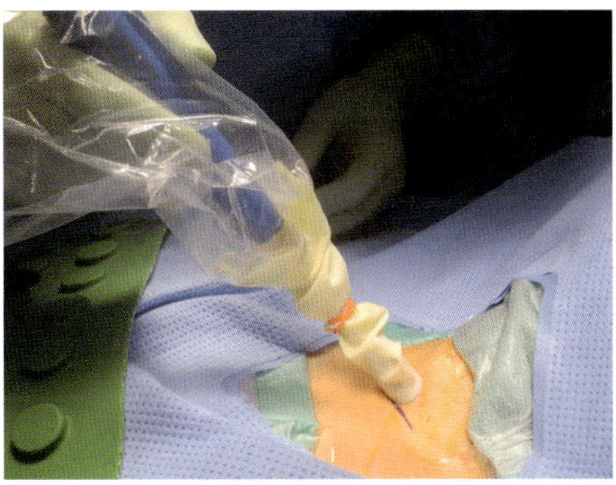

Fig. 13.1 Measuring background counts over the thyroid isthmus

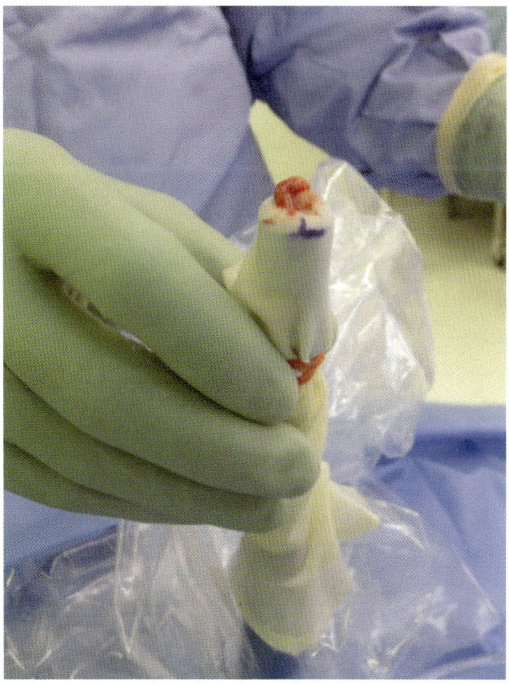

Fig. 13.2 Excised specimen placed on the tip of the gamma probe to obtain ex vivo counts

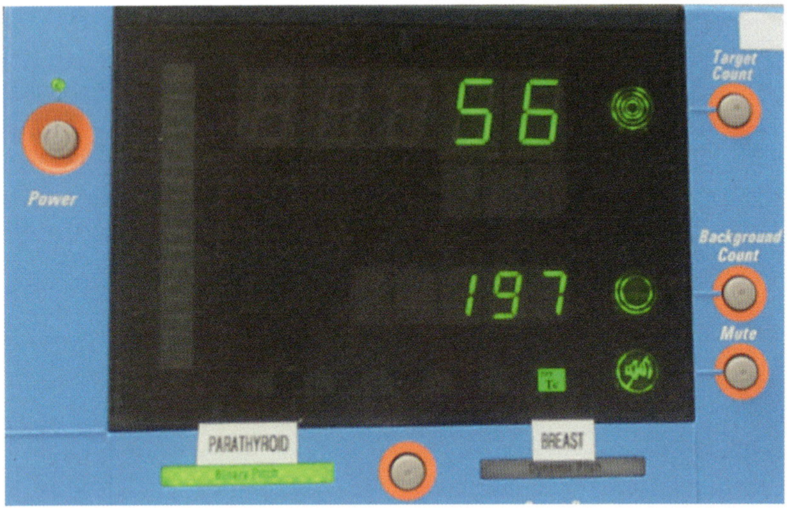

Fig. 13.3 Base unit displaying ratio of target (ex vivo) count over initial background count. In this instance the excised gland measured 28.4 % (56/197), meeting the 20 % rule diagnostic for parathyroid tissue

onstrate a 50 % decline in ioPTH from baseline at any time point [56, 60].

While waiting for the ioPTH results, we use this time to inject long-acting local anesthetic and proceed to closure of the wound. Once the ioPTH has returned to confirm no additional exploration is required, the patient is awoken and taken to recovery room.

13.4.3 Practical Pearls

The gamma probe measures emitted gamma rays based on the direction of the tip; therefore, the surgeon must be cognizant of the angle and direction of the tip when it is within the surgical incision. Increase background from the salivary glands, carotid arteries, heart, and liver can lead to false-positive readings. This is especially important when taking in vivo readings of the thymus and when looking for an upper mediastinal adenoma from a cervical incision. In addition, thyroid tissue has inconsistent uptake of the isotope in nodular disease. Taking measurements on the targeted tissue from various different angles optimizes the reliability of in vivo counts. Increased surgeon familiarity and consistent use of the probe also ensure more dependable results.

13.4.4 Postoperative Care

Patients can generally be discharged home from the recovery room after meeting criteria. All patients have a parathyroid hormone level drawn in the post-anesthesia recovery area. Based on these results, patients are kept on oral calcium ± vitamin D supplementation. They are also given clear instructions on the symptoms of hypocalcemia and what to do in the event these symptoms are experienced. Pain control is achieved with oral analgesia, and patients are advised to use topical ice packs to the anterior neck both for pain and to decrease swelling [61]. At the first postoperative visit, serum calcium and parathyroid hormone (PTH) levels are rechecked to document resolution of PTH elevation and hypercalcemia. These levels also help dictate the patient's clinical course in the event of hypocalcemia. An additional calcium and PTH should be checked at 6 months after surgery to document cure.

13.5 Case Examples

13.5.1 Case 1

A quadriplegic male in his 30s with a permanent tracheostomy has a history of multiple urinary tract infections and nephrocalcinosis. He is diagnosed with primary hyperparathyroidism but experiences a delay to surgery due to his multiple medical comorbidities including morbid obesity with a body mass index over 40 kg/m^2. In the operating room, the patient had a very short neck and excessive soft tissue. The gamma probe was able to focus the area of dissection, especially in light of previous scar tissue from his tracheostomy, and identify his parathyroid adenoma. Cure was confirmed with ioPTH. He recovered well from anesthesia and was discharged in excellent condition.

13.5.2 Case 2

A 39-year-old otherwise healthy schoolteacher is diagnosed with primary hyperparathyroidism, with negative preoperative localization studies. She is taken to the operating room and the gamma probe identifies a hot area in a high cervical position, several fingerbreadths above the traditional collar incision. A small 3 cm transverse incision is made high in the neck based on the area of highest intensity of the gamma probe. The patient was found to have an undescended parathyroid gland, which was successfully identified and removed with the aid of the probe via a minimally invasive incision.

13.5.3 Case 3

A 52-year-old female has a history of parathyroid carcinoma and as a result has had four previous neck operations. She is found to have local recurrence of her cancer necessitating another neck exploration. In the operating room, she has extensive scar tissue and obscured tissue planes. With the aid of the gamma probe, an area of high intensity signal was localized and resected from surrounding scar, both focusing and limiting the extent of dissection.

Conclusion

There are several intraoperative adjuncts in parathyroid surgery; however, the availability of these options varies. Radioguided parathyroidectomy is a helpful tool in the armamentarium of parathyroid surgeons and is applicable to nearly all patients. With practice and repetition, optimal results can be achieved. Familiarity with all of the available tools increases surgeon adaptability and acumen.

Conflicts of Interest and Source of Funding Irene Lou is currently receiving grant support from NIH T32 CA090217-14.

For the remaining authors, none are declared.

References

1. Irvin 3rd GL, Carneiro DM, Solorzano CC. Progress in the operative management of sporadic primary hyperparathyroidism over 34 years. Ann Surg. 2004; 239(5):704–8; discussion 708–11.
2. Irvin 3rd GL, Dembrow VD, Prudhomme DL. Operative monitoring of parathyroid gland hyperfunction. Am J Surg. 1991;162(4):299–302.
3. Sfakianakis GN, Irvin 3rd GL, Foss J, et al. Efficient parathyroidectomy guided by SPECT-MIBI and hormonal measurements. J Nucl Med. 1996;37(5): 798–804.
4. Sporn V, Perez Balino N, Holman BL, et al. Simultaneous measurement of ventricular function and myocardial perfusion using the technetium-99m isonitriles. Clin Nucl Med. 1988;13(2):77–81.
5. Hetrakul N, Civelek AC, Stagg CA, et al. In vitro accumulation of technetium-99m-sestamibi in human parathyroid mitochondria. Surgery. 2001;130(6): 1011–8.
6. Coakley AJ, Kettle AG, Wells CP, et al. 99Tcm sestamibi--a new agent for parathyroid imaging. Nucl Med Commun. 1989;10(11):791–4.
7. Ubhi CS, Hardy JG, Pegg CA. Mediastinal parathyroid adenoma: a new method of localization. Br J Surg. 1984;71(11):859–60.
8. Martinez DA, King DR, Romshe C, et al. Intraoperative identification of parathyroid gland pathology: a new approach. J Pediatr Surg. 1995; 30(9):1306–9.
9. Chen H, Mack E, Starling JR. Radioguided parathyroidectomy is equally effective for both adenomatous and hyperplastic glands. Ann Surg. 2003;238(3):332–7; discussion 337–8.
10. Norman J, Chheda H. Minimally invasive parathyroidectomy facilitated by intraoperative nuclear mapping. Surgery. 1997;122(6):998–1003; discussion 1003–4.
11. Murphy C, Norman J. The 20% rule: a simple, instantaneous radioactivity measurement defines cure and allows elimination of frozen sections and hormone

assays during parathyroidectomy. Surgery. 1999; 126(6):1023–8; discussion 1028–9.
12. Wang TS, Pasieka JL, Carty SE. Techniques of parathyroid exploration at North American endocrine surgery fellowship programs: what the next generation is being taught. Am J Surg. 2014;207(4):527–32.
13. Flynn MB, Bumpous JM, Schill K, et al. Minimally invasive radioguided parathyroidectomy. J Am Coll Surg. 2000;191(1):24–31.
14. Goldstein RE, Blevins L, Delbeke D, et al. Effect of minimally invasive radioguided parathyroidectomy on efficacy, length of stay, and costs in the management of primary hyperparathyroidism. Ann Surg. 2000;231(5):732–42.
15. McGreal G, Winter DC, Sookhai S, et al. Minimally invasive, radioguided surgery for primary hyperparathyroidism. Ann Surg Oncol. 2001;8(10):856–60.
16. Shabtai M, Ben-Haim M, Muntz Y, et al. 140 consecutive cases of minimally invasive, radio-guided parathyroidectomy: lessons learned and long-term results. Surg Endosc. 2003;17(5):688–91.
17. Takeyama H, Shioya H, Mori Y, et al. Usefulness of radio-guided surgery using technetium-99m methoxyisobutylisonitrile for primary and secondary hyperparathyroidism. World J Surg. 2004;28(6):576–82.
18. Rubello D, Pelizzo MR, Boni G, et al. Radioguided surgery of primary hyperparathyroidism using the low-dose 99mTc-sestamibi protocol: multiinstitutional experience from the Italian Study Group on Radioguided Surgery and Immunoscintigraphy (GISCRIS). J Nucl Med. 2005;46(2):220–6.
19. Caudle AS, Brier SE, Calvo BF, et al. Experienced radio-guided surgery teams can successfully perform minimally invasive radio-guided parathyroidectomy without intraoperative parathyroid hormone assays. Am Surg. 2006;72(9):785–9; discussion 790.
20. Chen H, Sippel RS, Schaefer S. The effectiveness of radioguided parathyroidectomy in patients with negative technetium tc 99m-sestamibi scans. Arch Surg. 2009;144(7):643–8.
21. Norman J, Politz D. 5,000 parathyroid operations without frozen section or PTH assays: measuring individual parathyroid gland hormone production in real time. Ann Surg Oncol. 2009;16(3):656–66.
22. Pitt SC, Panneerselvan R, Sippel RS, et al. Radioguided parathyroidectomy for hyperparathyroidism in the reoperative neck. Surgery. 2009; 146(4):592–8; discussion 598–9.
23. Chen J, Wang JD. Radioguided parathyroidectomy in patients with secondary hyperparathyroidism due to chronic renal failure. Nucl Med Commun. 2014;35(4):391–7.
24. Somnay YR, Weinlander E, Alfhefdi A, et al. Radioguided parathyroidectomy for tertiary hyperparathyroidism. J Surg Res. 2015;195(2):406–11.
25. Chen H. Radioguided Parathyroid surgery. Adv Surg. 2004;38:377–92.
26. Nichol PF, Mack E, Bianco J, et al. Radioguided parathyroidectomy in patients with secondary and tertiary hyperparathyroidism. Surgery. 2003;134(4):713–7.
27. International Agency of Atomic Energy. Pregnancy and radiation protection in nuclear medicine 2013. https://rpop.iaea.org/RPOP/RPoP/Content/SpecialGroups/1_PregnantWomen/PregnancyNuclearMedicine.htm Accessed 27 Apr 2015.
28. Commission USNR. Title 10, code of federal regulations, part 20, standards for the protection against radiation. In: Commission USNR, editor. http://www.nrc.gov/reading-rm/doc-collections/cfr/part020/. Accessed 27 Apr 2015.
29. Oltmann SC, Brekke AV, Macatangay JD, et al. Surgeon and staff radiation exposure during radioguided parathyroidectomy at a high-volume institution. Ann Surg Oncol. 2014;21(12):3853–8.
30. Bekis R, Celik P, Uysal B, et al. Exposure of surgical staff in surgical probe applications in radioguided parathyroidectomy. Eur Arch Otorhinolaryngol. 2008;265(12):1545–8.
31. Burke JF, Jacobson K, Gosain A, et al. Radioguided parathyroidectomy effective in pediatric patients. J Surg Res. 2013;184(1):312–7.
32. Rubello D, Casara D, Giannini S, et al. Minimally invasive radioguided parathyroidectomy: an attractive therapeutic option for elderly patients with primary hyperparathyroidism. Nucl Med Commun. 2004;25(9):901–8.
33. Rubello D, Al-Nahhas A, Mariani G, et al. Feasibility and long-term results of focused radioguided parathyroidectomy using a "low" 37 MBq (1 mCi) 99mTc-sestamibi protocol. Int Semin Surg Oncol. 2006;3:30.
34. Oltmann SC, Schneider D, Sippel RS, et al. Presentation, management and outcomes of hyperparathyroidism in octogenarians and nonagenarians. Ann Surg Oncol. 2013;20:4195-9
35. Wang TS, Roman SA, Sosa JA. Predictors of outcomes following pediatric thyroid and parathyroid surgery. Curr Opin Oncol. 2009;21(1):23–8.
36. Lambert LA, Shapiro SE, Lee JE, et al. Surgical treatment of hyperparathyroidism in patients with multiple endocrine neoplasia type 1. Arch Surg. 2005;140(4): 374–82.
37. Durkin ET, Nichol PF, Lund DP, et al. What is the optimal treatment for children with primary hyperparathyroidism? J Pediatr Surg. 2010;45(6):1142–6.
38. Oltmann SC, Rajaei MH, Sippel RS, et al. Primary hyperparathyroidism across the ages: presentation and outcomes. J Surg Res. 2014;190(1):185–90.
39. Kebebew E, Duh QY, Clark OH. Parathyroidectomy for primary hyperparathyroidism in octogenarians and nonagenarians: a plea for early surgical referral. Arch Surg. 2003;138(8):867–71.
40. Kundel A, Thompson GB, Richards ML, et al. Pediatric endocrine surgery: a 20-year experience at the Mayo Clinic. J Clin Endocrinol Metab. 2014;99(2): 399–406.
41. Rubello D, Casara D, Pagetta C, et al. Determinant role of Tc-99m MIBI SPECT in the localization of a retrotracheal parathyroid adenoma successfully treated by radioguided surgery. Clin Nucl Med. 2002;27(10):711–5.

42. Rubello D, Piotto A, Pagetta C, et al. Ectopic parathyroid adenomas located at the carotid bifurcation: the role of preoperative Tc-99m MIBI scintigraphy and the intraoperative gamma probe procedure in surgical treatment planning. Clin Nucl Med. 2001;26(9):774–6.
43. O'Herrin JK, Weigel T, Wilson M, et al. Radioguided parathyroidectomy via VATS combined with intraoperative parathyroid hormone testing: the surgical approach of choice for patients with mediastinal parathyroid adenomas? J Bone Miner Res. 2002;17(8): 1368–71.
44. Weigel TL, Murphy J, Kabbani L, et al. Radioguided thoracoscopic mediastinal parathyroidectomy with intraoperative parathyroid hormone testing. Ann Thorac Surg. 2005;80(4):1262–5.
45. Pitt SC, Panneerselvan R, Sippel RS, et al. Influence of morbid obesity on parathyroidectomy outcomes in primary hyperparathyroidism. Am J Surg. 2010;199(3):410–4; discussion 414–5.
46. Adam MA, Untch BR, Danko ME, et al. Severe obesity is associated with symptomatic presentation, higher parathyroid hormone levels, and increased gland weight in primary hyperparathyroidism. J Clin Endocrinol Metab. 2010;95(11):4917–24.
47. Norman J, Aronson K. Outpatient parathyroid surgery and the differences seen in the morbidly obese. Otolaryngol Head Neck Surg. 2007;136(2):282–6.
48. Perrier ND, Edeiken B, Nunez R, et al. A novel nomenclature to classify parathyroid adenomas. World J Surg. 2009;33(3):412–6.
49. Powell AC, Alexander HR, Chang R, et al. Reoperation for parathyroid adenoma: a contemporary experience. Surgery. 2009;146(6):1144–55.
50. Cutress RI, Manwaring-White C, Dixon K, et al. Gamma probe radioguided parathyroid forearm surgery in recurrent hyperparathyroidism. Ann R Coll Surg Engl. 2009;91(7):W1–3.
51. Ardito G, Revelli L, Giustozzi E, et al. Radioguided parathyroidectomy in forearm graft for recurrent hyperparathyroidism. Br J Radiol. 2012;85(1009): e1–3.
52. Sippel RS, Bianco J, Chen H. Radioguided parathyroidectomy for recurrent hyperparathyroidism caused by forearm graft hyperplasia. J Bone Miner Res. 2003;18(5):939–42.
53. Shane E. Clinical review 122: parathyroid carcinoma. J Clin Endocrinol Metab. 2001;86(2):485–93.
54. Placzkowski K, Christian R, Chen H. Radioguided parathyroidectomy for recurrent parathyroid cancer. Clin Nucl Med. 2007;32(5):358–60.
55. Udelsman R, Lin Z, Donovan P. The superiority of minimally invasive parathyroidectomy based on 1650 consecutive patients with primary hyperparathyroidism. Ann Surg. 2011;253(3):585–91.
56. Chen H, Mack E, Starling JR. A comprehensive evaluation of perioperative adjuncts during minimally invasive parathyroidectomy: which is most reliable? Ann Surg. 2005;242(3):375–80; discussion 380–3.
57. Olson J, Repplinger D, Bianco J, et al. Ex vivo radioactive counts and decay rates of tissues resected during radioguided parathyroidectomy. J Surg Res. 2006;136(2):187–91.
58. Chen H, Pruhs Z, Starling JR, et al. Intraoperative parathyroid hormone testing improves cure rates in patients undergoing minimally invasive parathyroidectomy. Surgery. 2005;138(4):583–7; discussion 587–90.
59. Ahmed K, Alhefdhi A, Schneider DF, et al. Minimal benefit to subsequent intraoperative parathyroid hormone testing after all four glands have been identified. Ann Surg Oncol. 2013;20(13):4200–4.
60. Irvin 3rd GL, Deriso 3rd GT. A new, practical intraoperative parathyroid hormone assay. Am J Surg. 1994;168(5):466–8.
61. Watkins AA, Johnson TV, Shrewsberry AB, et al. Ice packs reduce postoperative midline incision pain and narcotic use: a randomized controlled trial. J Am Coll Surg. 2014;219(3):511–7.

14 Radioguided Surgery of Thyroid Carcinoma Recurrences

Christina Bluemel, Ken Herrmann, Gerhard Wolf, Giorgo Castagnola, and Carlo Bellotti

Contents

Abstract

Thyroid cancer is the most common endocrine malignancy. The most frequent subtypes are differentiated thyroid cancer arising from the thyroid follicular epithelial cells and medullary thyroid cancer. The overall prognosis of patients with thyroid cancer is good, but more than one-third of patients experience recurrent disease. Patients with local recurrence in the thyroid bed or cervical lymph node metastases are usually treated with surgery, which may be complicated by the distorted anatomy due to total thyroidectomy and lymph node dissection for primary treatment. Especially in recurrent disease, exact localization of the diseased tissue or nodes may help to reduce the extent of the operative procedure. In this chapter the role of radioguided surgery for completion thyroidectomy in patients with differentiated and medullary thyroid cancer, and for reoperation in cases of recurrence, will be discussed; both iodine-guided and non-iodine-guided procedures will be considered.

Radioguided surgery is a very useful tool to administer minimal-invasive surgery in thyroid cancer.

C. Bluemel (✉) • K. Herrmann, MD
Department of Nuclear Medicine,
University Hospital of Würzburg,
Oberdürrbacher Str. 6, Würzburg Germany
e-mail: bluemel_c@ukw.de; herrmann_k1@ukw.de

G. Wolf
Endocrine Surgery, University of Graz, Graz, Austria

G. Castagnola • C. Bellotti
Operative Unit Surgery of Thyroid and Parathyroid,
Sapienza University of Rome, S. Andrea Hospital,
Rome, Italy

K. Herrmann et al. (eds.), *Radioguided Surgery: Current Applications and Innovative Directions in Clinical Practice*, DOI 10.1007/978-3-319-26051-8_14

14.1 Introduction

Thyroid cancer is the most common endocrine malignancy and in recent decades its incidence has increased worldwide. Nevertheless, thyroid cancer is rare [1]. In the United States only 1.0–1.5 % of all newly diagnosed malignancies are cancer of the thyroid [2]. The incidence in Europe is about 6.3 per 100,000 people per year [3]. Ninety percent of thyroid malignancies arise from the thyroid follicular epithelial cells. The papillary subtype accounts for 85 % of cases, the follicular subtype accounts for 10 %, and the remainder are Hürthle cell cancer and oxyphil tumors [4]. Papillary thyroid cancer (PTC) and follicular thyroid cancer (FTC) show a good overall prognosis, with the 10-year survival rate exceeding 90 % in cases of PTC [5, 6]. In more than 30 % of patients, however, locoregional recurrence occurs; recurrence is particularly frequent in patients with primary lymph node metastases and is predictive of long-term survival [7–10]. Especially lymph node recurrence is associated with a poor prognosis and such disease cannot be eradicated in 30 % of patients [7, 11]. Patients with medullary thyroid cancer and Hürthle cell thyroid carcinoma have an overall reduced disease-specific 10-year survival rate [12, 13].

As most recurrences in thyroid cancer occur within the neck, radical surgery is usually the preferred treatment [4]; it can, however, be challenging since most patients will have undergone surgery as primary treatment, including total extracapsular thyroidectomy with or without lymphadenectomy of the central/lateral compartment for cervical lymph nodes. Owing to the complex and distorted anatomy of the cervical region and the presence of scar tissue with possibly tenacious adhesions and fibrotic tissue, reoperations are accompanied by a higher complication rate and are often difficult even for skilled surgeons. Accordingly, while the morbidity of thyroid surgery is generally low, risks increase in cancer patients undergoing reoperative intervention for completion thyroidectomy or recurrence [14, 15].

With a view to reducing the risks of reoperation and ensuring complete resection, the potential role of radioguided surgery in detecting and safely resecting residual or recurrent disease in patients with thyroid cancer has been investigated.

14.2 Differentiated Thyroid Cancer: Completion Thyroidectomy

In DTC, radioguided surgery is mainly performed for sentinel lymph node biopsy [16, 17] and detection of locoregional recurrent disease. However, guidance of surgery with radiopharmaceuticals may also be beneficial for completion of thyroidectomy after a subtotal thyroid resection due to a (multi)nodular goiter or an incidental finding of DTC in the histopathologic examination [18–22]. In patients with an incidental PTC of >1 cm or an FTC, reintervention with (near) total thyroidectomy is recommended because of the risk of multifocal PTC (up to 88 % of cases) and the need to reduce the likelihood of locoregional recurrence and improve overall survival [20, 23–25]. Furthermore, total resection of thyroid tissue is required for the radioiodine ablation of thyroid bed remnants, facilitating postoperative follow-up.

It is to be borne in mind that reinterventions performed later than 24 h after the first resection may be associated with an increased complication rate. For example, the risk of injury to the recurrent laryngeal nerve in patients with thyroid malignancies rises from 0.3–3 % at initial surgery to 2–30 % at reoperation [26]. The early postoperative ultrasound for determination of remnant tissue might be misleading. The distinction between scar tissue and thyroid remnants may be difficult even for experienced surgeons. Therefore, radioguided completion thyroidectomy has been investigated by several groups. One group reported on the use of orally administered ^{131}I [21], while others have studied the potential value of intravenously injected ^{99m}Tc-pertechnetate [18–20, 22, 27]. ^{99m}Tc-pertechnetate is trapped by a nonspecific localization mechanism in thyroid tissue and maximal uptake is achieved 20–30 min later. ^{99m}Tc-pertechnetate is routinely used for diagnostic thyroid scintigraphy and is an "optimal" tracer

Table 14.1 Radioguided completion thyroidectomy (characteristics of trials)

	No. of patients	Radiopharmaceutical	Injected activity	Injection time
Erbil et al. (2005) [19]	11	^{99m}Tc-pertechnetate	[a]	[a]
Uludag et al. (2009) [22]	23	^{99m}Tc-pertechnetate	111 MBq	During anesthetic induction
Aras et al. (2009) [18]	14	^{99m}Tc-pertechnetate	185 MBq	5 min prior to surgery
Bender et al. (2009) [27]	50	^{99m}Tc-pertechnetate	[a]	[a]
Karyagar et al. (2010) [20]	27	^{99m}Tc-pertechnetate	185 MBq	10 min prior to surgery
Proczko et al. (2013) [21]	75	^{131}I	37–74 MBq	1 day prior to surgery

[a]Not reported in the available abstract/paper

because of the short half-life ($t_{1/2}$=6 h) and the 140-keV gamma photon emission, which can be easily detected by gamma cameras and probes. Furthermore, ^{99m}Tc-pertechnetate is easily available and also cheap.

The first study was reported by Erbil et al. in 2005 (Table 14.1). ^{99m}Tc-based radioguided completion thyroidectomy was performed in 11 patients who had undergone surgery for benign nodular goiter and an incidental finding of DTC [19]. The feasibility of this approach was confirmed in further studies [13, 18, 20, 22] in which between 111 and 185 MBq of ^{99m}Tc-pertechnetate was intravenously injected 5–10 min prior to surgery. All groups were spared preoperative scintigraphy.

For intraoperative localization of the thyroid remnant, the background activity has to be measured in addition to the counts in the region of interest. Aras et al. measured the counts over 10 s in the right, left, and pyramidal thyroid lobes and compared the count rates with the background activity measured over the strap muscles [18]. Karyagar et al. measured the background activity over the contralateral shoulder (non-injection arm) and performed three measurements over the thyroid bed on each side (upper, middle, and lower parts; each 10 s) [20]. Since physiologic uptake may be present in the adjacent salivary glands or thymus and may interfere with tumor detection, the probe tip should not be pointed at this region. In most studies, the tissue-to-background ratio has been calculated and successful resection of thyroid tissue proved by comparing the ratio before and after tissue resection [19, 20, 22]. An ex vivo measurement of the resected tissue may also be helpful. Aras et al. proposed an exchange ratio calculated using the formula [(thyroid lobe region counts − background counts)/background counts × 100] [18]. Additional postoperative scintigraphy could serve as a reference to prove the success of completion thyroidectomy [18, 20].

Using ^{99m}Tc-pertechnetate, Aras et al. demonstrated that the described radioguided procedure facilitated the differentiation of functioning thyroid tissue from fibrotic and cicatricial tissue. In their study the gamma probe failed to detect thyroid remnants in one out of 14 patients [18]. Karyagar et al. achieved complete resection in all but two patients, in whom tissue had to be left in order to avoid a recurrent nerve injury [20]. ^{99m}Tc-guided surgery helped to identify tumoral lesions in difficult and unexpected areas, for example, behind vascular structures or within sclerotic tissue, which could not be detected at presurgical evaluation. In none of the studies were specific or increased side effects observed compared with the conventional approach [19, 27].

In 2013 Proczko et al. published a study on 75 patients with an incidental finding of DTC in subtotal thyroidectomy, who were randomized to radioguided completion thyroidectomy (n=43) or conventional completion thyroidectomy (n=32) [21]. They used the most thyroid-specific tracer, applying radioiodine (^{131}I) orally 90 min before surgery. The authors observed no impairment in the therapeutic ablative radioiodine application, which is necessary for ablation of remaining thyroid tissue and for diagnostic scintigraphy, performed 6 weeks after surgery.

The results of these studies using ^{131}I and ^{99m}Tc-pertechnetate are promising and suggest that the approach may reduce the risk of complications when performing a reintervention for completion thyroidectomy with or without lymph node dissection. When anatomic landmarks and planes are obliterated due to scar and fibrosis, intraoperative gamma probe detection helps to distinguish thyroid remnants from surrounding tissue. However, while surgeons have described the procedure as decisive and favorable, the results are preliminary and none of the studies conducted to date has proved an impact on patient outcome. In addition, no studies on the role of additional intraoperative imaging are as yet available.

14.3 Differentiated Thyroid Cancer: Recurrences

Recurrences of DTC occur in 6–30 % of patients [7, 8]. Serum thyroglobulin, ultrasonography, and ^{131}I whole-body scintigraphy are used for clinical follow-up and detection of recurrent disease [4]. In addition to its role in the detection of locoregional recurrence, ^{131}I can be used for radioguided resection of the malignant tissue. However, in 20 % of patients, the recurring tumor is already iodine negative; in these patients non-iodine tracers (e.g., ^{18}F-FDG or ^{99m}Tc-nanocolloids) may be helpful for intraoperative localization of recurrent DTC, which may be hampered by scarred and fibrotic tissue due to previous surgery.

14.3.1 Iodine-Guided Resection of Recurrent Disease

After initial treatment of DTC, including surgery and remnant ablation with ^{131}I, locoregional recurrences may appear in the thyroid bed, soft tissue, or lymph nodes. Several treatment options are available, including surgery, external radiotherapy, and repeat iodine treatment. Surgery is the preferred option, especially in patients who do not respond to radioiodine treatment and have residual disease, mostly lymph node metastases of larger diameter (>1 cm). In these patients, reintervention with resection of tumor tissue may be the only curative option.

^{131}I-radioguided surgery for residual thyroid tissue was first described by Harris et al. in 1956 [28] and was taken up again by Morris et al. in 1971 [29] for gamma probe-guided localization of recurrent thyroid cancer during neck exploration. In 1998, Travagli et al. proposed a high-dose protocol using ^{131}I, performed over 1 week, in patients with recurrence of well-differentiated thyroid cancer [30]. All patients were initially treated with thyroidectomy and one to seven ^{131}I treatment cycles for remnant ablation and treatment of metastases. Radioiodine-guided surgery was applied on average 5 years (range, 5 months to 49 years) after primary treatment. In all patients, L-thyroxine was withdrawn to enhance the iodine uptake in the metastatic lesions (TSH >30 μIU/ml). The protocol proposed by the Institut Gustave-Roussy started on day 0 with the oral administration of a therapeutic dose of ^{131}I (3.7 GBq). Four days later a whole-body scan was performed using a gamma camera equipped with a high-energy collimator and a neck spot scan was carried out using a rectilinear scanner. The information provided by these two scans was employed for intraoperative navigation to the tumor lesions using a handheld gamma probe (day 5). The probe was directly placed over the iodine-avid lesions for the activity measurement and background activity values (vessels, normal soft tissue) were also assessed to allow calculation of the lesion-to-background ratio. After resection, the lesion bed was once again scanned for any residual activity, to prove that resection had been successful. In addition to the intraoperative measurements, a neck scan was performed on day 2 after surgery (day 7 after iodine administration) to prove complete resection of recurrent or residual functioning disease.

The protocol was slightly adapted by Lippi et al. [31], Salvatori et al. [32], and Rubello et al. [33], who investigated 6, 10, and 31 patients, respectively. They performed the preoperative whole-body scan on day 3 instead of day 4, while radioguided surgery was also performed on day 5. Scurry et al. reported that residual activity after therapeutic high-dose iodine (16.65 GBq) can guide neck dissection even 3 weeks later [34]. The radioguided procedure was shown to be feasible and safe [33]. Despite the hypothyroidism, no specific side effects of surgery and anesthesia were observed; however, Negele et al. proposed the intermittent administration of triiodothyronine during surgery [35].

Salvatori et al. reported that 41 of 78 lymph node metastases were detected only by the intraoperative use of the gamma probe and were not seen on the preoperative whole-body scan; of the remaining 37 lymph node metastases, 33 were detected by both whole-body scan and gamma probe but four were detected neither by intraoperative gamma probe nor by whole-body scan [32]. Their rate of false-negative lesions was higher in the study by Travagli et al. (14 of 46 lesions) [30].

A few years later Rubello et al. [33] published their results obtained in 31 patients with iodine-positive locoregional disease who had previously undergone thyroidectomy and two ineffective ^{131}I treatment cycles. Histopathologic evaluation showed 184 metastatic lesions in this patient cohort, approximately half of which (53.2 %) were detected by both whole-body scan and gamma probe. Of the metastatic foci, 5.4 % could not be detected by radioiodine. A reason for iodine-negative lesions in this patient cohort may have been the loss of cell differentiation and selection or induction of iodine-negative tumor cells after multiple treatment cycles with iodine. During the follow-up period (range, 8 months to 4.9 years), investigations including diagnostic whole-body scintigraphy, thyroglobulin measurement in hypothyroidism, and ultrasound showed no disease in 80.6 % of patients and persistent disease in the others [33].

All studies using a high-dose protocol concluded that radioguided surgery enables the detection of additional lymph node metastases in scarred and hidden areas. However, the acceptance of an intraoperative procedure depends on the opinion of the responsible surgeons. In the study by Salvatori et al., surgeons rated the radioguided procedure as decisive in two patients, favorable in six, and of negligible significance in two [32]. Rubello et al. judged the ^{131}I-guided operation technique as favorable or decisive in 83.8 % of patients [33]. No radioactive contamination of surfaces or surgical tools was observed, and radiation exposure of surgeons' hands was low (<40 μSv).

A low-dose protocol was first described by Littmann et al. in 1980 [36]. Negele et al. reported on this issue in four further patients with persistent lymph node metastases of PTC. In this cohort, 70–350 MBq ^{131}I was administered and a whole-body scan performed within 48 h to detect suspicious lesions. Surgery was performed 7–9 days after administration, similar to the timing in the high-dose protocol. On the preoperative day (6–8 days after radioiodine administration), residual activity in the hot spots detected by scintigraphy was confirmed with the handheld gamma probe in order to permit a decision on whether the surgery could be guided by ^{131}I. Despite the long time interval after administration of only a small dose of ^{131}I, successful and limited surgery was achieved in all four patients and no iodine-negative tumor lesions were observed. Although a larger number of patients have been investigated after administration of a therapeutic dose of radioiodine, the low-dose approach also seems feasible and can avoid hospitalization in some countries.

In summary, ^{131}I is affordable, needs no preparation process, and has a long half-time and therefore a good tumor-to-background ratio. Radioiodine was the first radionuclide to be investigated for radioguided surgery in DTC. Both therapeutic dosage and a low-dose approach are feasible when performing surgery 5–9 days after administration of radioiodine. ^{131}I-guided surgery accordingly represents a suitable means of individualized therapy for residual or recurrent disease in patients with DTC that enables complete resection and may reduce morbidity by limiting the extent of the surgical procedure.

In a few case reports, a ^{123}I-based approach has been investigated in patients with recurrent DTC [37–39] and primary thyroidectomy with lymph node dissection [40]. ^{123}I has a shorter half-life (13.2 h) than ^{131}I, allowing surgery to be performed within 4 h after administration of 74 MBq. This approach does not necessitate hospitalization of the patient and the gamma energy is easier to detect (^{123}I has a 159-keV photopeak vs 364 keV for ^{131}I). Khandelwal et al. reported that administration of only 12 MBq ^{123}I is also feasible and allows for radioguided surgery on the next day [39]. Besides a shorter time interval between oral administration of ^{123}I and surgery, further advantages are absence of the stunning effect on subsequent radioiodine uptake and reduced radiation exposure of the patient and surgeons due to the pure gamma emission. However, compared with ^{131}I, ^{123}I is more expensive and its availability is limited.

14.3.2 Non-iodine-Guided Resection of Recurrent Disease

Twenty percent of cases of recurrent disease in patients with well-differentiated thyroid cancer are iodine negative [41–43]. In these patients, diagnostic scintigraphy with various ^{99m}Tc-labeled tracers [^{99m}Tc-hexakis 2-methoxy isobutyl isonitrile (MIBI), ^{99m}Tc-pentavalent dimercaptosuccinic acid (^{99m}Tc-(V)-DMSA), and ^{99m}Tc-tetrafosmin] [44–50] and ^{18}F-FDG positron emission tomography/computed tomography (PET/CT) have been investigated. Furthermore, ^{99m}Tc-MIBI and ^{99m}Tc-(V)-DMSA scintigraphy and ^{18}F-FDG PET/CT have been demonstrated to be promising tools for intraoperative localization of recurrent disease and also guidance of surgery.

14.3.2.1 ^{99m}Tc-MIBI-Guided Surgery

^{99m}Tc-MIBI scintigraphy is a sensitive imaging method in patients with iodine-negative recurrence of DTC [44, 51, 52]. Alam et al. reported the sensitivity and negative and positive predictive values to be 94.4 %, 97.7 %, and 96.3 %, respectively, for the detection of locoregional metastases [51].

^{99m}Tc-MIBI-guided surgery procedures were first described in 2001 by Boz et al. [53], who reported the case of a 30-year-old woman with a FTC who had undergone two previous operations and ablative therapy with ^{131}I (3.33 GBq). Because of a rising thyroglobulin level 7 years after the primary diagnosis, a ^{99m}Tc-MIBI scan was performed and showed focal tracer uptake in the neck. Surgery, guided by a gamma probe, was performed 2 h after the intravenous injection of 740 MBq ^{99m}Tc-MIBI. A tumor-to-background ratio of 4:1 enabled safe resection of tumor tissue within scar tissue.

In 2002 Rubello et al. reported on eight patients [54], all of whom had elevated thyroglobulin levels, a positive ^{99m}Tc-MIBI scan, and evidence for locoregional recurrence on high-resolution ultrasound, which was proven by fine-needle aspiration cytology. Unlike in the study of Boz et al., in these patients low-dose ^{99m}Tc-MIBI (37 MBq) was injected in the operating room 10 min before the start of surgery. The authors decided to inject the tracer in the operating room to avoid false-negative results as fast washout had previously been reported in DTC metastases [44]. This approach has the further advantage of reducing the radiation exposure of the surgeons. Using 37 MBq of ^{99m}Tc-MIBI for radioguided surgery, the surgeon receives 1.2 μSv/h, which is 25- to 30-fold less than with the protocols using ^{131}I [44, 54]. During the wide bilateral neck exploration, the surgeon was guided intraoperatively by a gamma probe and the preoperative ^{99m}Tc-MIBI scan. The radioactivity deposits were measured in vivo and ex vivo. In addition, the background activity (apex of the lung contralateral to the injection site) and the activity in the tumor bed after excision were assessed, and tumor-to-background ratios were calculated. The tumor-to-background ratio was higher than 2.0 in all patients. One patient had a persistent high background activity after the tumor extirpation, leading the surgeon to another tumor deposit [54].

These promising results were confirmed in a further study [55]. In 37 patients the detection of all 66 nodules ranging in size from 6 mm up to 45 mm was possible. A correlation between tumor size and uptake was not found. A four-point scale was used to rate the usefulness of the radioguided technique: very useful, useful, moderately useful, or not useful. In eight patients the procedure was very useful because the metastatic foci were hidden in fibrotic tissues or located behind the vessels. In 17 patients the radioguided procedure was rated as useful and in ten as moderately useful, while in two it was deemed not useful. In the final report [56], 58 patients with a local recurrence in the thyroid bed ($n=14$) or lymph node metastases ($n=37$) or both ($n=7$) were included. The intraoperative gamma probe detected more metastatic foci than did preoperative imaging. However, 16 % (24/147) of the metastatic lesions identified by histopathologic evaluation were missed. In the final report the procedure was rated as useful or very useful in 62 % of the patients ($n=58$).

14.3.2.2 ^{18}F-FDG-Guided Surgery

In the postoperative follow-up of patients with ^{131}I-negative DTC and elevated thyroglobulin, ^{18}F-FDG PET/CT is also recommended for restaging [4]. In these patients, ^{18}F-FDG PET/CT has been reported to have a sensitivity of 93.5 %, which is superior to that of other conventional imaging methods as well as ^{99m}Tc-MIBI scan [57–59]. The feasibility of ^{18}F-FDG-directed surgery had previously been described for other tumor entities, in the first instance for colorectal cancer [60, 61].

In 2005, Kraeber-Bodere et al. [62] described ^{18}F-FDG-guided surgery in nine patients with PTC and one with Hürthle cell tumor, who had between one and five lesions suspicious for lymph node metastases and no distant metastases (Table 14.2). All patients received recombinant human thyroid-stimulating hormone (rhTSH) 2 days before surgery to increase the tracer uptake in metastatic lesions. This approach was subsequently adopted by other groups [64, 65]. On

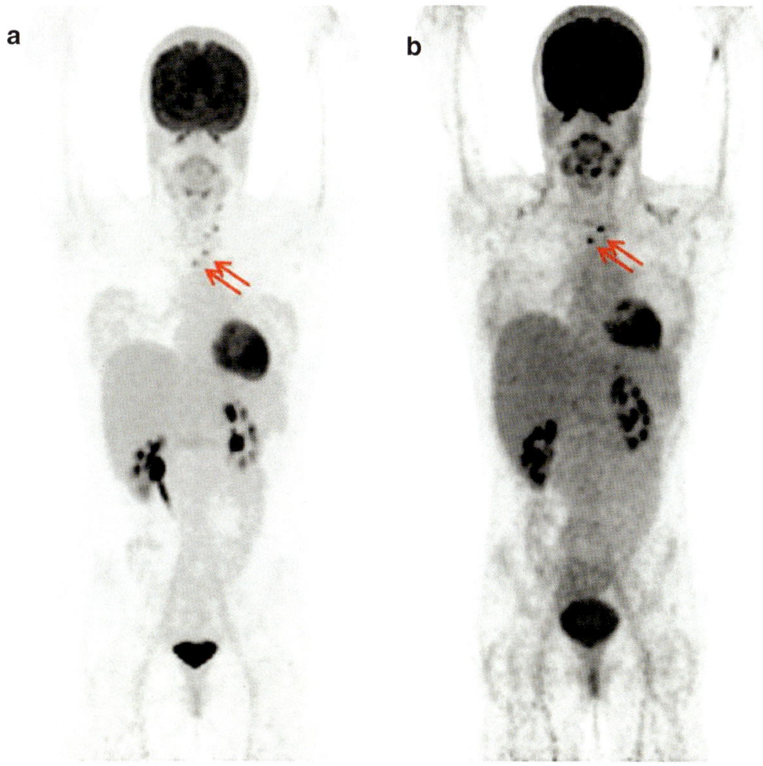

Fig. 14.1 Residual lymph node metastasis after reoperation. This 32-year-old female patient with bilateral PTC had been treated with thyroidectomy combined with central lymph node dissection and radioiodine therapy. (**a**) ^{18}F-FDG-PET/CT (MIP) 5 months after radioiodine ablation: the ^{131}I whole-body scan was negative, but the thyroglobulin level (16.1 ng/ml) was still elevated. Before reintervention, imaging with FDG-PET/CT was performed and showed multiple cervical lymph node metastases on the left side and also lymph node metastasis in the upper mediastinum. (**b**) ^{18}F-FDG PET/CT (MIP) 6 months after reoperation: Because of the still elevated thyroglobulin (12.5 ng/ml), FDG-PET/CT was repeated and still showed two unresected lymph node metastases in the upper mediastinum

Table 14.2 ^{18}F-FDG-guided surgery (characteristics of trials)

	No. of patients	Radiopharmaceutical	Injected activity	Injection time (prior to surgery)	Lesions
Kraeber-Bodere et al. (2005) [62]	10	^{18}F-FDG	265 MBq (range, 165–526)	30 min	LNM
Meller et al. (2005)[a] [63]	[a]	^{18}F-FDG vs ^{99m}Tc-MIBI	[a]	[a]	[a]
Curtet et al. (2007) [64]	7	^{18}F-FDG	211 MBq (range, 165–231)	60 min	LNM
Gulec et al. (2007) [65]	4	^{18}F-FDG	185–555 MBq	2–4 h	LNM
Agrawal et al. (2008) [66]	2	^{18}F-FDG	555–740 MBq	20 min	LNM
Francis et al. (2012) [67]	13	^{18}F-FDG	[a]	[a]	LNM

LNM lymph node metastases, *^{18}F-FDG* fluorine-18 fluorodeoxyglucose
[a]Not reported in the available abstract

average, 265 MBq of ^{18}F-FDG was injected intravenously 30 min prior to surgery. The activity was measured with a gamma probe using the 511-keV channel. Counts were collected for 10 s over the metastatic lesions and also normal tissue (head and neck region and the shoulder) in vivo, and in addition ex vivo counts of the resected tissue were obtained. Tumor-to-normal tissue ratios were calculated, whereby the tumor-to-neck ratios were found to be lower than the tumor-to-shoulder ratios (mean 1.40 vs 1.73). The authors attributed the low tumor-to-background ratio to the high vascular uptake observed 1–2 h after injection. All lesions identified as suspicious preoperatively ($n=12$) could also be detected intraoperatively and were confirmed as metastases at histopathologic evaluation. No additional lesions were found with the gamma probe. All patients in this study underwent a completion lymph node dissection and, in accordance with findings in other studies (e.g., ^{131}I guided), additional lymph node metastases were detected in five patients. These nodes were non-radioactive owing to microscopic disease.

The radiation exposure of the surgeons' hands ranged from 90 to 270 μSv. Nalley et al. reported on this topic in more detail in a case series of three patients with iodine-negative thyroid cancer [68]. After injection of an activity ranging from 278 to 303 MBq ^{18}F-FDG and commencement of surgery 3–5 h later, the corresponding highest measured radiation exposure was 53 μSv/h.

^{18}F-FDG-guided surgery is challenging because of the high energy of the emitted photons (511 keV). In 2007, Curtet et al. investigated the performance of two different gamma probes for ^{18}F-FDG-guided surgery in seven patients with iodine-negative DTC [64]. A mean activity of 211 MBq was injected 60 min before surgery. The study demonstrated that high-energy photon detection is feasible with a conventional scintillator equipped with a collimator. Detection of metastatic lesions was possible using a tumor-to-background ratio of 1.5.

In the same year Gulec et al. [65] reported on 25 patients with various tumor entities, including four with recurrent DTC, with the purpose of assessing the feasibility of PET probe-guided surgery using ^{18}F-FDG for tumor detection. Between 185 and 555 MBq ^{18}F-FDG was injected 2–6 h prior to surgery. Using the PET probe, all preoperatively assessed lesions (diameter, 0.8–4 cm) could be localized with a satisfactory in vivo lesion count rate of ≥1.5 and in addition in eight patients non-palpable and non-obvious lesions could be found in regions with adhesions or scar tissue during surgical exploration.

A multimodality approach for detection and resection of recurrent cancer was described by Agrawal et al. in two patients with well-differentiated thyroid cancer. Both patients received recombinant human TSH 48 and 24 h prior to surgery [66]. After thyroid simulation with rhTSH, 555–740 MBq of ^{18}F-FDG was injected and both patients underwent: (1) preoperative patient imaging, specimen imaging and postoperative patient imaging, (2) ultrasonography, and (3) gamma probe detection using the three-sigma criteria for threshold determination. The approach was feasible and allowed for successful resection of recurrent thyroid cancer tissue.

Recently, Francis et al. [67] reported on 13 patients with recurrent well-differentiated thyroid cancer. The patients were divided into two groups, iodine-positive vs iodine-negative (9 and 4 patients, respectively), in whom ^{18}F-FDG-directed surgery was performed. This study confirmed the feasibility of the technique and former results.

In summary, PET-guided surgery is feasible and detects the preoperatively found FDG-avid lesions (Fig. 14.1), but it is also challenging owing to the high energy (511 keV) of the photons emitted by ^{18}F-FDG. Up to now no PET tracers (e.g., ^{124}I) other than ^{18}F-FDG have been evaluated for radioguided surgery of recurrent DTC.

14.3.2.3 Intralesional Injection of ^{99m}Tc-Labeled Colloids

The technique of intraoperative radioguided occult lesion localization (ROLL), developed for use in non-palpable breast cancer, has been transferred to locoregional recurrent thyroid cancer. Its feasibility was first described in two patients with non-palpable thyroid lymph node metastases after previous operation on the neck compartment for treatment of PTC and medullary thyroid cancer, respectively [69].

The intralesional injection of ^{99m}Tc-labeled colloids provides an alternative to intraoperative ultrasound examination, wire-guided excision, or intraoperative ultrasound-guided dye injection. The method has mainly been investigated for excision of recurrent non-palpable lymph node metastases.

In 2010 Erbil et al. reported on a further 46 patients with recurrent or persistent PTC detected by elevated thyroglobulin level, positive radioiodine whole-body scan, or PET and confirmed by fine-needle aspiration cytology and fine-needle aspiration thyroglobulin measurement [70] (Table 14.3). Under ultrasound guidance, 20 MBq of ^{99m}Tc-labeled rhenium colloid was injected directly into the pathologic node. Most other groups reporting on this topic used ^{99m}Tc-macroaggregated albumin (MAA) [71–73, 75]. In order to prove successful injection, Erbil et al. performed preoperative scintigraphy 30 min and 12 h after injection [70]. Additional preoperative SPECT/CT may be used as a road map and to speed up the identification of radiolabeled tissue [77]. For intraoperative lesion detection, Erbil et al. measured the activity counts 3 times for 20 s each and calculated a mean count rate. The background count rate was derived from a measurement over the normal adjacent tissue.

Besides radioguided lymph node dissection, the feasibility of intralesional injection has also been investigated for perioperative identification of residual thyroid tissue and parathyroid adenoma using a very small amount (7.4 MBq) of ^{99m}Tc-MAA, injected 90 min prior to surgery. Terzioglu et al. showed that despite the low injected activity, measurement over 10 s is sufficient [71]. An advantage of this protocol is the reduction of radiation exposure to surgeons. Both colloid tracers allowed the dedicated intraoperative detection of preoperatively assessed suspicious lesions, even in patients with extensive scar tissue. Recently, Giles et al. published the results of the first randomized study using low-dose ^{99m}Tc-MAA injection [75]. Patients with non-palpable lymph node metastatic disease were randomized to radioguided lesion localization or intraoperative ultrasound localization (IOUS). Both approaches had a high rate of safe and successful excision of recurrent lymph nodes in patients with PTC. Radioguided surgery may be preferred by surgeons unskilled in IOUS because it is very easy to perform.

For radioguided lesion localization, the radioiodine avidity of the tumor lesions is not relevant. In 2013 Borso et al. [74] described the intralesional injection of ^{99m}Tc-MAA in patients with iodine-negative DTC. In 12 out of 35 cases, a minimally invasive excision could be performed, whereas the other patients underwent an additional modified radical neck dissection. Ninety-five percent of the marked lesions could be easily detected during surgery by use of a gamma probe. Detection of the remaining three lesions was also possible, but was hindered by tracer leakage.

Table 14.3 Surgery guided by ^{99m}Tc-labeled colloids (characteristics of trials)

	No. of patients	Radiopharmaceutical	Injected activity	Lesions
Tukenmez et al. (2007) [69]	2	^{99m}Tc-rhenium colloid	20 MBq	LNM
Erbil et al. (2010) [70]	46	^{99m}Tc-rhenium colloid	20 MBq	LNM
Terzioglu et al. (2010) [71]	21	^{99m}Tc-MAA	7.4 MBq	LNM, thyroid tissue, parathyroid adenoma
Martino et al. (2010) [72]	20	^{99m}Tc-MAA	14.8 MBq	LNM
Ilgan et al. (2010) [73]	8	^{99m}Tc-MAA	7.4–14.8 MBq	Local recurrence and lateral compartment
Borso et al. (2013) [74]	32	^{99m}Tc-MAA	7.4 MBq	[a]
Bellotti et al. (2013) [13]	22	^{99m}Tc-MAA	20 MBq	LNM
Giles et al. (2014) [75]	20	^{99m}Tc-MAA	7.4 MBq	LNM
Jung et al. (2014) [76]	7	^{99m}Tc-TIGMA	0.1 ml of TIGMA	Not specified

TIGMA ^{99m}Tc-macroaggregated human serum albumin and indocyanine green, *^{99m}Tc-MAA* ^{99m}Tc-marcoaggregated albumin, *LNM* lymph node metastases
[a]Not reported in the available abstract

Recurrence rates were similar in both groups (33 % for ROLL vs 40 % for additional neck dissection).

In the same year Bellotti et al. [78] reported on 22 patients with recurrent DTC in whom a gamma probe was used for intraoperative lesion detection and a small-field gamma camera for intraoperative imaging. All included patients had undergone radical surgery including central and/or lateral neck dissection for primary treatment and suffered from locoregional lymph node recurrences of PTC in the follow-up. Recurrent disease was detected by thyroglobulin measurement, ultrasound, radioiodine whole-body scan, and fine-needle aspiration cytology. In a 1-day protocol, 20 MBq of ^{99m}Tc-MAA (0.2 ml) was directly injected into the suspicious lesions under ultrasound guidance before surgery. Thirty-nine pathologic nodes were injected and 61 nodes removed, including 22 additional nodes not injected by radiotracer. Of these additional lymph nodes, seven (31.8 %) were metastatic. Similarly, Erbil et al. and Giles et al. reported metastatic disease in 32–40 % of additionally resected nodes [70, 75]. Bellotti et al. avoided preoperative imaging because intraoperative images of the cervical region were acquired with the gamma camera. After imaging, the thyroid bed was explored using the acoustic gamma probe, enabling lesion localization. Complete excision was proven by measuring the count rate of the lesions and the surgical bed after resection on the one hand and by intraoperative imaging on the other. Bellotti et al. demonstrated that this technique is feasible without complications and does not prolong the operation significantly. Intraoperative imaging allowed for a minimally invasive approach and fast lesion localization and was of additional value if lesion detection with the gamma probe was difficult [78].

Recently, a radiofluorescence approach combining ^{99m}Tc-MAA with indocyanine green (TIGMA) was reported in seven patients with a recurrent DTC [76]. The maximum excitation light wavelength of indocyanine green is 780 nm and the highest emission light wavelength, 800 nm, generating a low background signal as this light is not absorbed by tissue and is invisible to human eye [79]. Jung et al. reported that preoperative hybrid tracer preparation required about 20 min. Under ultrasound guidance, 0.1 ml of the mixture was injected. For intraoperative imaging, a near-infrared fluorescence (NIRF) camera was necessary in addition to a gamma probe. Prior to incision, a scan with the gamma probe was performed and confirmed by use of the NIRF camera, enabling NIRF observation in real time. The fluorescence could be easily detected at a depth of 3.25 mm and the hybrid tracer was retained at the injection site without spreading to adjacent tissue, resulting in better imaging than was possible with indocyanine green alone. The authors reported that TIGMA is safe (low toxicity) and facilitates the detection of recurrent lesions. However, fluorescence imaging requires further surgical equipment (NIRF camera) and may be influenced by surgical lights.

It has to be kept in mind that the intralesional injection of a radiotracer has one major limitation: the technique is only suitable in lesions which can be localized by ultrasound. This may be the reason for the unexpected lymph node metastasis at non-injected nodes [75] and the appearance of suspicious nodes during follow-up [34, 74]. Therefore, radioguided resection may be combined with compartment-oriented lymph node dissection [75].

14.4 Medullary Thyroid Cancer

Sporadic or hereditary medullary thyroid cancer (MTC) is a rare disease and only 3–10 % of thyroid cancers are of medullary origin [80, 81]. However, this thyroid cancer has a recurrence rate of up to 50 % [80], and resection seems to be the only promising treatment option for achievement of locoregional disease control in patients with recurrent disease. For detection of recurrent disease, besides calcitonin and CEA measurement or ultrasonography, use of various radiotracers has been described, e.g., ^{99m}Tc-(V)-DMSA, thallium-201, ^{99m}Tc-MIBI, ^{18}F-L-dihydroxyphenylalanine (DOPA), and ^{68}Ga-labeled somatostatin analogs [82]. The value of radioguided surgery in facilitating tumor detection has been investigated, but not for all available radiotracers.

14.4.1 ^{99m}Tc-(V)-DMSA-Guided Surgery

^{99m}Tc-(V)-DMSA scintigraphy is a diagnostic tool for detection of recurrent medullary cancer, but ^{99m}Tc-(V)-DMSA is no longer commercially available. The reported sensitivity of this imaging method varies and it has reduced sensitivity for bone metastases [83–85]. The variation in detection rate may be attributable to the use of different commercial kits and their instability [82].

Adams et al. investigated 35 patients with previously operated MTC and suspicion for recurrence due to elevated calcitonin levels [86, 87]. These patients underwent CT scanning and diagnostic double-nuclide scintigraphy. First 180 or 222 MBq ^{111}In-DTPA octreotide was injected, followed by 500 MBq ^{99m}Tc-(V)-DMSA. Image acquisition was performed 4 and 24 h later for ^{111}In-DTPA octreotide and 6 h later for ^{99m}Tc-(V)-DMSA imaging including whole-body scintigraphy and SPECT. In the first study (n = 10), double-nuclide scintigraphy revealed 20 of 30 suspicious lesions, while radiologic imaging (CT and sonography) revealed 15 of the lesions. Intraoperative use of a gamma probe detected all lesions, but three lesions proved false positive, showing lymphadenitis on histopathology [86]. In the second study (n = 25), the sensitivity of preoperative CT, ^{111}In-DTPA-octreoitide scintigraphy, and ^{99m}Tc-(V)-DMSA was 32 %, 34 %, and 65 %, respectively [87]. For radioguided surgery the tracer with the highest detection rate was reinjected preoperatively. During surgery, a tumor-to-non-tumor count ratio of 2:1 was considered positive. Detection rates were compared with preoperative imaging and intraoperative palpation. The smallest detected metastasis within the entire cohort was a lymph node with a diameter of 5 mm. The sensitivity of radioguided surgery was superior to that of surgical palpation (97 % vs 65 %) [87], and radioguided surgery allowed detection of 30 % more lesions compared with preoperative conventional imaging [88].

14.4.2 Radioimmunoguided Surgery

^{123}I-, ^{131}I-, and ^{111}In-labeled monoclonal antibodies have been investigated for imaging of MTC [89–91]. Only three reports are available on radioimmunoguided surgery in MTC [92–94].

In 1993, Peltier et al. [94] described two-step radioimmunotargeting in patients with recurrent MTC and performed radioguided surgery in five patients. This group injected a bispecific antibody (anti-CEA monoclonal IgG coupled with anti-In-DTPA monoclonal IgG) and ^{111}In-labeled DTPA dimer (diDTPA-TL). The procedure of tumor radioimmunotargeting consisted of two steps: first 1 mg/10 kg of body weight non-radiolabeled specific antibody was injected intravenously over 20 min. Four days later 1 nmol/10 kg ^{111}In-labeled diDTPA-TL was injected. Preoperative scintigraphy including SPECT was performed after 5 and 24 h. In three of the five patients who underwent surgery, intraoperative use of the gamma probe detected suspicious lesions not identified by the surgeon. Two further studies confirmed the feasibility of this technique [92, 93]. De Labriolle-Vaylet et al. pointed out the additional value of the technique compared with physical examination and conventional imaging. In their cohort of 13 patients, 22 of 34 metastases would have been missed using the latter methods. Radioimmunoguided surgery had an accuracy of 86 % (sensitivity 75 %, specificity 90 %). The limitations of this promising technique are the time delay and the availability of competing radiolabeled compounds.

14.4.3 ^{123}I- MIBG-Guided Surgery

^{123}Iodine-123-labeled MIBG can be used for diagnostic purposes in patients with MTC. However, there has been only one published case in which ^{123}I-MIBG guided surgery was used in MTC. Shimotake et al. reported on a MEN2B 14-year-old girl suffering from recurrent MTC in whom reoperation on the cervical and upper mediastinal regions was hampered by fibrotic scar tissue due to four previous neck operations. Twenty-four hours after injection of 100 MBq ^{123}I-MIBG, successful tumor resection in the cervical region and upper mediastinum was possible without side effects. However, because many recurrent MTCs are not MIBG avid, somatostatin receptor scintigraphy imaging may have greater potential.

14.4.4 Somatostatin Receptor-based Surgery

Medullary thyroid cancer often expresses somatostatin receptors, which can be visualized with somatostatin receptor scintigraphy. Radioguided surgery has also been investigated using radiolabeled somatostatin analogs. As long ago as 1995, Wangberg et al. investigated ten patients with residual MTC using ^{111}In-DTPA-octreotide-guided surgery [95]. Injection of the radiotracer (140–300 MBq) was performed 24–168 h prior to surgery. Eight of the ten patients had positive lesions on preoperative scintigraphy performed 24 h after injection. At surgery, in situ measurements of macroscopically identified tumors were false negative in 4 out of 37 lesions.

In summary, MTC is rare and therefore only a limited number of reports are available on radioguided surgery in patients with recurrent disease. However, the results are promising and further studies are necessary to investigate new tracers (e.g., ^{68}Ga-labeled somatostatin analogs) and the ROLL concept.

14.5 Outlook

Currently the experience gained in the application of radioguided surgery techniques in residual or recurrent (differentiated) thyroid cancer is still limited. Despite promising results in this challenging setting, radioguided approaches have not yet become established in daily clinical routine or in guidelines. One reason may be the existence of multiple competing tracers, which may hamper selection of the "optimal" tracer. Furthermore, no studies exist on very novel tracers like ^{68}Ga-labeled somatostatin analogs in MTC. In future studies the role of intraoperative imaging needs to be investigated, and evaluation of radioguided surgery for non-locoregional metastases would also be of interest.

References

1. Torre LA, Bray F, Siegel RL, Ferlay J, Lortet-Tieulent J, Jemal A. Global cancer statistics, 2012. CA Cancer J Clin. 2015;65:87–108.
2. Pellegriti G, Frasca F, Regalbuto C, Squatrito S, Vigneri R. Worldwide increasing incidence of thyroid cancer: update on epidemiology and risk factors. J Cancer Epidemiol. 2013;2013:965212.
3. Ferlay J, Steliarova-Foucher E, Lortet-Tieulent J, Rosso S, Coebergh JW, Comber H, et al. Cancer incidence and mortality patterns in Europe: estimates for

40 countries in 2012. Eur J Cancer. 2013;49(6):1374–403.
4. Cooper DS, Doherty GM, Haugen BR, Kloos RT, Lee SL, Mandel SJ, et al. Revised American Thyroid Association management guidelines for patients with thyroid nodules and differentiated thyroid cancer. Thyroid. 2009;19(11):1167–214.
5. Davies L, Welch HG. Thyroid cancer survival in the United States: observational data from 1973 to 2005. Arch Otolaryngol Head Neck Surg. 2010;136(5):440–4.
6. Yu XM, Schneider DF, Leverson G, Chen H, Sippel RS. Follicular variant of papillary thyroid carcinoma is a unique clinical entity: a population-based study of 10,740 cases. Thyroid. 2013;23(10):1263–8.
7. Mazzaferri EL. An overview of the management of papillary and follicular thyroid carcinoma. Thyroid. 1999;9(5):421–7.
8. Rouxel A, Hejblum G, Bernier MO, Boelle PY, Menegaux F, Mansour G, et al. Prognostic factors associated with the survival of patients developing loco-regional recurrences of differentiated thyroid carcinomas. J Clin Endocrinol Metab. 2004;89(11):5362–8.
9. Leboulleux S, Rubino C, Baudin E, Caillou B, Hartl DM, Bidart JM, et al. Prognostic factors for persistent or recurrent disease of papillary thyroid carcinoma with neck lymph node metastases and/or tumor extension beyond the thyroid capsule at initial diagnosis. J Clin Endocrinol Metab. 2005;90(10):5723–9.
10. Mazzaferri EL, Kloos RT. Clinical review 128: current approaches to primary therapy for papillary and follicular thyroid cancer. J Clin Endocrinol Metab. 2001;86(4):1447–63.
11. Mirallie E, Hamy A, Floch I, Sagan C, Paineau J, Murat A, et al. Outcome in cervical recurrences of papillary or follicular thyroid cancer. Ann Chir. 1999;53(7):577–82. Devenir des recidives cervicales de cancer papillaire ou vesiculaire de la thyroide.
12. Goffredo P, Roman SA, Sosa JA. Hurthle cell carcinoma: a population-level analysis of 3311 patients. Cancer. 2013;119(3):504–11.
13. de Groot JW, Plukker JT, Wolffenbuttel BH, Wiggers T, Sluiter WJ, Links TP. Determinants of life expectancy in medullary thyroid cancer: age does not matter. Clin Endocrinol (Oxf). 2006;65(6):729–36.
14. Bergamaschi R, Becouarn G, Ronceray J, Arnaud JP. Morbidity of thyroid surgery. Am J Surg. 1998;176(1):71–5.
15. Shah MD, Harris LD, Nassif RG, Kim D, Eski S, Freeman JL. Efficacy and safety of central compartment neck dissection for recurrent thyroid carcinoma. Arch Otolaryngol Head Neck Surg. 2012;138(1):33–7.
16. Carcoforo P, Portinari M, Feggi L, Panareo S, De Troia A, Zatelli MC, et al. Radio-guided selective compartment neck dissection improves staging in papillary thyroid carcinoma: a prospective study on 345 patients with a 3-year follow-up. Surgery. 2014;156(1):147–57.
17. Dhepnorrarat RC, Witterick IJ. New technologies in thyroid cancer surgery. Oral Oncol. 2013;49(7):659–64.
18. Aras G, Gultekin SS, Kucuk NO, Demirer S, Tug T. Intraoperative gamma probe guidance with 99mTc-pertechnetate in the completion thyroidectomy. Ann Nucl Med. 2009;23(5):421–6.
19. Erbil Y, Barbaros U, Deveci U, Kaya H, Bozbora A, Ozbey N, et al. Gamma probe-guided surgery for revision thyroidectomy: in comparison with conventional technique. J Endocrinol Invest. 2005;28(7):583–8.
20. Karyagar S, Karatepe O, Bender O, Mulazimoglu M, Ozpacaci T, Uyanik E, et al. Tc-99m radio-guided completion thyroidectomy for differentiated thyroid carcinoma. Indian J Nucl Med. 2010;25(1):12–5.
21. Proczko M, Stefaniak T, Sworczak K, Kobiela J, Lachinski AJ, Stepaniak P, et al. Completion thyroidectomy of well-differentiated thyroid cancer – a prospective, randomised study. Endokrynol Pol. 2013;64(5):335–9.
22. Uludag M, Yetkin G, Citgez B, Isgor A, Atay M, Kebudi A, et al. Contribution of gamma probe-guided surgery to lateral approach completion thyroidectomy. Endocr Pract. 2009;15(3):213–9.
23. Pacini F, Elisei R, Capezzone M, Miccoli P, Molinaro E, Basolo F, et al. Contralateral papillary thyroid cancer is frequent at completion thyroidectomy with no difference in low- and high-risk patients. Thyroid. 2001;11(9):877–81.
24. Pasieka JL, Thompson NW, McLeod MK, Burney RE, Macha M. The incidence of bilateral well-differentiated thyroid cancer found at completion thyroidectomy. World J Surg. 1992;16(4):711–6. discussion 6–7.
25. Kim ES, Kim TY, Koh JM, Kim YI, Hong SJ, Kim WB, et al. Completion thyroidectomy in patients with thyroid cancer who initially underwent unilateral operation. Clin Endocrinol (Oxf). 2004;61(1):145–8.
26. Hayward NJ, Grodski S, Yeung M, Johnson WR, Serpell J. Recurrent laryngeal nerve injury in thyroid surgery: a review. ANZ J Surg. 2013;83(1–2):15–21.
27. Bender O, Karyagar S, Levent Balci F, Yuney E, Kamali S, Ozpacaci T, et al. Gamma probe (99m) Tc-pertechnetate assisted completion thyroidectomy vs conventional thyroidectomy in differentiated thyroid carcinoma. Hell J Nucl Med. 2009;12(2):138–41.
28. Harris C, Bigelow R, Francis J, Kelly G, Bell P. A Cis(Ti)-crystal surgical scintillation probe. Nucleonics. 1956;14:102–8.
29. Morris Jr AC, Barclay TR, Tanida R, Nemcek JV. A miniaturized probe for detecting radioactivity at thyroid surgery. Phys Med Biol. 1971;16(3):397–404.
30. Travagli JP, Cailleux AF, Ricard M, Baudin E, Caillou B, Parmentier C, et al. Combination of radioiodine (131I) and probe-guided surgery for persistent or recurrent thyroid carcinoma. J Clin Endocrinol Metab. 1998;83(8):2675–80.
31. Lippi F, Capezzone M, Miccoli P, Traino C, Di Martino F, Angelini F, et al. Use of surgical gamma probe for

the detection of lymph node metastases in differentiated thyroid cancer. Tumori. 2000;86(4):367–9.
32. Salvatori M, Rufini V, Reale F, Samanes Gajate AM, Maussier ML, Revelli L, et al. Radio-guided surgery for lymph node recurrences of differentiated thyroid cancer. World J Surg. 2003;27(7):770–5.
33. Rubello D, Salvatori M, Ardito G, Mariani G, Al-Nahhas A, Gross MD, et al. Iodine-131 radio-guided surgery in differentiated thyroid cancer: outcome on 31 patients and review of the literature. Biomed Pharmacother. 2007;61(8):477–81.
34. Scurry WC, Lamarre E, Stack B. Radioguided neck dissection in recurrent metastatic papillary thyroid carcinoma. Am J Otolaryngol. 2006;27(1):61–3.
35. Negele T, Meisetschlager G, Bruckner T, Scheidhauer K, Schwaiger M, Vogelsang H. Radio-guided surgery for persistent differentiated papillary thyroid cancer: case presentations and review of the literature. Langenbecks Arch Surg. 2006;391(3):178–86.
36. Littmann K, Magdsick G, Strotges MW, Eigler FW. Intraoperative localization measurement following preoperative radioiodine marking to facilitate the treatment of differentiated thyroid carcinoma. Chirurg. 1980;51(6):389–94. Intraoperative Lokalisationsmessung nach praoperativer Radiojodmarkierung zur Verbesserung der Behandlung differenzierter Schilddrusencarcinome.
37. Gallowitsch HJ, Fellinger J, Mikosch P, Kresnik E, Lind P. Gamma probe-guided resection of a lymph node metastasis with I-123 in papillary thyroid carcinoma. Clin Nucl Med. 1997;22(9):591–2.
38. Mansberg R, Crawford B, Uren RF, Thompson JF. Minimally invasive radio-guided surgery for recurrent thyroid cancer using iodine-123. Clin Nucl Med. 2005;30(1):43–4.
39. Khandelwal S, Sener SF, Purdy L, Perlman RM. I-123-guided excision of metastatic papillary thyroid cancer. J Surg Oncol. 2007;96(2):173–5.
40. Gulec SA, Eckert M, Woltering EA. Gamma probe-guided lymph node dissection ('gamma picking') in differentiated thyroid carcinoma. Clin Nucl Med. 2002;27(12):859–61.
41. Helal BO, Merlet P, Toubert ME, Franc B, Schvartz C, Gauthier-Koelesnikov H, et al. Clinical impact of (18) F-FDG PET in thyroid carcinoma patients with elevated thyroglobulin levels and negative (131)I scanning results after therapy. J Nucl Med. 2001;42(10):1464–9.
42. Frilling A, Tecklenborg K, Gorges R, Weber F, Clausen M, Broelsch EC. Preoperative diagnostic value of [(18)F] fluorodeoxyglucose positron emission tomography in patients with radioiodine-negative recurrent well-differentiated thyroid carcinoma. Ann Surg. 2001;234(6):804–11.
43. Pacini F, Agate L, Elisei R, Capezzone M, Ceccarelli C, Lippi F, et al. Outcome of differentiated thyroid cancer with detectable serum Tg and negative diagnostic (131)I whole body scan: comparison of patients treated with high (131)I activities versus untreated patients. J Clin Endocrinol Metab. 2001;86(9): 4092–7.
44. Rubello D, Mazzarotto R, Casara D. The role of technetium-99m methoxyisobutylisonitrile scintigraphy in the planning of therapy and follow-up of patients with differentiated thyroid carcinoma after surgery. Eur J Nucl Med. 2000;27(4):431–40.
45. Elser H, Henze M, Hermann C, Eckert W, Mende U. 99m-Tc-MIBI for recurrent and metastatic differentiated thyroid carcinoma. Nuklearmedizin. 1997;36(1): 7–12. 99mTc-MIBI zur Rezidiv- und Metastasensuche bei differenzierten Schilddrusenkarzinomen.
46. Rubello D, Saladini G, Carpi A, Casara D. Nuclear medicine imaging procedures in differentiated thyroid carcinoma patients with negative iodine scan. Biomed Pharmacother. 2000;54(6):337–44.
47. Wu HS, Liu FY, Huang WS, Liu YC, Chang CT, Kao CH. Technetium-99m tetrofosmin single photon emission computed tomography to detect metastatic papillary thyroid carcinoma in patients with elevated human serum thyroglobulin levels but negative I-131 whole body scan. Clin Radiol. 2003;58(10):787–90.
48. Fujie S, Okumura Y, Sato S, Akaki S, Katsui K, Himei K, et al. Diagnostic capabilities of I-131, TI-201, and Tc-99m-MIBI scintigraphy for metastatic differentiated thyroid carcinoma after total thyroidectomy. Acta Med Okayama. 2005;59(3):99–107.
49. Kucuk NO, Kulak HA, Aras G. Clinical importance of technetium-99m-methoxyisobutylisonitrile (MIBI) scintigraphy in differentiated thyroid carcinoma patients with elevated thyroglobulin levels and negative I-131 scanning results. Ann Nucl Med. 2006;20(6):393–7.
50. Iwata M, Kasagi K, Misaki T, Matsumoto K, Iida Y, Ishimori T, et al. Comparison of whole-body 18F-FDG PET, 99mTc-MIBI SPET, and post-therapeutic 131I-Na scintigraphy in the detection of metastatic thyroid cancer. Eur J Nucl Med Mol Imaging. 2004;31(4):491–8.
51. Alam MS, Kasagi K, Misaki T, Miyamoto S, Iwata M, Iida Y, et al. Diagnostic value of technetium-99m methoxyisobutyl isonitrile (99mTc-MIBI) scintigraphy in detecting thyroid cancer metastases: a critical evaluation. Thyroid. 1998;8(12):1091–100.
52. Hsu CH, Liu FY, Yen RF, Kao CH. Tc-99m MIBI SPECT in detecting metastatic papillary thyroid carcinoma in patients with elevated human serum thyroglobulin levels but negative I-131 whole body scan. Endocr Res. 2003;29(1):9–15.
53. Boz A, Arici C, Gungor F, Yildiz A, Colak T, Karayalcin B. Gamma probe-guided resection and scanning with TC-99m MIBI of a local recurrence of follicular thyroid carcinoma. Clin Nucl Med. 2001;26(10):820–2.
54. Rubello D, Piotto A, Pagetta C, Pelizzo MR, Casara D. (99m)Tc-MIBI radio-guided surgery for recurrent thyroid carcinoma: technical feasibility and procedure, and preliminary clinical results. Eur J Nucl Med Mol Imaging. 2002;29(9):1201–5.
55. Rubello D, Pelizzo MR, Casara D, Piotto A, Toniato A, Fig L, et al. Radio-guided surgery for non-131I-avid thyroid cancer. Thyroid. 2006;16(11):1105–11.
56. Rubello D, Salvatori M, Casara D, Piotto A, Toniato A, Gross MD, et al. 99mTc-sestamibi radio-guided

surgery of loco-regional 131Iodine-negative recurrent thyroid cancer. Eur J Surg Oncol. 2007;33(7):902–6.

57. Dong MJ, Liu ZF, Zhao K, Ruan LX, Wang GL, Yang SY, et al. Value of 18F-FDG-PET/PET-CT in differentiated thyroid carcinoma with radioiodine-negative whole-body scan: a meta-analysis. Nucl Med Commun. 2009;30(8):639–50.
58. Weber T, Ohlhauser D, Hillenbrand A, Henne-Bruns D, Reske SN, Luster M. Impact of FDG-PET computed tomography for surgery of recurrent or persistent differentiated thyroid carcinoma. Horm Metab Res. 2012;44(12):904–8.
59. Seo JH, Lee SW, Ahn BC, Lee J. Recurrence detection in differentiated thyroid cancer patients with elevated serum level of antithyroglobulin antibody: special emphasis on using (18)F-FDG PET/CT. Clin Endocrinol (Oxf). 2010;72(4):558–63.
60. Essner R, Hsueh EC, Haigh PI, Glass EC, Huynh Y, Daghighian F. Application of an [(18)F] fluorodeoxyglucose-sensitive probe for the intraoperative detection of malignancy. J Surg Res. 2001;96(1):120–6.
61. Zervos EE, Desai DC, DePalatis LR, Soble D, Martin EW. 18F-labeled fluorodeoxyglucose positron emission tomography-guided surgery for recurrent colorectal cancer: a feasibility study. J Surg Res. 2001;97(1):9–13.
62. Kraeber-Bodere F, Cariou B, Curtet C, Bridji B, Rousseau C, Dravet F, et al. Feasibility and benefit of fluorine 18-fluoro-2-deoxyglucose-guided surgery in the management of radioiodine-negative differentiated thyroid carcinoma metastases. Surgery. 2005;138(6):1176–82. discussion 82.
63. Meller B, Sahlmann C, Horstmann O, Gerl J, Baehre M, Meller J. Conventional gamma and high energy probe for radioguided dissection of metastases in a patient with recurrent thyroid carcinoma with (99m) Tc-MIBI and (18)F-FDG. Nuklearmedizin. 2005; 44(3):N23–5.
64. Curtet C, Carlier T, Mirallie E, Bodet-Milin C, Rousseau C, Barbet J, et al. Prospective comparison of two gamma probes for intraoperative detection of 18F-FDG: in vitro assessment and clinical evaluation in differentiated thyroid cancer patients with iodine-negative recurrence. Eur J Nucl Med Mol Imaging. 2007;34(10):1556–62.
65. Gulec SA, Hoenie E, Hostetter R, Schwartzentruber D. PET probe-guided surgery: applications and clinical protocol. World J Surg Oncol. 2007;5:65.
66. Agrawal A, Hall NC, Ringel MD, Povoski SP, Martin Jr EW. Combined use of perioperative TSH-stimulated (18)F-FDG PET/CT imaging and gamma probe radioguided surgery to localize and verify resection of iodine scan-negative recurrent thyroid carcinoma. Laryngoscope. 2008;118(12): 2190–4.
67. Francis CL, Nalley C, Fan C, Bodenner D, Stack Jr BC. 18F-fluorodeoxyglucose and 131I radioguided surgical management of thyroid cancer. Otolaryngol Head Neck Surg. 2012;146(1):26–32.
68. Nalley C, Wiebeck K, Bartel TB, Bodenner D, Stack Jr BC. Intraoperative radiation exposure with the use of (18)F-FDG-guided thyroid cancer surgery. Otolaryngol Head Neck Surg. 2010;142(2):281–3.
69. Tukenmez M, Erbil Y, Barbaros U, Dural C, Salmaslioglu A, Aksoy D, et al. Radio-guided nonpalpable metastatic lymph node localization in patients with recurrent thyroid cancer. J Surg Oncol. 2007;96(6):534–8.
70. Erbil Y, Sari S, Agcaoglu O, Ersoz F, Bayraktar A, Salmaslioglu A, et al. Radio-guided excision of metastatic lymph nodes in thyroid carcinoma: a safe technique for previously operated neck compartments. World J Surg. 2010;34(11):2581–8.
71. Terzioglu T, Senyurek YG, Tunca F, Turkmen C, Mudun A, Salmaslioglu A, et al. Excision efficiency of radioguided occult lesion localization in reoperative thyroid and parathyroid surgery. Thyroid. 2010;20(11):1271–8.
72. Martino A, Monaco L, Golia R, Miletto P, Capasso P, Lombardi C, et al. A new radioguided procedure for localization and surgical treatment of neck node metastasis of papillary thyroid cancer. J Endocrinol Invest. 2010;33(5):339–42.
73. Ilgan S, Ozturk E, Yildiz R, Emer O, Ayan A, Gorgulu S, et al. Combination of preoperative ultrasonographic mapping and radioguided occult lesion localization in patients with locally recurrent/persistent papillary thyroid carcinoma: a practical method for central compartment reoperations. Clin Nucl Med. 2010;35(11):847–52.
74. Borso E, Grosso M, Boni G, Manca G, Bianchi P, Puccini M, et al. Radioguided occult lesion localization of cervical recurrences from differentiated thyroid cancer: technical feasibility and clinical results. Q J Nucl Med Mol Imaging. 2013;57(4):401–11.
75. Giles YS, Sarici IS, Tunca F, Sormaz IC, Salmaslioglu A, Adalet I, et al. The rate of operative success achieved with radioguided occult lesion localization and intraoperative ultrasonography in patients with recurrent papillary thyroid cancer. Surgery. 2014;156:1116–26.
76. Jung YS, Kim SK, Park I, Ryu J, Kim SW, Lee CY, et al. Surgical targeting of recurrent thyroid cancer using a novel mixture of 99m-technetium macroaggregated albumin and indocyanine green. Surg Innov. 2014;21:622–9.
77. Giovanella L, Suriano S, Lunghi L, Bongiovanni M, Ceriani L. Radioguided surgery of thyroid carcinoma recurrences: the role of preoperative (99m)Tc-labeled human serum albumin macroaggregates-SPECT/CT mapping. Clin Nucl Med. 2013;38(4):e207–9.
78. Bellotti C, Castagnola G, Tierno SM, Centanini F, Sparagna A, Vetrone I, et al. Radioguided surgery with combined use of gamma probe and hand-held gamma camera for treatment of papillary thyroid cancer locoregional recurrences: a preliminary study. Eur Rev Med Pharmacol Sci. 2013;17(24):3362–6.
79. Alander JT, Kaartinen I, Laakso A, Patila T, Spillmann T, Tuchin VV, et al. A review of indocyanine green fluorescent imaging in surgery. Int J Biomed Imaging. 2012;2012:940585.

80. Kloos RT, Eng C, Evans DB, Francis GL, Gagel RF, Gharib H, et al. Medullary thyroid cancer: management guidelines of the American Thyroid Association. Thyroid. 2009;19(6):565–612.
81. Leboulleux S, Baudin E, Travagli JP, Schlumberger M. Medullary thyroid carcinoma. Clin Endocrinol (Oxf). 2004;61(3):299–310.
82. Skoura E. Depicting medullary thyroid cancer recurrence: the past and the future of nuclear medicine imaging. Int J Endocrinol Metab. 2013;11(4), e8156.
83. Ugur O, Kostakglu L, Guler N, Caner B, Uysal U, Elahi N, et al. Comparison of 99mTc(V)-DMSA, 201Tl and 99mTc-MIBI imaging in the follow-up of patients with medullary carcinoma of the thyroid. Eur J Nucl Med. 1996;23(10):1367–71.
84. Reiners C. Imaging methods for medullary thyroid cancer. Recent Results Cancer Res. 1992;125:125–45.
85. Arslan N, Ilgan S, Yuksel D, Serdengecti M, Bulakbasi N, Ugur O, et al. Comparison of In-111 octreotide and Tc-99m (V) DMSA scintigraphy in the detection of medullary thyroid tumor foci in patients with elevated levels of tumor markers after surgery. Clin Nucl Med. 2001;26(8):683–8.
86. Adams S, Baum RP, Hertel A, Wenisch HJ, Staib-Sebler E, Herrmann G, et al. Intraoperative gamma probe detection of neuroendocrine tumors. J Nucl Med. 1998;39(7):1155–60.
87. Adams S, Acker P, Lorenz M, Staib-Sebler E, Hor G. Radioisotope-guided surgery in patients with pheochromocytoma and recurrent medullary thyroid carcinoma: a comparison of preoperative and intraoperative tumor localization with histopathologic findings. Cancer. 2001;92(2):263–70.
88. Adams S, Baum RP. Intraoperative use of gamma-detecting probes to localize neuroendocrine tumors. Q J Nucl Med. 2000;44(1):59–67.
89. Sandrock D, Blossey HC, Steinroeder M, Munz DL. Contribution of different scintigraphic techniques to the management of medullary thyroid carcinoma. Henry Ford Hosp Med J. 1989;37(3–4):173–4.
90. Behr TM, Gratz S, Markus PM, Dunn RM, Hufner M, Schauer A, et al. Anti-carcinoembryonic antigen antibodies versus somatostatin analogs in the detection of metastatic medullary thyroid carcinoma: are carcinoembryonic antigen and somatostatin receptor expression prognostic factors? Cancer. 1997;80(12 Suppl):2436–57.
91. Busnardo B, Girelli ME, Simioni N, Nacamulli D, Busetto E. Nonparallel patterns of calcitonin and carcinoembryonic antigen levels in the follow-up of medullary thyroid carcinoma. Cancer. 1984;53(2):278–85.
92. Barbet J, Peltier P, Bardet S, Vuillez JP, Bachelot I, Denet S, et al. Radioimmunodetection of medullary thyroid carcinoma using indium-111 bivalent hapten and anti-CEA x anti-DTPA-indium bispecific antibody. J Nucl Med. 1998;39(7):1172–8.
93. de Labriolle-Vaylet C, Cattan P, Sarfati E, Wioland M, Billotey C, Brocheriou C, et al. Successful surgical removal of occult metastases of medullary thyroid carcinoma recurrences with the help of immunoscintigraphy and radioimmunoguided surgery. Clin Cancer Res. 2000;6(2):363–71.
94. Peltier P, Curtet C, Chatal JF, Le Doussal JM, Daniel G, Aillet G, et al. Radioimmunodetection of medullary thyroid cancer using a bispecific anti-CEA/anti-indium-DTPA antibody and an indium-111-labeled DTPA dimer. J Nucl Med. 1993;34(8):1267–73.
95. Wangberg B, Forssell-Aronsson E, Tisell LE, Nilsson O, Fjalling M, Ahlman H. Intraoperative detection of somatostatin-receptor-positive neuroendocrine tumours using indium-111-labelled DTPA-D-Phe1-octreotide. Br J Cancer. 1996;73(6):770–5.

Part VII

Clinical Application: Urogenital Tract

Radioguided Sentinel Lymph Node Biopsy and Lymphatic Mapping in Urogenital Malignancies

15

Henk G. van der Poel, Joost A.P. Leijte, and Simon Horenblas

Contents

H.G. van der Poel (✉) • J.A.P. Leijte • S. Horenblas
Department of Urology, Netherlands Cancer Institute, Amsterdam, NL, USA
e-mail: h.vd.poel@nki.nl

Abstract

Radioguided sentinel lymph node (SLN) detection is applied in the management of several urogenital malignancies. International guidelines recommend SLN detection in men with penile cancer and increased risk of nodal metastases. For several other urogenital malignancies, SLN detection is considered experimental: prostate cancer, testicular cancer, bladder cancer, and renal cancer. Largest series are published on prostate cancer management. No randomized studies are available for review. Although SLN detection was shown to provide detection of nodal metastases outside standard nodal dissection templates in prostate and bladder cancer, the lack of standard methodology and definitions of SLN may explain why SLN detection is still considered experimental. Only few studies discuss the use of SLN detection in renal and testicular cancer. With improved intraoperative imaging modalities, better anatomical localization of SLN in particular in the retroperitoneum is feasible. This may boost the design of appropriately designed prospective comparative trials to study the oncological benefit of SLN detection in urogenital malignancies.

K. Herrmann et al. (eds.), *Radioguided Surgery: Current Applications and Innovative Directions in Clinical Practice*, DOI 10.1007/978-3-319-26051-8_15

15.1 Introduction

The "sentinel node concept" was first described by Gould et al. in 1960 for parotid gland cancer [1]. Later, in 1977, Cabanas utilized this same concept in urological surgery for penile cancer, as based upon lymphangiographic studies in 100 men (including 10 healthy volunteers and 10 patients with a benign penile lesion) to identify the first draining lymph node [2]. Cabanas found this sentinel lymph node (SLN) to be anatomically located in a fixed, predetermined location close to the superficial epigastric vein. In this initial experience, Cabanas reported that a SLN biopsy was performed in 64 penile cancer patients, of whom 15 patients had a lymph node metastasis within the SLN and 12 patients had a lymph node metastasis only within the SLN. From that point forward in time, SLN surgery in penile cancer surgery subsequently consisted of removal of the lymph node in this fixed, predetermined location, not taking into account possible individual variations in lymphatic drainage patterns. However, secondary to false-negative results, this fixed, predetermined anatomical location technique for identification of the SLN fell into disfavor and was subsequently abandoned and has been replaced by radioguided SLN biopsy methodologies [3].

In current urological surgery practice, radioguided SLN biopsy has also been used or clinically been evaluated in other urologic tumor types, such as prostate, bladder, testicular, and renal cancer. However, no consensus exists on the value of radioguided SLN biopsy in these urologic malignancies, and its use is not a standard of care currently. Even in penile cancer, the use of radioguided SLN biopsy remains subject to much discussion, and its use is not as widespread in the USA as it is in Europe.

Novel technical approaches such as image-guided surgery using fluorophores in the near-infrared (NIR) spectrum and improved scintigraphic staging with SPECT-CT have drawn attention towards the SLN approach in abovementioned cancers. The lack of consensus of the value of the SLN approach in urological cancers is mainly due to the scarcity of high-level clinical studies. In this chapter, we will present the available literature on SLN biopsy in urological cancers and define the state-of-the-art approaches and recommendations in the urological guidelines.

15.2 Penile Cancer

About 95 % of penile tumors are squamous cell carcinomas. It has a predominantly lymphogenic dissemination pattern. The first draining nodes are the inguinal lymph nodes. Occult inguinal metastases occur in around 20 % of patients with clinically node-negative groins. A prophylactic bilateral inguinal lymph node dissection may thus be unnecessary in the majority of patients, while this procedure has high morbidity – a possible explanation for its reported underutilization [4]. SLN biopsy plays an important role reducing overtreatment and morbidity. The complication rate of SLN biopsy is around 5–7 %, while complication rates of inguinal lymph node dissection are up to 74 %, even in contemporary series [5–8].

Although survival in men with cN0 penile cancer improved in recent years, nodal metastases are seen in a large portion of men [9]. With improvements in lymphatic mapping techniques and the gradual acceptance of radioguided SLN biopsy techniques in melanoma and breast cancer, SLN biopsy, using radioguided techniques (combined blue dye and radioactive technetium-99m (99mTc) tracer utilization), was introduced into penile cancer surgery in 2000 [10]. Since then, several modifications to the procedure have been made to improve its reliability [7, 11–46]. Unfortunately, no randomized trials exist, and all reported studies contain a limited number of cases or are case reports. A meta-analysis from 2012 containing 18 studies showed a 88.3 % pooled detection rate increasing to 90.1 % when blue dye was added to the radiotracer; no report on false-negative rate was available from this analysis [47]. A review of 10 studies published in 2011 showed a 3.5 % false-negative rate for the SLN biopsy [48].

According to the EAU guidelines, SLN biopsy is indicated in men with cN0 and at least cT1G2 disease [49]. In low-risk penile cancer patients with larger exophytic tumor, the yield of positive SLN is high and maybe therefore considered [50]. In intermediate-risk patients with microscopic SLN biopsy metastases, Akduman et al. found no further metastases in completing inguinal node dissection, but additional inguinal node dissection is still recommended in all men with nodal metastases on SLN biopsy [49, 51]. In a recently updated prognostic scoring system, SLN biopsy added predictive value [52]. Currently, several centers in Europe have confirmed the reliability and reproducibility of SLN biopsy in penile cancer. Reported false-negative rates of contemporary series vary between 3 and 15 % [28, 29, 37, 53]. In combination with inguinal ultrasound, SLN biopsy had a sensitivity of 94 % in a large series [53, 54].

15.2.1 Preoperative Visualization of Lymphatic Drainage

The day before SLN surgery, a radioactive tracer (^{99m}Technetium-nanocolloid), is injected around the tumor subcutaneously in 2–3 injection at a total dose of 50–90 MBq in 0.2–0.4 cc volume [14, 24]. Subsequently, timed planar scintigraphic imaging is performed at 10–20 min and 2 h postinjection (Fig. 15.1) [7, 16, 18]. Some centers add single-photon emission computed tomography-computed tomography (SPECT-CT) imaging to the preoperative imaging to acquire additional anatomical information of the SLN and drainage patterns (Fig. 15.2) [55].

Interestingly, SLN detection seems feasible even after removal of the primary penile cancer by partial penectomy, allowing for rapid removal of the primary tumor where needed and subsequent SLN dissection in a specialized center in a separate procedure [35]. Moreover, repeat SLN after an initial negative SLN procedure in patients with a local (penile) recurrence is possible [56]. Proper pathological node evaluation is essential to avoid

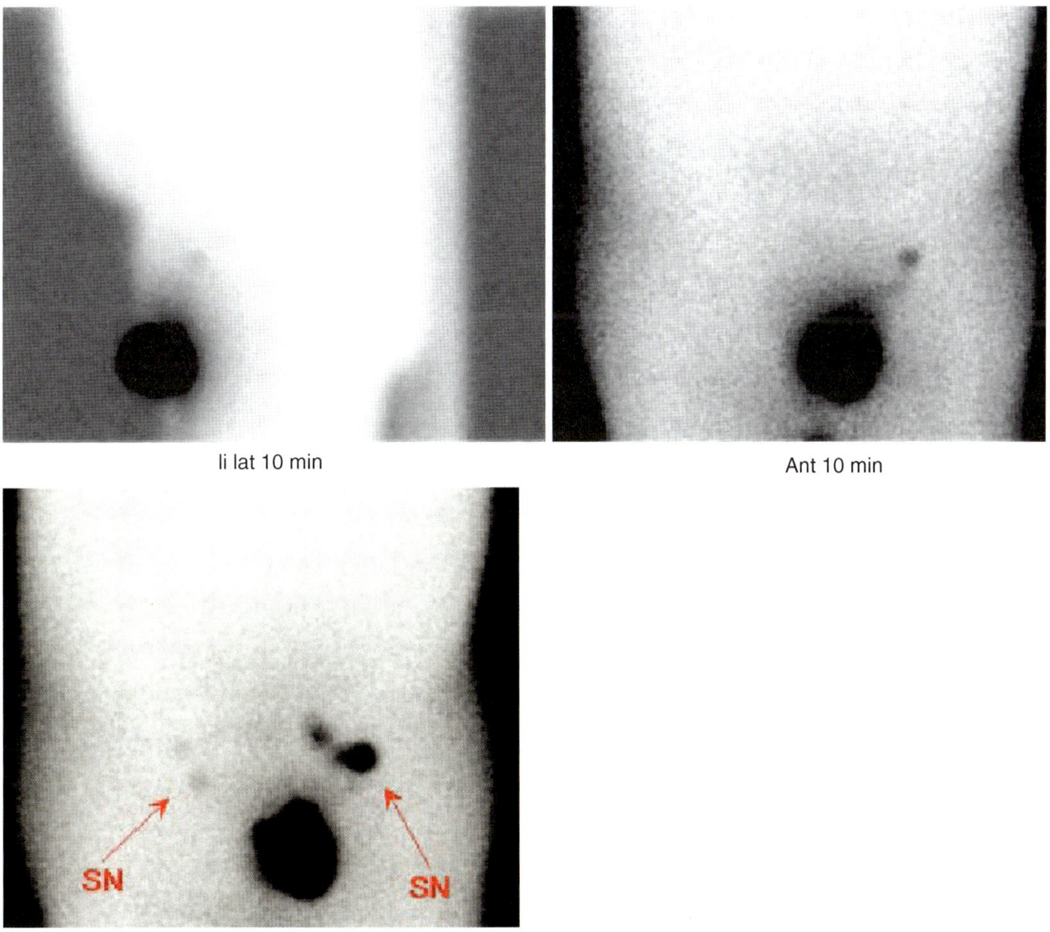

Fig. 15.1 Early scintigram for penile cancer SLN detection

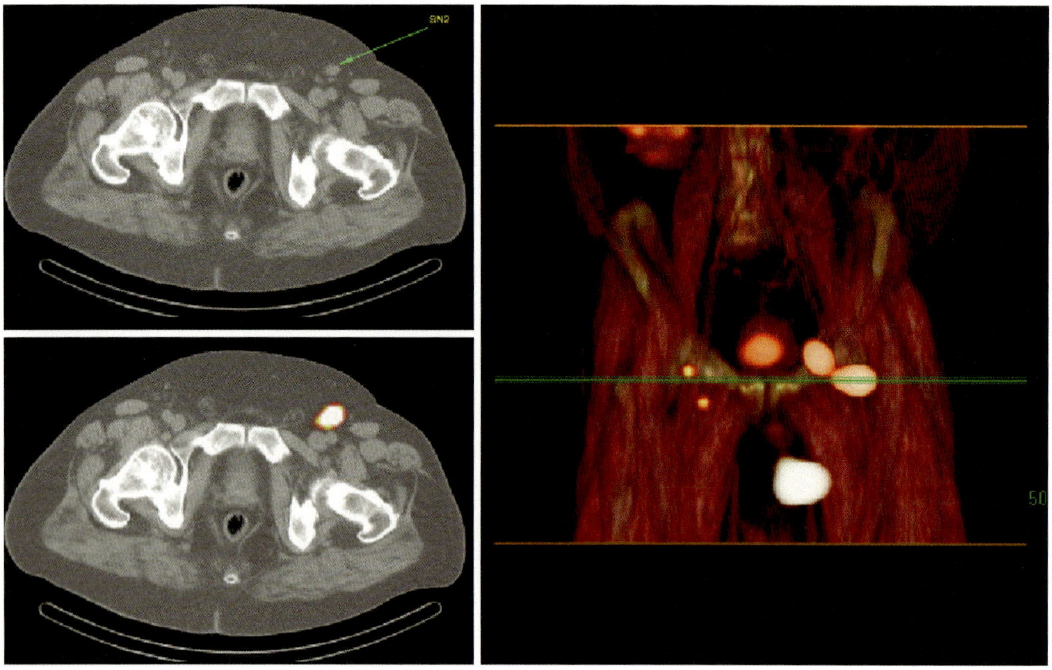

Fig. 15.2 SPECT/CT for SLN detection in penile cancer

false-negative SLN removal [11]. The reproducibility of preoperative imaging of SLN is high [57]. Preoperative inguinal ultrasound improves the clinical diagnosis of nodal metastases, in particular when combined with a cytological aspiration biopsy of suspicious lymph nodes [12]. It also seems to improve the false-negative rate of SLN biopsy by reducing the chance of tumor blockage [58]. In men with a tumor-positive cytological aspiration, SLN should only be considered to detect contralateral inguinal metastases, and an ipsilateral inguinal node dissection is recommended [11].

15.2.2 Intraoperative SLN Detection Using Gamma Tracing

Based on the preoperative scintigraphic imaging, the location of the SLN is marked on the skin. Directly before the SLN procedure, patent blue is injected into the skin surrounding the tumor as an additional tracer. A small incision (3–4 cm) is then made, preferably just below the inguinal plica. The incision is made preferably somewhat lower than the inguinal plica, since this allows for a lower incision in cases where an additional inguinal node dissection is required because of a positive SLN. A lower inguinal incision in these men is associated with more favorable wound healing.

The SLN is then identified using the combination of blue dye and a handheld gamma probe to identify the radioactive nodes. Preoperative imaging using SPECT/CT was shown to improve inguinal detection of SLN by providing superior 3D information on lymph node location as compared to conventional scintigraphy imaging [13, 59]. Interestingly, SLN location was found to be limited to the superior and central inguinal lymph nodes. This knowledge could be used to determine the extent of a lymph node dissection when the SLN method is not used [60].

15.2.3 Optical Tracers and SLN Detection in Penile Cancer

As mentioned before, the most widely used visual marker is blue dye. The visualization rate of lymph nodes with blue dye alone is between 55 and 70 % [14, 18]. An advantage of blue dye is the visualization of the lymphatic ducts what aids in a more rapid identification of the SLN.

Near infrared (NIR) imaging options have become available as an additional visual tracer. Fluorescent tracers in the NIR spectrum of light provide the benefit of visualization of lymph drainage without obscuring anatomical planes in the white light surgical setting. Indocyanine green (ICG) is a fluorophore that can be visualized by using NIR imaging systems and emits light at 820 nm when excitated by 770 nm light, both in the invisible spectrum of the NIR light. When injected locally, ICG rapidly migrates through the lymphatic system enabling intraoperative visualization of tracts and nodes. Hybrid tracers, comprised of the fluorescent dye ICG covalently attached to the ^{99m}Tc nanocolloid, have been developed that can be used to provide both preoperative SPECT imaging and intraoperative fluorescence guidance for surgery [14]. Intraoperative visualization of ICG is superior to the visualization of SLNs with blue dye [14].

15.2.4 Clinical Outcome

Similar to many other tumors, the lymph node status is the most important prognostic factor in penile carcinoma [61]. Prediction of nodal metastases based on clinical factors is inaccurate, and prophylactic inguinal lymph node dissection would imply overtreatment in the majority of patients [34, 62]. Early detection and treatment of inguinal nodal metastases by SLN biopsy improved survival in comparison to a cohort that was observed (albeit retrospectively) [17, 63].

Staging has improved and survival of men with cN0 disease has increased after the introduction of the SLN method [9]. In the majority of cases, the SLN was the only node containing metastases [18]. Size of the nodal metastases in SLNs was the best predictor of additional positive nodes [64].

Close follow-up is therefore indicated in men with SLNpN0 penile cancer in particular in centers with limited experience in SLN detection [65]. In a series of men with recurrent disease, nonpalpable tumor-positive lymph nodes were frequently detected using ultrasound methods, and therefore, the role of ultrasound in the follow-up of these men is useful [66].

15.3 Prostate Cancer

Prostate cancer initially metastasizes to the lymph nodes, and intermediate- and high-risk prostate cancer patients have a risk of 5–70 % to develop nodal metastases. Predictive nomograms are generally used to define the indication for a nodal dissection concomitant to a prostatectomy in men with localized prostate cancer [67–69]. Guidelines recommend nodal dissection when nomograms predict a risk of more than 5 % on the presence of nodal metastases. For optimal nodal yield, an extended nodal dissection is recommended, and recent retrospective data suggest that removal of less than 14 nodes resulted in poorer outcome when compared to removal of more lymph nodes [70]. Prognosis of men with nodal metastases from prostate cancer is relatively good with the majority surviving more than 10 years [71, 72]. However, an extended nodal dissection is not without morbidity, and complications of the procedure are strongly correlated with the number of nodes removed [73]. Despite extended nodal dissection, pelvic recurrences do occur, and the false-negative rate of extended pelvic nodal dissection for prostate cancer was estimated to be around 12.5 % [74, 75].

The first results of SLN biopsy in prostate cancer have been published in 1999 [76–80]. Unlike in penile cancer, the routine use of SLN dissection in prostate cancer is still topic of debate. Although the SLN can be detected, some studies have found that metastases are frequently occurring in nodes besides the tumor-bearing SLN. Lymph drainage targeting therapy rather than SLN-targeted diagnostics has therefore been proposed [81–85]. A recent meta-analysis in prostate cancer was supportive of the use of SLN, despite the lack of high-level evidence, for the reason that it may reduce morbidity of the extended nodal dissection often propagated [86].

15.3.1 Preoperative Imaging

Most studies use the transperineal or transrectal tracer injection method. One study described intraoperative optical tracer injection transperitoneally [87], but in general, preoperative injection is used and allows preoperative imaging by SPECT/CT (Figs. 15.3 and 15.4). Buckle et al. showed variable tracer distribution within the prostate [88]. Ongoing studies should reveal whether intratumoral injection is superior to several tracer depots within the entire prostate. After injection, imaging with scintigraphy and SPECT/CT is applied. Both open [78, 89–95] and laparoscopic [96–99] gamma probe SLN detection has been extensively studied in prostate cancer, and over 7000 cases were reported in the literature. The 99m technetium tracer is either bound to sulfur [100], phylate [101, 102], or nanocolloid with varying sizes from 80 nm [78, 97] to 1500 nm [101–103]. The amount of radioactive tracer injected varied from 60 MBq [100] to 267 MBq [104]. No comparative studies are available on the optimal dose and injection volume.

15.3.2 Intraoperative Detection

Various groups distinguished SLNs and higher-echelon LNs based on the (dynamic) lymphatic drainage routes, enabling selective removal. During open surgical procedures, standard gamma probes can be used to detect activity and identify the draining patterns during open prostatectomy [78, 105, 106]. In most studies, the SLN or landing site resection is combined with a routine or extended nodal dissection. Since a secondary resection of lymph nodes in the small pelvis is cumbersome, most studies combine SLN resection with more extensive pelvic node dissection. A novel portable gamma camera (Sentinella, Oncovision; Valencia, Spain) has provided intraoperative imaging of 99mTc containing lymph nodes [107]. This two-dimensional imaging system was shown to aid in confirmation of accurate SLN removal in the laparoscopic setting [108]. Besides gamma probe and camera tracing, visual detection of SLN is applied using fluorophore dyes (Fig. 15.5). As described earlier, these tracers are injected intraprostatically and allow for visual confirmation of the gamma

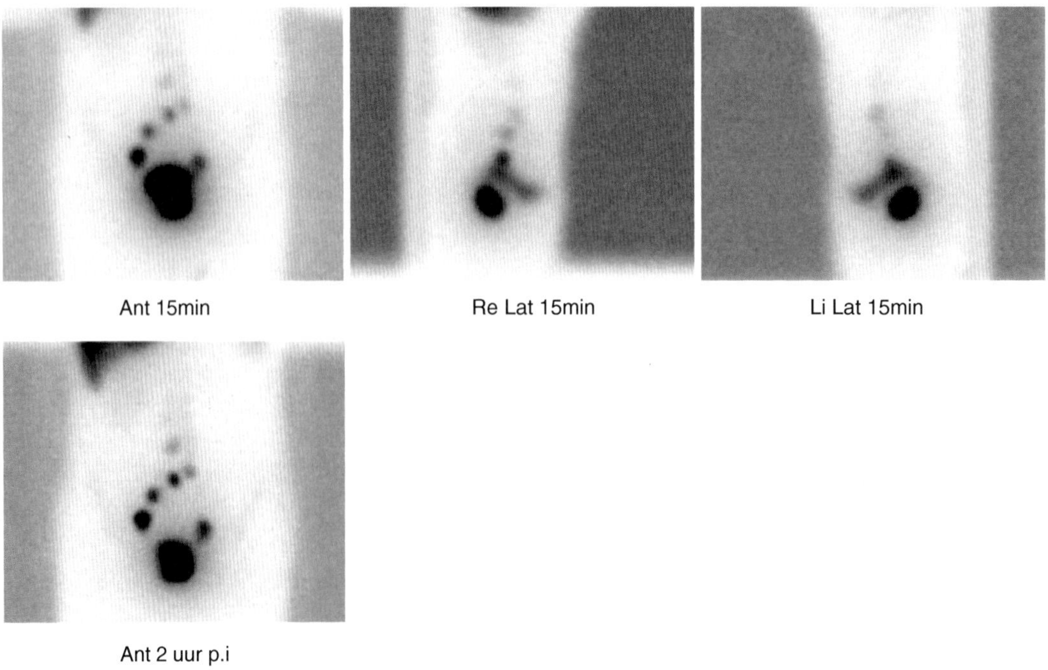

Fig. 15.3 Scintigraphy for prostate cancer SLN detection

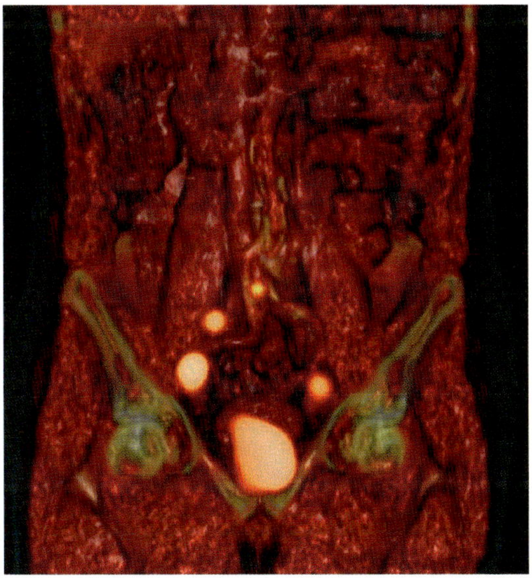

Fig. 15.4 SPECT/CT for SLN detection in prostate cancer

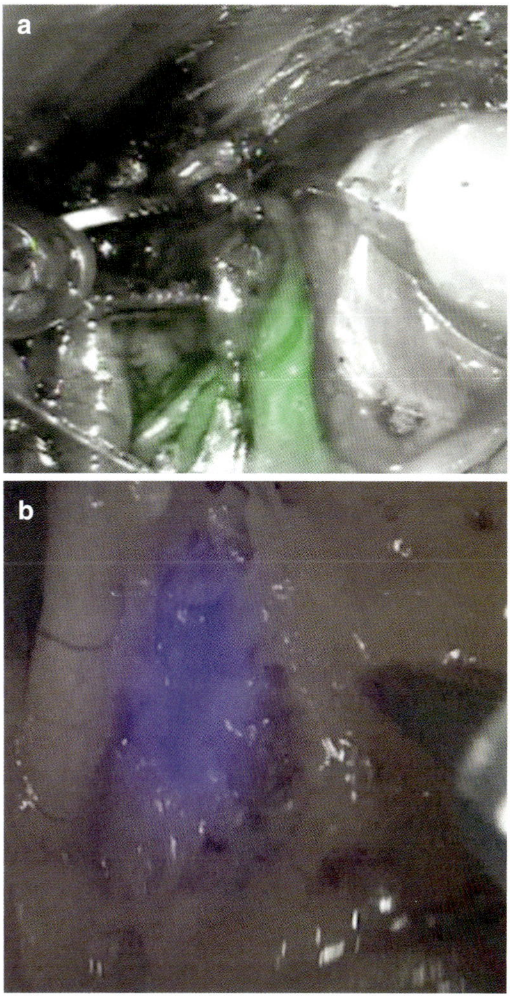

Fig. 15.5 Intraoperative image of sentinel lymph node. (**a**) SPIES system from Storz (Tuttlingen, Germany). (**b**) FireFly system from Intuitive Surgical (Sunnyvale, USA)

probe signal. The relatively low penetrance of NIR light systems does still require close-up resection often guided by the gamma probe. Initial studies used ICG bound to nanocolloid to retain the optical tracer in the lymph nodes and allow combined pre- and perioperative imaging [98]. More recently, free ICG was used as tracer. Free-ICG has the benefit of rapid migration into the lymph nodes draining the prostate after intraprostatic injection. Retention of tracer in lymph nodes, however, is much lower than with the use of nanocolloid bound ICG. Injection of free ICG, therefore, is applied briefly (10–30 min) prior to the nodal dissection. Moreover, at longer intervals or damage of lymphatic ducts due to surgical manipulation, ICG may leak from the lymphatic system and stain surrounding tissue rendering identification of draining lymph nodes more difficult. Several groups have successfully used free ICG to identify lymph nodes draining the prostate. Jeschke et al. compared free ICG to preoperatively injected and imaged gamma tracer and found high correlation between both tracing methods [109]. Manny et al. reported a 100 % sensitivity for predicting nodal metastases by SLN detection using an intraoperative ICG injection during robot-assisted radical prostatectomy [87]. Although free ICG seems to provide a practical alternative gamma tracing, it lacks the preoperative option of anatomical location of alternative lymph draining patterns that may be missed due to the low penetrance of the NIR signal of ICG. A study is ongoing to confirm the value of free ICG in comparison for nanocolloid bound multimodal tracer (NL41285.031.12).

Nanocolloid bound ICG has the advantage that it remains in the prostate at the injection site. This allows for postoperative localization of the injection site inside the prostate. Analysis of 19 prostatectomy specimen showed remarkable variation of location of ICG deposits inside the prostate after ultrasound-guided tracer injection [88]. Interestingly, draining patterns of tracer in the lymphatic system seemed dependent on location of the tracer inside the prostate [88]. To evaluate the effects of tracer injection location, a randomized study between intraprostatic and intratumoral injections is ongoing (NL46580.031.13).

Ultrasmall superparamagnetic nanoparticle MRI has been described to improve nodal metastases detection in prostate cancer [110, 111]. A handheld magnetometer was used to detect intraprostatically injected superparamagnetic iron oxide in 20 men with prostate cancer. Metastases were found only in lymph nodes detected using the magnetometer and identified as SLNs in this analysis [112]. The role of this new tracer for intraoperative detection of lymphatic drainage patterns needs further evaluation but holds promise.

15.3.3 Outcome

Different studies report different outcome of SLN approaches in prostate cancer. The median number of resected SLNs was 6 (range 2–26) per patient. The detection rate of SLN ranged 76–100 % [87, 91, 96–98, 100, 101, 104, 108, 113–119]. In 13–75 % of patients, one or more SLN(s) outside the limited pelvic lymph node dissection (PLND) template were found. In addition, tumor-bearing SLNs were detected outside the standard PLND in 51.8–76.9 % of the patients. In 4.1–25 % of patients, SLNs outside the extended PLND template were found, whereas 3.5–17 % of patients with positive LNs had SLN metastases outside the extended PLND template [75, 76, 78, 91, 96, 98–102, 113–116, 119–125]. In these studies, the median percentage of positive LNs was 20.4 % (range 4.7–50) with a false-negative rate of 1 % (range 0–20), respectively (Table 15.1).

15.4 Bladder Cancer

Lymph drainage from the bladder shows a wide variation [136] and contralateral drainage is frequent [137]. The application of SLN detection in bladder cancer is complicated by the complexity of tracer injection. Both intraoperative [138] and transurethral injection [137] may yield different draining patterns. In a study on 60 patients with radioactive tracer injections in the nontumor-bearing bladder site, extended nodal dissection included 92 % of the active nodes. In a more limited resection of external and obturator template, only 50 % of the radioactive lymph nodes were included [137]. In a smaller series of bladder cancer patients, SLN were detected in 85 % of cases suggesting that diagnostic yield of the SLN approach in bladder cancer may be lower than generally found in penile cancer [136]. The method of injection did influence drainage in a study using ICG tracers [136, 138, 139]. Moreover, multiple tumors may result in false-negative SLN biopsies [140], reported as high as 19 % [141]. Interestingly, one report introduces the use of SLN biopsy to harvest T-cells for immunotherapy for bladder cancer [142]. The complexity of injection and additional need of an extended nodal dissection has so far prohibited the extensive use of SLN for bladder cancer management.

15.5 Testis and Renal Cancer

Experience with the application of SLN methods for testis [143–146] and renal cancer [147–151] is limited. For testicular cancer, injection of tracer into the funiculus of the tumor-bearing testis resulted in visualization of a retroperitoneal SLN in 16 of 17 men with clinically node-negative testicular cancer. A median number of 2 lymph nodes were laparoscopically removed. Nodal metastasis was found in 1 men with testis cancer. Treatment in this case consisted of additional bleomycin, etoposide, and cisplatin chemotherapy. Whereas men with a negative SLN were followed according to guidelines, none of the men with a negative SLN developed a retroperitoneal recurrence at a median follow-up of 43 months. In renal cancer, SLN visualization was possible in 70–77 % of cases. In one small series, 2 of 20 patients had SLN outside the retroperitoneal region. These observations in small groups

Table 15.1 Results

Authors	Number of patients	SLN dissection method	Patient features (D'Amico risk classification)	Primary treatment	Excised SLN (*n*) (median)	Percentage of SLN detection	Percentage of positive lymph node (% patients)	Percentage of false negative lymph node (%)	Percentage of SLN outside of limited LND plate (% patients)	Percentage of SLN outside of extended LND plate (% patients)	Complications
Wawroschek et al. [78]	117	Open	All risk groups	NR	4	96 (in LN(+) patients)	23.9	4	51.8 (in LN(+) patients)	7.4 (in LN(+) patients)	No complication
Wawroschek et al. [104]	350	Open	All risk groups	RRP and radiotherapy	5.6 (mean)	97.1	24.5	0.5	59.3 (in LN(+) patients)	3.5 (in LN(+) patients)	NR
Takashima et al. [102]	24	Open	All risk groups	NR	4.2 (mean)	87.5	12.5	0	25	4.1	NR
Bastide et al. [93]	34	Open	All risk groups	RRP		85.3	11.7			66.6	NR
Brenot-Rossi et al. [100]	27	Open	All risk groups	RRP	3.5 (mean)	100	14.8	0	55.5	11.1	NR
Silva et al. [126]	23	Open	All risk groups	NR	3	95.6	13	4.3	13	NR	NR
Jeschke et al. [108]	71	Laparoscopic	All risk groups	LRP	4.7 (mean)	97.2	12.7	0	54.7	NR	1 prostatitis 2 ext. iliac artery injury 3 pulmonary embolism
Kizu et al. [127]	11	Open	NR	NR	3	100	9	0	45.4	NR	NR
Häcker et al. [113]	20	Laparoscopic	Intermediate- and high-risk groups	LRP	NR	70 (in LN(+) patients)	50	20	62	10	1 neuropraxia 1 deep vein thrombosis 3 lymphoceles

(continued)

Table 15.1 (continued)

Authors	Number of patients	SLN dissection method	Patient features (D'Amico risk classification)	Primary treatment	Excised SLN (*n*) (median)	Percentage of SLN detection	Percentage of positive lymph node (% patients)	Percentage of false negative lymph node (%)	Percentage of SLN outside of limited LND plate (% patients)	Percentage of SLN outside of extended LND plate (% patients)	Complications
Krengli et al. [128]	23	Open	16 patients pT2N0M0, 7 patients pT3-4N0M0	RRP	1.6 (mean)	87	NR	NR	NR	25	No complication
Corvin et al. [96]	28	Laparoscopic	Intermediate- and high-risk groups	Radiotherapy	2.1 (mean)	93	23	3.5	52	35.7	No complication
Weckermann et al. [118]	1055	Open	All risk groups	RRP	7	100	19.6	1	76(in LN(+) patients)	NR	NR
Weckermann et al. [129]	564	Open	All risk groups with presumed unilateral disease	RRP	6	100	9.2	0	75 (in LN(+) patients)	NR	NR
Fukuda et al. [101]	42	Open	All risk groups with/without NHT	RRP or radiotherapy	26	97.6	30.9	4.8	76.9 (in LN(+) patients)	15.3 (in LN(+) patients)	NR
Warncke et al. [90]	36	Open	Low- and intermediate-risk groups with/without the surgeon knowing imaging findings	RRP	8/10	99.5/98.5	4.7/6.6	0	NR	NR	1 retroperitoneal bleeding
Meinhardt et al. [97]	35	Laparoscopic	Intermediate- and high-risk groups	Radiotherapy	13.5 (mean)	81.5	40	0	NR	17.1	5 lymphocele 2 mild leg edema

Hautmann et al. [95]	108	Open	All risk groups	RRP	13.4 (mean)	91	15	0	NR	0	NR
eschke et al. [99]	140	Laparoscopic	Low- and intermediate-risk groups	LRP	4	95.3	13.5	NR	55.7	5.7	2 prostatitis 1 external iliac vein injury 1 neuropraxia 1 deep venous thrombosis 3 lymphoceles
Brenot-Rossi et al. [120]	100	Open	All risk groups	87 patients RRP 13 patients radiotherapy	7	76	12	0	69.3	4.1	NR
Vermeeren et al. [130]	46	Laparoscopic	Intermediate-risk group	Radiotherapy	4.3 (mean)	98	33	NR	NR	35	NR
Holl et al. [91]	2020	Open	All risk groups	RRP	9	98	16.7	5.8	NR	NR	NR
Vermeeren et al. [131]	16	Laparoscopic	Intermediate- and high-risk groups	NR	3	100	43.1	NR	NR	6.2	NR
Schilling et al. [132]	463	Open and laparoscopic	All risk groups for open PLND and high-risk group for laparoscopic PLND	RRP (418 patients) and laparoscopic PLND (45 patients) for staging procedure	3	89.3	6.1	2.1	76.7	NR	18 (3.9 %) lymphoceles 3 (0.6 %) ureteral injuries
Vermeeren et al. [107]	80	Laparoscopic	10 patients with recurrent prostate cancer 70 patients with intermediate-risk group	Salvage treatment and radiotherapy	3	100	50	NR	80	NR	NR

(continued)

Table 15.1 (continued)

Authors	Number of patients	SLN dissection method	Patient features (D'Amico risk classification)	Primary treatment	Excised SLN (*n*) (median)	Percentage of SLN detection	Percentage of positive lymph node (% patients)	Percentage of false negative lymph node (%)	Percentage of SLN outside of limited LND plate (% patients)	Percentage of SLN outside of extended LND plate (% patients)	Complications
Vermeeren et al. [133]	55	Laparoscopic	Intermediate-risk group	Radiotherapy	3.2 (mean)	84	40	NR	NR	NR	NR
Inoue et al. [114]	14	Open	All risk groups	RRP	11	100	14.2	NR	66.2	NR	NR
Van der Poel et al. [98]	11	Robot-assisted laparoscopic	Intermediate- and high-risk groups	RARP	2	91	18	NR	NR	36	NR
Ponholzer et al. [123]	54	Open and laparoscopic	Intermediate- and high-risk groups	RRP (38 patients) and LRP (16 patients)	NR	98	22.2	1.8	NR		NR
Jeschke et al. [109]	26	Laparoscopic	Intermediate- and high-risk groups	LRP	22	70.8	7.7	NR	42	20.3	No complication
Meinhardt et al. [122]	121	Laparoscopic	Intermediate- and high-risk groups, recurrent prostate cancer patients	Salvage treatment and radiotherapy	NR	100	40	0	NR	31	NR
Rousseau et al. [115]	93	Laparoscopic	All risk groups	LRP	5	92.5	20.4	10.5	79.7	3.6	No complication
De Bonilla-Damia et al. [75]	18	Laparoscopic	Intermediate- and high-risk groups,	Radiotherapy	3	100	33	0	44	19.8	NR

Joniau et al. [89]	74	Open	Intermediate- and high-risk groups	RRP	4	96	46	NR	75	13	8 (11 %) lymphoceles, 8 (11 %) limited lower limb edema 2(3 %) osteitis pubis 1(1 %) deep venous thrombosis 1 (1 %) transient obturator nerve malfunctioning
Manny et al. [87]	50	Robot-assisted laparoscopic	Low-risk group	RARP	14	100	8	24.4	47.4	10	NR
Stanik et al. [124]	80	Open	Intermediate- and high-risk groups	RRP	17	98	40	9	NR	28	1 major complication (%1): bleeding from ext. iliac vein 8 minor complications (%10): symptomatic lymphocele, pulmonary embolism and deep venous thrombosis

(continued)

Table 15.1 (continued)

Authors	Number of patients	SLN dissection method	Patient features (D'Amico risk classification)	Primary treatment	Excised SLN (*n*) (median)	Percentage of SLN detection	Percentage of positive lymph node (% patients)	Percentage of false negative lymph node (%)	Percentage of SLN outside of limited LND plate (% patients)	Percentage of SLN outside of extended LND plate (% patients)	Complications
Winter et al. [119]	1229	Open	All risk groups	RRP	10	99.8	17.1	2.4	NR	NR	NR
Yuen et al. [134]	66	Open	All risk groups	RRP	4 (median)	97	9	0	19	3	6 % lymphoceles
Van den Bergh et al. [135]	74	Open	>10 % N+ risk Partin nomogram	RRP	6 (median)	96/79	50	24	NR	44 (18 % outside seLND)	NR
Rousseau et al. [116]	203	Laparoscopic	Intermediate- and high-risk groups	LRP	5.6 (mean)	96	17.2	8.5	72.1	19.5	Complication rate: %4: 1 ureter injury, 1 bleeding from int. iliac vein 7 lymphoceles

suggest that lymph drainage of the kidney may be rapid and bypass lymph nodes nearby possibly through direct drainage of the lymph ducts into the thoracic duct.

15.6 Summary

Radioguided SLN procedures are clinically established in patients with penile cancer and increased risk of lymph node metastases. Limited clinical data is available for radioguided SLN procedures in prostate and bladder cancer, partially reporting reduced morbidity rates. However, convincing prospective clinical data is not available yet. For renal and testis cancer, only few pilot data has been published for radioguided SLN applications.

Recent improvement in intraoperative detection techniques allowing for better intraoperative anatomical SLN localization hopefully triggers prospectively designed randomized clinical trials investigating the impact of radioguided SLN procedures on outcome and morbidity in prostate, bladder, testis, and renal cancer.

References

1. Gould EA, Winship T, Philbin PH, Kerr HH. Observations on a "sentinel node" in cancer of the parotid. Cancer. 1960;13:77–8.
2. Cabanas RM. An approach for the treatment of penile carcinoma. Cancer. 1977;39(2):456–66.
3. Perinetti E, Crane DB, Catalona WJ. Unreliability of sentinel lymph node biopsy for staging penile carcinoma. J Urol. 1980;124(5):734–5.
4. Thuret R, Sun M, Lughezzani G, Budaus L, Liberman D, Abdollah F, Morgan M, Johal R, Jeldres C, Latour M, et al. A contemporary population-based assessment of the rate of lymph node dissection for penile carcinoma. Ann Surg Oncol. 2011;18(2):439–46.
5. Stuiver MM, Westerduin E, ter Meulen S, Vincent AD, Nieweg OE, Wouters MW. Surgical wound complications after groin dissection in melanoma patients – a historical cohort study and risk factor analysis. Eur J Surg Oncol. 2014;40(10):1284–90.
6. Wawroschek F, Vogt H, Bachter D, Weckermann D, Hamm M, Harzmann R. First experience with gamma probe guided sentinel lymph node surgery in penile cancer. Urol Res. 2000;28(4):246–9.
7. Valdes Olmos RA, Tanis PJ, Hoefnagel CA, Jansen L, Nieweg OE, Meinhardt W, Horenblas S. Penile lymphoscintigraphy for sentinel node identification. Eur J Nucl Med. 2001;28(5):581–5.
8. Perdona S, Autorino R, De Sio M, Di Lorenzo G, Gallo L, Damiano R, D'Armiento M, Gallo A. Dynamic sentinel node biopsy in clinically node-negative penile cancer versus radical inguinal lymphadenectomy: a comparative study. Urology. 2005;66(6):1282–6.
9. Djajadiningrat RS, Graafland NM, van Werkhoven E, Meinhardt W, Bex A, van der Poel HG, van Boven HH, Valdes Olmos RA, Horenblas S. Contemporary management of regional nodes in penile cancer-improvement of survival? J Urol. 2014;191(1):68–73.
10. Horenblas S, Jansen L, Meinhardt W, Hoefnagel CA, de Jong D, Nieweg OE. Detection of occult metastasis in squamous cell carcinoma of the penis using a dynamic sentinel node procedure. J Urol. 2000;163(1):100–4.
11. Kroon BK, Horenblas S, Estourgie SH, Lont AP, Valdes Olmos RA, Nieweg OE. How to avoid false-negative dynamic sentinel node procedures in penile carcinoma. J Urol. 2004;171(6 Pt 1):2191–4.
12. Kroon BK, Horenblas S, Deurloo EE, Nieweg OE, Teertstra HJ. Ultrasonography-guided fine-needle aspiration cytology before sentinel node biopsy in patients with penile carcinoma. BJU Int. 2005;95(4):517–21.
13. Brouwer OR, van den Berg NS, Matheron HM, Wendler T, van der Poel HG, Horenblas S, Valdes Olmos RA, van Leeuwen FW. Feasibility of intraoperative navigation to the sentinel node in the groin using preoperatively acquired single photon emission computerized tomography data: transferring functional imaging to the operating room. J Urol. 2014;192(6):1810–6.
14. Brouwer OR, van den Berg NS, Matheron HM, van der Poel HG, van Rhijn BW, Bex A, van Tinteren H, Valdes Olmos RA, van Leeuwen FW, Horenblas S. A hybrid radioactive and fluorescent tracer for sentinel node biopsy in penile carcinoma as a potential replacement for blue dye. Eur Urol. 2014;65(3):600–9.
15. Benejam Gual JM, García-Miralles Grávalos R, Hidalgo Pardo F, Muñoz Vélez D, Hellín Hellín D, Lago Rodríguez J. Usefulness of the dynamic sentinel node technique in patients with penile carcinoma. Actas Urol Esp. 2001;25(6):409–14.
16. Tanis PJ, Lont AP, Meinhardt W, Olmos RA, Nieweg OE, Horenblas S. Dynamic sentinel node biopsy for penile cancer: reliability of a staging technique. J Urol. 2002;168(1):76–80.
17. Lont AP, Horenblas S, Tanis PJ, Gallee MP, van Tinteren H, Nieweg OE. Management of clinically node negative penile carcinoma: improved survival after the introduction of dynamic sentinel node biopsy. J Urol. 2003;170(3):783–6.

18. Kroon BK, Horenblas S, Meinhardt W, van der Poel HG, Bex A, van Tinteren H, Valdes Olmos RA, Nieweg OE. Dynamic sentinel node biopsy in penile carcinoma: evaluation of 10 years experience. Eur Urol. 2005;47(5):601–6; discussion 606.
19. Perdona S, Autorino R, Gallo L, Di Lorenzo G, Cascini GL, Lastoria F, Marra L, De Sio M, Damiano R, Gallo A. Role of dynamic sentinel node biopsy in penile cancer: our experience. J Surg Oncol. 2006;93(3):181–5.
20. Leijte JA, Kroon BK, Valdes Olmos RA, Nieweg OE, Horenblas S. Reliability and safety of current dynamic sentinel node biopsy for penile carcinoma. Eur Urol. 2007;52(1):170–7.
21. Gonzaga-Silva LF, Tavares JM, Freitas FC, Tomas Filho ME, Oliveira VP, Lima MV. The isolated gamma probe technique for sentinel node penile carcinoma detection is unreliable. Int Braz J Urol. 2007;33(1):58–63; discussion 64–7.
22. Spiess PE, Izawa JI, Bassett R, Kedar D, Busby JE, Wong F, Eddings T, Tamboli P, Pettaway CA. Preoperative lymphoscintigraphy and dynamic sentinel node biopsy for staging penile cancer: results with pathological correlation. J Urol. 2007;177(6):2157–61.
23. Hernandez-Toris N, Quintero-Becerra J, Gallegos-Hernandez JF, Flores-Ojeda R, Alvarado-Cabrero I, Flores-Lopez D, Pichardo-Romero P. Lymphatic mapping and sentinel node biopsy in penis cancer. Feasibility study and preliminary report. Cir Cir. 2007;75(2):87–91.
24. Hadway P, Smith Y, Corbishley C, Heenan S, Watkin NA. Evaluation of dynamic lymphoscintigraphy and sentinel lymph-node biopsy for detecting occult metastases in patients with penile squamous cell carcinoma. BJU Int. 2007;100(3):561–5.
25. Rubi S, Vidal-Sicar S, Ortega M, Domenech B, Lafuente S, Corral JM, Gelabert-Mas A. Localization of sentinel node in squamous cell carcinoma of the penis. Initial experience. Rev Esp Med Nucl. 2008;27(1):3–7.
26. Heyns CF, Theron PD. Evaluation of dynamic sentinel lymph node biopsy in patients with squamous cell carcinoma of the penis and palpable inguinal nodes. BJU Int. 2008;102(3):305–9.
27. Ferreira U, Ribeiro MA, Reis LO, Prudente A, Matheus WE. Sentinel lymph node biopsy in penile cancer: a comparative study using modified inguinal dissection. Int Braz J Urol. 2008;34(6):725–30; discussion 730–3.
28. Kirrander P, Andren O, Windahl T. Dynamic sentinel node biopsy in penile cancer: initial experiences at a Swedish referral centre. BJU Int. 2013;111(3 Pt B):E48–53.
29. Fuchs J, Hamann MF, Schulenburg F, Knupfer S, Osmonov D, Lutzen U, Junemann KP, Naumann CM. Sentinel lymph node biopsy for penile carcinoma : assessment of reliability. Urologe A. 2013;52(10): 1447–50.
30. La-Touche S, Ayres B, Lam W, Alnajjar HM, Perry M, Watkin N. Trial of ligation versus coagulation of lymphatics in dynamic inguinal sentinel lymph node biopsy for staging of squamous cell carcinoma of the penis. Ann R Coll Surg Engl. 2012;94(5):344–6.
31. Bucher S, Guerra M, Ribuffo D. Selective lymphadenectomy for penile cancer. Eur Rev Med Pharmacol Sci. 2011;15(8):967–70.
32. Zhu Y, Ye DW. Repeat dynamic sentinel node biopsy in locally recurrent penile carcinoma. BJU Int. 2010;105(12):1732; author reply 1732–3.
33. Wood HM, Angermeier KW. Anatomic considerations of the penis, lymphatic drainage, and biopsy of the sentinel node. Urol Clin North Am. 2010;37(3):327–34.
34. Graafland NM, Lam W, Leijte JA, Yap T, Gallee MP, Corbishley C, van Werkhoven E, Watkin N, Horenblas S. Prognostic factors for occult inguinal lymph node involvement in penile carcinoma and assessment of the high-risk EAU subgroup: a two-institution analysis of 342 clinically node-negative patients. Eur Urol. 2010;58(5):742–7.
35. Graafland NM, Valdes Olmos RA, Meinhardt W, Bex A, van der Poel HG, van Boven HH, Nieweg OE, Horenblas S. Nodal staging in penile carcinoma by dynamic sentinel node biopsy after previous therapeutic primary tumour resection. Eur Urol. 2010;58(5):748–51.
36. Leijte JA, Graafland NM, Valdes Olmos RA, van Boven HH, Hoefnagel CA, Horenblas S. Prospective evaluation of hybrid 18F-fluorodeoxyglucose positron emission tomography/computed tomography in staging clinically node-negative patients with penile carcinoma. BJU Int. 2009;104(5):640–4.
37. Leijte JA, Hughes B, Graafland NM, Kroon BK, Olmos RA, Nieweg OE, Corbishley C, Heenan S, Watkin N, Horenblas S. Two-center evaluation of dynamic sentinel node biopsy for squamous cell carcinoma of the penis. J Clin Oncol. 2009;27(20): 3325–9.
38. Wespes E. The management of regional lymph nodes in patients with penile carcinoma and reliability of sentinel node biopsy. Eur Urol. 2007;52(1): 15–6; discussion 20–1.
39. Naumann CM, Hamann MF, Wefer B, Kaufmann S, Al Najar A, Seif C, Braun PM, Hautmann S, Junemann KP, van der Horst C. 30 Years of sentinel lymph node diagnostic in penile carcinoma: development of a diagnostic procedure and current results. Urologe A. 2007;46(11):1514–8.
40. Loughlin KR. Is sentinel node biopsy indicated in penile cancer? Nat Clin Pract Urol. 2007;4(2):80–1.
41. Kim S, Brock GB, Temple CL. Minimizing morbidity in the treatment of penile melanoma: Mohs micrographic surgery and sentinel lymph node biopsy. Can J Urol. 2007;14(1):3467–70.
42. Hautmann S. Sentinels and markers: new methods of examination and treatment in urology. Urologe A. 2007;46(11):1483–4.

43. Jensen JB, Jensen KM, Ulhoi BP, Nielsen SS, Lundbeck F. Sentinel lymph-node biopsy in patients with squamous cell carcinoma of the penis. BJU Int. 2009;103(9):1199–203.
44. Ficarra V, Galfano A. Should the dynamic sentinel node biopsy (DSNB) be considered the gold standard in the evaluation of lymph node status in patients with penile carcinoma? Eur Urol. 2007;52(1):17–9; discussion 20–1.
45. Izawa J, Kedar D, Wong F, Pettaway CA. Sentinel lymph node biopsy in penile cancer: evolution and insights. Can J Urol. 2005;12 Suppl 1:24–9.
46. Jakub JW, Pendas S, Reintgen DS. Current status of sentinel lymph node mapping and biopsy: facts and controversies. Oncologist. 2003;8(1):59–68.
47. Sadeghi R, Gholami H, Zakavi SR, Kakhki VR, Tabasi KT, Horenblas S. Accuracy of sentinel lymph node biopsy for inguinal lymph node staging of penile squamous cell carcinoma: systematic review and meta-analysis of the literature. J Urol. 2012;187(1):25–31.
48. Neto AS, Tobias-Machado M, Ficarra V, Wroclawski ML, Amarante RD, Pompeo AC, Del Giglio A. Dynamic sentinel node biopsy for inguinal lymph node staging in patients with penile cancer: a systematic review and cumulative analysis of the literature. Ann Surg Oncol. 2011;18(7):2026–34.
49. Hakenberg OW, Comperat EM, Minhas S, Necchi A, Protzel C, Watkin N. EAU guidelines on penile cancer: 2014 update. Eur Urol. 2015;67(1):142–50.
50. Brennhovd B, Johnsrud K, Berner A, Bogsrud T, Waehre H, Giercksky KE, Axcrona K. Sentinel node procedure in low-stage/low-grade penile carcinomas. Scand J Urol Nephrol. 2006;40(3): 204–7.
51. Akduman B, Fleshner NE, Ehrlich L, Klotz L. Early experience in intermediate-risk penile cancer with sentinel node identification using the gamma probe. Urology. 2001;58(1):65–8.
52. Sun M, Djajadiningrat RS, Alnajjar HM, Trinh QD, Graafland NM, Watkin N, Karakiewicz PI, Horenblas S. Development and external validation of a prognostic tool for prediction of cancer-specific mortality after complete loco-regional pathological staging for squamous cell carcinoma of the penis. BJU Int. 2014;116:734–43.
53. Lam W, Alnajjar HM, La-Touche S, Perry M, Sharma D, Corbishley C, Pilcher J, Heenan S, Watkin N. Dynamic sentinel lymph node biopsy in patients with invasive squamous cell carcinoma of the penis: a prospective study of the long-term outcome of 500 inguinal basins assessed at a single institution. Eur Urol. 2013;63(4):657–63.
54. Crawshaw JW, Hadway P, Hoffland D, Bassingham S, Corbishley CM, Smith Y, Pilcher J, Allan R, Watkin NA, Heenan SD. Sentinel lymph node biopsy using dynamic lymphoscintigraphy combined with ultrasound-guided fine needle aspiration in penile carcinoma. Br J Radiol. 2009;82(973):41–8.
55. Vermeeren L, van der Ploeg IM, Olmos RA, Meinhardt W, Klop WM, Kroon BB, Nieweg OE. SPECT/CT for preoperative sentinel node localization. J Surg Oncol. 2010;101(2):184–90.
56. Graafland NM, Leijte JA, Olmos RA, Van Boven HH, Nieweg OE, Horenblas S. Repeat dynamic sentinel node biopsy in locally recurrent penile carcinoma. BJU Int. 2010;105(8):1121–4.
57. Kroon BK, Valdes Olmos RA, van Tinteren H, Nieweg OE, Horenblas S. Reproducibility of lymphoscintigraphy for lymphatic mapping in patients with penile carcinoma. J Urol. 2005;174(6):2214–7.
58. Leijte JA, van der Ploeg IM, Valdes Olmos RA, Nieweg OE, Horenblas S. Visualization of tumor blockage and rerouting of lymphatic drainage in penile cancer patients by use of SPECT/CT. J Nucl Med. 2009;50(3):364–7.
59. Kroon BK, Valdes Olmos R, Nieweg OE, Horenblas S. Non-visualization of sentinel lymph nodes in penile carcinoma. Eur J Nucl Med Mol Imaging. 2005;32(9):1096–9.
60. Leijte JA, Valdes Olmos RA, Nieweg OE, Horenblas S. Anatomical mapping of lymphatic drainage in penile carcinoma with SPECT-CT: implications for the extent of inguinal lymph node dissection. Eur Urol. 2008;54(4):885–90.
61. Ornellas AA, Kinchin EW, Nobrega BL, Wisnescky A, Koifman N, Quirino R. Surgical treatment of invasive squamous cell carcinoma of the penis: Brazilian National Cancer Institute long-term experience. J Surg Oncol. 2008;97(6):487–95.
62. Hughes BE, Leijte JA, Kroon BK, Shabbir MA, Swallow TW, Heenan SD, Corbishley CM, van Boven HH, Perry MJ, Watkin NA, et al. Lymph node metastasis in intermediate-risk penile squamous cell cancer: a two-centre experience. Eur Urol. 2010; 57(4):688–92.
63. Kroon BK, Horenblas S, Lont AP, Tanis PJ, Gallee MP, Nieweg OE. Patients with penile carcinoma benefit from immediate resection of clinically occult lymph node metastases. J Urol. 2005;173(3):816–9.
64. Kroon BK, Nieweg OE, van Boven H, Horenblas S. Size of metastasis in the sentinel node predicts additional nodal involvement in penile carcinoma. J Urol. 2006;176(1):105–8.
65. Leijte JA, Kirrander P, Antonini N, Windahl T, Horenblas S. Recurrence patterns of squamous cell carcinoma of the penis: recommendations for follow-up based on a two-centre analysis of 700 patients. Eur Urol. 2008;54(1):161–8.
66. Djajadiningrat RS, Teertstra HJ, van Werkhoven E, van Boven HH, Horenblas S. Ultrasound examination and fine needle aspiration cytology-useful for followup of the regional nodes in penile cancer? J Urol. 2014;191(3):652–5.
67. Briganti A, Chun FK, Salonia A, Gallina A, Farina E, Da Pozzo LF, Rigatti P, Montorsi F, Karakiewicz PI. Validation of a nomogram predicting the probability of lymph node invasion based on the extent of

pelvic lymphadenectomy in patients with clinically localized prostate cancer. BJU Int. 2006; 98(4):788–93.
68. Cagiannos I, Karakiewicz P, Eastham JA, Ohori M, Rabbani F, Gerigk C, Reuter V, Graefen M, Hammerer PG, Erbersdobler A, et al. A preoperative nomogram identifying decreased risk of positive pelvic lymph nodes in patients with prostate cancer. J Urol. 2003;170(5):1798–803.
69. Eifler JB, Feng Z, Lin BM, Partin MT, Humphreys EB, Han M, Epstein JI, Walsh PC, Trock BJ, Partin AW. An updated prostate cancer staging nomogram (Partin tables) based on cases from 2006 to 2011. BJU Int. 2013;111(1):22–9.
70. Abdollah F, Gandaglia G, Suardi N, Capitanio U, Salonia A, Nini A, Moschini M, Sun M, Karakiewicz PI, Shariat SF, et al. More extensive pelvic lymph node dissection improves survival in patients with node-positive prostate cancer. Eur Urol. 2015;67:212–9.
71. Touijer KA, Mazzola CR, Sjoberg DD, Scardino PT, Eastham JA. Long-term outcomes of patients with lymph node metastasis treated with radical prostatectomy without adjuvant androgen-deprivation therapy. Eur Urol. 2013;65(1):20–5.
72. Da Pozzo LF, Cozzarini C, Briganti A, Suardi N, Salonia A, Bertini R, Gallina A, Bianchi M, Fantini GV, Bolognesi A, et al. Long-term follow-up of patients with prostate cancer and nodal metastases treated by pelvic lymphadenectomy and radical prostatectomy: the positive impact of adjuvant radiotherapy. Eur Urol. 2009;55(5):1003–11.
73. Briganti A, Blute ML, Eastham JH, Graefen M, Heidenreich A, Karnes JR, Montorsi F, Studer UE. Pelvic lymph node dissection in prostate cancer. Eur Urol. 2009;55(6):1251–65.
74. Weckermann D, Dorn R, Holl G, Wagner T, Harzmann R. Limitations of radioguided surgery in high-risk prostate cancer. Eur Urol. 2007;51(6):1549–56; discussion 1556–8.
75. de Bonilla-Damia A, Roberto Brouwer O, Meinhardt W, Valdes-Olmos RA. Lymphatic drainage in prostate carcinoma assessed by lymphoscintigraphy and SPECT/CT: its importance for the sentinel node procedure. Rev Esp Med Nucl Imagen Mol. 2012;31(2):66–70.
76. Wawroschek F, Vogt H, Weckermann D, Wagner T, Harzmann R. The sentinel lymph node concept in prostate cancer – first results of gamma probe-guided sentinel lymph node identification. Eur Urol. 1999;36(6):595–600.
77. Wengenmair H, Kopp J, Vogt H, Wawroschek F, Grober S, Dorn R, Heidenreich P. Sentinel lymph node diagnosis in prostatic carcinoma: II. Biokinetics and dosimetry of 99mTc-Nanocolloid after intraprostatic injection. Nuklearmedizin. 2002; 41(2):102–7.
78. Wawroschek F, Vogt H, Weckermann D, Wagner T, Hamm M, Harzmann R. Radioisotope guided pelvic lymph node dissection for prostate cancer. J Urol. 2001;166(5):1715–9.
79. Vogt H, Wawroschek F, Wengenmair H, Wagner T, Kopp J, Dorn R, Grober S, Heidenreich P. Sentinel lymph node diagnosis in prostatic carcinoma: I: method and clinical evaluation. Nuklearmedizin. 2002;41(2):95–101.
80. Rudoni M, Sacchetti GM, Leva L, Inglese E, Monesi G, Minocci D, Frea B. Recent applications of the sentinel lymph node concept: preliminary experience in prostate cancer. Tumori. 2002;88(3):S16–7.
81. Vees H, Dipasquale G, Nouet P, Zilli T, Cozzi L, Miralbell R. Pelvic lymph node irradiation including pararectal sentinel nodes for prostate cancer patients: treatment optimization comparing intensity modulated X-rays, volumetric modulated arc therapy, and intensity modulated proton therapy. Technol Cancer Res Treat. 2015;14:181–9.
82. Ganswindt U, Paulsen F, Corvin S, Hundt I, Alber M, Frey B, Stenzl A, Bares R, Bamberg M, Belka C. Optimized coverage of high-risk adjuvant lymph node areas in prostate cancer using a sentinel node-based, intensity-modulated radiation therapy technique. Int J Radiat Oncol Biol Phys. 2007;67(2):347–55.
83. Ganswindt U, Schilling D, Muller AC, Bares R, Bartenstein P, Belka C. Distribution of prostate sentinel nodes: a SPECT-derived anatomic atlas. Int J Radiat Oncol Biol Phys. 2011;79(5):1364–72.
84. Janetschek G. Can sentinel pelvic lymph node dissection replace extended pelvic lymph node dissection in patients with prostate cancer? Nat Clin Pract Urol. 2007;4(12):636–7.
85. Janetschek G, Hruby S. Prostate cancer: how to manage prostate cancer with lymph node metastases? Nat Rev Urol. 2014;11(3):137–8.
86. Sadeghi R, Tabasi KT, Bazaz SM, Kakhki VR, Massoom AF, Gholami H, Zakavi SR. Sentinel node mapping in the prostate cancer. Meta-analysis. Nuklearmedizin. 2011;50(3):107–15.
87. Manny TB, Patel M, Hemal AK. Fluorescence-enhanced robotic radical prostatectomy using real-time lymphangiography and tissue marking with percutaneous injection of unconjugated indocyanine green: the initial clinical experience in 50 patients. Eur Urol. 2013;65(6):1162–8.
88. Buckle T, Brouwer OR, Valdes Olmos RA, van der Poel HG, van Leeuwen FW. Relationship between intraprostatic tracer deposits and sentinel lymph node mapping in prostate cancer patients. J Nucl Med. 2012;53(7):1026–33.
89. Joniau S, Van den Bergh L, Lerut E, Deroose CM, Haustermans K, Oyen R, Budiharto T, Ameye F, Bogaerts K, Van Poppel H. Mapping of pelvic lymph node metastases in prostate cancer. Eur Urol. 2013;63(3):450–8.
90. Warncke SH, Mattei A, Fuechsel FG, Z'Brun S, Krause T, Studer UE. Detection rate and operating time required for gamma probe-guided sentinel

lymph node resection after injection of technetium-99m nanocolloid into the prostate with and without preoperative imaging. Eur Urol. 2007;52(1):126–32.
91. Holl G, Dorn R, Wengenmair H, Weckermann D, Sciuk J. Validation of sentinel lymph node dissection in prostate cancer: experience in more than 2,000 patients. Eur J Nucl Med Mol Imaging. 2009;36(9):1377–82.
92. Egawa M, Fukuda M, Takashima H, Imao T, Namiki M. Application of sentinel node navigation surgery to prostate cancer. Gan To Kagaku Ryoho. 2005;32(1):117–20.
93. Bastide C, Brenot-Rossi I, Garcia S, Dumas S, Anfossi E, Ragni E, Rossi D. Feasibility and value of the isotope sentinel node mapping technique in prostate cancer. Prog Urol. 2004;14(4):501–6.
94. Weckermann D, Hamm M, Dorn R, Wagner T, Wawroschek F, Harzmann R. Sentinel lymph node dissection in prostate cancer. Experience after more than 800 interventions. Urologe A. 2006;45(6):723–7.
95. Hautmann S, Beitz S, Naumann M, Lutzen U, Seif C, Stubinger SH, van der Horst C, Braun PM, Leuschner I, Henze E, et al. Extended sentinel lymph node dissection in radical prostatectomy for prostate cancer: a study in the Kiel risk population. Urologe A. 2008;47(3):299–303.
96. Corvin S, Schilling D, Eichhorn K, Hundt I, Hennenlotter J, Anastasiadis AG, Kuczyk M, Bares R, Stenzl A. Laparoscopic sentinel lymph node dissection--a novel technique for the staging of prostate cancer. Eur Urol. 2006;49(2):280–5.
97. Meinhardt W, Valdes Olmos RA, van der Poel HG, Bex A, Horenblas S. Laparoscopic sentinel node dissection for prostate carcinoma: technical and anatomical observations. BJU Int. 2008;102(6):714–7.
98. van der Poel HG, Buckle T, Brouwer OR, Valdes Olmos RA, van Leeuwen FW. Intraoperative laparoscopic fluorescence guidance to the sentinel lymph node in prostate cancer patients: clinical proof of concept of an integrated functional imaging approach using a multimodal tracer. Eur Urol. 2011;60(4):826–33.
99. Jeschke S, Beri A, Grull M, Ziegerhofer J, Prammer P, Leeb K, Sega W, Janetschek G. Laparoscopic radioisotope-guided sentinel lymph node dissection in staging of prostate cancer. Eur Urol. 2008;53(1):126–32.
100. Brenot-Rossi I, Bastide C, Garcia S, Dumas S, Esterni B, Pasquier J, Rossi D. Limited pelvic lymphadenectomy using the sentinel lymph node procedure in patients with localised prostate carcinoma: a pilot study. Eur J Nucl Med Mol Imaging. 2005;32(6):635–40.
101. Fukuda M, Egawa M, Imao T, Takashima H, Yokoyama K, Namiki M. Detection of sentinel node micrometastasis by step section and immunohistochemistry in patients with prostate cancer. J Urol. 2007;177(4):1313–7; discussion 1317.
102. Takashima H, Egawa M, Imao T, Fukuda M, Yokoyama K, Namiki M. Validity of sentinel lymph node concept for patients with prostate cancer. J Urol. 2004;171(6 Pt 1):2268–71.
103. Egawa M, Fukuda M, Takashima H, Misaki T, Kinuya K, Terahata S. The sentinel node concept in prostate cancer: present reality and future prospects. Indian J Urol. 2008;24(4):451–6.
104. Wawroschek F, Vogt H, Wengenmair H, Weckermann D, Hamm M, Keil M, Graf G, Heidenreich P, Harzmann R. Prostate lymphoscintigraphy and radio-guided surgery for sentinel lymph node identification in prostate cancer. Technique and results of the first 350 cases. Urol Int. 2003;70(4):303–10.
105. Grasso M, Blanco S, Grasso AA, Crespi A, De Ponti E, Zucchini N, Bovo G, Arosio M, Marcelli S, Messa C. Radio guided radical prostatectomy. Evaluation of feasibility, safety and clinical outcomes. Minerva Urol Nefrol. 2014. http://www.minervamedica.it/en/journals/minerva-urologica-nefrologica/article.php?cod=R19Y9999N00A140012.
106. Mattei A, Fuechsel FG, Bhatta Dhar N, Warncke SH, Thalmann GN, Krause T, Studer UE. The template of the primary lymphatic landing sites of the prostate should be revisited: results of a multimodality mapping study. Eur Urol. 2008;53(1):118–25.
107. Vermeeren L, Meinhardt W, van der Poel HG, Valdes Olmos RA. Lymphatic drainage from the treated versus untreated prostate: feasibility of sentinel node biopsy in recurrent cancer. Eur J Nucl Med Mol Imaging. 2010;37(11):2021–6.
108. Jeschke S, Nambirajan T, Leeb K, Ziegerhofer J, Sega W, Janetschek G. Detection of early lymph node metastases in prostate cancer by laparoscopic radioisotope guided sentinel lymph node dissection. J Urol. 2005;173(6):1943–6.
109. Jeschke S, Lusuardi L, Myatt A, Hruby S, Pirich C, Janetschek G. Visualisation of the lymph node pathway in real time by laparoscopic radioisotope- and fluorescence-guided sentinel lymph node dissection in prostate cancer staging. Urology. 2012;80(5):1080–6.
110. Harisinghani MG, Barentsz J, Hahn PF, Deserno WM, Tabatabaei S, van de Kaa CH, de la Rosette J, Weissleder R. Noninvasive detection of clinically occult lymph-node metastases in prostate cancer. N Engl J Med. 2003;348(25):2491–9.
111. Turkbey B, Hoyt Jr RF, Agarwal HK, Bernardo M, Sankineni S, Johnson L, Grant KB, Rais-Bahrami S, Kobayashi H, Wood BJ, et al. Magnetic resonance sentinel lymph node imaging of the prostate with gadofosveset trisodium-albumin: preliminary results in a canine model. Acad Radiol. 2015;22:646–52.
112. Winter A, Woenkhaus J, Wawroschek F. A novel method for intraoperative sentinel lymph node detection in prostate cancer patients using superparamagnetic iron oxide nanoparticles and a handheld magnetometer: the initial clinical experience. Ann Surg Oncol. 2014;21(13):4390–6.

113. Hacker A, Jeschke S, Leeb K, Prammer K, Ziegerhofer J, Sega W, Langsteger W, Janetschek G. Detection of pelvic lymph node metastases in patients with clinically localized prostate cancer: comparison of [18F] fluorocholine positron emission tomography-computerized tomography and laparoscopic radioisotope guided sentinel lymph node dissection. J Urol. 2006;176(5):2014–8; discussion 2018–9.
114. Inoue S, Shiina H, Arichi N, Mitsui Y, Hiraoka T, Wake K, Sumura M, Honda S, Yasumoto H, Urakami S, et al. Identification of lymphatic pathway involved in the spreading of prostate cancer by fluorescence navigation approach with intraoperatively injected indocyanine green. Can Urol Assoc J. 2011; 5(4):254–9.
115. Rousseau C, Rousseau T, Bridji B, Pallardy A, Lacoste J, Campion L, Testard A, Aillet G, Mouaden A, Curtet C, et al. Laparoscopic sentinel lymph node (SLN) versus extensive pelvic dissection for clinically localized prostate carcinoma. Eur J Nucl Med Mol Imaging. 2012;39(2):291–9.
116. Rousseau C, Rousseau T, Campion L, Lacoste J, Aillet G, Potiron E, Lacombe M, Le Coguic G, Mathieu C, Kraeber-Bodere F. Laparoscopic sentinel lymph node versus hyperextensive pelvic dissection for staging clinically localized prostate carcinoma: a prospective study of 200 patients. J Nucl Med. 2014;55:753–8.
117. Vermeeren L, Muller SH, Meinhardt W, Valdes Olmos RA. Optimizing the colloid particle concentration for improved preoperative and intraoperative image-guided detection of sentinel nodes in prostate cancer. Eur J Nucl Med Mol Imaging. 2010; 37(7):1328–34.
118. Weckermann D, Dorn R, Trefz M, Wagner T, Wawroschek F, Harzmann R. Sentinel lymph node dissection for prostate cancer: experience with more than 1,000 patients. J Urol. 2007;177(3):916–20.
119. Winter A, Kneib T, Henke RP, Wawroschek F. Sentinel lymph node dissection in more than 1200 prostate cancer cases: Rate and prediction of lymph node involvement depending on preoperative tumor characteristics. Int J Urol. 2014;21(1):58–63.
120. Brenot-Rossi I, Rossi D, Esterni B, Brunelle S, Chuto G, Bastide C. Radioguided sentinel lymph node dissection in patients with localised prostate carcinoma: influence of the dose of radiolabelled colloid to avoid failure of the procedure. Eur J Nucl Med Mol Imaging. 2008;35(1):32–8.
121. Krag DN, Weaver DL, Alex JC, Fairbank JT. Surgical resection and radiolocalization of the sentinel lymph node in breast cancer using a gamma probe. Surg Oncol. 1993;2(6):335–9; discussion 340.
122. Meinhardt W, van der Poel HG, Valdes Olmos RA, Bex A, Brouwer OR, Horenblas S. Laparoscopic sentinel lymph node biopsy for prostate cancer: the relevance of locations outside the extended dissection area. Prostate Cancer. 2012;2012:751753.
123. Ponholzer A, Lamche M, Klitsch M, Kraischits N, Hiess M, Schenner M, Brossner C, Schramek P. Sentinel lymphadenectomy compared to extended lymphadenectomy in men with prostate cancer undergoing prostatectomy. Anticancer Res. 2012; 32(3):1033–6.
124. Stanik M, Capak I, Macik D, Vasina J, Lzicarova E, Jarkovsky J, Sustr M, Miklanek D, Dolezel J. Sentinel lymph node dissection combined with meticulous histology increases the detection rate of nodal metastases in prostate cancer. Int Urol Nephrol. 2014;46(8):1543–9.
125. van der Poel HG, de Blok W, Tillier C, van Muilekom E. Robot-assisted laparoscopic prostatectomy: nodal dissection results during the first 440 cases by two surgeons. J Endourol. 2012;26(12):1618–24.
126. Silva Jr N, Anselmi CE, Anselmi OE, Madke RR, Hunsche A, Souto JS, Souto CA, Sica FD, Pioner GT, Macalos EC, et al. Use of the gamma probe in sentinel lymph node biopsy in patients with prostate cancer. Nucl Med Commun. 2005;26(12):1081–6.
127. Kizu H, Takayama T, Fukuda M, Egawa M, Tsushima H, Yamada M, Ichiyanagi K, Yokoyama K, Onoguchi M, Tonami N. Fusion of SPECT and multidetector CT images for accurate localization of pelvic sentinel lymph nodes in prostate cancer patients. J Nucl Med Technol. 2005;33(2):78–82.
128. Krengli M, Ballare A, Cannillo B, Rudoni M, Kocjancic E, Loi G, Brambilla M, Inglese E, Frea B. Potential advantage of studying the lymphatic drainage by sentinel node technique and SPECT-CT image fusion for pelvic irradiation of prostate cancer. Int J Radiat Oncol Biol Phys. 2006;66(4):1100–4.
129. Weckermann D, Holl G, Dorn R, Wagner T, Harzmann R. Reliability of preoperative diagnostics and location of lymph node metastases in presumed unilateral prostate cancer. BJU Int. 2007;99(5): 1036–40.
130. Vermeeren L, Valdes Olmos RA, Meinhardt W, Bex A, van der Poel HG, Vogel WV, Sivro F, Hoefnagel CA, Horenblas S. Value of SPECT/CT for detection and anatomic localization of sentinel lymph nodes before laparoscopic sentinel node lymphadenectomy in prostate carcinoma. J Nucl Med. 2009;50(6): 865–70.
131. Vermeeren L, Valdes Olmos RA, Meinhardt W, Bex A, van der Poel HG, Vogel WV, Sivro F, Hoefnagel CA, Horenblas S. Intraoperative radioguidance with a portable gamma camera: a novel technique for laparoscopic sentinel node localisation in urological malignancies. Eur J Nucl Med Mol Imaging. 2009;36(7):1029–36.
132. Schilling D, Boekeler U, Gakis G, Schwentner C, Corvin S, Sotlar K, Muller AC, Bares R, Stenzl A. Modified concept for radioisotope-guided sentinel lymph node dissection in prostate cancer. World J Urol. 2010;28(6):715–20.
133. Vermeeren L, Valdes Olmos RA, Meinhardt W, Horenblas S. Intraoperative imaging for sentinel node identification in prostate carcinoma: its use in combination with other techniques. J Nucl Med. 2011;52(5):741–4.

134. Yuen K, Miura T, Sakai I, Kiyosue A, Yamashita M. Intraoperative fluorescence imaging for detection of sentinel lymph nodes and lymphatic vessels during open prostatectomy using indocyanine green. J Urol. 2015;194:371–7.
135. Van den Bergh L, Joniau S, Haustermans K, Deroose CM, Isebaert S, Oyen R, Mottaghy FM, Ameye F, Berkers J, Van Poppel H, et al. Reliability of sentinel node procedure for lymph node staging in prostate cancer patients at high risk for lymph node involvement. Acta Oncol. 2015;54(6): 896–902.
136. Sherif A, De La Torre M, Malmstrom PU, Thorn M. Lymphatic mapping and detection of sentinel nodes in patients with bladder cancer. J Urol. 2001;166(3):812–5.
137. Roth B, Wissmeyer MP, Zehnder P, Birkhauser FD, Thalmann GN, Krause TM, Studer UE. A new multimodality technique accurately maps the primary lymphatic landing sites of the bladder. Eur Urol. 2010;57(2):205–11.
138. Schaafsma BE, Verbeek FP, Elzevier HW, Tummers QR, van der Vorst JR, Frangioni JV, van de Velde CJ, Pelger RC, Vahrmeijer AL. Optimization of sentinel lymph node mapping in bladder cancer using near-infrared fluorescence imaging. J Surg Oncol. 2014;110(7):845–50.
139. Sherif A, Garske U, de la Torre M, Thorn M. Hybrid SPECT-CT: an additional technique for sentinel node detection of patients with invasive bladder cancer. Eur Urol. 2006;50(1):83–91.
140. Liedberg F, Chebil G, Davidsson T, Malmstrom PU, Sherif A, Thorn M, De La Torre M. Mansson W: [Bladder cancer and the sentinel node concept]. Aktuelle Urol. 2003;34(2):115–8.
141. Liedberg F, Chebil G, Davidsson T, Gudjonsson S, Mansson W. Intraoperative sentinel node detection improves nodal staging in invasive bladder cancer. J Urol. 2006;175(1):84–8; discussion 88–9.
142. Sherif A, Hasan MN, Marits P, Karlsson M, Winqvist O, Thorn M. Feasibility of T-cell-based adoptive immunotherapy in the first 12 patients with advanced urothelial urinary bladder cancer. Preliminary data on a new immunologic treatment based on the sentinel node concept. Eur Urol. 2010;58(1):105–11.
143. Brouwer OR, Valdes Olmos RA, Vermeeren L, Hoefnagel CA, Nieweg OE, Horenblas S. SPECT/CT and a portable gamma-camera for image-guided laparoscopic sentinel node biopsy in testicular cancer. J Nucl Med. 2011;52(4):551–4.
144. Tanis PJ, Horenblas S, Valdes Olmos RA, Hoefnagel CA, Nieweg OE. Feasibility of sentinel node lymphoscintigraphy in stage I testicular cancer. Eur J Nucl Med Mol Imaging. 2002;29(5):670–3.
145. Ohyama C, Chiba Y, Yamazaki T, Endoh M, Hoshi S, Arai Y. Lymphatic mapping and gamma probe guided laparoscopic biopsy of sentinel lymph node in patients with clinical stage I testicular tumor. J Urol. 2002;168(4 Pt 1):1390–5.
146. Satoh M, Ito A, Kaiho Y, Nakagawa H, Saito S, Endo M, Ohyama C, Arai Y. Intraoperative, radio-guided sentinel lymph node mapping in laparoscopic lymph node dissection for Stage I testicular carcinoma. Cancer. 2005;103(10):2067–72.
147. Bex A, Vermeeren L, Meinhardt W, Prevoo W, Horenblas S, Valdes Olmos RA. Intraoperative sentinel node identification and sampling in clinically node-negative renal cell carcinoma: initial experience in 20 patients. World J Urol. 2011;29(6): 793–9.
148. Sherif AM, Eriksson E, Thorn M, Vasko J, Riklund K, Ohberg L, Ljungberg BJ. Sentinel node detection in renal cell carcinoma. A feasibility study for detection of tumour-draining lymph nodes. BJU Int. 2012;109(8):1134–9.
149. Karmali RJ, Suami H, Wood CG, Karam JA. Lymphatic drainage in renal cell carcinoma: back to the basics. BJU Int. 2014;114(6):806–17.
150. Bex A, Vermeeren L, de Windt G, Prevoo W, Horenblas S, Olmos RA. Feasibility of sentinel node detection in renal cell carcinoma: a pilot study. Eur J Nucl Med Mol Imaging. 2010;37(6):1117–23.
151. Brouwer OR, Noe A, Olmos RA, Bex A. Lymphatic drainage from renal cell carcinoma along the thoracic duct visualized with SPECT/CT. Lymphat Res Biol. 2013;11(4):233–8.

Radioguided Sentinel Lymph Node Mapping and Biopsy in Gynaecological Malignancies

16

Pilar Paredes and Sergi Vidal-Sicart

Contents

Abstract

The application of radioguided surgery to gynaecological tumours is more complex than in other fields such as breast cancer or melanoma, where its use is widespread. That complexity probably explains the current lack of applications.

The most easily accessible of gynaecological tumours, cancer of the vulva, is where sentinel lymph node biopsy (SLNB) is most in use. However, this cancer has a low incidence. In cervical cancer, radioguided surgery is well established, with a globally accepted methodology. But, thanks to new vaccines against the human papilloma virus, its occurrence is reducing. In the case of endometrial cancer, a methodological consensus is still pending. There is a scarcity of data regarding vaginal tumours (due to its low frequency) and ovarian cancer (technically controversial).

Over the past years, near-infrared (NIR) fluorescence imaging has emerged as a promising complimentary technique for intraoperative visualisation of tumour tissue, SLN and vital structures. This technology provides real-time images, which allows accurate guidance during surgery. In gynaecological oncology, NIR fluorescence imaging has been used for intraoperative identification of SLN vulvar, cervical and endometrial cancer.

P. Paredes
Nuclear Medicine Department, Hospital Clínic Barcelona, Barcelona, Spain
e-mail: pparedes@clinic.ub.es

S. Vidal-Sicart (✉)
Nuclear Medicine Department, Hospital Clínic Barcelona. Institut d'Investigació Biomèdica August Pi I Sunyer (IDIBAPS), Barcelona, Spain
e-mail: SVIDAL@clinic.ub.es

K. Herrmann et al. (eds.), *Radioguided Surgery: Current Applications and Innovative Directions in Clinical Practice*, DOI 10.1007/978-3-319-26051-8_16

16.1 Clinical Value and Relevance of Radioguided Sentinel Lymph Node Mapping and Biopsy in Gynaecological Malignancies

The clinical value and relevance of radioguided sentinel lymph node (SLN) mapping and biopsy to the treatment of gynaecological malignancies is very dependent upon the gynaecological tumour type being treated [1–50]. The indications and contraindications for radioguided SLN biopsy (SLNB) in gynaecological malignancies are outlined in Table 16.1. The most relevant clinical studies which have evaluated radioguided SLNB in gynaecological malignancies are outlined in Table 16.2. For vulvar cancer [1, 2] and endometrial cancer [3], SLNB allows for a significant reduction in patient-related morbidity, leading to a decrease in both intraoperative and early postoperative complications, as well as reduces the length of total time under anaesthesia. For cervical cancer, SLNB represents a useful tool for helping to determine the best postoperative adjuvant therapeutic approach. During cervical cancer surgery, the finding of a positive SLN allows the surgeon to consider foregoing a hysterectomy or trachelectomy, while proceeding forward with a para-aortic lymphadenectomy secondary to the higher risk of further lymph node involvement. The use of this methodological approach in cervical cancer can spare the patient from unnecessary further surgery (i.e., removal of the primary cervical tumour), and then chemoradiation therapy becomes the primary postoperative adjuvant treatment of choice. In contrast, if the SLN is negative for tumor involvement, then hysterectomy or trachelectomy can be performed as planned. Finally, for ovarian cancer [4–6] and vaginal cancer [20–22], the utility of SLNB has only been evaluated in an extremely limited fashion, and therefore, its clinical value and relevance for ovarian cancer and vaginal cancer remains unclear.

16.2 Preoperative Imaging

In malignancies with intra-abdominal lymphatic drainage, we need a preoperative lymphoscintigraphic image to draw the lymphatic map of the tumour. The acquisition of this lymphatic map can be performed between 12 and 18 h before surgery, on either the previous or the same day. A time delay between preoperative lymphoscintigraphy and surgery is advisable so that enough views can be acquired to precisely define the location and number of SLNs. For this purpose, a tomographic SPECT/CT study may be necessary at times.

Some methodological aspects will affect the choice of radiotracer to be injected, such as the experience of the surgical team and the medical devices available. In terms of accuracy in intraoperative detection of SLN, radiotracers have excelled, and in the hands of an experienced surgical team, gamma probes detect a higher number of SLN than does preoperative lymphoscintigraphy. Nonetheless, in some tumours, such as cervical cancer, the combined technique of radiotracer plus blue dyes offers the highest sensitivity [11]. Nowadays, the use of blue dye alone is not recommended for any gynaecological malignancy. While use of blue dye obviates the need for lymphoscintigraphy,

Table 16.1 Indications and contraindications for radioguided sentinel lymph node biopsy in gynaecological malignancies

<table>
<tr><th>Tumour</th><th>Indications</th><th>Contraindications</th></tr>
<tr><td>Vulvar SCC cancer</td><td>SCC Ib–II
T1–T2 < 4 cm</td><td rowspan="6">Pregnancy (relative contraindication)
Previous surgery on the present surgical field (e.g. inguinofemoral lymphadenectomy in vulvar cancer)[a]
Node involvement based on other image modalities</td></tr>
<tr><td>Vulvovaginal melanoma</td><td>Breslow 1–4 mm (T1b-T4b)</td></tr>
<tr><td>Cervical cancer</td><td>SCC Ia2-Ib1 (IA1 + LVI)</td></tr>
<tr><td>Endometrial cancer</td><td>Not established</td></tr>
<tr><td>Vaginal cancer</td><td>Not established</td></tr>
<tr><td>Ovarian cancer</td><td>Not indicated</td></tr>
</table>

SCC squamous cell carcinoma, *LVI* lymphovascular invasion

[a]Cone biopsy is not a contraindication for cervical sentinel lymph node detection

Table 16.2 Summary of the most relevant studies for radioguided sentinel lymph node biopsy in gynaecological malignancies

Tumour	Author	*n*	Stage	Injection type	Tracer	Surgical approach	Detection rate (DR)	Radiotracer DR	Blue DR	ICG DR
Endometrial	Frati, 2014 [7]	118	I–II	Cervical	RT + BD	–	89 %	86 %	N/A	–
Endometrial	Robova, 2009 [8]	91		Subserous vs. HSC	RT + BD vs. RT	LT	73 % vs. 50 %			
Endometrial	Rossi, 2013 [9]	29	?	Cervical vs. HSC	ICG		82 % vs. 33 %	–	–	82 %
Endometrial	Holloway, 2012 [10]	35	–	Cervical	BD + ICG	LSC robotical	100 %	–	77 %	97 %
Cervical	Bats, 2013 [11]	139	IA1 (VLI+)-IB1	–	RT + BD	LSC	98 %	94 %	90 %	–
Cervical	Altgassen, 2008 [12]	590	all	–	RT + BD	LSC or LT	90 %	82 %	82 %	–
Cervical	Crane, 2011 [13]	10	IA2–IIA	–	BD + ICG	LT	90 %	–	N/A	90 %
Cervical+ Endometrial	Plante, 2015 [14]	50	Early stages	–	ICG	LSC	96 %	–	–	96 %
Vulvar	van der Zee, 2008 [1]	403	T1–T2 < 4 cm	NP	RT + BD	–	–	–	–	–
Vulvar	Hampl, 2008 [15]	127	T1–T3	NP	RT + BD	–	100 %	94 %	63 %	–
Vulvar	Levenback, 2012 [16]	452	T1–T2 < 6 cm	NP	RT + BD	–	92.5 %	76 %	85 %	–
Vulvar	Matheron, 2013 [17]	15	–	NP	RT + BD + ICG	–	98 %	97 %	85 %	–
Vulvar	Hutteman, 2012 [18]	14	I–II	NP	RT + BD + ICG	–	100 %	98 %	65 %	96 %
Ovarian	Kleppe, 2014 [6]	21	–	Ovarian ligaments	RT + BD	LT	96 %	100 %	79 %	100 %
Vaginal	Hertel, 2013 [19]	7	–	–	RT + BD	–	100 %	–	–	–

HSC hysteroscopy, *LT* laparotomy, *LSC* laparoscopy, *N/A* non-available some lymph nodes located within unexpected lymphatic areas can be missed due to the lack of a lymphatic map of the tumour. Clinical situations in which the use of blue dye is indicated in a combined technique are SLN detection in vulvar cancer by a non-trained team, all cases of SLN detection in cervical cancer, and patients with faint drainage seen on preoperative lymphoscintigraphy [2].

16.2.1 Vulvar Cancer

16.2.1.1 Preoperative Imaging and Lymphatic Drainage

The normal distribution pattern of drainage for vulvar cancer is bilateral inguinofemoral lymph nodes, first to the superficial lymph nodes and then onto the deep lymph nodes. Some midline structures, such as the clitoris, can drain directly to deep lymph nodes.

In vulvar cancer, due to its superficial drainage and easy access to the primary lesion, performing the radiotracer injection under the gamma camera and acquisition of a dynamic study is advisable. This allows visualisation of lymph pathways and helps establish which is the first lymph node to receive the radiotracer, i.e. the SLN. Preoperative lymphoscintigraphy should include an early and late planar study, at 10 min and 2 h after radiotracer injection, to accurately differentiate the SLN from second echelon lymph nodes. Bilateral drainage is expected in vulvar tumours placed on midline or until 2 cm from the midline. That means that a lack of drainage to one of the two sides of the inguinofemoral regions requires further actions to ensure the bilateral drainage. The first option is to perform a second injection of the radiotracer, considering the superficial location of the vulva. The injection dose can be lower or equal than the previous injection dose, but an increase in the volume provides higher intercellular pressure that facilitates the drainage. Another option is the acquisition of a SPECT/CT study (Fig. 16.1) to increase the number of SLN and lymphatic echelons visualised [24, 25]. It can be performed after radiotracer reinjection or directly after the first preoperative lymphoscintigraphy. If unilateral drainage is confirmed on tomographic images, radiotracer reinjection can then be administered. As mentioned before, lateralised vulvar tumours are considered as an exception when located in the labia majora, 2 cm away from the midline. In these cases, unilateral drainage is accepted and a second radiotracer injection is not required. But if bilateral drainage is found, all SLNs must be removed, including those on contralateral region.

16.2.1.2 Tracers and Route of Administration

Standard tracers used for SLN mapping in vulvar cancer are blue dye and radiotracers. They are usually combined, with the administration of radiotracer previous to surgery and the blue dye at the onset of surgery. Radiotracers have demonstrated excellent detection rate if used alone, but blue dyes can provide an additional degree of confidence to the surgical team in such superficial drainage as vulvar's [2]. The use of blue dye as the only tracer is not recommended because of its lower rate of detection. Fluorescent tracers, such as indocyanine green, appear as an alternative to radioguided surgery, as have developed later.

16.2.1.3 Preoperative Imaging: Role of Planar and Tomographic Images

As mentioned before, early and late planar acquisitions during preoperative imaging are essential to distinguish which lymph nodes are SLN and which are second echelon nodes. In vulvar cancer, an early study is performed immediately after the dynamic study, at 10 min after tracer injection, and a late study will be acquired 2-h post-injection. The lymph node that first receives direct drainage from the tumour or shows an increase of uptake in the latter images will be considered to be an SLN as opposed to the other lymph nodes detected. Inguinofemoral regions will be considered as two independent lymphatic echelons. The role of SPECT/CT in this malignancy is limited [17] because of the low rate of cases with aberrant drainage and the superficial location of SLNs.

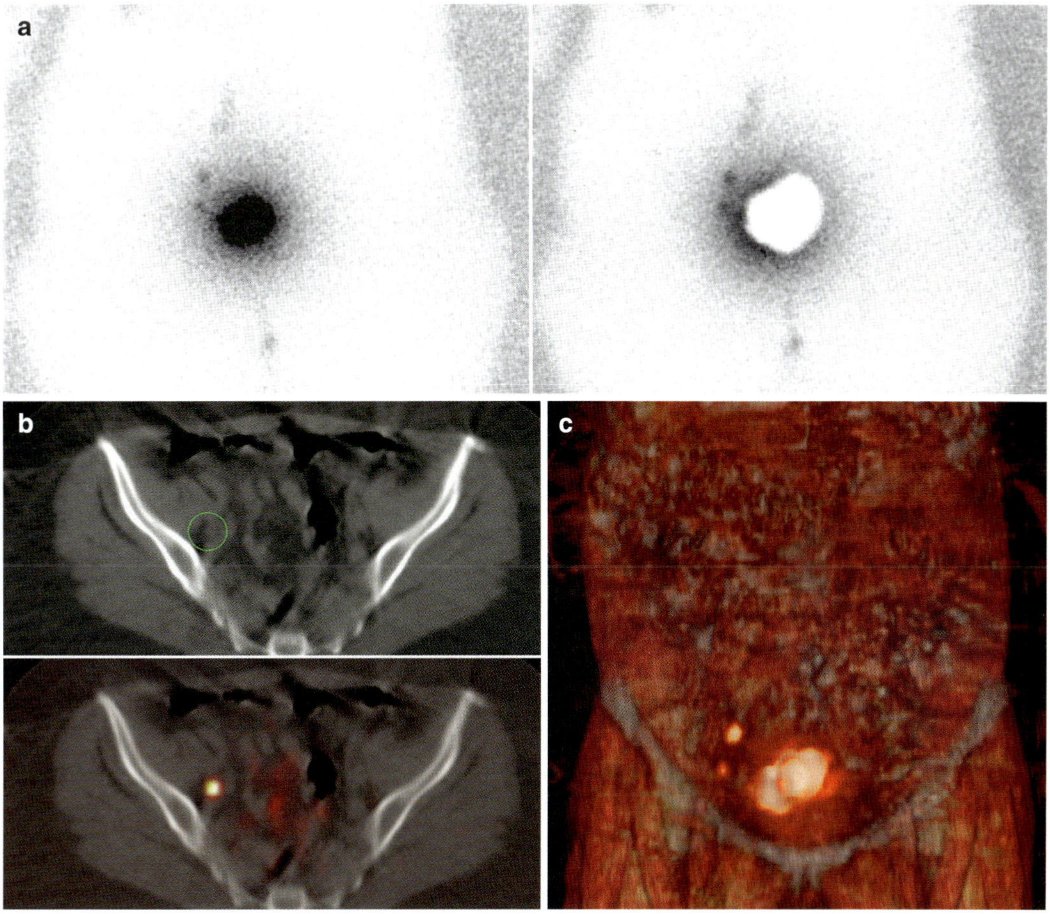

Fig. 16.1 *Lymphatic drainage from a cervix uteri tumour (Ib2).* Seventy-six-year-old woman diagnosed of cervical cancer (Ib2) who was submitted to SLNB. Planar views (**a**) show unilateral drainage to the right pelvic nodes. A lead shield (*right*) was used to avoid activity from the injection site. A SPECT/CT study (**b**, **c**) was performed 2 h after tracer injection to confirm the lack of left drainage. Two SLNs are shown on volume-rendering image (**c**) at the right side; one of them was localised in the external iliac chain on CT (**b**) and fusion (**c**) images

16.2.1.4 Alternatives to Radioguided Surgery

The main alternative to using radiotracers for identifying SLNs during radioguided surgery is to use blue dyes. However, the use of blue dye alone (without concomitant use of a radiotracer) is not recommended. Due to its rapid flow through the lymphatic system, blue dye administration must be done in the operating room shortly before the start of the operation. This short time detection window may partially explain why approximately 35 % of the time that SLNs identified with radiotracer fail to accumulate any blue dye. On a per groin basis, in 55–75 % of groins, at least one blue SLN could be detected.

Other recently introduced alternatives to radioguided surgery are fluorescent tracers, such as indocyanine green (ICG) [26], with its near-infrared (NIR) emission, which can be detected by special intraoperative devices. They have been most commonly used in the treatment of malignant melanoma and breast cancer. Due to its superficial drainage, the detection of fluorescent lymph nodes is easy seen in vulvar cancer [17, 18, 27], the first gynaecological tumour to be evaluated with a fluorescent tracer. The use of a fluorescent tracer does not contraindicate the simultaneous injection of other tracers, blue dyes or radiotracers. The injection must be performed at the onset of the surgery, and the fluorescent tracer can be seen to migrate along the lymph pathways until it reaches a SLN.

The main disadvantage of fluorescent tracers is that intraoperative detection must be carried out in the dark to appreciate the fluorescence, which may impair the surgeon's ability to adequately see the surgical field for actively performing tissue dissection for identification and removal of SLNs.

An optimisation of ICG dosage has been tested in vulvar [28] and uterine [29] cancers. Schaafsma et al. developed a tracer combining ICG and human serum albumin (HSA). While the intraoperative rate of detection of this new molecule reaches 78 % for cervical cancer [29], the results are similar to those of ICG alone, and the authors conclude that it can be used as a stand-alone tracer [28, 29].

Intraoperative fluorescence imaging allows the visualisation of at least one SLN in 86 % of groins with a total of 96 % of SLNs visualised intraoperatively. Despite the improved tissue penetration compared to that of blue dye, visualisation of ICG is still limited to a depth below 10 mm. For this reason, a hybrid tracer which combines the advantages of radiotracers (99mTc- albumin nanocolloid) and fluorescence has been developed [30]. The main advantage is to add the functional properties of radiotracers while allowing fluorescence-based SLN detection during surgery. It has been widely used in other pelvic tumours having similar characteristic to gynaecological tumours, such as prostate cancer [31]. Results show a high intraoperative detection rate secondary to the advantages of using dual tracers. Nonetheless, in gynaecology to date, there is only two published studies, in vulvar cancer [17, 32], with a 98 % intraoperative SLN detection rate.

16.2.2 Cervical Cancer

16.2.2.1 Preoperative Imaging and Lymphatic Drainage

The expected drainage for cervical cancer is bilateral migration to the external iliac lymph nodes. Obturator is the commonest group, followed by a progression to common iliac and para-aortic nodes as the second echelon group [33]. However, direct para-aortic drainage has been observed in 1 % of cases [34]. So, if para-aortic drainage is visualised on early lymphoscintigraphic images, these SLNs require a surgical approach.

As explained for vulvar cancer, in cervical tumours, bilateral drainage is also expected, so new acquisitions are required when a lack of tracer migration is observed. A second injection is less feasible than for vulvar tumours, but possible. The best option is the acquisition of a SPECT/CT study (Fig. 16.1), preferably included in clinical routine, to increase the number of SLN and lymphatic echelons visualised [24, 25].

16.2.2.2 Tracers and Route of Administration

In cervical cancer, the combination of blue dye and radiotracer is recommended because of the added advantages it offers to both techniques. The radiotracer allows for rapid localization of SLNs and allows the surgeon to minimize the extent of necessary soft tissue dissection for successful identification of SLNs. While, in turn, blue dye paper visual cues for instantaneous visual recognition of an SLN during the identification process. The detection rate with using dual tracers is superior to that of either of them alone [12, 35], even the radiotracer.

16.2.2.3 Preoperative Imaging: Role of Planar and Tomographic Images

As mentioned before, early and late planar acquisitions are essential to distinguish which lymph nodes are SLN and which are second echelon nodes. In vulvar cancer, an early study is performed immediately after the dynamic study, but in other tumour types, it will be acquired at 30 min after injection. Late study will be acquired 2-h post-injection.

Lymph nodes seen on preoperative lymphoscintigraphy from different lymphatic chains are regarded as independent SLNs (Fig. 16.2), including para-aortic lymph nodes. In cervical and endometrial cancer, at least three lymphatic echelons have to be considered: right pelvic lymph nodes, left pelvic lymph nodes and para-aortic lymph nodes. The lack of hot spots in any of these areas required dissection of the contralateral lym-

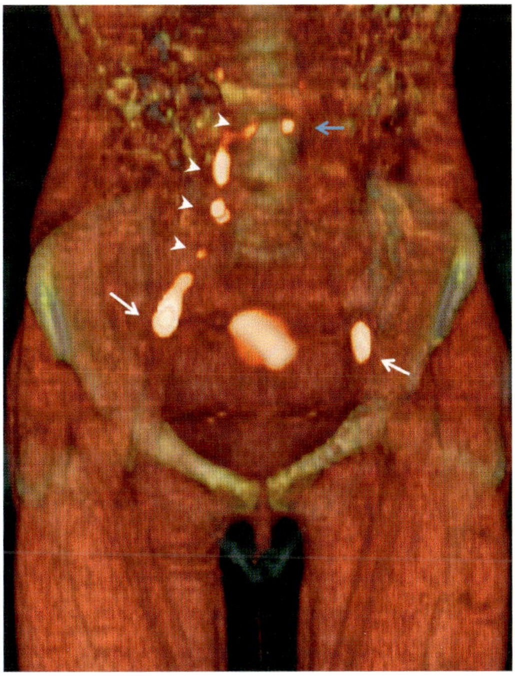

Fig. 16.2 *SPECT/CT in cervical cancer.* Volume-rendering image shows bilateral pelvic drainage in the external iliac chains (*arrows*) and in the left para-aortic region (*blue arrow*). Secondary lymphatic nodes are represented on the right side (*head arrow*)

phatic area, due to the possibility of a metastatic blockage [36]. The lack of para-aortic drainage is not a requisite for lymphadenectomy. If unilateral drainage is seen, a prior surgical or radiotherapeutic intervention must be ruled out. In such cases, the injection of blue dye prior to lymphatic dissection will allow the detection of SLNs not detected on preoperative lymphoscintigraphy and can help avoid a lymphadenectomy.

To decide on the best surgical approach, interpretation of preoperative lymphatic map images by nuclear medicine specialists, together with surgeons, prior to surgery, is highly recommended.

16.2.2.4 Alternatives to Radioguided Surgery

For tumours from the cervix, the best methodology is to combine blue dyes and radiotracers, with the highest detection rate, greater than radiotracer or blue dye alone [12].

An increase in the use of fluorescence in intra-abdominal tumours, cervical and endometrial cancer, has been dependent on the development of fluorescent optics for use inside laparoscopic devices, so advances are very recent. So far, results are promising, with an intraoperative detection of 75 % for the first series of patients, which increases to 95 % in later series [37, 38].

As a non-radioactive tracer, it has been compared to blue dyes, with generally similar results [38, 39] for intraoperative detection. However, the fluorescent tracer ICG can be beneficial in patients with increased body mass index (BMI), since the identification of SLNs in this patient population can be challenging and suboptimal. Generally speaking, ICG seems to have a higher detection rate than blue dye [13, 39] (Fig. 16.3). The first feasibility study was done by Crane et al. [13] in a small series of 10 patients. They observed real-time NIR fluorescence lymphatic pathway mapping in 60 % of cases.

16.2.3 Endometrial Cancer

16.2.3.1 Preoperative Imaging and Lymphatic Drainage

Drainage from corpus uteri differs from cervical drainage. The two lower thirds of the corpus is similar to the cervix. However, the upper third drains directly to the para-aortic area. Establishing this pattern of drainage is essential for a correct interpretation of preoperative lymphoscintigraphic images and identifying the best approach to SLNB. The main obstacle to endometrial SLN detection is the difficulty in reaching the lesion. Although cervical injection provides an easy injection route, without complications, it only offers partial information, because drainage in the upper third of the endometrium remains unstudied [40]. Therefore, a deeper, subendometrial, serous or myometrial injection is required to ensure complete characterization of this lymphatic drainage pathways of the uterus [8].

The methodology of preoperative imaging acquisition is similar than those for cervical cancer and includes early and late planar images and, if possible, a tomographic study. In absence of radiotracer migration in one of the expected echelons (two pelvic sides and para-aortic region), metastatic blockage has to be suspected and further image acquisitions performed.

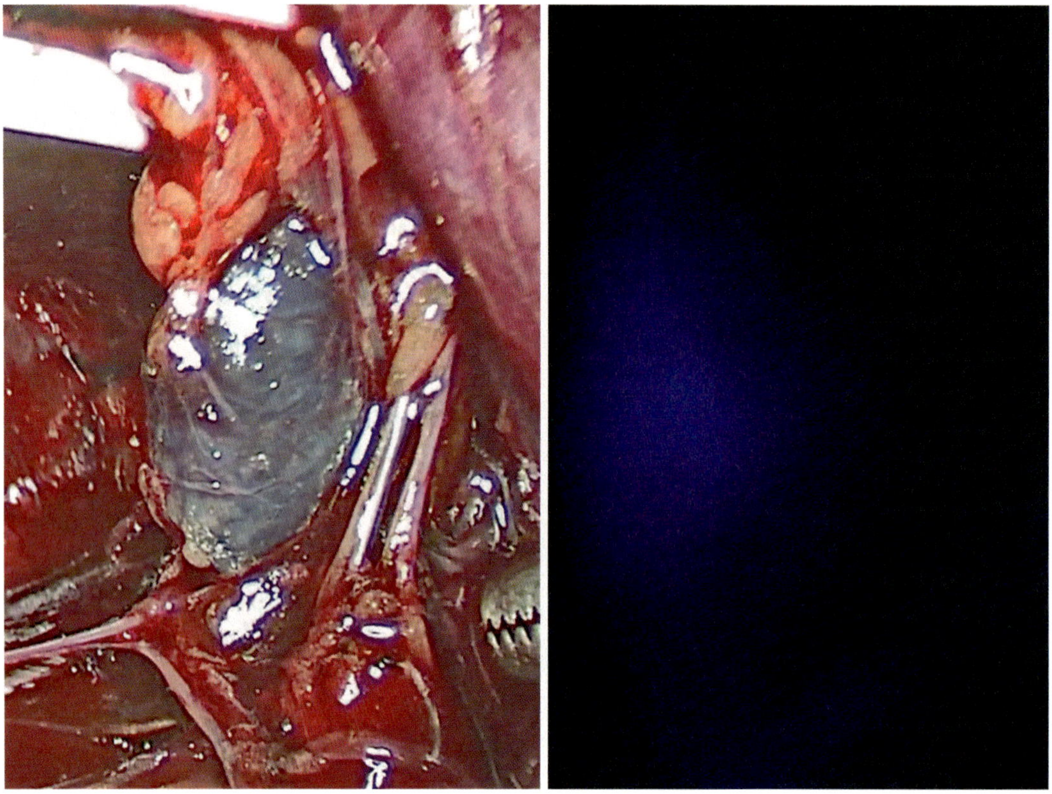

Fig. 16.3 *Radioguided surgery with ^{99m}Tc-colloid + ICG and blue dye*. An external iliac SLN detected by fluorescent emission on NIR spectrum (*right*) and, once localised, by blue dye stain with ambient light (*left*)

16.2.3.2 Tracers and Route of Administration

The choice of tracer depends on the type of injection used. *Cervical injection* is the most accessible, reporting the highest rate of drainage [7, 41]. With this "superficial" injection, both tracers give good results, although lymphatic tracks are sometimes difficult to identify, due to an increase in fatty tissue in these patients. With deeper injections, however, performed during surgery, prior to hysterectomy, the use of dyes such as blue dye or fluorescent tracers gives the surgeon more guarantees, as is described at the end of this section. The deep injection of the tracer can be performed by laparotomy, laparoscopy or hysteroscopy. Injection by laparotomy or laparoscopy offer instantaneous SLN detection during the same surgical procedure. But unexpected lymph nodes that are not in the usual drainage territories can be missed due to the lack of a lymphatic map. Hysteroscopy enjoys the benefits of the other techniques: the injection can be performed in advance, prior to surgery (up to 18 h before), so as to obtain a lymphatic map of the tumour on lymphoscintigraphy; and the endometrial tumour drainage can be assessed rather than that of the cervix alone. The rate of detection reaches 100 % in some centres [42], exceeding that of intraoperative injections [8]. But morbidity is grearter than with cervical or intraoperative injection, as two surgical interventions are required. In terms of morbidity, injection by hysteroscopy is the least recommended. A recent technique, known as *TUMIR* [43], is a transvaginal myometrial injection guided by ultrasonography; consisting of a myometrial injection in the corpus uteri the day before surgery, and reports a low morbidity for the patient. Ultrasonography can be carried out in advance, allowing for preoperative lymphoscintigraphy and a planned surgical approach. Results match or even exceed hysteroscopy [44], with less morbidity. The use of blue dyes in endometrial cancer does not increase SLN detection due to the amount of fatty tissue surrounding lymphatic chains and impairing the identification of blue stained lymph nodes.

16.2.3.3 Preoperative Imaging: Role of Planar and Tomographic Images

See Sect. 16.2.2.3.

16.2.3.4 Alternatives to Radioguided Surgery

The use of blue dye alone is not recommended for any gynaecological malignancy, especially in endometrial cancer, due to the amount of fat tissue surrounding the nodes. This disadvantage is also present for fluorescent tracers, but ICG seems to have higher detection rate than blue dye [10, 29, 37, 39] (Fig. 16.3). Rossi et al. used ICG fluorescence with robot-assisted laparoscopic surgery in patients with cervical or endometrial cancer, with higher detection (85 %), although there was one false-negative result after lymphadenectomy. Bilateral SLN detection is more frequently seen using ICG fluorescence (97 %) as opposed to using blue dye (77 %) [10]. In these patients, the combination of ICG with a radiotracer may be a good alternative.

16.3 Intraoperative Detection (and Resection of SLNs/Tumour)

Intraoperative detection includes the use of blue dyes or the latest fluorescent tracers, either hybrid or alone, as has been explained above. Blue dyes require only visual inspection but a greater extent of dissection of the lymphatic pathways to reach the blue stained lymph node, meaning the SLN. However, the aim of reducing morbidity is compromised due to the need for greater dissection of soft tissue.

The detection of fluorescent tracers requires near-infrared devices to localise the source of the emission of fluorescence. As has already been mentioned, a dimly lit room is necessary to visualise the light emission. This problem has been addressed with the addition of an NIR optic in the laparoscopic instruments that allows the surgeon to switch easily from normal light view to NIR view. The sensitivity of the devices varies from centre to centre and, in some cases, a low level of ambient light has to be maintained in order to facilitate the dissection of soft tissues around the targeted SLN.

Nowadays, in the intraoperative detection of SLNs, 1D gamma probes are supplemented by the use of portable gamma cameras (PGCs) or intraoperative SPECT, called freehand SPECT (fhSPECT). These devices are not an alternative to gamma probes in the operating theatre but offer extra visual information. Currently, the gamma probe is still the best tool for locating SLNs. But in gynaecological tumours, the greater anatomical complexity and the process of physiological radiotracer elimination can mask activity coming from the SLN, making intraoperative visual information more useful. Examples of this are the detection of an inguino-femoral SLN adjacent to the radiotracer injection site in vulvar cancer or for parametrial lymph nodes in cervical cancer. Moreover, in the case of intra-abdominal drainage, the slight activity coming from inside the ureter can mask detection of retroperitoneal and common iliac SLNs. As the liver is an organ with high colloid uptake, hepatic activity hampers the localisation of a retroperitoneal SLN with laparoscopic probe, especially in its retroperitoneal approach from the left side, due to the limitation of movement.

Therefore, intraoperative gamma camera imaging devices can positively impact upon the success of radioguided surgery procedures for gynaecologic malignancies.

16.3.1 Portable Gamma Cameras

Portable gamma cameras (PGCs) are small-sized devices capable of acquiring an intraoperative image during surgery. The image can be obtained in a short space of time and as many views as are necessary can be acquired during the surgical procedure. Once the SLNs are harvested, obtaining a post-excision intraoperative image (showing the absence of any residual hot spots) can help to

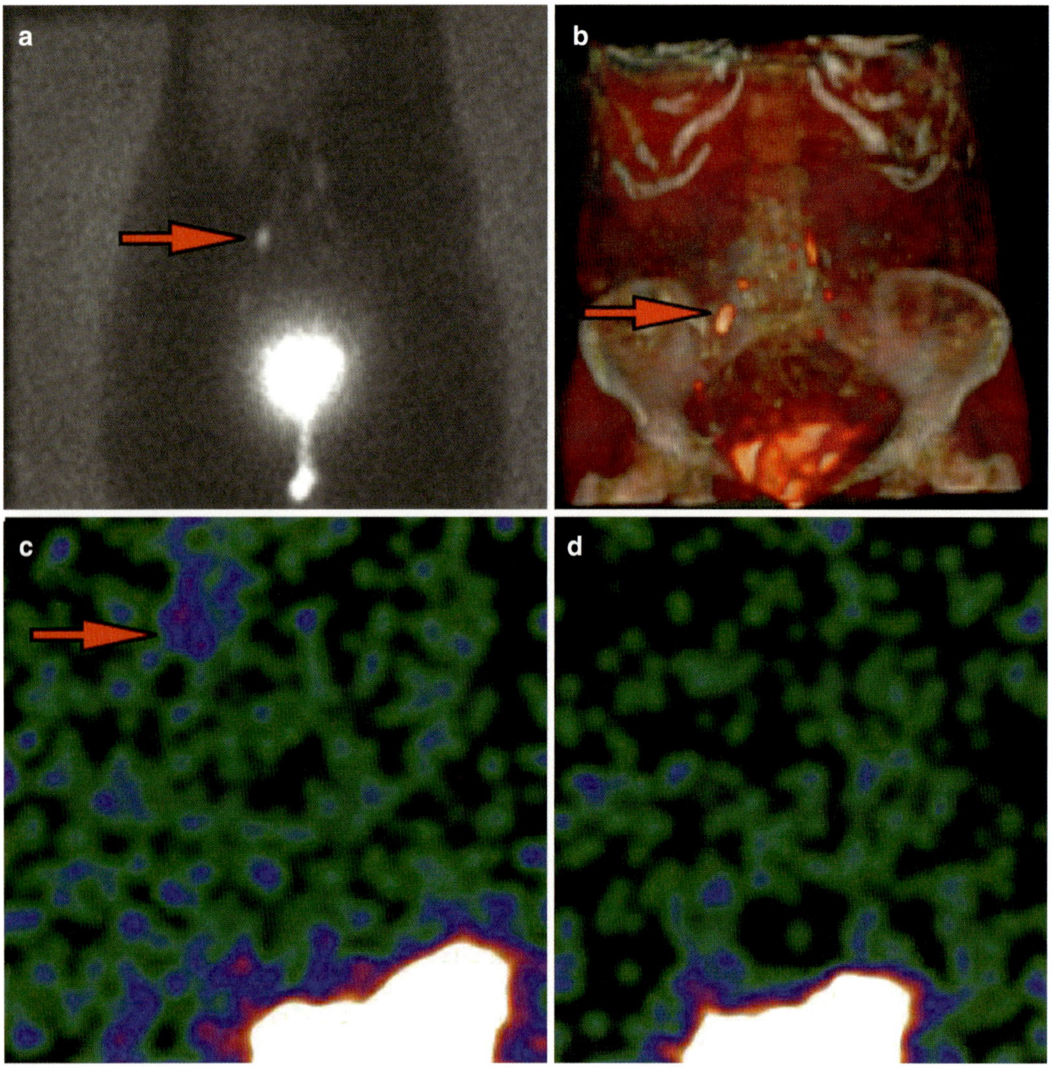

Fig. 16.4 *Portable gamma camera guiding the biopsy of a right iliac SLN (arrows)*. Planar preoperative lymphoscintigraphic view (**a**) shows bilateral pelvic drainage, confirmed on volume-rendering image from SPECT/CT (**b**). During surgery, a new acquisition (2 min lasting) with PGC shows the exact location of the iliac SLN (**c**) and the lack of activity after SLN biopsy (**d**), that confirms the correct resection

confirm appropriate excision of the target lesions (Fig. 16.4). As PGCs are small devices, the images they offer are located in a limited area and are no substitute for conventional diagnostic gamma cameras [45] because PGCs do not show more global drainage nor can they show SLNs in unexpected regions. Their high spatial resolution allows the discrimination of two adjacent hot spots [46]. This advantage is useful in vulvar cancer, in which the SLN is always very close to the injection site, and especially for SLNs of low activity. In pelvic tumours, where SLN detection using PGC can reach 92 %, the PGC is used differently than in other regions, because the greater overall distance between the position of the intraoperative imaging device and the hot spot decreases the spatial resolution. This situation could reduce the rate of intraoperative localisation, but can be overcome with a dual-energy acquisition. Some PGCs are capable of detecting more than one photopeak, one to create the image (99mTc) and another to create a marker. Some centres introduced the use of 125I seeds at the tip of the laparoscopic probe [47], and the matching of both hot spots ensures the placement of the SLN, which is especially useful in endometrial cancer due to the amount of fat tissue around the lymphatic drainage pathways (Fig. 16.4).

While the main use is these imaging devices are intraoperative, they can be used to acquire a preoperative image in centres without conventional diagnostic gamma cameras [45] or as a preparation for surgery, where deciding the best view for SLN identification can reduce the time spent in the operating room.

16.3.2 Intraoperative SPECT (fhSPECT)

The most recent advance in radioguided surgery is intraoperative SPECT, known as freehand SPECT (fhSPECT), a device capable of creating a three-dimensional image in a few minutes during a surgical procedure.

Freehand SPECT collects image projections of a definite area of interest from different directions/angles and reconstructs them into a 3D tomographic image. The difference between freehand SPECT and regular diagnostic SPECT is the fact that instead of a 2D gamma camera mounted to a gantry, the detector uses a handheld gamma probe. Since the position and orientation of the handheld gamma probe are arbitrary, a freehand SPECT imaging unit includes a positioning system, which is able to record the position of the handheld gamma probe relative to that of the patient. The imaging procedure for this device differs from conventional diagnostic SPECT. Instead of being acquired at known positions along a specific and predefined orbit, the different projections are generated by the operator using the handheld gamma probe through the operative field. In our own experience in gynaecological cancers (cervix and endometrium), a freehand SPECT system declipse SPECT (SurgicEye GmbH, Munich, Germany) connected to a 45° angled laparoscopic Tc-99 m-optimised Crystal Probe (Crystal Photonics, Berlin, Germany) was used. The declipse SPECT system includes an optical positioning system, updating the relative position of the handheld gamma probe 20 times per second with an accuracy of less than 0.5 mm. The handheld gamma probe is connected to a sterile reference target (gamma probe reference target) which includes reflective spheres (Navigation I-Spheres, SurgicEye GmbH, Munich, Germany) and is compatible with the positioning system. At least one reference target is attached to the patient (reference target), which makes it possible to move the positioning system.

Dependent on lymphatic basin drainage, different positions are selected as patient reference targets (pubis, iliac). Ideally, the chosen reference target is unchanged in its position relative to the SLN basin during patient movements (Fig. 16.5). Generally, the closer the reference target is to the SLN site, the more accurate the positioning, but this may cause more disturbances to the surgical workflow. The position of the optical imaging camera is optimised in such way that the handheld gamma probe and patient reference targets are visible during image acquisition and visualisation. Care must be taken to avoid interference with the system recognition of different references as this can hamper correct data collection and analysis.

The freehand SPECT system provides several potential advantages:

1. It provides precise depth information in a nearly real time fashion, thereby facilitating SLN detection. It may therefore reduce the trauma and the risk of lymphatic fistulas.
2. Intraoperative nearly real-time image acquisition is usually fast and does not delay the surgical procedure significantly (in our experience about 15–20 min). It can be done beforehand after the resection of SLNs and may be repeated as often as required if the post-incision findings suggest remnant activity.
3. Freehand SPECT offers confirmation of complete SLN removal and provides a reliable source of documentation as images can be printed or saved electronically and may be added to the patient's record.
4. Previous SPECT/CT data must be uploaded and included in the image display to give anatomic surroundings and the possibility of a mixed reality intraoperative navigation.

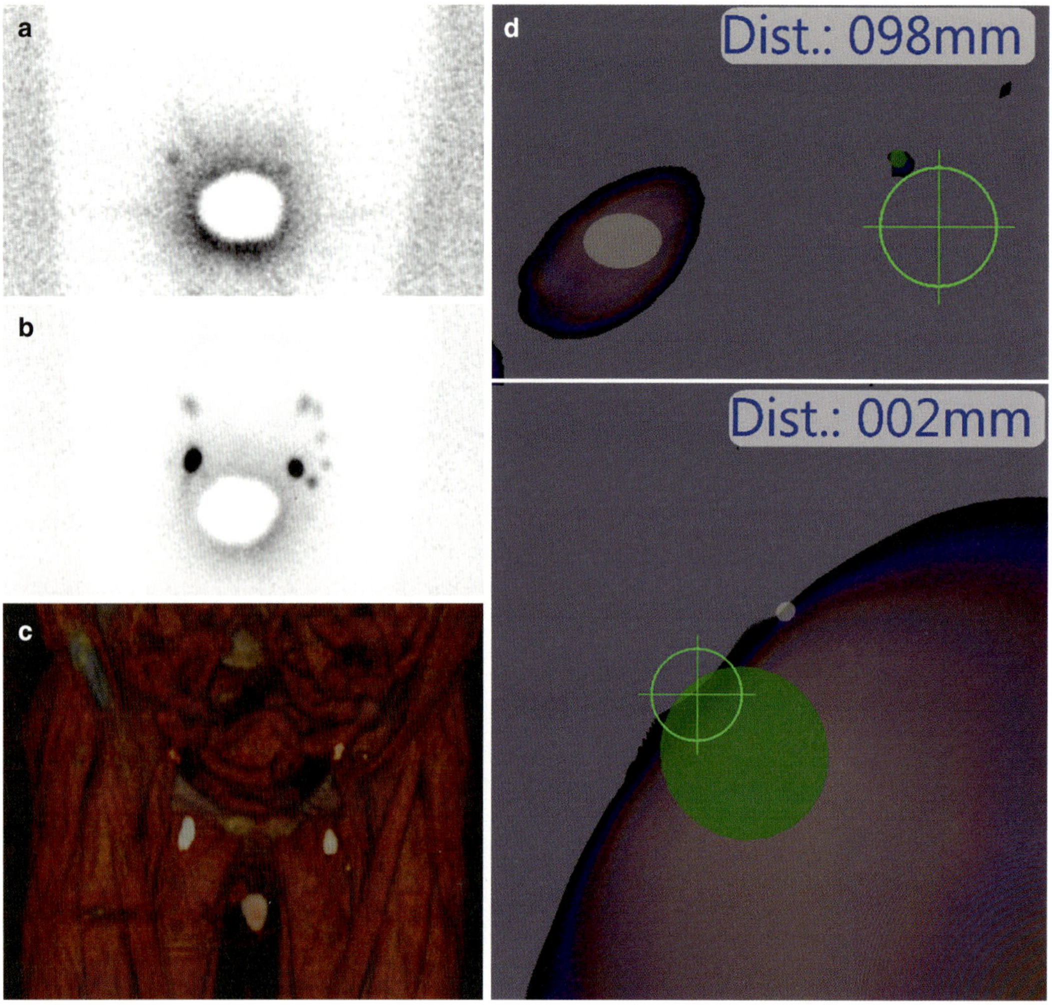

Fig. 16.5 Radioguided surgery using fhSPECT. Seventy-nine-year-old patient diagnosed of vulvar cancer. Bilateral inguinofemoral drainage was observed on late (**b**) lymphoscintigraphy and confirmed in SPECT/CT images (**c**). Early planar views (**a**) show only one SLN in the right inguinal area. During surgery fhSPECT was used to guide the SLN biopsy (**d**). First scan (*up*) indicates the best approach to reach the SLN, which is at a great distance (*green spot*). The injection site is represented on the left. Once soft tissues are dissected, the target is nearer (*bottom*), 2-mm away the probe. The *green circle* with the *cross-over the green spot* confirms the correct placement of the probe over the SLN

16.4 Other Gynaecological Tumours

16.4.1 Ovarian Cancer

The experience of SLN mapping in ovarian cancer is limited because of the high risk of tumour spread. There are two series describing the lymphatic drainage from the ovaries in patients without ovarian malignancy, but with malignancy of the endometrial or fallopian tube [4, 5]. Only one surgical team has evaluated the feasibility of SLN mapping in 21 women with ovarian cancer [6], with the administration of blue dye and radiotracer into the proper of ovarian and suspensory ligaments. The detection rate was 100 %, with ipsilateral drainage in 90.4 % of patients. The most frequent location was para-aortic region (67 %) followed by pelvic or a combination of both (9 % and 24 %, respectively).

Therefore, ovarian cancer remains as one of the gynaecologic malignancies for which there is much room for exploring the use of novel hybrid tracers and intraoperative detection and imaging devices.

16.4.2 Vaginal Cancer

There are very few studies regarding sentinel node in vaginal cancer, but they report successful SLN detection in isolated cases [20, 21, 22]. Frumovitz et al. [23] used the lymphatic mapping of lymphoscintigraphy for radiotherapy planning in 14 patients. They found lymphatic drainage in 79 % of patients, with bilateral lymph nodes in 55 % of cases. The most frequent location was the inguinal basin (45 %). There are only 3 reported cases, all in vulvovaginal melanoma, where detection was higher due to the increase of SLN locations identified by SPECT/CT [48, 49].

16.5 Summary

The accurate harvesting of SLNs in gynaecological cancer (i.e. vulvar, vaginal, cervical, endometrial, or ovarian cancer) is a complex process that can involve the coordination of several procedural components to successfully accomplish. These issues have been covered in a recent general guideline from EANM-SNMMI [50]. There are some well-established indications for SLNB (especially in vulvar and cervical cancers), but some further clarification issues still remain (SLN detection in endometrial, vaginal, and ovarian cancer is not a standard of care) and should be considered an investigational procedure. The use of new intraoperative detection and imaging devices, as well as hybrid tracers, may help to broaden the application of radioguided SLN biopsy in gynaecologic malignancies, and, therefore, warrant further clinical investigation.

References

1. Van der Zee AGJ, Oonk MH, De Hullu J a, Ansink AC, Vergote I, Verheijen RH, et al. Sentinel node dissection is safe in the treatment of early-stage vulvar cancer. J Clin Oncol [Internet]. 2008 Feb 20 [cited 2013 Dec 22];26(6):884–9. Available from: http://www.ncbi.nlm.nih.gov/pubmed/18281661.
2. Vidal-Sicart S, Puig-Tintoré LM, Lejárcegui JA, Paredes P, Ortega ML, Muñoz A, et al. Validation and application of the sentinel lymph node concept in malignant vulvar tumours. Eur J Nucl Med Mol Imaging [Internet]. 2007 Mar [cited 2013 Dec 30];34(3):384–91. Available from: http://www.ncbi.nlm.nih.gov/pubmed/17006693.
3. Abu-Rustum NR. Update on sentinel node mapping in uterine cancer: 10-year experience at Memorial Sloan-Kettering Cancer Center. J Obstet Gynaecol Res [Internet]. 2014 Feb [cited 2015 Feb 19]; 40(2):327–34. Available from: http://www.ncbi.nlm.nih.gov/pubmed/24620369.
4. Negishi H, Takeda M, Fujimoto T, Todo Y, Ebina Y, Watari H, et al. Lymphatic mapping and sentinel node identification as related to the primary sites of lymph node metastasis in early stage ovarian cancer. Gynecol Oncol [Internet]. 2004 Jul [cited 2013 Dec 30];94(1):161–6. Available from: http://www.ncbi.nlm.nih.gov/pubmed/15262135
5. Nyberg RH, Korkola P, Mäenpää J. Ovarian sentinel node: is it feasible? Int J Gynecol Cancer [Internet]. 2011 Apr [cited 2013 Dec 30];21(3):568–72. Available from: http://www.ncbi.nlm.nih.gov/pubmed/21436705.
6. Kleppe M, Brans B, Van Gorp T, Slangen BFM, Kruse AJ, Pooters INA, et al. The detection of sentinel nodes in ovarian cancer: a feasibility study. J Nucl Med [Internet]. 2014 Nov [cited 2015 Apr 1]; 55(11):1799–804. Available from: http://www.ncbi.nlm.nih.gov/pubmed/25332439.
7. Frati A, Ballester M, Dubernard G, Bats AS, Heitz D, Mathevet P, et al. Contribution of Lymphoscintigraphy for Sentinel Lymph Node Biopsy in Women with Early Stage Endometrial Cancer: Results of the SENTI-ENDO Study. Ann Surg Oncol [Internet]. 2014 Nov 13 [cited 2015 Feb 15]; Available from: http://www.ncbi.nlm.nih.gov/pubmed/25391264.
8. Robova H, Charvat M, Strnad P, Hrehorcak M, Taborska K, Skapa P, et al. Lymphatic mapping in endometrial cancer: comparison of hysteroscopic and subserosal injection and the distribution of sentinel lymph nodes. Int J Gynecol Cancer [Internet]. 2009 May [cited 2013 Dec 31];19(3):391–4. Available from: http://www.ncbi.nlm.nih.gov/pubmed/19407565.
9. Rossi EC, Jackson A, Ivanova A, Boggess JF. Detection of sentinel nodes for endometrial cancer with robotic assisted fluorescence imaging: cervical versus hysteroscopic injection. Int J Gynecol Cancer [Internet]. 2013 Nov [cited 2015 Mar 19];23(9):1704–11. Available from: http://www.ncbi.nlm.nih.gov/pubmed/24177256.
10. Holloway RW, Bravo RAM, Rakowski JA, James JA, Jeppson CN, Ingersoll SB, et al. Detection of sentinel lymph nodes in patients with endometrial cancer undergoing robotic-assisted staging: a comparison of colorimetric and fluorescence imaging. Gynecol Oncol [Internet]. 2012 Jul [cited 2013 Dec

31];126(1):25–9. Available from: http://www.ncbi.nlm.nih.gov/pubmed/22507531.

11. Bats A-S, Mathevet P, Buenerd A, Orliaguet I, Mery E, Zerdoud S, et al. The sentinel node technique detects unexpected drainage pathways and allows nodal ultrastaging in early cervical cancer: insights from the multicenter prospective SENTICOL study. Ann Surg Oncol [Internet]. 2013 Feb [cited 2014 Jan 9];20(2):413–22. Available from: http://www.ncbi.nlm.nih.gov/pubmed/22911367.
12. Altgassen C, Hertel H, Brandstädt A, Köhler C, Dürst M, Schneider A. Multicenter validation study of the sentinel lymph node concept in cervical cancer: AGO Study Group. J Clin Oncol [Internet]. 2008 Jun 20 [cited 2013 Dec 30];26(18):2943–51. Available from: http://www.ncbi.nlm.nih.gov/pubmed/18565880.
13. Crane LM, Themelis G, Pleijhuis RG, Harlaar NJ, Sarantopoulos A, Arts HJG, et al. Intraoperative multispectral fluorescence imaging for the detection of the sentinel lymph node in cervical cancer: a novel concept. Mol Imaging Biol [Internet]. 2011 Oct [cited 2015 Mar 8];13(5):1043–9. Available from: http://www.pubmedcentral.nih.gov/articlerender.fcgi?artid=3179588&tool=pmcentrez&rendertype=abstract.
14. Plante M, Touhami O, Trinh X-B, Renaud M-C, Sebastianelli A, Grondin K, et al. Sentinel node mapping with indocyanine green and endoscopic near-infrared fluorescence imaging in endometrial cancer. A pilot study and review of the literature. Gynecol Oncol [Internet]. 2015 Mar 11 [cited 2015 Apr 12]; Available from: http://www.ncbi.nlm.nih.gov/pubmed/25771495.
15. Hampl M, Hantschmann P, Michels W, Hillemanns P. Validation of the accuracy of the sentinel lymph node procedure in patients with vulvar cancer: results of a multicenter study in Germany. Gynecol Oncol [Internet]. Elsevier Inc.; 2008 Nov [cited 2013 Dec 30];111(2):282–8. Available from: http://www.ncbi.nlm.nih.gov/pubmed/18804850.
16. Levenback CF, Ali S, Coleman RL, Gold MA, Fowler JM, Judson PL, et al. Lymphatic mapping and sentinel lymph node biopsy in women with squamous cell carcinoma of the vulva: a gynecologic oncology group study. J Clin Oncol [Internet]. 2012 Nov 1 [cited 2015 Mar 19];30(31):3786–91. Available from: http://www.pubmedcentral.nih.gov/articlerender.fcgi?artid=3478573&tool=pmcentrez&rendertype=abstract.
17. Mathéron HM, van den Berg NS, Brouwer OR, Kleinjan GH, van Driel WJ, Trum JW, et al. Multimodal surgical guidance towards the sentinel node in vulvar cancer. Gynecol Oncol [Internet]. 2013 Dec [cited 2015 Mar 2];131(3):720–5. Available from: http://www.ncbi.nlm.nih.gov/pubmed/24051219.
18. Hutteman M, van der Vorst JR, Gaarenstroom KN, Peters AAW, Mieog JSD, Schaafsma BE, et al. Optimization of near-infrared fluorescent sentinel lymph node mapping for vulvar cancer. Am J Obstet Gynecol. 2013;206(206):89.e1–5.
19. Hertel H, Soergel P, Muecke J, Schneider M, Papendorf F, Laenger F, et al. Is there a place for sentinel technique in treatment of vaginal cancer?: feasibility, clinical experience, and results. Int J Gynecol Cancer [Internet]. 2013 Nov [cited 2015 Apr 26];23(9):1692–8. Available from: http://www.ncbi.nlm.nih.gov/pubmed/24177255.
20. Dhar KK, DAS N, Brinkman DA, Beynon JL, Woolas RP. Utility of sentinel node biopsy in vulvar and vaginal melanoma: report of two cases and review of the literature. Int J Gynecol Cancer [Internet]. [cited 2014 Jan 1];17(3):720–3. Available from: http://www.ncbi.nlm.nih.gov/pubmed/17343569
21. Descheemaeker V, Garin E, Morcel K, Lesimple T, Burtin F, Levêque J. Radioisotopic location of the sentinel node in vaginal mucous melanoma before laparoscopic sampling. Surg Laparosc Endosc Percutan Tech [Internet]. 2008 Apr [cited 2014 Jan 1];18(2):195–6. Available from: http://www.ncbi.nlm.nih.gov/pubmed/18427341.
22. Van Dam P, Sonnemans H, van Dam P-J, Verkinderen L, Dirix LY. Sentinel node detection in patients with vaginal carcinoma. Gynecol Oncol [Internet]. 2004 Jan [cited 2014 Jan 1];92(1):89–92. Available from: http://www.ncbi.nlm.nih.gov/pubmed/14751143.
23. Frumovitz M, Ramirez PT, Levenback CF. Lymphatic mapping and sentinel lymph node detection in women with cervical cancer. Gynecol Oncol [Internet]. 2008 Sep [cited 2013 Dec 30];110(3 Suppl 2):S17–20. Available from: http://www.ncbi.nlm.nih.gov/pubmed/18502488.
24. Perissinotti A, Paredes P, Vidal-Sicart S, Torné A, Albela S, Navales I, et al. Use of SPECT/CT for improved sentinel lymph node localization in endometrial cancer. Gynecol Oncol [Internet]. 2013 May [cited 2013 Dec 31];129(1):42–8. Available from: http://www.ncbi.nlm.nih.gov/pubmed/23376806.
25. Martínez a, Zerdoud S, Mery E, Bouissou E, Ferron G, Querleu D. Hybrid imaging by SPECT/CT for sentinel lymph node detection in patients with cancer of the uterine cervix. Gynecol Oncol [Internet]. Elsevier Inc.; 2010 Dec [cited 2013 Dec 30];119(3):431–5. Available from: http://www.ncbi.nlm.nih.gov/pubmed/20822803.
26. Crane LMA, Themelis G, Buddingh KT, Buddingh T, Harlaar NJ, Pleijhuis RG, et al. Multispectral real-time fluorescence imaging for intraoperative detection of the sentinel lymph node in gynecologic oncology. J Vis Exp [Internet]. 2010 Jan [cited 2013 Dec 31];(44). Available from: http://www.pubmedcentral.nih.gov/articlerender.fcgi?artid=3185642&tool=pmcentrez&rendertype=abstract.
27. Crane LMA, Themelis G, Arts HJG, Buddingh KT, Brouwers AH, Ntziachristos V, et al. Intraoperative near-infrared fluorescence imaging for sentinel lymph node detection in vulvar cancer: first clinical results. Gynecol Oncol [Internet]. 2011 Feb [cited 2013 Dec 18];120(2):291–5. Available from: http://www.ncbi.nlm.nih.gov/pubmed/21056907.
28. Schaafsma BE, Verbeek FPR, Peters AAW, van der Vorst JR, de Kroon CD, van Poelgeest MIE, et al. Near-infrared fluorescence sentinel lymph node biopsy in vulvar cancer: a randomised comparison of lymphatic tracers. BJOG [Internet]. 2013 May [cited 2015 Feb 14];120(6):758–64. Available

from: http://www.pubmedcentral.nih.gov/articlerender.fcgi?artid=3622799&tool=pmcentrez&rendertype=abstract.

29. Schaafsma BE, van der Vorst JR, Gaarenstroom KN, Peters AAW, Verbeek FPR, de Kroon CD, et al. Randomized comparison of near-infrared fluorescence lymphatic tracers for sentinel lymph node mapping of cervical cancer. Gynecol Oncol [Internet]. 2012 Oct [cited 2013 Dec 31];127(1):126–30. Available from: http://www.pubmedcentral.nih.gov/articlerender.fcgi?artid=3432653&tool=pmcentrez&rendertype=abstract.
30. Brouwer OR, Buckle T, Vermeeren L, Klop WMC, Balm AJM, van der Poel HG, et al. Comparing the hybrid fluorescent-radioactive tracer indocyanine green-99mTc-nanocolloid with 99mTc-nanocolloid for sentinel node identification: a validation study using lymphoscintigraphy and SPECT/CT. J Nucl Med [Internet]. 2012 Jul [cited 2013 Dec 17];53(7):1034–40. Available from: http://www.ncbi.nlm.nih.gov/pubmed/22645297.
31. Van den Berg NS, Valdés-Olmos R a, van der Poel HG, van Leeuwen FWB. Sentinel lymph node biopsy for prostate cancer: a hybrid approach. J Nucl Med [Internet]. 2013 Apr [cited 2015 Feb 15];54(4):493–6. Available from: http://www.ncbi.nlm.nih.gov/pubmed/23492883.
32. Verbeek FPR, Tummers QRJG, Rietbergen DDD, Peters AAW, Schaafsma BE, van de Velde CJH, et al. Sentinel Lymph Node Biopsy in Vulvar Cancer Using Combined Radioactive and Fluorescence Guidance. Int J Gynecol Cancer [Internet]. 2015 Mar 12 [cited 2015 Apr 27]; Available from: http://www.ncbi.nlm.nih.gov/pubmed/25768079.
33. Sakuragi N, Satoh C, Takeda N, Hareyama H, Takeda M, Yamamoto R, et al. Incidence and distribution pattern of pelvic and paraaortic lymph node metastasis in patients with Stages IB, IIA, and IIB cervical carcinoma treated with radical hysterectomy. Cancer [Internet]. 1999 May 1 [cited 2013 Dec 31];85(7):1547–54. Available from: http://www.ncbi.nlm.nih.gov/pubmed/10193945.
34. Bader AA, Winter R, Haas J, Tamussino KF. Where to look for the sentinel lymph node in cervical cancer. Am J Obstet Gynecol [Internet]. 2007 Dec [cited 2013 Dec 30];197(6):678.e1–7. Available from: http://www.ncbi.nlm.nih.gov/pubmed/18060980.
35. Marnitz S, Köhler C, Bongardt S, Braig U, Hertel H, Schneider A. Topographic distribution of sentinel lymph nodes in patients with cervical cancer. Gynecol Oncol [Internet]. 2006 Oct [cited 2013 Dec 31];103(1):35–44. Available from: http://www.ncbi.nlm.nih.gov/pubmed/16600355.
36. Domenech B, Paredes P, Rubí S, Pahisa J, Vidal-Sicart S, Pons F. Mirror-image lymph node in FDG PET/CT and SPECT/CT for sentinel node detection. Clin Nucl Med [Internet]. 2014 Mar [cited 2015 Mar 6];39(3):e241–2. Available from: http://www.ncbi.nlm.nih.gov/pubmed/24458175.
37. Rossi EC, Ivanova A, Boggess JF. Robotically assisted fluorescence-guided lymph node mapping with ICG for gynecologic malignancies: a feasibility study. Gynecol Oncol [Internet]. 2012 Jan [cited 2015 Feb 14];124(1):78–82. Available from: http://www.ncbi.nlm.nih.gov/pubmed/21996262.
38. Jewell EL, Huang JJ, Abu-Rustum NR, Gardner GJ, Brown CL, Sonoda Y, et al. Detection of sentinel lymph nodes in minimally invasive surgery using indocyanine green and near-infrared fluorescence imaging for uterine and cervical malignancies. Gynecol Oncol [Internet]. 2014 May [cited 2015 Feb 14];133(2):274–7. Available from: http://www.ncbi.nlm.nih.gov/pubmed/24582865.
39. Sinno AK, Fader AN, Roche KL, Giuntoli RL, Tanner EJ. A comparison of colorimetric versus fluorometric sentinel lymph node mapping during robotic surgery for endometrial cancer. Gynecol Oncol [Internet]. 2014 Aug [cited 2015 Feb 14]; 134(2):281–6. Available from: http://www.ncbi.nlm.nih.gov/pubmed/24882555.
40. Perrone AM, Casadio P, Formelli G, Levorato M, Ghi T, Costa S, et al. Cervical and hysteroscopic injection for identification of sentinel lymph node in endometrial cancer. Gynecol Oncol [Internet]. 2008 Oct [cited 2013 Dec 30];111(1):62–7. Available from: http://www.ncbi.nlm.nih.gov/pubmed/18625518.
41. Daraï E, Dubernard G, Bats A-S, Heitz D, Mathevet P, Marret H, et al. Sentinel node biopsy for the management of early stage endometrial cancer: Long-term results of the SENTI-ENDO study. Gynecol Oncol [Internet]. 2015 Jan [cited 2015 Feb 15];136(1):54–9. Available from: http://www.ncbi.nlm.nih.gov/pubmed/25450151.
42. Maccauro M, Lucignani G, Aliberti G, Villano C, Castellani MR, Solima E, et al. Sentinel lymph node detection following the hysteroscopic peritumoural injection of 99mTc-labelled albumin nanocolloid in endometrial cancer. Eur J Nucl Med Mol Imaging [Internet]. 2005 May [cited 2015 Mar 2];32(5):569–74. Available from: http://www.ncbi.nlm.nih.gov/pubmed/15625604.
43. Torné A, Pahisa J, Vidal-Sicart S, Martínez-Roman S, Paredes P, Puerto B, et al. Transvaginal ultrasound-guided myometrial injection of radiotracer (TUMIR): a new method for sentinel lymph node detection in endometrial cancer. Gynecol Oncol [Internet]. Elsevier Inc.; 2013 Jan [cited 2013 Dec 30];128(1):88–94. Available from: http://www.ncbi.nlm.nih.gov/pubmed/23085461.
44. Gien LT, Covens A. Lymph node assessment in cervical cancer: prognostic and therapeutic implications. J Surg Oncol [Internet]. 2009 Mar 15 [cited 2013 Dec 30];99(4):242–7. Available from: http://www.ncbi.nlm.nih.gov/pubmed/19048600.
45. Vidal-Sicart S, Vermeeren L, Solà O, Paredes P, Valdés-Olmos R a. The use of a portable gamma camera for preoperative lymphatic mapping: a comparison with a conventional gamma camera. Eur J Nucl Med Mol Imaging [Internet]. 2011 Apr [cited 2013 Dec 17];38(4):636–41. Available from: http://www.ncbi.nlm.nih.gov/pubmed/21174091.
46. Vidal-Sicart S, Paredes P, Zanón G, Pahisa J, Martinez-Román S, Caparrós X, et al. Added value of intraoperative real-time imaging in searches for difficult-to-locate sentinel nodes. J Nucl Med [Internet]. 2010 Aug [cited

2013 Dec 17];51(8):1219–25. Available from: http://www.ncbi.nlm.nih.gov/pubmed/20660385.
47. Olmos R a V, Vidal-Sicart S, Nieweg OE. SPECT-CT and real-time intraoperative imaging: new tools for sentinel node localization and radioguided surgery? Eur J Nucl Med Mol Imaging [Internet]. 2009 Jan [cited 2013 Dec 20];36(1):1–5. Available from: http://www.ncbi.nlm.nih.gov/pubmed/18931842.
48. Kim W, Menda Y, Willis J, Bartel TB, Graham MM. Use of lymphoscintigraphy with SPECT/CT for sentinel node localization in a case of vaginal melanoma. Clin Nucl Med [Internet]. 2006 Apr;31(4):201–2. Available from: http://www.ncbi.nlm.nih.gov/pubmed/16550011.
49. Kobayashi K, Ramirez PT, Kim EE, Levenback CF, Rohren EM, Frumovitz M, et al. Sentinel node mapping in vulvovaginal melanoma using SPECT/CT lymphoscintigraphy. Clin Nucl Med [Internet]. 2009 Dec [cited 2014 Jan 2];34(12):859–61. Available from: http://www.ncbi.nlm.nih.gov/pubmed/20139817.
50. Giammarile F, Bozkurt M, Cibula D, Pahisa J, Oyen W, Paredes P, et al. The EANM clinical and technical guidelines for lymphoscintigraphy and sentinel node localization in gynaecological cancers. Eur J Nucl Med Mol Imaging [Internet]. 2014 [cited 2015 Apr 28];41:1463–77. Available from: http://link.springer.com/article/10.1007/s00259-014-2732-8.

Part VIII

Clinical Application: Gastrointestinal Tract

17 Radioguided Sentinel Lymph Node Mapping and Biopsy in Esophagogastric Cancer

Hiroya Takeuchi and Yuko Kitagawa

Contents

H. Takeuchi, MD, PhD (✉) • Y. Kitagawa, MD, PhD
Department of Surgery,
Keio University School of Medicine,
35 Shinanomachi, Shinjuku-ku,
Tokyo 160-8582, Japan
e-mail: htakeuchi@a6.keio.jp

Abstract

Clinical application of sentinel lymph node (SLN) mapping and biopsy for early esophageal or gastric cancer had been controversial for years. However, single-institutional results of SLN mapping and biopsy for these cancers are almost acceptable in terms of detection rate and accuracy to determine the lymph node status. SLN mapping and biopsy may play a key role to obtain individual metastatic information and allows modification of the surgical procedures for early upper gastrointestinal (GI) cancer.

Radioguided, endoscopic SLN biopsy using preoperative lymphoscintigraphy and intraoperative gamma-probe has been established for early esophageal cancer. Previous reports suggest that the SLN concept seems to be valid, and radioguided SLN biopsy may be feasible in cT1N0 esophageal cancer. Radioguided SLN mapping and biopsy has proven to be a promising strategy for a less invasive individualized surgery for early-stage esophageal cancer.

For early gastric cancer, the Japan Society of Sentinel Node Navigation Surgery conducted a prospective multicenter trial of SLN mapping and biopsy by a dual-tracer method with radioactive colloid and blue dye. Corresponding detection rates of hot and/or blue lymph node were 98 %, respectively. The sensitivity to detect metastasis based on SLN

K. Herrmann et al. (eds.), *Radioguided Surgery: Current Applications and Innovative Directions in Clinical Practice*, DOI 10.1007/978-3-319-26051-8_17

status was 93 % and the accuracy 99 %. Based on these results, minimized gastrectomy (such as proximal gastrectomy, segmental gastrectomy, and pylorus-preserving gastrectomy), with individualized selective and modified lymphadenectomy for early gastric cancer with negative SLN are now being performed in specialized institutions. More recently, the combination of endoscopic resection with SLN biopsy also appears attractive.

The SLN concept for cN0 early upper GI cancer has been validated, and modified esophagectomy/gastrectomy with individualized minimally invasive surgery, which might retain the patients' quality of life, should be established as the next surgical challenge.

17.1 Introduction

Clinical application of sentinel lymph node (SLN) mapping and biopsy for early esophageal or gastric cancer had been controversial for years. However, previous results of SLN biopsy for these cancers are almost acceptable in terms of detection rate and accuracy to determine lymph node status. SLN biopsy may play a key role to obtain individual metastatic information and allows modification of the surgical procedures for early upper gastrointestinal cancer.

17.2 Esophageal Cancer

Esophageal cancer has one of the highest malignant potentials of any tumor. Lymph node metastasis has been recognized as one of the useful indicators for predicting the outcome of esophageal cancer. Specific characteristics of esophageal cancer are multidirectional lymphatic flow from the primary lesion and the widespread and random patterns of lymph node metastasis from cervical to abdominal areas [1]. Moreover lymph node metastasis is not a rare event in esophageal cancer even in pT1b tumors [1]. Based on these clinical observations, radical esophagectomy with two- or three-field lymph node dissection has become recognized as a standard procedure, even for clinically node-negative cases [1, 2]. However, the esophagectomy with extended lymph node dissection is one of the most invasive procedures in gastrointestinal surgeries even by thoracoscopic and laparoscopic approaches as minimally invasive esophagectomy [3–5]. To eliminate the necessity of uniform application of highly invasive surgery, SLN biopsy may play a significant role by obtaining individual information to permit adjustments and modifications of the surgical procedure for that specific patient [6].

17.2.1 Sentinel Lymph Node (SLN) Mapping and Biopsy Procedures in Esophageal Cancer

In general, radioguided method rather than the conventional blue dye method is preferred to detect the SLN in esophageal cancer [7–9]. In our procedures, a 2.0-ml volume of technetium-99m tin colloid solution (150 MBq) is injected at four quadrants into the submucosal layer around the primary tumor using an endoscopic puncture needle the day before surgery. Preoperative lymphoscintigraphy is usually obtained 3–4 h after the radiotracer injection (Fig. 17.1). Distribution of SLN was widely spread from cervical to abdominal areas.

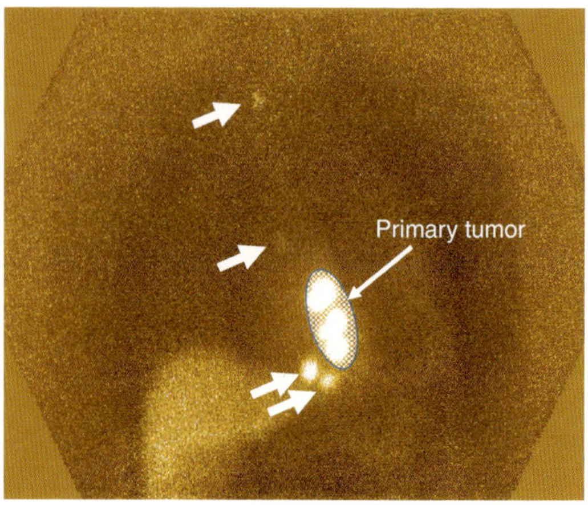

Fig. 17.1 Preoperative lymphoscintigraphy in thoracic esophageal cancer. *Arrows*, sentinel nodes

Intraoperative SLN (i.e., radiolabeled lymph nodes) sampling is performed using a handheld gamma-probe (GPS Navigator; RMD Instruments LLC, Watertown, MA, USA). Gamma probing is also feasible in thoracoscopic or laparoscopic sampling of SLNs using the special gamma-detector, which is introducible from trocar ports. SLN located in the cervical area could be identified by percutaneous gamma-probing. On the back table, the search for residual SLNs in the resected specimen is carefully investigated using the gamma-probe, and all SLNs are sent for intraoperative pathology examination.

For abdominal esophageal cancer or adenocarcinoma of gastroesophageal (GE) junction, a dual-tracer method of the radioactive tracer and blue dye (isosulfan blue or indocyanine green) is primarily used for SLN detection [10]. The blue dye is injected into the submucosal layer of the primary lesion endoscopically right after the start of surgery. Subsequently, the radiotracer passes through the afferent lymphatics, and blue-stained lymph nodes are identified as the SLNs approximately 15 min after the injection.

We believe that dye-only-guided SLN mapping is not suitable for thoracic esophageal cancer secondary to the fact that regional lymph nodes of the thoracic esophagus in the mediastinum are frequently pigmented by anthracosis. Furthermore, real-time observation of the lymphatic route using blue dye is impossible without operative mobilization and dissection of the esophagus; however, mobilization and dissection itself may interfere with active lymphatic flow from the primary lesion. Intraoperative SLN sampling using gamma-probe is considerably accurate and useful for prediction of lymph node metastasis in esophageal cancer.

17.2.2 Results of SLN Biopsy for Esophageal Cancer

There have been relatively less number of studies demonstrating the feasibility and validity of the SLN concept in esophageal cancer, compared to those in gastric cancer (Table 17.1). To date, however, a number of single-institutional studies,

Table 17.1 Representative results of sentinel node biopsy for esophageal cancer using radioguided methods

Author (Ref.)	Year	Radiotracers	Tumor depth	Number of patients	SLN detection rate (%)	Sensitivity (%)	Accuracy (%)
Kato [35]	2003	RI (^{99m} technetium rhenium sulfide)	pT1–T4	25 SCC	23/25 (92)	13/15 (87)	21/23 (91)
Yasuda [36]	2003	RI (^{99m} technetium tin colloid)	pT1–T3	23	23/23 (100)	9/12 (75)	20/23 (87)
Lamb [12]	2005	RI(^{99m} technetium nanocolloid)	N.D.	57 Adeno	57/57 (100)	35/37 (95)	55/57 (96)
Takeuchi [9]	2009	RI (^{99m} technetium tin colloid)	cT1–T2	75 SCC+ Adeno	71/75 (95)	29/33 (88)	67/71 (94)
Thompson [14]	2011	RI (^{99m} technetium antimony colloid)	pT1a–T3	16 SCC+ Adeno	14/16 (88)	3/3 (100)	16/16 (100)
Kim [37]	2011	RI (^{99m} technetium neomannosyl HSA)	cT1–T4	23 ESCC	21/23 (91)	8/8 (100)	21/21 (100)
Uenosono [15]	2011	RI (^{99m} technetium tin colloid)	cT1–T3	134 SCC+ Adeno	cT1: 56/60 (93)	cT1: 11/12 (92)	cT1: 55/56 (98)
					cT2: 31/31 (100)	cT2: 12/18 (67)	cT2: 25/31 (81)
					cT3: 28/32 (88)	cT3: 13/24 (54)	cT3: 17/28 (61)
					CRT: 5/11 (46)	CRT: 0/3 (0)	CRT: 2/5 (40)

RI radioisotope, *N.D.* not determined, *HSA* human serum albumin, *SCC* squamous cell carcinoma, *Adeno* adenocarcinoma, *SLN* sentinel lymph node including us, have demonstrated acceptable outcomes of SLN biopsy for early esophageal cancer. In particular, radioguided method seems superior in terms of the SLN detection rate and accuracy of determination of lymph node status to the conventional blue dye method (Table 17.1).

Cases with clinically apparent lymph node metastasis should be excluded from SLN biopsy because the purpose of this technique is to identify clinically undetectable lymph node involvement. Clinically T1 esophageal cancers were suitable targets of the SLN biopsy. On the other hand, clinically T3 or T4 tumors, in which original lymphatic drainage routes might be obstructed and altered, result in high incidence of false-negative cases. Therefore, clinically T3 or T4 tumors should be also excluded from the indication for SLN biopsy.

In our previous study, we have performed radioguided SLN biopsy for clinically T1N0 or T2N0 esophageal cancer to verify the feasibility of the SLN mapping [9]. Our data indicates successful SLN detection in 71 (95 %) of 75 patients, and the diagnostic accuracy based on SLN status was 94 %. The SLN biopsy was successful even during thoracoscopic esophagectomy, along with conventional surgical procedures [9]. The mean number of identified SLNs per case was 4.7, and not 1 or 2 in our study [9].

Also in our study, distribution of identified SLNs was widely spread from cervical to abdominal areas [9]. In more than 85 % of cases with thoracic esophageal cancer, at least one SLN was found to be located in the second or third compartment of regional lymph nodes [9]. In general, the stations which were frequently identified as SLNs tended to have high incidence of metastasis pathologically.

Most of the SLN studies have shown that in the squamous cell carcinoma (SCC), the distribution of SLNs is randomized (cervical, thoracic, and abdominal); however, in the adenocarcinoma (AC), the distribution is relatively located in periesophageal tissue and abdominal area. Grotenhuis et al. [11] found a high false-negative rate (15 %) in SLNs in the AC; however, perhaps it was related to dye-only-guided SLN biopsy in the study and transhiatal operation which had limited lymphadenectomy of supracarinal lymph nodes and the fact that it was high number of T3 tumors (65 %), which could supplied to low accuracy rate. On the other hand, Lamb et al. [12] reported excellent results of SLN biopsy in 57 patients with AC. Burian et al. [13] also demonstrated that SLN biopsy is feasible and reliable in patients with adenocarcinoma of GE junction. We think that the SLN mapping and biopsy will also be adaptable and reliable to AC of distal esophagus or GE junction [10].

In general, lymphadenectomy is still necessary at least for staging purposes even after neoadjuvant therapy, such as neoadjuvant chemotherapy or chemoradiotherapy, and the distribution of nodal metastasis after neoadjuvant therapy could be useful information in planning the operative techniques. Therefore, if we could use the SLN to study the remained pathologic lymph nodes after neoadjuvant therapy, this could avoid extended lymphadenectomy or using SLN to establish a new pathologic staging disease. Thompson et al. [14] did not find any difference between patients who received neoadjuvant therapy, as well did not have and increased difficulty in identifying SLNs in these patients. On the other hand, Uenosono et al. [15] agreed that SLN navigation surgery also is unacceptable for patients who have had neoadjuvant chemoradiotherapy.

17.2.3 Future Application of SLN Biopsy in Esophageal Cancer

SLN biopsy would provide significant information to perform individualized selective lymphadenectomy for esophageal cancer that might reduce the morbidity without having a negative impact on the prognosis. For instance, if the SLNs were identified only in the mediastinum or abdominal area and all SLNs were pathologically negative in patients with cT1N0 middle or lower thoracic esophageal cancer, the cervical lymph node dissection would be unnecessary [9].

SLN mapping and biopsy will also be adaptable and reliable to adenocarcinomas of distal esophagus or GE junction [10]. We think that the SLN mapping and biopsy for adenocarcinomas of distal esophagus or GE junction is useful to adjust and modify the surgical procedures. For instance, if the SLNs were identified only in the abdominal area and pathologically negative in the case with cT1N0 adenocarcinoma of distal esophagus, the patient would be treated with limited resection of distal esophagus by transhiatal approach without extensive mediastinal lymph node dissection [9, 10]. On the other hand, if the SLNs were positive for metastasis by intraoperative diagnosis, the patient should be treated with extended transthoracic lymphadenectomy. The new surgical procedure might reduce the morbidity and mortality without having a negative impact on the quality of life (QOL) for early-stage esophageal cancer patients with pathologically negative SLN.

Previous reports suggest that the SLN concept seems to be valid, and radioguided SLN biopsy may be feasible in cT1N0 esophageal cancer. SLN mapping and biopsy surgery has proven to be a promising strategy for a less invasive individualized surgery for early-stage esophageal cancer.

17.3 Gastric Cancer

Many patients with early gastric cancer are currently treated with advanced laparoscopic gastrectomy procedures, such as laparoscopy-assisted distal gastrectomy (LADG) and laparoscopy-assisted total gastrectomy in Asian countries [16–19]. Advanced laparoscopic gastrectomy contributes to both better esthetics and early postoperative recovery [20]. However, patients' QOL is mainly affected by late phase complications, such as dumping syndrome and body weight loss resulting from oral intake disturbance. Therefore, both minimal invasiveness for early phase recovery and satisfactory late phase function after gastric cancer surgery should be carefully considered in patients indicated for these procedures.

Although function-preserving gastrectomy such as partial gastrectomy, segmental gastrectomy, and proximal gastrectomy, with limited stomach resection and lymph node dissection, may help in improving postoperative late phase function, a certain incidence of skip metastasis in the 2nd or 3rd compartment of regional lymph nodes remains an obstacle to the wider application of these procedures. To overcome these issues, the concept of SLN mapping and biopsy is anticipated to become a novel diagnostic tool for the identification of clinically undetectable lymph node metastasis in patients with early gastric cancer.

The clinical application of SLN biopsy for early gastric cancer has been controversial for years. However, single-institutional results, including ours and those from a recent multicenter trial of SLN mapping for early gastric cancer, are considered acceptable in terms of the SLN detection rate and accuracy of determination of lymph node status [7, 21]. On the basis of these results, we are developing a novel, laparoscopic, minimally invasive gastrectomy technique combined with SLN mapping and biopsy.

17.3.1 Laparoscopic SLN Mapping and Biopsy Procedures

A dual-tracer method that utilizes radioactive colloids and blue dyes is currently considered the most reliable method for the detection of SLNs in patients with early gastric cancer [21, 22]. An accumulation of radioactive colloids facilitates the identification of SLNs, even in resected specimens, by using a handheld gamma-probe, and the blue dye is effective for intraoperative visualization of lymphatic flow, even during laparoscopic surgery. Technetium-99m tin colloid, technetium-99m sulfur colloid, and technetium-99m antimony sulfur colloid are preferentially used as the radioactive tracers. Isosulfan blue, patent blue, and indocyanine green (ICG) are the currently preferred choices as the dye tracers.

In general, patients with clinical T1 (or T2) tumors, primary lesions less than approximately 4 cm in diameter, and clinical N0 gastric cancer undergo SLN mapping and biopsy. In our procedures, 2.0 ml (150 MBq) of technetium-99m tin colloid solution is injected the day before surgery into four quadrants of the submucosal layer of the primary tumor site using an endoscopic puncture needle. Endoscopic injections facilitate accurate tracer injection. Technetium-99m tin colloid with relatively large particle size accumulates in the SLNs after local administration.

The blue dye is injected into four quadrants of the submucosal layer of the primary site using an endoscopic puncture needle at the beginning of surgery. Blue lymphatic vessels and blue-stained lymph nodes can be identified by laparoscopy within 15 min after the injection of the blue dye. Simultaneously, a handheld gamma-probe is used to locate the radioactive SLNs, similar to esophageal SLN biopsy. Intraoperative gamma-probing is feasible in laparoscopic gastrectomy using a special gamma-detector introducible through trocar ports.

During radioguided SLN biopsy for breast-cancer and melanoma, individual SLNs are excised from the in situ lymph node basin tissue. However, it is recommended that the clinical application of intraoperative SLN sampling for gastric cancer should include SLN lymphatic basin lymph node dissection, which is a sort of focused lymph node dissection involving hot and blue nodes [21, 22]. The gastric lymphatic basins are considered to be divided in the following five directions along the main arteries: left gastric artery area, right gastric artery area, left gastroepiploic artery area, right gastroepiploic artery area, and posterior gastric artery area [23].

ICG is known to have excitation and fluorescence wavelengths in the near-infrared range [24]. To date, some investigators have used infrared ray electronic endoscopy (IREE) to demonstrate the clinical utility of intraoperative ICG infrared imaging as a new tracer for laparoscopic SLN biopsy [24, 25]. IREE might be a useful tool to improve visualization of ICG-stained lymphatic vessels and SLNs even in the fat tissues. More recently, ICG fluorescence imaging has been developed as another promising novel technique for SLN biopsy [26, 27]. SLNs could be clearly visualized by ICG fluorescence imaging compared to the naked eye (Fig. 17.2). Further studies would be needed to evaluate the clinical efficacy of ICG infrared or fluorescence imaging and to compare those with radioguided methods in established prospective studies. However, these new technologies might revolutionize the SLN mapping and biopsy procedures not only in gastric cancer, but also in many other solid tumors.

17.3.2 Results of SLN Biopsy for Gastric Cancer

To date, more than 50 single-institutional studies have demonstrated acceptable outcomes of SLN biopsy for early gastric cancer in terms of the

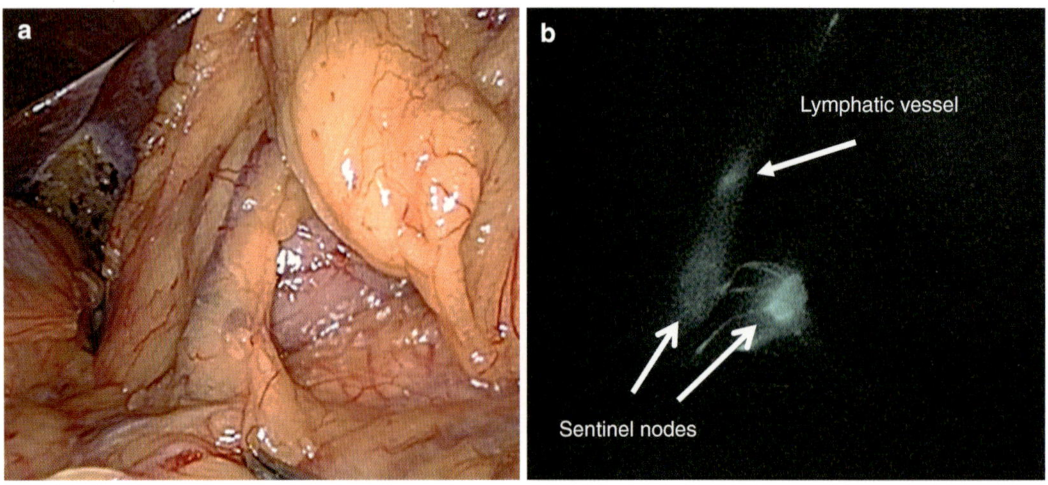

Fig. 17.2 Indocyanine green fluorescence imaging using infrared ray electronic endoscopy for laparoscopic sentinel lymph node biopsy. (**a**) Normal light, (**b**) infrared ray electronic endoscopy. Infrared ray electronic endoscopy can visualize SLNs and lymphatics clearly

SLN detection rate (90–100 %) and accuracy (85–100 %) of determination of lymph node status; these outcomes are comparable to those of SLN biopsy for melanoma and breast cancer [22]. Recently, Wang et al. reported a systematic review that evaluated the diagnostic value of SLN biopsy for gastric cancer [28]. The results of their large-scale meta-analysis, which included 38 relevant studies with 2128 patients, demonstrated that the SLN detection rate and accuracy of prediction of lymph node metastasis based on SLN status were 94 % and 92 %, respectively [28]. They concluded that the SLN concept is technically feasible for gastric cancer, especially cases with early T stage (T1), with the use of combined tracers and submucosal injection methods during the SLN biopsy procedures.

A study group in the Japan recently conducted a multicenter prospective trial of SLN biopsy using a dual-tracer method with a radioactive colloid and blue dye [21]. In the trial, SLN biopsy was performed between 2004 and 2008 for approximately 400 patients with early gastric cancer at 12 comprehensive hospitals, including our institution. Eligibility criteria were that patients had cT1N0M0 or cT2N0M0 single tumor with diameter of primary lesion less than 4 cm, without any previous treatments. As results, the SLN detection rate was 98 %, and the accuracy of determination of metastatic status was 99 % [21]. The results of that clinical trial are expected to provide us with perspectives on the future of SLN navigation surgery for early gastric cancer.

17.3.3 Clinical Application of Laparoscopic SLN Biopsy for Early Gastric Cancer

The distribution of SLN lymphatic basins and the pathological status of SLNs would be useful in deciding on the minimized extent of gastric resection and in avoiding the universal application of distal or total gastrectomy with D2 dissection. Appropriate indications for laparoscopic surgeries such as partial (wedge) resection, segmental gastrectomy, pylorus-preserving gastrectomy, and proximal gastrectomy (LAPG) for cT1N0 gastric cancer could be individually determined on the basis of SLN status (Fig. 17.3) [29, 30]. Earlier recovery after surgery and preservation of QOL in the late phase can be achieved by laparoscopic limited gastrectomy with SLN navigation. Our study group in Japan currently started the multicenter prospective trial which will

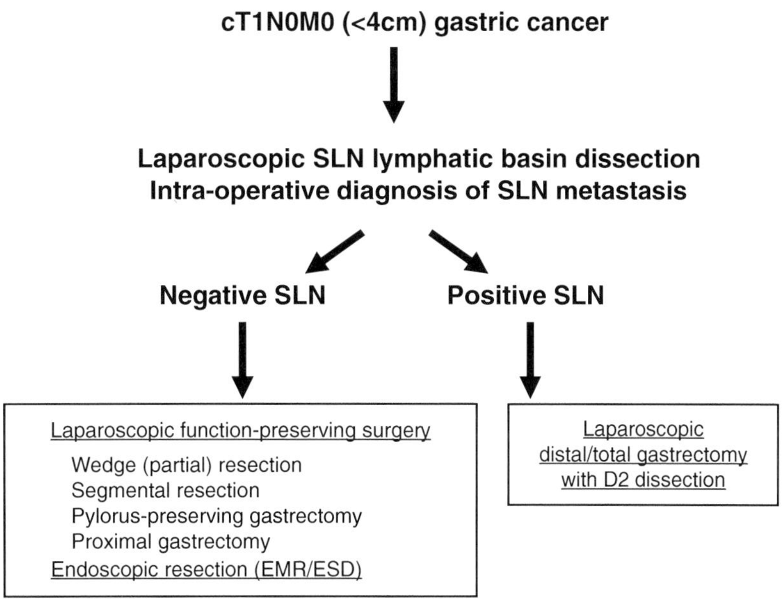

Fig. 17.3 Individualized function-preserving approaches for cT1N0M0 gastric cancer based on SLN mapping. *EMR* endoscopic mucosal resection, *ESD* endoscopic submucosal dissection

evaluate the function-preserving gastrectomy with SLN biopsy in terms of long-term survival and patients' QOL as the next step.

A combination of laparoscopic SLN biopsy and endoscopic mucosal resection (EMR)/endoscopic submucosal dissection (ESD) for early gastric cancer is another attractive option as a novel, whole stomach-preserved, minimally invasive approach. If all SLNs are pathologically negative for cancer metastasis, theoretically, EMR/ESD instead of gastrectomy may be sufficient for the curative resection of cT1 gastric cancer beyond the EMR criteria [11, 20]. However, further studies are required to verify the safety and effectiveness of combined treatments involving laparoscopic SLN biopsy and EMR/ESD.

Nowadays, LADG or LAPG are frequently applied to the patients with early gastric cancer according to the results of pathological assessment of primary tumor resected by EMR/ESD in clinical practices. To date, it has not been clarified whether the SLN biopsy is feasible even after EMR/ESD. One of the most important issues is whether lymphatic flow from the primary tumor to the original SLNs may change after EMR/ESD. In our preliminary study, however, at least the sentinel lymphatic basin is not markedly affected by previous EMR/ESD [31, 32]. Modified gastrectomy according to SLN distribution and metastatic status might be feasible even for the patients who underwent EMR/ESD prior to surgery.

The recent appearance of a new technique, referred to as non-exposed endoscopic wall-inversion surgery (NEWS), is a technique of full-thickness resection using endoscopy and laparoscopic surgery without transluminal access mainly designed to treat gastric cancer. We have been accumulating cases of NEWS with SLN biopsy for early gastric cancer with the risk of lymph node metastasis in the clinical trial (Fig. 17.4a–f) [33, 34]. The combination of NEWS with SLN biopsy is expected to become a promising, ideal minimally invasive, function-preserving surgery to cure cases of cN0 early gastric cancer.

For early-stage gastric cancer, for which a better prognosis can be achieved through conventional surgical approaches, the establishment of individualized, minimally invasive treatments that may retain the patients' QOL should be the next surgical challenge. Although further studies are needed for careful validation, SLN navigation surgery could be a promising strategy to achieve this goal.

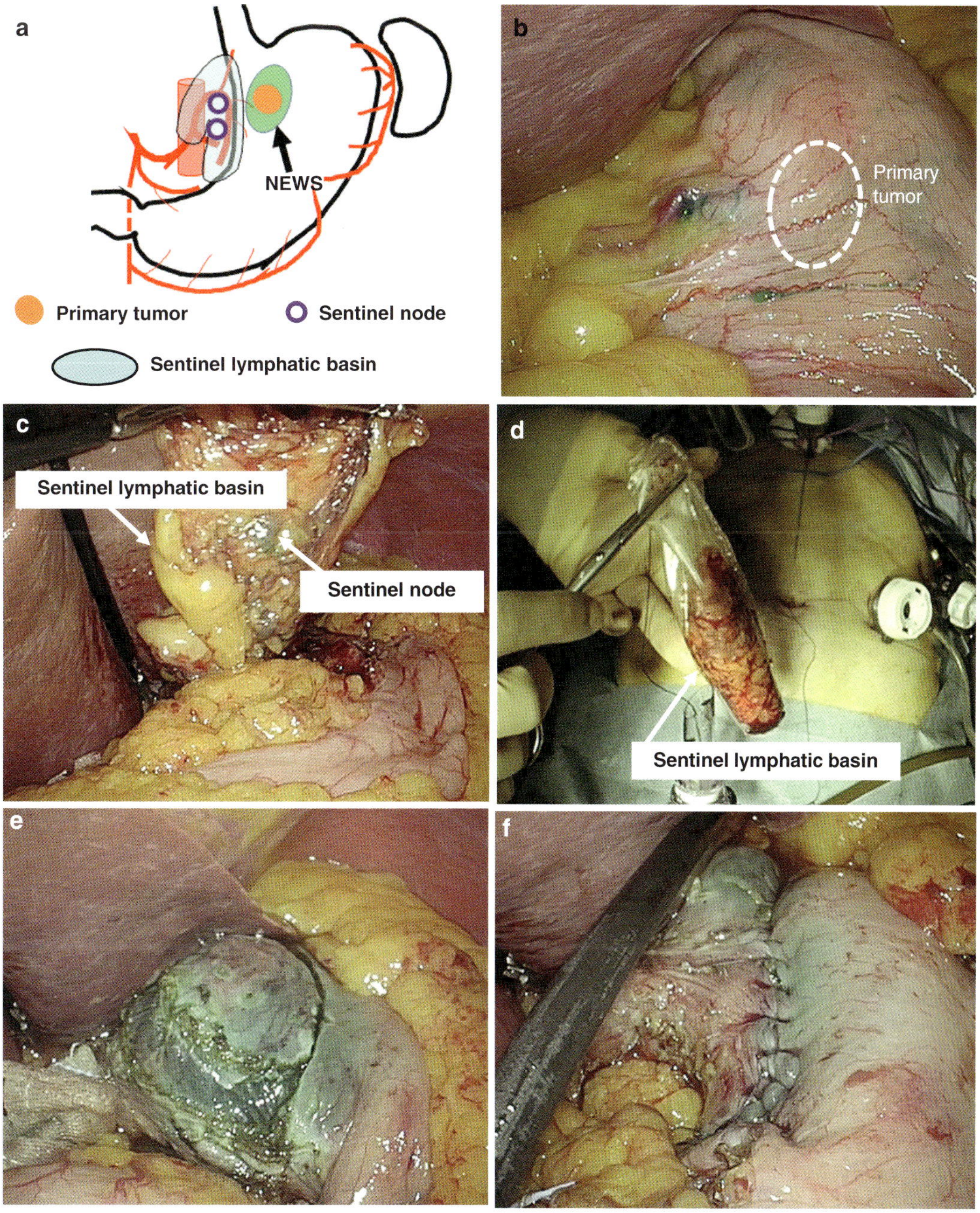

Fig. 17.4 (**a**) Schema of non-exposed endoscopic wall-inversion surgery (NEWS) with SLN biopsy and SLN lymphatic basin dissection. (**b**) Injected indocyanine green to the gastric wall surrounding the primary tumor. (**c**) SLN lymphatic basin resection. (**d**) Retrieved sentinel lymphatic basin. (**e**) Laparoscopic circumferential seromuscular incision. (**f**) Laparoscopic seromuscular suturing and inversion of the primary lesion. Subsequently, endoscopic circumferential mucosal and remnant submucosal tissue incision was performed. Finally, the detached primary lesion was retrieved perorally. By the new surgical approaches, the patients could avoid total gastrectomy and preserve almost all stomach

Conclusion

Radioguided SLN mapping and biopsy in esophagogastric cancer has been now validated in early upper gastrointestinal tumors. Correspondingly less extensive surgeries in SLN negative patients hopefully increase the patient's quality of life. However, the implementation of this technique into daily clinical practice represents the next surgical challenge.

References

1. Ando N, Ozawa S, Kitagawa Y, Shinozawa Y, Kitajima M. Improvement in the results of surgical treatment of advanced squamous esophageal carcinoma during 15 consecutive years. Ann Surg. 2000;232:225–32.
2. Akiyama H, Tsurumaru M, Udagawa H, Kajiyama Y. Radical lymph node dissection for cancer of the thoracic esophagus. Ann Surg. 1994;220:360–73.
3. Fujita H, Kakegawa T, Yamana H, Shima I, Toh Y, et al. Mortality and morbidity rates, postoperative course, quality of life, and prognosis after extended radical lymphadenectomy for esophageal cancer. Comparison of three-field lymphadenectomy with two-field lymphadenectomy. Ann Surg. 1995;222:654–62.
4. Kinugasa S, Tachibana M, Yoshimura H, Ueda S, Fujii T, et al. Postoperative pulmonary complications are associated with worse short- and long-term outcomes after extended esophagectomy. J Surg Oncol. 2004;88:71–7.
5. Fang WT, Chen WH, Chen Y, Jiang Y. Selective three-field lymphadenectomy for thoracic esophageal squamous carcinoma. Dis Esophagus. 2007;20:206–11.
6. Morton DL, Wen DR, Wong JH, Economou JS, Cagle LA, et al. Techinical details of intraoperative lymphatic mapping for early stage melanoma. Arch Surg. 1992;127:392–9.
7. Kitagawa Y, Fujii H, Mukai M, Kubota T, Ando N, et al. The role of the sentinel lymph node in gastrointestinal cancer. Surg Clin North Am. 2000;80:1799–809.
8. Kitagawa Y, Fujii H, Mukai M, Kubota T, Ando N, et al. Intraoperative lymphatic mapping and sentinel lymph node sampling in esophageal and gastric cancer. Surg Oncol Clin North Am. 2002;11:293–304.
9. Takeuchi H, Fujii H, Ando N, Oyama T, Mukai M, et al. Validation study of radio-guided sentinel lymph node navigation in esophageal cancer. Ann Surg. 2009;249:757–63.
10. Matsuda T, Takeuchi H, Tsuwano S, Nakahara T, Mukai M, Kitagawa Y. Sentinel node mapping in adenocarcinoma of the esophagogastric junction. World J Surg. 2014;38:2337–44.
11. Grotenhuis BA, Wijnhoven BP, van Marion R, van Dekken H, Hop WC, et al. The sentinel node concept in adenocarcinoma of the distal esophagus and gastroesophageal junction. J Thorac Cardiovasc Surg. 2009;138:608–12.
12. Lamb PJ, Griffin SM, Burt AD, Lloyd J, Karat D, et al. Sentinel node biopsy to evaluate the metastatic dissemination of oesophageal adenocarcinoma. Br J Surg. 2005;92:60–7.
13. Burian M, Stein HJ, Sendler A, Piert M, Nährig J, et al. Sentinel node detection in Barrett's and cardia cancer. Ann Surg Oncol. 2004;3:255S–8.
14. Thompson SK, Bartholomeusz D, Devitt PG, Lamb PJ, Ruszkiewicz AR, et al. Feasibility study of sentinel lymph node biopsy in esophageal cancer with conservative lymphadenectomy. Surg Endosc. 2011;25:817–25.
15. Uenosono Y, Arigami T, Yanagita S, Kozono T, Arima H, et al. Sentinel node navigation surgery is acceptable for clinical T1 and N0 esophageal cancer. Ann Surg Oncol. 2011;18:2003–9.
16. Kitano S, Iso Y, Moriyama M, Sugimachi K. Laparoscopy-assisted Billroth I gastrectomy. Surg Laparosc Endosc. 1994;4:146–8.
17. Adachi Y, Shiraishi N, Shiromizu A, Shiromizu A, Bandoh T, Aramaki M, Kitano S. Laparoscopy-assisted Billroth I gastrectomy compared with conventional open gastrectomy. Arch Surg. 2000;135:806–10.
18. Shinohara T, Kanaya S, Taniguchi K, Fujita T, Yanaga K, Uyama I. Laparoscopic total gastrectomy with D2 lymph node dissection for gastric cancer. Arch Surg. 2009;144:1138–42.
19. Hur H, Jeon HM, Kim W. Laparoscopy-assisted distal gastrectomy with D2 lymphadenectomy for T2b advanced gastric cancers: three years' experience. J Surg Oncol. 2008;98:515–9.
20. Kim YW, Baik YH, Yun YH, Nam BH, Kim DH, Choi IJ, Bae JM. Improved quality of life outcomes after laparoscopy-assisted distal gastrectomy for early gastric cancer: results of a prospective randomized clinical trial. Ann Surg. 2008;248:721–7.
21. Kitagawa Y, Takeuchi H, Takagi Y, Natsugoe S, Terashima M, Murakami N, Fujimura T, Tsujimoto H, Hayashi H, Yoshimizu N, Takagane A, Mohri Y, Nabshima K, Uenosono Y, Kinami S, Sakamoto J, Morita S, Aikou T, Miwa K, Kitajima M. Sentinel node mapping for gastric cancer: a prospective multicenter trial in Japan. J Clin Oncol. 2013;31: 3704–10.
22. Takeuchi H, Kitagawa Y. New sentinel node mapping technologies for early gastric cancer. Ann Surg Oncol. 2013;20:522–32.
23. Kinami S, Fujimura T, Ojima E, Fushida S, Ojima T, Funaki H, Fujita H, Takamura H, Ninomiya I, Nishimura G, Kayahara M, Ohta T, Yoh Z. PTD classification: proposal for a new classification of gastric cancer location based on physiological lymphatic flow. Int J Clin Oncol. 2008;13:320–9.

24. Tajima Y, Murakami M, Yamazaki K, Masuda Y, Kato M, Sato A, Goto S, Otsuka K, Kato T, Kusano M. Sentinel node mapping guided by indocyanine green fluorescence imaging during laparoscopic surgery in gastric cancer. Ann Surg Oncol. 2010;17:1787–93.
25. Ishikawa K, Yasuda K, Shiromizu T, Etoh T, Shiraishi N, Kitano S. Laparoscopic sentinel node navigation achieved by infrared ray electronic endoscopy system in patients with gastric cancer. Surg Endosc. 2007;21:1131–4.
26. Nimura H, Narimiya N, Mitsumori N, Yamazaki Y, Yanaga K, Urashima M. Infrared ray electronic endoscopy combined with indocyanine green injection for detection of sentinel nodes of patients with gastric cancer. Br J Surg. 2004;91:575–9.
27. Miyashiro I, Miyoshi N, Hiratsuka M, Kishi K, Yamada T, Ohue M, Ohigashi H, Yano M, Ishikawa O, Imaoka S. Detection of sentinel node in gastric cancer surgery by indocyanine green fluorescence imaging: comparison with infrared imaging. Ann Surg Oncol. 2008;15:1640–3.
28. Wang Z, Dong ZY, Chen JQ, Liu JL. Diagnostic value of sentinel lymph node biopsy in gastric cancer: a meta-analysis. Ann Surg Oncol. 2012;19:1541–50.
29. Takeuchi H, Saikawa Y, Kitagawa Y. Laparoscopic sentinel node navigation surgery for early gastric cancer. Asian J Endosc Surg. 2009;2:13–7.
30. Takeuchi H, Oyama T, Kamiya S, Nakamura R, Takahashi T, Wada N, Saikawa Y, Kitagawa Y. Laparoscopy-assisted proximal gastrectomy with sentinel node mapping for early gastric cancer. World J Surg. 2011;35:2463–71.
31. Takeuchi H, Kitagawa Y. Sentinel node navigation surgery in patients with early gastric cancer. Dig Surg. 2013;30:104–11.
32. Mayanagi S, Takeuchi H, Kamiya S, Niihara M, Nakamura R, Takahashi T, Wada N, Kawakubo H, Saikawa Y, Omori T, Nakahara T, Mukai M, Kitagawa Y. Suitability of sentinel node mapping as an index of metastasis in early gastric cancer following endoscopic resection. Ann Surg Oncol. 2014;21:2987–93.
33. Goto O, Takeuchi H, Kawakubo H, Sasaki M, Matsuda T, Matsuda S, Kigasawa Y, Kadota Y, Fujimoto A, Ochiai Y, Horii J, Uraoka T, Kitagawa Y, Yahagi N. First case of non-exposed endoscopic wall-inversion surgery with sentinel node basin dissection for early gastric cancer. Gastric Cancer. 2015;18:440–5.
34. Takeuchi H, Kitagawa Y. Sentinel lymph node biopsy in gastric cancer. Cancer J. 2015;21:21–4.
35. Kato H, Miyazaki T, Nakajima M, Takita J, Sohda M, Fukai Y, Masuda N, Fukuchi M, Manda R, Ojima H, Tsukada K, Asao T, Kuwano H, Oriuchi N, and Endo K. Sentinel lymph nodes with technetium-99m colloidal rhenium sulfide in patients with esophageal carcinoma. Cancer 2003;98:932–9.
36. Yasuda S, Shimada H, Chino O, Tanaka H, Kenmochi T, Takechi M, Nabeshima K, Okamoto Y, Kato Y, Kijima H, Suzuku Y, Ogoshi K, Tajima T, and Makuuchi H. Sentinel lymph node detection with Tc-99m tin colloids in patients with esophagogastric cancer. Jpn J Clin Oncol. 2003;33:68–72.
37. Kim HK, Kim S, Park JJ, Jeong JM, Mok YJ, and Choi YH. Sentinel node identification using technetium-99m neomannosyl human serum albumin in esophageal cancer. Ann Thorac Surg. 2011;91:1517–22.

Radioguided Sentinel Lymph Node Mapping and Biopsy in Colorectal Cancer

18

Dawid Murawa, Piotr Nowaczyk, and Armin Wiegering

Contents

D. Murawa (✉)
1st Department of Surgical Oncology and General Surgery, Greater Poland Cancer Center, ul. Garbary 15, Poznan 61-866, Poland

Regional Specialist Hospital in Wroclaw, Research and Development Centre, ul. Kamieńskiego 73a, Wrocław 51-124, Poland
e-mail: dmurawa@gmail.com

P. Nowaczyk
1st Department of Surgical Oncology and General Surgery, Greater Poland Cancer Center, ul. Garbary 15, Poznan 61-866, Poland

A. Wiegering
Department of General, Visceral, Vascular and Pediatric Surgery, University Hospital of Wuerzburg, Oberduerrbacher Strasse 6, Wuerzburg 97080, Germany

Department of Biochemistry and Molecular Biology, Theodor-Boveri-Institute, Biocenter, University of Wuerzburg, Wuerzburg 97070, Germany

Abstract

Colorectal cancer is the most frequent malignancy of the gastrointestinal tract. After distant metastasis, the presence of metastases in regional lymph nodes is the main prognostic factor. Examination of only a selected group of lymph nodes harvested separately during the surgical procedure and containing the highest probability of metastatic cells – the sentinel lymph nodes (SLNs) – could be useful in this context given that SLN biopsy allows a more comprehensive analysis of the status of the regional lymph nodes. In this context, it is to be noted that standard H&E histopathology analysis can potentially underestimate the degree of lymph node involvement by failing to recognize micrometastatic disease that may be apparent only at H&E histopathology analysis of

K. Herrmann et al. (eds.), *Radioguided Surgery: Current Applications and Innovative Directions in Clinical Practice*, DOI 10.1007/978-3-319-26051-8_18

serial sections and/or immunohistochemistry. To date, in colorectal cancer, the SLN procedure has only diagnostic relevance. En bloc resection of the tumor and regional lymph node dissection remains the standard treatment.

The most commonly used tracers in lymphatic mapping in colon cancer are colorimetric dyes. The in vivo use of colorimetric dyes does not require any additional technology, does not prolong the procedure significantly, and shows several advantages over the use of a radioisotope. The in vivo administration of dye allows the detection of aberrant lymphatic drainage of the regional lymph nodes. Because of the principle of oncological radicality associated with total mesorectal excision, lymphatic mapping in rectal cancer is frequently done on the specimen ex vivo. Accordingly, there is no impact on intraoperative strategy. In anal cancer (for which radiochemotherapy is the treatment of choice), in selected cases, SLN biopsy has been indicated as a tool for precise and minimally invasive assessment of the regional inguinal lymphatic system and also for further therapeutic decision making (regarding the use of radiotherapy).

18.1 Value and Relevance of Sentinel Lymph Node (SLN) Biopsy in Clinical Practice

18.1.1 Conceptual Background in Relation to Colorectal Cancer

Colorectal cancer is the most common malignancy of the gastrointestinal tract, the third most common malignancy, and the fourth leading cause of cancer death (with an incidence of 1.36 million and 694,000 deaths worldwide in 2012). Epidemiological estimates indicate that around 6 % of the population will develop colorectal cancer during the course of their lives, of whom 40 % will die. Presently, the number of colorectal cancer cases is on the rise in countries with a lower incidence, but is stabilizing or even decreasing in countries with a higher incidence, especially among younger patients. On average, around 70 % of colorectal cancer patients are over 65 years old [1, 2].

After distant metastasis, the most important prognostic factor in colorectal cancer is the presence of metastases in the regional lymph nodes, with 5-year survival of approximately 70–90 % in patients with stage I and II diseases but only 40–60 % in those with stage III disease. Thus, the regional lymph node status is the principal influence on all decision making regarding the need for additional treatment, such as adjuvant chemotherapy. Accordingly, appropriate selection of diagnostic methods for the determination of regional lymph node involvement is highly relevant to long-term patient outcome and prognosis [3–19].

Another important clinical finding is the fact that up to 30 % of patients with colorectal cancer diagnosed as pN0 following surgery will die within 5 years owing to regional recurrence or distant metastases [4–6, 8–11, 15, 17, 20–23]. The results of MOSAIC and NSABP C-07 research initiated a lively debate over establishing a so-called high-risk stage 2 group, which would potentially benefit from adjuvant treatment. Presently, the high-risk group, according to ESMO and NCCN treatment standards, comprises patients with T4 tumors (especially T4b), a high grade of histological malignancy in the tumor, infiltration of vessels and perineural tissue, tumor budding, a small number of removed lymph nodes (<12), emergency surgery caused by obstruction, tumor hemorrhage, or perforation [5, 8, 10, 12, 14, 24, 25]. When selecting such a group of high-risk patients, none of these prognostic factors seems more significant than the presence of regional lymph node involvement. Therefore, the problem is to find diagnostic methods that could improve selection based on this criterion in terms of both cost and effectiveness [9, 10, 12, 20, 26]. The relevant literature shows that examination of only one lymph node slide using hematoxylin and eosin (H&E) stain leaves up to 33 % of metastases unidentified. A single slide with H&E stain through the center of a node 1 cm in diameter provides information on <1 % of its volume [4, 8, 14, 27].

Additional H&E histopathologic analysis of serial sections allows for the identification of micrometastatic disease in up to 20 % of lymph nodes determined to be negative by standard H&E methods [13]. However, performing H&E histopathologic analysis of sections can be technically challenging and time consuming, as well as entailing significantly greater cost. Other histopathologic methods utilized for more accurate assessment of the status of the regional lymph nodes, such as immunohistochemistry using antibodies against human cytokeratins or RT-PCR, require even more time and incur an even higher cost. Therefore, what would be most useful and relevant is a more careful evaluation of a selected group of lymph nodes that have the highest probability of containing metastatic cells, i.e., the sentinel lymph nodes (SLNs) [4, 6–10, 14–16, 20–23, 27, 28].

The concept of SLN biopsy in colorectal cancer is currently not analogous to the similar procedure employed in cases of melanoma, breast cancer, or Merkel cell carcinoma, where it has direct implications for further therapy. En bloc resection of the tumor with systematic lymph node resection and central vessel ligation is the gold standard in colorectal cancer. SLN biopsy would allow a more comprehensive diagnosis of the status of the lymphatic system, which, as already stated, may be underestimated during the normal staining. This benefit is attributable to the identification of cancer cell foci that are impossible to verify when using the H&E procedure [4–6, 8, 9, 17, 22]. The identification of micrometastases in SLNs during the more thorough analysis may suggest the presence of metastases in non-SLNs. This idea was originally put forward in single studies, but in a meta-analysis by Des Guetz et al. in 2007, it was emphasized that standard histopathology of lymph nodes in colorectal cancer delivers less diagnostic and prognostic information than does thorough examination of the lymph nodes identified during lymphatic mapping [7, 14, 29]. Presently, SLN biopsy is recommended as an examination that provides some additional, prognostically relevant information, despite its not entirely satisfying sensitivity. The results of the procedure depend on a series of conditions that influence the quality of the procedure [18, 19, 30].

Performance of lymphatic mapping in the rectum is less reliable than in the colon owing to the different anatomy. The principle of oncological radicality associated with TME requires the mesorectal fascia to remain intact during surgery. This makes it impossible to apply the dye and to search for lymph nodes intraoperatively. Another issue is neoadjuvant radio- or radiochemotherapy, which affects the vessels and lymph nodes in the vicinity of the tumor. In principle, patients with rectal cancer should be excluded from the analyzed material, or the procedural calculations presented for them should be presented separately [10, 11, 20].

Table 18.1 provides a short overview of studies of the use of SLN biopsy in colorectal cancer.

18.1.2 Inclusion Criteria

In order to qualify for SLN biopsy, patients typically have to meet the following criteria: provision of patient consent, age over 18, satisfactory general condition (ASA I–III), primary histopathologically confirmed resectable colorectal cancer, no previous surgical interventions in the colon or its mesentery (including appendectomy in the superior proximal right half of the colon), and no allergies to contrast agents. Patients with previous lymphadenectomy (regardless of the reasons), pregnant women, patients who have lymph nodes intraoperatively suspected of harboring metastases, tumors infiltrating neighboring organs, remote metastases, or synchronous cancer and patients undergoing emergency procedures (obstruction, massive bleeding, perforation) are excluded.

In some studies, several further factors have been taken into consideration in assessing whether patients qualify for SLN biopsy, i.e., anthropometric data, intraoperative appearance of the tumor, and macroscopic and microscopic characteristics at histopathology [5, 7, 17–20, 29, 35, 37, 40, 46–51].

Table 18.1 Parameters achieved in SLN biopsy in colon cancer, published by selected authors after the year 2000

Author	Year	Journal	No. of patients with CC	% of patients with CC	DR (%)	Accuracy (%)	Sensitivity (%)	FNR (%)	NPV (%)	Upstaging (%)	IHC/ RT-PCR
Saha [31]	2000	*Ann Surg Oncol*	74	86	99	96	91	9	–	18	No
Wiese [22]	2000	*Arch Pathol Lab Med*	70	70	99	96	91	9	–	–	Yes
Bilchik [32]	2001	*J Clin Oncol*	33	83	100	100	100	0	100	50	Yes
Esser [27]	2001	*Dis Colon Rectum*	26	84	58	94	67	33	94	7	No
Wood [8]	2002	*J Gastrointest Surg*	78	78	97	95	92	8	–	24	Yes
Bilchik [33]	2002	*Eur J Cancer*	100	100	97	95	91	5	–	24	Yes
Feig [34]	2001	*Am J Surg*	48	100	98	79	38	62	76	8	Yes
Bilchik [14]	2003	*J Clin Oncol*	102	85	96	96	92	8	–	29	Yes
Viehl [35]	2003	*World J Surg*	31	100	87	78	50	50	71	11	Yes
Saha [11]	2004	*Dis Colon Rectum*	336	83	99	–	88	12	–	13	Yes
Dan [21]	2004	*Arch Surg*	106	88	99	96	86	16	–	5	Yes
Bertagnolli [15]	2004	*Ann Surg*	72	100	92	80	46	54	75	0	no
Saha [36]	2004	*Semin Oncol*	209	80	100	96	92	8	–	13	Yes
Bilchik [4]	2006	*Arch Surg*	97	73	100	95	88	12	–	23	Yes
Saha [10]	2006	*Am J Surg*	408	82	98	96	90	10	93	–	Yes
Thomas [37]	2006	*Am Surg*	69	100	93	20	46	54	73	5	Yes
Kelder [38]	2007	*Int J Colorectal Dis*	69	100	97	96	89	11	93	–	Yes
Murawa [39]	2007	*Acta Chir Belg*	13	48	93	84	83	17	–	8	Yes
Bembenek [40]	2007	*Ann Surg*	315	100	85	86	54	46	80	21	Yes
Lim [6]	2008	*Ann Surg Oncol*	120	100	99	83	59	41	78	–	Yes
Quadros [20]	2008	*J Surg Oncol*	22	42	91	80	67	33	67	25	Yes
Ivanov [41]	2009	*Hepatogastroenterology*	48	47	100	97	–	–	95	19	Yes
Retter [42]	2011	*Colorectal Dis*	31	100	90	71	33	67	46	5	Yes
Albayrak [43]	2011	*Turk J Gastroenterol*	38	100	95	100	100	0	100	–	No
Murawa [44]	2011	*Int J Colorectal Dis*	100	100	99	94	83	17	91	10	Yes
Vilcea [45]	2011	*Rom J Morphol Embryol*	43	51	74	84	62	38	–	10	No
Viehl [46]	2013	*World J Surg*	74	100	89	84	55	45	80	15	Yes

CC colon cancer, *DR* detection rate, *FNR* false-negative results, *NPV* negative predictive value, *IHC* immunochemistry

18.1.3 Prognostic Significance of Micrometastases in SLNs

The prognostic significance of micrometastases has not yet been definitively established. What has been proven is the lack of clinical relevance of isolated cancer cells found in lymph nodes [10, 52–59]. Furthermore, few studies have analyzed the issue of prognosis in colon cancer patients in whom micrometastases have been detected in the SLN. In the Sirop et al. study in 2011, 109 patients with colorectal cancer were investigated, with a follow-up of at least 5 years. The SLN was analyzed through serial dissections and immunohistochemistry. In 14 patients, micrometastases were confirmed in the SLNs. All of these patients received adjuvant treatment. 5-year survival in the group with micrometastases after chemotherapy was 100 %, compared with 96.2 % in the pN0 group and 75 % in the pN+ group. Owing to the small group size, this analysis did not achieve statistical significance ($p=0.07$) [3].

In a study in 2014, 55 patients with colon cancer after SLN biopsy were compared with a control group of 110 patients adjusted for tumor-related factors and operated on without SLN biopsy. The average number of examined lymph nodes in the clinical and control group differed significantly, being nine and seven, respectively ($p=0.03$). Immunochemistry resulted in upstaging owing to the detection of metastases in 3 of 38 SLNs initially considered true negative. The 5-year survival rates differed significantly in the two groups: 83 % in the SLN biopsy group vs. 69 % in the control group with no SLN biopsy ($p=0.03$). Furthermore, within the SLN group, the 5-year survival rate was higher in SLN-negative patients (91 % vs. 76 %; $p=0.04$). The authors emphasized the excellent prognosis in SLN-negative patients when using H&E stain and immunochemistry together with automated microscopy [60].

The studies utilizing molecular biology techniques (RT-PCR) have revealed that the frequency of discovery of small tumor deposits is statistically higher in the SLN than in other analyzed lymph nodes [4, 26].

One of the largest studies analyzed 192 patients with colon cancer. In 42 (22 %) patients, aberrant lymphatic drainage was observed which changed the scope of the resection. In 19 patients with extended scope of resection, metastases were found in lymph nodes located beyond the standard resection margin, and in two of these patients, these lymph nodes were the only sites of metastases. Furthermore, metastases to lymph nodes were detected in 62 % of patients in whom the scope of resection was extended after lymphatic mapping, compared with only 43 % of those who underwent standard resection. In the extended resection group, an average of 17.6 lymph nodes was examined, while in the standard resection group, the average was 15.8. Analysis of the data indicates that aberrant lymphatic drainage influences disease management, assessment of the disease stage, and, to a limited extent, survival [66].

18.2 Lymphatic Drainage of the Colon and Rectum

Lymphatic vessels in the colon run together with blood vessels (Fig. 18.1), which is the reason why colon resection should be accompanied by resection of the regional lymph nodes from the vicinity of the superior and inferior mesenteric vessels. The regional lymph nodes associated with the colon are divided into four groups:

1. Lymph nodes, located subserously in the intestinal wall.
2. Paracolic lymph nodes, located along the marginal artery.
3. Mesocolic lymph nodes, located along arteries. These include:
   - Ileocolic lymph nodes, which are divided into prececal, retrocecal, and appendicular lymph nodes. Lymph flows along the ileocolic artery toward the superior mesenteric lymph nodes.
   - Left, middle, and right colic lymph nodes transport lymph to the superior and inferior mesenteric lymph nodes.

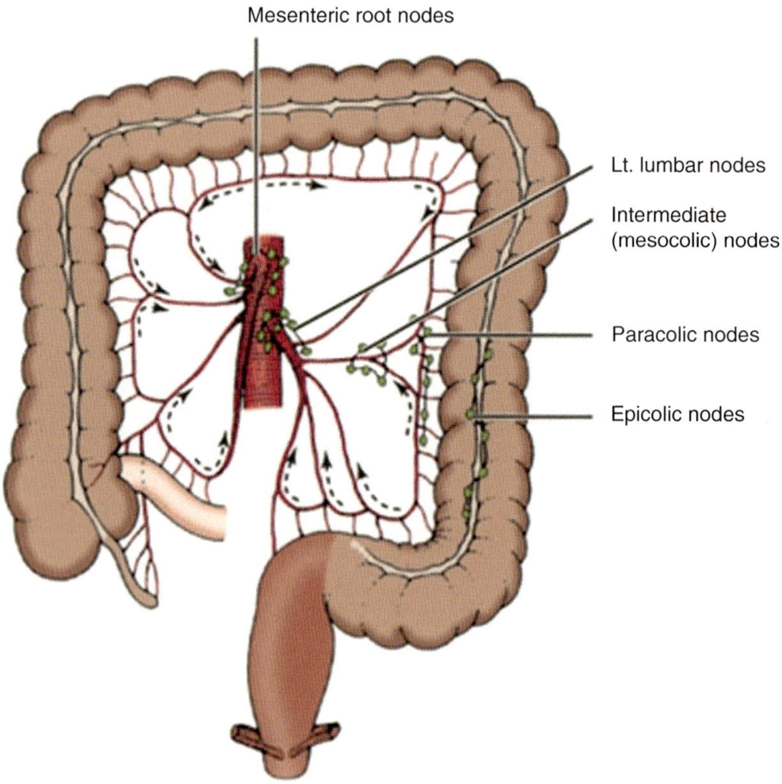

Fig. 18.1 Lymphatic drainage and regional lymph nodes associated with the colon (Source: Skandalakis et al. [61])

- Inferior mesenteric lymph nodes, which are located in the sigmoid colon mesentery and along the superior rectal artery. They gather lymph from the sigmoid colon and the superior part of the rectum.

4. Major lymph nodes located by the inferior and superior mesenteric arteries bifurcation. These include inferior mesenteric lymph nodes, periaortic lymph nodes, and left perilumbar lymph nodes [61, 62].

Several studies show that in more than 80 % of cases, the first metastatic lymph node in colorectal cancer is a paracolic lymph node located 5 cm or less from the tumor (Fig. 18.2) [8, 11, 29, 47, 63, 64].

Beside this classic lymphatic drainage, aberrant drainage within the regional lymph nodes can exist. Such drainage leads directly to main lymph node stations near the superior and inferior mesenteric vessels or to colic and paracolic lymph nodes located at a significant distance from the tumor.

The prevalence of aberrant lymphatic drainage has generally been reported to be up to 20 % [32, 65, 66]. Drainage of this nature influences the scope of lymphadenectomy since "aberrant" lymph nodes are potential locations for "skip metastases" [5, 8, 11, 16, 22, 67]. In some cases, the first lymph nodes to become dyed are those on the opposite side of the colon. Instances of lymphatic drainage from the transverse colon through the greater omentum to the splenic hilar lymph nodes have also been published [8, 11]. Moreover, tumors located in the hepatic flexure can, in about 5 % of cases, metastasize to lymph nodes located around the head of pancreas and in about 4 % of cases to omental lymph nodes [68].

In some individual studies, a higher rate of aberrant lymphatic drainage reaching up to 29 % has been observed in patients undergoing lymphatic mapping. Sometimes, however, the

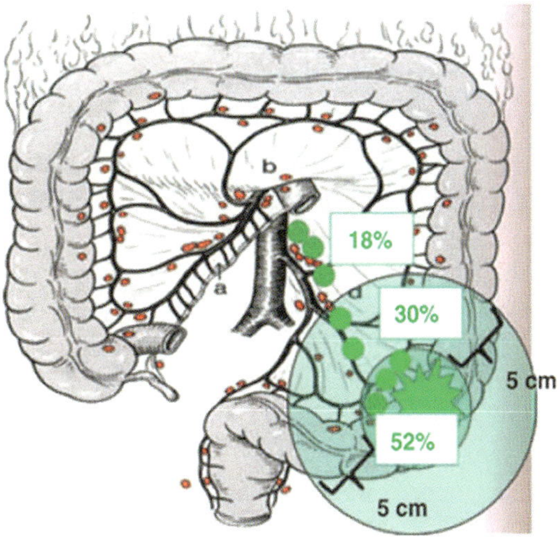

Fig. 18.2 Distribution of the first metastatic lymph node in colorectal cancer (Source: Bembenek [51])

identification of such drainage results from methodological shortcomings, such as dye migration during the procedure or administration of the tracer into the intestinal lumen (rather than intermurally), where it is absorbed by the mucous membrane at a location remote from the primary tumor [23].

The introduction of modern techniques, such as lymphoscintigraphy, has allowed more precise determination of the clinical anatomy of lymphatic drainage of the rectum, whose pattern does not fully match the vascular pattern (Fig. 18.3). Lymph from the superior third of the rectum is drained from the pararectal lymph nodes into the superior rectal lymph nodes and then into the inferior mesenteric lymph nodes. These lymph nodes are often the first sites of metastases: in

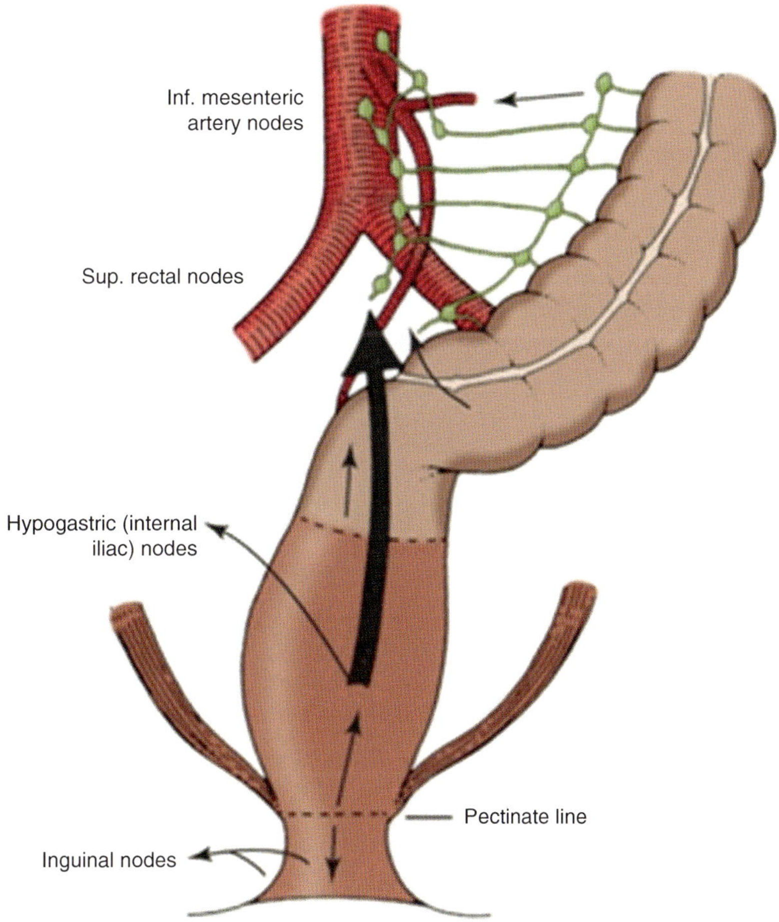

Fig. 18.3 Lymphatic drainage and regional lymph nodes associated with the rectum (Source: Skandalakis et al. [61])

most cases, metastases are located 3 or fewer centimeters from the primary tumor, but in 25 % of patients, they are situated very close to the superior rectal vessel bifurcation. Drainage from the remaining part of the rectum, located below the superior third but proximal to the mucocutaneous junction, takes place parallel to the middle rectal artery and its branches on the lateral pelvic wall or through the levator ani muscle along the inferior rectal artery; both these routes end in the internal iliac lymph nodes, common iliac lymph nodes, and lumbar trunk. Metastases to these lymph nodes are found in up to 12 % of patients. Drainage from tissues located below the mucocutaneous junction (anal canal) is not typical and does not take place in parallel to vessels. Lymph ducts run anterior and posterior to the perineum, together with ducts draining the nearby skin, and terminate in the superficial inguinal lymph nodes. Drainage via the external iliac lymph nodes takes place toward the lumbar trunk [61, 62, 69–73]; this route of spread is significant in tumors located in the inferior part of the rectum (possible metastases to inguinal lymph nodes) and above all in squamous cell carcinoma of the anal canal [74–77].

18.3 Colorimetric Markers: Mode of Administration and Limitations

The most commonly used tracers in lymphatic mapping in colorectal cancer are colorimetric markers. In Europe, Patent Blue V (sulfan blue, E131) is used most frequently in SLN marking, while in North America, the most frequently used dye is isosulfan blue – Lymphazurin. Less frequently used tracers include Evans Blue (T-1824), methylene blue, and indigo carmine. Soluble blue dyes are lymphotropic; they bond with endogenous protein through sulfonation and are retained in lymph ducts [7, 9, 20, 21, 26, 27, 78, 79]. The use of colorimetric dyes does not require any additional technology, nor does it prolong the procedure significantly (it does so by 5–10 min on average) [22, 26, 27]. A potential complication in the case of blue dyes, such as isosulfan blue and Patent Blue V, is allergic reactions, which occur in 1–1.5 % of cases [80–82]. These reactions include urticaria (hives), itching, nausea, hypotension, and, in very rare instances, life-endangering anaphylaxis. An additional problem is interference with pulse oximeter readings during the procedure [83–86].

As an alternative to blue dyes, fluorescent dyes such as indocyanine green can be used. These dyes yield satisfactory results in terms of detection and sensitivity in both open surgery and laparoscopy. However, additional technological assistance is required in the form of an infrared light camera to allow observation and analysis of the fluorescence. The rare occurrence of severe allergic reactions to indocyanine green needs to be underlined [87, 88].

Technical aspects of dye administration are very important. In the vast majority of cases, dye is administered intraoperatively via subserosal injection. No advantage of submucosal injection during colonoscopy has been demonstrated [5, 7, 26]. It needs to be underlined that unskilled administration of the dye – with injection into the intestinal lumen – may result in its absorption at a remote location (as described in Sect. 18.2). Spilling the dye outside the tumor is also problematic, since it makes it impossible to find the right node after the mesentery has been stained [7, 10, 16, 21, 26].

Dyes should be administered intraoperatively, with in vivo lymphatic mapping. From a technical standpoint, the staining and mapping of the lymph nodes ex vivo is simpler. Ex vivo mapping, however, may be considered reliable only when the section and the mesentery have remained intact during the resection (operating in exact anatomic planes). Identification ex vivo alone, done after the administration of dye during the operation, without marking the lymph node with, for example, a suture or a clamp, has a satisfactory detection rate but entails a significantly higher rate of false-negative results. This is especially true when the duration of studies following dye injection extends toward 100 min. The false-negative rate may then even reach 45–60 %, rendering the SLN biopsy clinically useless [89, 90]. In the prolonged interval between dye administration and lymph node identification, the marker relocates, sometimes resulting in loss of staining of the primary nodal station or in the marking of other nodal groups which are not composed of SLNs [4, 8, 9, 14, 17, 21, 26, 33, 36, 48, 91].

18.4 Role of Radiocolloids in Lymphatic System Mapping

The use of radiocolloids is restricted by various attendant problems and limitations, most of which are due to the complexity of dealing with radioisotopes. Further problems are of a legal nature. In many countries, formal authorization is required from medical personnel, which limits the number of people allowed to inject the isotope [26, 47, 94]. The advantage of radiocolloids is the absence of allergic reactions and lack of interference with equipment monitoring vital signs [78].

The radiotracers most often used are ^{99m}Tc-tin (especially in Japan) and ^{99m}Tc-sulfur colloid (especially in North America) [92], but ^{99m}Tc-albumin may also be administered [93]. In some cases, endoscopic examination with submucosal injection can be performed a day before the operation [7, 16, 20, 26, 47, 63, 94]. Here it must be emphasized that only about 10 % of the administered ^{99m}Tc migrates from the site of injection to lymph nodes. Taking into account the half-life of ^{99m}Tc, which is 6 h, the activity in the lymph nodes at 12 h after administration during preoperative endoscopy (via submucosal injection) may be too weak to enable SLN identification [47]. From this perspective, intraoperative administration of the radiocolloid (at a suitably set dose) seems advantageous; however, administration of the radiocolloid on the day of surgery (preferably no more than 2 h before the operation) will also be adequate [47, 95].

Owing to the size of the molecules, radiocolloids may be expected to travel more slowly in lymph channels than do blue dyes, thereby permitting more precise identification of SLNs. Moreover, the larger size of radiocolloids, compared with blue dyes, causes them to remain longer within the first draining lymph node [78, 94, 96]. A real problem, however, is the fact that radiocolloid migrates more rapidly in intestinal lymphatic channels than in breast cancer or melanoma, thus increasing the probability of observing more "hot" lymph nodes [63]. The use of handheld gamma probes means that, to a certain degree, radiocolloids allow for easier identification of lymph nodes located deep within the intestinal mesentery, where blue dye may not be readily visible. It should be emphasized, however, that the SLN identification process can be imprecise and is sometimes more indicative of the general pattern of lymphatic flow through the lymphatic channels rather than any particular lymph node. Another problem is the "shine through" effect that results from the overlap of radioactivity which can be encountered when the tumor is in close proximity to the SLN candidates. The minimum cutoff value for the identification of any given SLN candidate with the gamma detection probe is generally defined as a count rate greater than twice the background count rate. This background radiation is described as radiation of tissues located remotely from the site of injection and from the intestinal mesentery, measured in three independent places [14, 78, 93, 96]. Therefore, when performing submucosal injections, it is necessary to repeat lymphoscintigraphy 2 or 3 times before the operation, to exclude spillage of the marker or contamination of the abdominal cavity [63]. It should be noted that when performing intraoperative subserosal administration, all contaminated materials (needles, syringes, gloves, swabs, setons) must be removed from the operation site both to ensure adequate radiation protection and to exclude the possibility of interference in the process of lymphatic mapping [78].

Some studies have concluded that lymphatic mapping using radiocolloids does not improve SLN biopsy in colorectal cancer, whereas others [47] have indicated that the combined radiocolloid/blue dye method is associated with improvement of quality and results in this setting [7, 14, 16, 20, 21, 23, 26, 29, 94, 97]. Importantly, in comparison with the use of dye only, double mapping leads to a statistically significant increase in the probability of finding an SLN and of identifying metastasis within that SLN [78].

18.5 Intraoperative Detection and Harvesting the SLN in Colorectal Cancer

18.5.1 Standard SLN Biopsy Method in Colon Cancer with the Use of Blue Dye

According to the most commonly accepted protocol, after the abdominal cavity has been opened, the fragment of colon to be resected is delicately mobilized to avoid potential extensive damage to lymphatic and vascular structures. Next, blue dye (e.g., 2 ml of Patent Blue V dye) is administered subserosally around the tumor by means of four or more injections (Fig. 18.4). After 5–10 min, the lymph ducts become dyed and visible (Fig. 18.5), as do the first lymph nodes (most often 1–4) (Fig. 18.6). Lymph nodes are marked with a suture (Fig. 18.7). At the end of the operation, they are harvested separately to be examined as SLNs (Fig. 18.8). The whole procedure of lymphatic mapping, from administration of the dye to marking the SLNs with a suture, takes place intraoperatively, in vivo. In the further operation, a standard en bloc resection is performed with a margin of healthy tissues and mesenteric lymphatic system.

The method of administration and mapping is similar when using fluorescent dye. To make the lymph flow visible and detect the lymph node, however, special equipment is required that permits in vivo analysis of intraoperative images in infrared (Figs. 18.9 and 18.10).

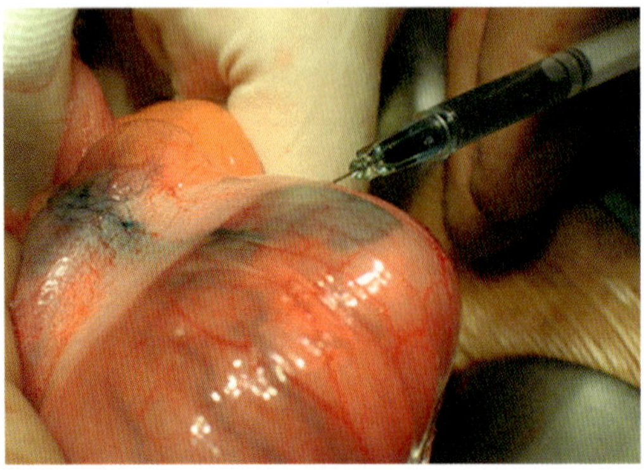

Fig. 18.4 Subserous injection of the dye in the area around the tumor (Source: author's materials)

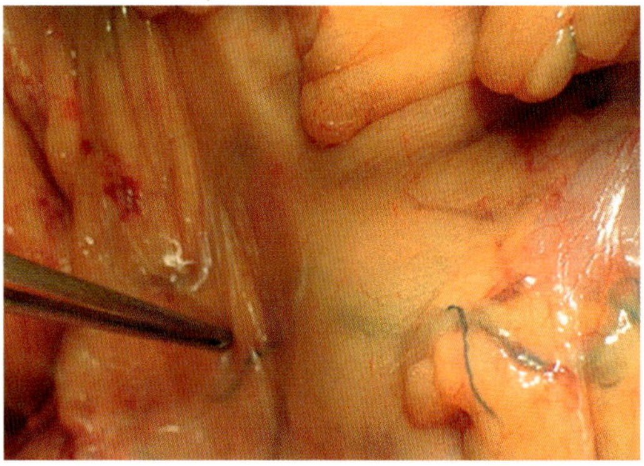

Fig. 18.5 Identification of a dyed lymphatic channel (Source: author's materials)

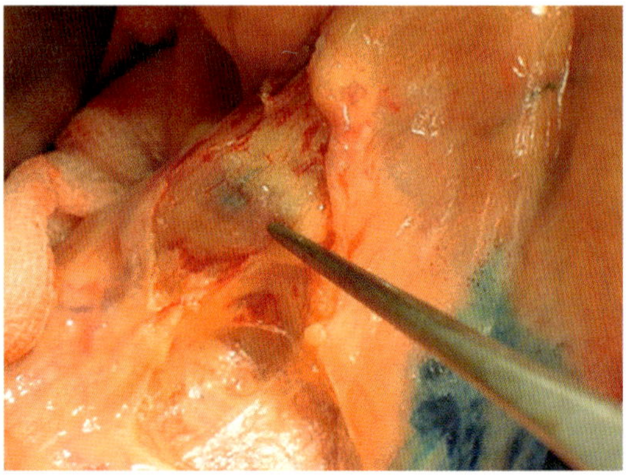

Fig. 18.6 SLN in the process of dyeing (Source: author's materials)

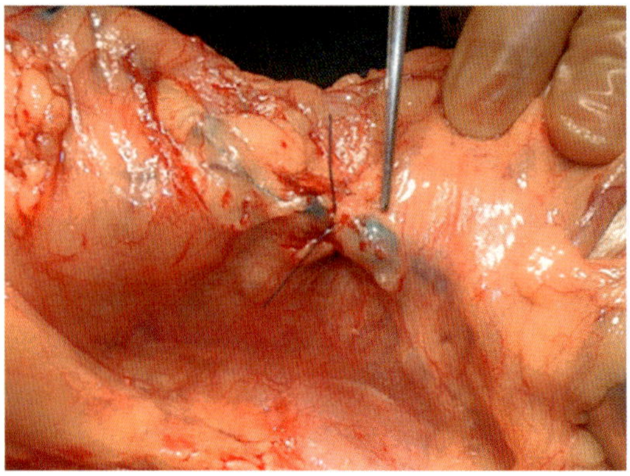

Fig. 18.7 Dyed SLN and lymphatic channel marked with a suture (Source: author's materials)

The results of SLN biopsy in colorectal cancer using mapping with colorimetric tracers are described in Table 1.1.

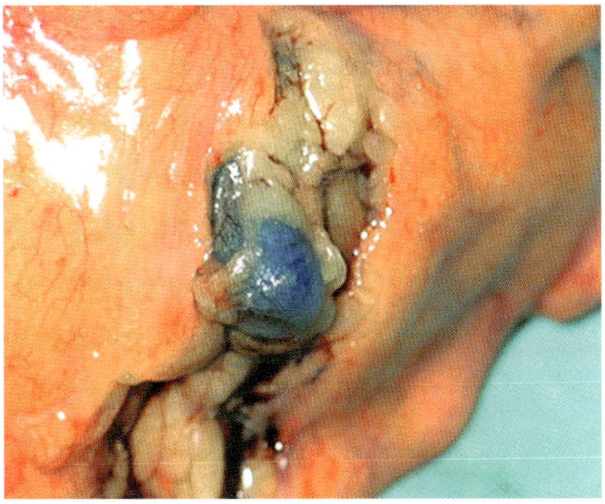

Fig. 18.8 Dyed SLN (Source: author's materials)

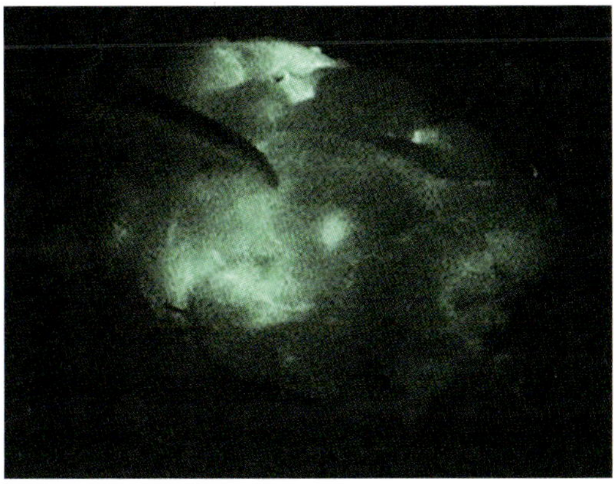

Fig. 18.9 Lymphatic mapping procedure in colon cancer using indocyanine green and a Pulsion camera (Source: author's materials)

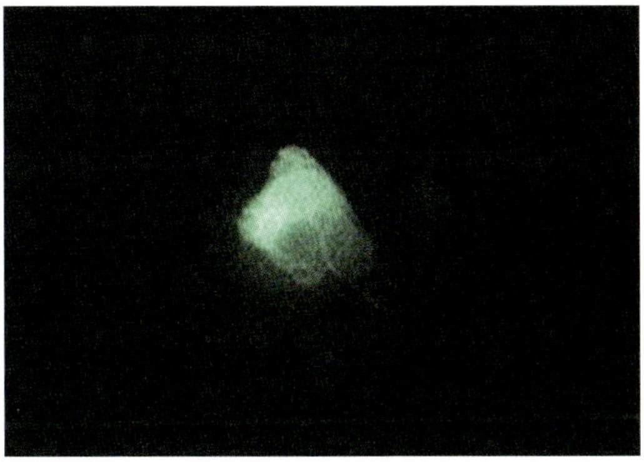

Fig. 18.10 SLN harvested using the indocyanine green method; image in infrared light (Source: author's materials)

18.5.2 Clinical Use of Radiocolloids in SLN Biopsy in Colon Cancer

Most of the available literature on SLN biopsies performed at major colon cancer centers relates to the blue dye method alone, without the combined use of radiocolloid. Due to the already mentioned problems and limitations, as well as the fact that they often provide diverging results, methods using ^{99m}Tc-sulfur colloid and intraoperative gamma probe detection have been described relatively rarely [98]. During surgery, 0.5–2.0 ml (or, in some cases, 3–5 ml) of 1 % isosulfan blue and then 1 ml of ^{99m}Tc-sulfur colloid in saline solution with an activity of 0.5–1.0 μCi [6, 14, 78, 96, 97] are administered subserously via several injections around the tumor. The doses are increased significantly (three- to fourfold) if the injection is performed submucosally during endoscopy on the day before surgery [47]. During combined radiocolloid/blue dye mapping, blue dye (1–2 ml) and ^{99m}Tc-labeled albumin are used [93]. In patients undergoing total endoscopic polypectomy, the expected difficulties in intraoperative localization of the site of polypectomy usually lead to a decision to perform submucosal injection of radiocolloid during endoscopy prior to surgery, in combination with the preoperative lymphoscintigraphy. Endoscopic administrations are also described as standard procedures when combined with lymphoscintigraphy performed around 4-h post injection. The injection is typically performed submucosally in four rectangles around the tumor, but in the event of technical difficulties, it is limited to the tumor's posterior edge. It is worth noting that performance of endoscopy shortly before or during the surgery will entail intestinal distension, complicating the whole surgical procedure [47]. The potential benefit of administering radiocolloids before surgery is the possibility of performing lymphoscintigraphy and visualizing potentially aberrant lymph flow prior to surgery. Furthermore, due to complementary planar mapping, it is also possible to determine the depth of the lymph nodes. Lymphoscintigraphy enables identification of the nodes before surgery in more than 75 % of patients; however, in around 10 % of cases, the nodes are not found in vivo. In the 25 % of patients in whom the lymph nodes have not been identified before surgery, this is done during intraoperative mapping while using the gamma detection probe [47, 78].

Intraoperatively, dyed lymph nodes are usually identified approximately 1–10 min after the administration of the dye, and they are then marked with a suture. Next, the identification is performed using a handheld gamma detection probe (usually within 30 min following intraoperative radiocolloid administration). As previously mentioned, the minimum cutoff value for identification of any given SLN candidate with the gamma detection probe is generally defined as twice the background count rate [6, 14, 78, 93, 96]. In the majority of studies utilizing the combined radiocolloid/blue dye method of SLN biopsy, the SLN identification rate approaches 100 %, exceeding the rate achieved by the blue dye approach alone by several percentage points [6, 14, 47, 78, 96]. Less optimal results, approximately in the 90 % range, are reported using the radiocolloid SLN biopsy approach alone with the gamma detection probe [47, 78]. The accuracy of the combined radiocolloid/blue dye method of SLB biopsy in predicting the status of the regional lymph nodes is generally >90 %, barring some methodological flaws [14, 78, 96]. The relative numbers of blue-dyed, radioactive, and blue/radioactive SLNs identified by the combined radiocolloid/blue dye method vary: several studies have indicated the detection of significantly more blue-dyed lymph nodes than radioactive or radioactive/blue lymph nodes, while others indicate a greater number of radioactive or radioactive/blue lymph nodes than blue-dyed lymph nodes [14, 78, 96, 97]. In general, it has been found that the combined radiocolloid/blue dye method more accurately recognizes SLNs with metastases [47, 78].

Several recent studies have described the use of radiocolloid alone for SLN mapping and biopsy in patients with colon cancer [94, 95]. The first study utilized the submucosal injection of radiocolloid 2 h before surgery, with intraoperative identification performed with a gamma detection probe. The authors demonstrated good results, with a detection rate of 91 % and an accuracy of 97 % [95].

Taking into account the abovementioned data, the various technical difficulties, the need for additional medical equipment, the required team of medical specialists, the specificity of lymph flow in the intestinal mesentery, and, of course, the added costs, it remains clear that at present there is no consensus on the standard use of radiocolloid in lymphatic mapping and SLN biopsy for colon cancer [94, 97, 98].

18.5.3 Clinical Use of Radiocolloids in SLN Biopsy in Rectal Cancer

Because of the anatomic specificity, the possibilities and technique of lymphatic mapping in the rectum are different. In the case of rectal cancer, intraoperative lymphatic mapping is very difficult owing to the anatomic conditions and the limited space within the lower pelvis [93]. Additionally, the neoadjuvant radiochemotherapy for locally advanced rectal cancer causes sclerosis and fibrosis of the lymphatic system, changing and disturbing the patterns of lymphatic flow [100]. Furthermore, lymphatic mapping during the surgery results in damage to the mesorectal fascia, which is at odds with the purpose of total mesorectal excision, acknowledged to be the gold standard in rectal cancer. Therefore, the blue dye methods are predominantly used ex vivo, most often by folding the rectum and administering 1–2 ml of blue dye submucosally around the tumor. The combined radiocolloid/blue dye method is also used, especially for tumors located in the middle and lower parts of the rectum. In these cases, administration of the blue dye and radiocolloid is done submucosally prior to surgery with the use of a rigid rectoscope [78, 100]. This method of applying the tracers seems acceptable [10, 17, 69, 99, 100–104]. The ease of access to rectal cancer via the rectoscope facilitates trials in SLN biopsy with the use of radiocolloids. The radiocolloid may be administered about 16–18 h (or more) before surgery, during endoscopy (most often 1 ml ^{99m}Tc solution is applied submucosally around the tumor). If it is possible to go cephalad, beyond the tumor, the radiocolloid is administered as four injections; otherwise, it is administered as three injections (from the two sides lateral and distal to the tumor). At 1–2 h before surgery, lymphoscintigraphy is performed. The main issue regarding the use of radiocolloids is the direct proximity of the main nodal stations (pararectal lymph nodes) and the primary rectal tumor, the result of which is an overlap of radioactivity and more problematic identification of SLNs than in cases of colon cancer.

In publications on the ex vivo lymphatic mapping of rectal cancer, the authors often underline the advantages of this approach, from the perspective of both blue dye administration and lymph node identification. They point out the relatively short duration of the procedure (around 10 min) and the lack of allergic reactions. However, they often do not take into account the limitations ensuing from such a method of dye application [17, 100, 102, 104, 109]. Accurate ex vivo lymphatic mapping of the total mesorectum specimen is only possible if there is truly no disruption of the intrinsic vascular and lymphatic anatomy of the specimen, including the small lymphatic channels leading to the lymph nodes harvested within the specimen. Another issue is that the disruption of the intact total mesorectum specimen during surgery can lead to intravasation of radiocolloid from the specimen, thus causing a mismatch in the post-resection imaging as compared with the preoperative lymphoscintigraphy imaging. Likewise, ex vivo lymphatic mapping may entail discrepancies between the pattern of lymphatic flow within the total mesorectum specimen and that observed in vivo in the native mesorectum secondary to aberrant lymphatic flow. The conclusion from ex vivo mapping is that the analysis of other, non-SLNs is more important and forces intricate analysis of the SLN into the background [17, 69, 100–102, 104, 109]. Details and results of studies of SLN biopsy in rectal cancer are summarized in Table 18.2.

18.5.4 Clinical Use of Radiocolloids in SLN Biopsy in Anal Cancer

According to current recommendations, the initial therapeutic approach to anal squamous cell carcinoma is radiochemotherapy, with surgical management generally being considered only in selected cases of local recurrent disease. Synchronous regional lymph node metastases are found in 10–25 % of patients, but as surgical treatment is not the standard procedure, the true state of lymph nodes is not a key issue. The lymphatic drainage from tumors around the anal canal depends on their location in reference to the Z-line. For tumors located below this line, the main route of lymphatic drainage is to the inguinal lymph nodes and further along the femoral artery. However, around 15–35 % of metastases to the inguinal lymph nodes are encountered in patients with tumors located above the Z-line. This indicates that the Z-line does not represent an exact borderline for the lymphatic system and metastatic spread [69, 101, 109]. Drainage is often bilateral, which significantly increases the importance of preoperative lymphoscintigraphy. Furthermore, in most cases the inguinal region is the predominant lymphatic drainage pathway [98]. Hence, if the inguinal lymph nodes seem clinically or radiologically suspicious, or histopathologic evidence of metastasis is available, the primary treatment is radiation. In selected cases, radiation treatment is combined with inguinal lymphadenectomy. In cases that are not clinically suspicious, some medical centers advise strict control and observation. Others, however, propose elective radiation therapy of the inguinal region with the exclusion of early cases, i.e., stages T1 and T2 (which have a 5–10 % frequency of inguinal lymph node invasion). Hence, SLN biopsy has been proposed as a tool for precise and minimally invasive assessment of the regional inguinal lymph nodes and also for further therapeutic decision making (radiotherapy). The method applicable is first and foremost the radiocolloid procedure, sometimes in combination with the blue dye method. Radiotracers such as ^{99m}Tc-sulfur colloid, ^{99m}Tc-colloidal human albumin, ^{99m}Tc-colloidal

Table 18.2 Details and results of studies of SLN biopsy in rectal cancer, performed after the year 2000

Main author	Year	Journal	No. of patients	N(+) in H&E (%)	Technique	Injection	Identification	DR (%)	Sensitivity (%)	Upstaging (%)	ALD (%)
Kitagawa [99]	2000	*Surg Clin North Am*	56	29	RC	Pre-op	In vivo	91	81	–	–
Bembenek [100]	2004	*Surgery*	48	33	RC	Pre-op	Ex vivo	96	44	0	4
Saha [11]	2004	*Dis Colon Rectum*	71	32	BD	Intraop	In vivo	92	96	7	4
Baton [102]	2005	*World J Surg*	31	23	BD	Post-op	Ex vivo	97	57	13	–
Braat [103]	2005	*Br J Surg*	34	32	BD	Post-op	Ex vivo	76	40	6	–
Saha [10]	2006	*Am J Surg*	92	29	BD	Intraop + post-op	In vivo+ex vivo	91	93	26	7
Yagci [104]	2007	*Int J Colorectal Dis*	47	43	BD	Post-op	Ex vivo	98	80	15	–
van der Zaag [17]	2009	*Eur J Surg Oncol*	32	53	BD	Post-op	Ex vivo	78	57	27	–

N(+) in H&E (%),the percentage of patients with infiltrated lymph nodes at H&E staining
DR detection rate, *RC* radiocolloid, *BD* blue dye, *Pre-op* preoperative, *Intraop*, intraoperative, *Post-op* postoperative

Table 18.3 Details and results of studies of SLN biopsy in anal cancer, performed after the year 2000

Main author	Year	Journal	No. of pts	Technique	Injection	DR (%)	Pts with SLN in the inguinal region (%)	Pts with positive SLN in the inguinal region (%)
Perera [108]	2003	*Dis Colon Rectum*	12	RC+BD	Pre-op + intraop	67	67	29
Damin [106]	2003	*Dis Colon Rectum*	14	RC+BD	Pre-op + intraop	100	100	7
Bobin [105]	2003	*Cancer Radiother*	33	RC+BD	Pre-op + intraop	100	100	21
Ulmer [109]	2004	*Ann Surg Oncol*	17	RC	Pre-op	76	71	43
Gretschel [107]	2008	*Eur J Surg Oncol*	40	RC	Pre-op	90	56	30
Mistrangelo [110]	2009	*Q J Nucl Med Mol Imaging*	35	RC	Pre-op	97	97	20

DR detection rate, *RC* radiocolloid, *BD* blue dye, *Pre-op* preoperative, *Intraop*, intraoperative, *pts* patients, *SLN* sentinel lymph node

rhenium sulfide, and ^{99}Tc-antimony trisulfide are used. The radiocolloid is administered into the subcutaneous or submucosal tissue from the four injection sites around the primary tumor in a total dose ranging from 5 MBq (0.135 mCi) to 37 MBq (1.0 mCi). The frequency of localization is 75–100 %, and identification of metastases in the inguinal lymph nodes is successfully achieved in 10–40 % of patients, with a low rate of complications of between 3 % and 7 % [98, 103–110]. The results of selected studies concerning the application of SLN biopsy in anal cancer are shown in Table 18.3.

References

1. IARC, WHO. Cancer Incidence, Mortality and Prevalence Worldwide in 2008. http://globocan.iarc.fr/.
2. Labianca R, Nordlinger B, Beretta GD, et al. Primary colon cancer: ESMO Clinical Practice Guidelines for diagnosis, adjuvant treatment and follow-up. Ann Oncol. 2010;21 Suppl 5:v70–7.
3. Sirop S, Kanaan M, Korant A, et al. Detection and prognostic impact of micrometastasis in colorectal cancer. J Surg Oncol. 2011;103:534–7.
4. Bilchik AJ, DiNome M, Saha S, et al. Prospective multicenter trial of staging adequacy in colon cancer: preliminary results. Arch Surg. 2006;141:527–33.
5. Iddings D, Bilchik A. The biologic significance of micrometastatic disease and sentinel lymph node technology on colorectal cancer. J Surg Oncol. 2007;96:671–7.
6. Lim SJ, Feig BW, Wang H, et al. Sentinel lymph node evaluation does not improve staging accuracy in colon cancer. Ann Surg Oncol. 2008;15:46–51.
7. Des Guetz G, Uzzan B, Nicolas P, et al. Is sentinel lymph node mapping in colorectal cancer a future prognostic factor? A meta-analysis. World J Surg. 2007;31:1304–12.
8. Wood TF, Nora DT, Morton DL, et al. One hundred consecutive cases of sentinel lymph node mapping in early colorectal carcinoma: detection of missed micrometastases. J Gastrointest Surg. 2002;6:322–9.
9. Broderick-Villa G, Ko A, O'Connell TX, et al. Does tumor burden limit the accuracy of lymphatic mapping and sentinel lymph node biopsy in colorectal cancer? Cancer J. 2002;8:445–50.
10. Saha S, Seghal R, Patel M, et al. A multicenter trial of sentinel lymph node mapping in colorectal cancer: prognostic implications for nodal staging and recurrence. Am J Surg. 2006;191:305–10.
11. Saha S, Monson KM, Bilchik A, et al. Comparative analysis of nodal upstaging between colon and rectal cancers by sentinel lymph node mapping: a prospective trial. Dis Colon Rectum. 2004;47:1767–72.
12. Wright FC, Law CH, Berry S, et al. Clinically important aspects of lymph node assessment in colon cancer. J Surg Oncol. 2009;99:248–55.
13. Dionigi G, Castano P, Rovera F, et al. The application of sentinel lymph node mapping in colon cancer. Surg Oncol. 2007;16 Suppl 1:S129–32.
14. Bilchik AJ, Nora DT, Sobin LH, et al. Effect of lymphatic mapping on the new tumor-node-metastasis classification for colorectal cancer. J Clin Oncol. 2003;21:668–72.
15. Bertagnolli M, Miedema B, Redston M, et al. Sentinel node staging of resectable colon cancer: results of a multicenter study. Ann Surg. 2004;240:624–8.
16. Bianchi PP, Ceriani C, Rottoli M, et al. Laparoscopic lymphatic mapping and sentinel lymph node detection in colon cancer: technical aspects and preliminary results. Surg Endosc. 2007;21:1567–71.
17. van der Zaag ES, Buskens CJ, Kooij N, et al. Improving staging accuracy in colon and rectal

cancer by sentinel lymph node mapping: a comparative study. Eur J Surg Oncol. 2009;35:106570.
18. van der Pas MH, Meijer S, Hoekstra OS, et al. Sentinel-lymph-node procedure in colon and rectal cancer: a systematic review and meta-analysis. Lancet Oncol. 2011;12:540–50.
19. van der Zaag ES, Bouma WH, Tanis PJ, et al. Systematic review of sentinel lymph node mapping procedure in colorectal cancer. Ann Surg Oncol. 2012;19:3449–59.
20. Quadros CA, Lopes A, Araujo I, et al. Upstaging benefits and accuracy of sentinel lymph node mapping in colorectal adenocarcinoma nodal staging. J Surg Oncol. 2008;98:324–30.
21. Dan AG, Saha S, Monson KM, et al. 1% lymphazurin vs. 10% fluorescein for sentinel node mapping in colorectal tumors. Arch Surg. 2004;139:1180–4.
22. Wiese DA, Saha S, Badin J, et al. Pathologic evaluation of sentinel lymph nodes in colorectal carcinoma. Arch Pathol Lab Med. 2000;124:1759–63.
23. Bilchik AJ, Trocha SD. Lymphatic mapping and sentinel node analysis to optimize laparoscopic resection and staging of colorectal cancer: an update. Cancer Control. 2003;10:219–23.
24. Andre T, Boni C, Mounedji-Boudiaf L, et al. Oxaliplatin, fluorouracil, and leucovorin as adjuvant treatment for colon cancer. N Engl J Med. 2004;350:2343–51.
25. Kuebler JP, Wieand HS, O'Connell MJ, et al. Oxaliplatin combined with weekly bolus fluorouracil and leucovorin as surgical adjuvant chemotherapy for stage II and III colon cancer: results from NSABP C-07. J Clin Oncol. 2007;25:2198–204.
26. Bembenek A, String A, Gretschel S, et al. Technique and clinical consequences of sentinel lymph node biopsy in colorectal cancer. Surg Oncol. 2008;117:183–93.
27. Esser S, Reilly WT, Riley LB, et al. The role of sentinel lymph node mapping in staging of colon and rectal cancer. Dis Colon Rectum. 2001;44:850–4.
28. Wiese D, Sirop S, Yestrepsky B, et al. Ultrastaging of sentinel lymph nodes (SLNs) vs. non-SLNs in colorectal cancer-do we need both? Am J Surg. 2010;199:354–8.
29. Cahill RA, Bembenek A, Sirop S, et al. Sentinel node biopsy for the individualization of surgical strategy for cure of early-stage colon cancer. Ann Surg Oncol. 2009;16:2170–80.
30. Viehl CT, Guller U, Cecini R, et al. Sentinel lymph node procedure leads to upstaging of patients with resectable colon cancer: results of the Swiss prospective, multicenter study sentinel lymph node procedure in colon cancer. Ann Surg Oncol. 2013;19:1959–65.
31. Saha S, Wiese D, Badin J, et al. Technical details of sentinel lymph node mapping in colorectal cancer and its impact on staging. Ann Surg Oncol. 2000;7:120–4.
32. Bilchik AJ, Saha S, Wiese D, et al. Molecular staging of early colon cancer on the basis of sentinel node analysis: a multicenter phase II trial. J Clin Oncol. 2001;19:1128–36.
33. Bilchik AJ, Nora D, Tollenaar RA, et al. Ultrastaging of early colon cancer using lymphatic mapping and molecular analysis. Eur J Cancer. 2002;38:977–85.
34. Feig BW, Curley S, Lucci A, et al. Caution regarding lymphatic mapping in patients with colon cancer. Am J Surg. 2001;182:707–12.
35. Viehl CT, Hamel CT, Marti WR, et al. Identification of sentinel lymph nodes in colon cancer depends on the amount of dye injected relative to tumor size. World J Surg. 2003;27:1285–90.
36. Saha S, Dan AG, Beutler T, et al. Sentinel lymph node mapping technique in colon cancer. Semin Oncol. 2004;31:374–81.
37. Thomas KA, Lechner J, Shen P, et al. Use of sentinel node mapping for cancer of the colon: 'to map or not to map". Am Surg. 2006;72:606–11.
38. Kelder W, Braat AE, Karrenbeld A, et al. The sentinel node procedure in colon carcinoma: a multicentre study in The Netherlands. Int J Colorectal Dis. 2007;22:1509–14.
39. Murawa D, Filas V, Breborowicz J, et al. Evaluation of the sentinel node biopsy in colorectal carcinoma including the results of immunohistochemical examinations. Acta Chir Belg. 2007;107:45–8.
40. Bembenek AE, Rosenberg R, Wagler E, et al. Sentinel lymph node biopsy in colon cancer: a prospective multicenter trial. Ann Surg. 2007;245:858–63.
41. Ivanov K, Kolev N, Ignatov V, et al. Intraoperative sentinel lymph node mapping in patients with colorectal cancer. Hepatogastroenterology. 2009;56:99–105.
42. Retter SM, Herrmann G, Schiedeck TH. Clinical value of sentinel node mapping in carcinoma of the colon. Colorectal Dis. 2011;13:855–9.
43. Albayrak Y, Oren D, Gündoğdu C, et al. Intraoperative sentinel lymph node mapping in patients with colon cancer: study of 38 cases. Turk J Gastroenterol. 2011;22:286–92.
44. Murawa D, Nowaczyk P, Hünerbein M, et al. One hundred consecutive cases of sentinel lymph node mapping in colon cancer-the results of prospective, single-centre feasibility study with implementation of immunohistochemical staining. Int J Colorectal Dis. 2011;26:897–902.
45. Vîlcea ID, Vasile I, Mirea CS, et al. Sentinel lymph node study in colorectal cancer using serial sectioning and Hematoxylin-Eosin staining: importance and limitations. Rom J Morphol Embryol. 2011;52(1 Suppl):379–83.
46. Viehl CT, Guller U, Langer I, et al. Factors influencing the success of in-vivo sentinel lymph node procedure in colon cancer patients: Swiss prospective, multicenter study sentinel lymph node procedure in colon cancer. World J Surg. 2013;37:873–7.
47. Tiffet O, Kaczmarek D, Chambonnière ML, et al. Combining radioisotopic and blue-dye technique does not improve the false-negative rate in sentinel

lymph node mapping for colorectal cancer. Dis Colon Rectum. 2007;50:962–70.
48. Cahill RA, Leroy J, Marescaux J. Could lymphatic mapping and sentinel node biopsy provide oncological providence for local resectional techniques for colon cancer? A review of the literature. BMC Surg. 2008;8:17.
49. Nowaczyk P, Murawa D, Połom K, et al. Analysis of sentinel lymph node biopsy results in colon cancer in regard of the anthropometric features of the population and body composition assessment formulas. Langenbecks Arch Surg. 2012;397:779–86.
50. Wood TF, Spirt M, Rangel D, et al. Lymphatic mapping improves staging during laparoscopic colectomy for cancer. Surg Endosc. 2001;15:715–9.
51. Bembenek A. Current clinical status of sentinel lymph nodes in colon and proximal rectal cancer. Colorectal Dis. 2011;13 Suppl 7:63–6.
52. Natsugoe S, Arigami T, Uenosono Y, et al. Lymph node micrometastasis in gastrointestinal tract cancer-a clinical aspect. Int J Clin Oncol. 2013;18: 752–61.
53. Fisher ER, Colangelo L, Wieand S, et al. Lack of influence of cytokeratin-positive mini micrometastases in "Negative Node" patients with colorectal cancer: findings from the national surgical adjuvant breast and bowel projects protocols R-01 and C-01. Dis Colon Rectum. 2003;46:1021–5.
54. Bilchik A, Nissan A, Wainberg Z, et al. Surgical quality and nodal ultrastaging is associated with long-term disease-free survival in early colorectal cancer: an analysis of 2 international multicenter prospective trials. Ann Surg. 2010;252:467–74.
55. Reggiani Bonetti L, Di Gregorio C, De Gaetani C, et al. Lymph node micrometastasis and survival of patients with Stage i (Dukes' A) colorectal carcinoma. Scand J Gastroenterol. 2011;46:881–6.
56. Märkl B, Herbst C, Cacchi C, et al. Prognostic significance of histologically detected lymph node micrometastases of sizes between 0.2 and 2 mm in colorectal cancer. Int J Colorectal Dis. 2013;28:977–83.
57. Bukholm IR, Bondi J, Wiik P, et al. Presence of isolated tumour cells in mesenteric lymph nodes predicts poor prognosis in patients with stage II colon cancer. Eur J Surg Oncol. 2003;29:862–6.
58. Bosch Roig CE, Rosello-Sastre E, Alonso Hernandez S, et al. Prognostic value of the detection of lymph node micrometastases in colon cancer. Clin Transl Oncol. 2008;10:572–8.
59. Faerden AE, Sjo OH, Bukholm IR, et al. Lymph node micrometastases and isolated tumor cells influence survival in stage I and II colon cancer. Dis Colon Rectum. 2011;54:200–6.
60. Braat AE, Pol RA, Oosterhuis JW, et al. Excellent prognosis of node negative patients after sentinel node procedure in colon carcinoma: a 5-year follow-up study. Eur J Surg Oncol. 2014;40:747–55.
61. Skandalakis JE, Colborn GL, Weidman TA. Skandalakis' Surgical Anatomy: The Embryologic and Anatomic Basis of Modern Surgery. Paschalidis Medical Publication Ltd. International Student Edition, Two Volumes. 2004.
62. Woźniak W. Anatomia człowieka. Podręcznik dla studentów i lekarzy. Elsevier Urban & Partner Wydawnictwo; Wrocław 2003, wyd.2.
63. Bianchi PP, Petz W, Casali L. Laparoscopic lymphatic roadmapping with blue dye and radioisotope in colon cancer. Colorectal Dis. 2011;13 Suppl 7:67–9.
64. Tan KY, Kawamura YJ, Mizokami K, et al. Distribution of the first metastatic lymph node in colon cancer and its clinical significance. Colorectal Dis. 2010;12:44–7.
65. Wood TF, Tsioulias GJ, Morton DL, et al. Focused examination of sentinel lymph nodes upstages early colorectal carcinoma. Am Surg. 2000;66:998–1003.
66. Saha S, Johnston G, Korant A, et al. Aberrant drainage of sentinel lymph nodes in colon cancer and its impact on staging and extent of operation. Am J Surg. 2013;205:302–5.
67. Tsioulias GJ, Wood TF, Spirt M, Morton DL, Bilchik AJ. A novel lymphatic mapping technique to improve localization and staging of early colon cancer during laparoscopic colectomy. Am Surg. 2002;68:561–5.
68. Hohenberger W, Weber K, Matzel K, et al. Standardized surgery for colonic cancer: complete mesocolic excision and central ligation-technical notes and outcome. Colorectal Dis. 2009;11: 354–64.
69. Bembenek A, Gretschel S, Schlag PM. Sentinel lymph node biopsy for gastrointestinal cancers. J Surg Oncol. 2007;96:342–52.
70. Simunovic M, Smith AJ, Heald RJ. Rectal cancer surgery and regional lymph nodes. J Surg Oncol. 2009;99:256–9.
71. Sakorafas GH, Zouros E, Peros G. Applied vascular anatomy of the colon and rectum: clinical implications for the surgical oncologist. Surg Oncol. 2006;15:243–55.
72. Leong SPL, Cady B, Jablons DM, Garcia-Aguilar J, Reintgen D, Jakub J, Pendas S, Duhaime L, Cassell R, Gardner M, Giuliano R, Archie V, Calvin D, Mensha L, Shivers S, Cox C, Werner JA, Kitagawa Y, Kitajima M. Clinical patterns of metastasis. Cancer Metastasis Rev. 2006;25:221–32.
73. Morón FE, Szklaruk J. Learning the nodal stations in the abdomen. Br J Radiol. 2007;80:841–8.
74. Bell S, Sasaki J, Sinclair G, Chapuis PH, Bokey EL. Understanding the anatomy of lymphatic drainage and the use of blue-dye mapping to determine the extent of lymphadenectomy in rectal cancer surgery: unresolved issues. Colorectal Dis. 2009;11:443–9.
75. Cutini G, Gesuelli GC, Sartelli M, Brianzoni E, Musolino G, Nestori M, Scibé R, Berbellini A. The role of lymphoscintigraphy in rectal laparoscopic surgery: can the sentinel node concept be applied to rectal carcinoma? Surg Endosc. 2001;15(12): 1440–3.

76. Funahashi K, Koike J, Shimada M, Okamoto K, Goto T, Teramoto T. A preliminary study of the draining lymph node basin in advanced lower rectal cancer using a radioactive tracer. Dis Colon Rectum. 2006;49:S53–8.
77. Topor B, Acland R, Kolodko V, Galandiuk S. Mesorectal lymph nodes: their location and distribution within the mesorectum. Dis Colon Rectum. 2003;46:779–85.
78. Saha S, Dan AG, Berman B, Wiese D, Schochet E, Barber K, Choudhri S, Kaushal S, Ganatra B, Desai D, Nagaraju M, Mannam S. Lymphazurin 1% versus 99mTc sulfur colloid for lymphatic mapping in colorectal tumors: a comparative analysis. Ann Surg Oncol. 2004;11(1):21–6.
79. Soni M, Saha S, Korant A, et al. A prospective trial comparing 1% lymphazurin vs. 1% methylene blue in sentinel lymph node mapping of gastrointestinal tumors. Ann Surg Oncol. 2009;16:2224–30.
80. Leong SP, Donegan E, Hefferson W, Dean S, Katz JA. Adverse reactions to isosulfan blue during selective sentinel lymph node dissection in melanoma. Ann Surg Oncol. 2000;7:361–6.
81. Longnecker SM, Guzzardo MM, Van Voris LP. Life-threatening anaphylaxis following subcutaneous administration of isosulfan blue 1%. Clin Pharmacol. 1985;4:219–21.
82. Kuerer HM, Wayne JD, Ross MI. Anaphylaxis during breast cancer lymphatic mapping. Surgery. 2001;129:119–20.
83. Coleman RL, Whitten CW, O' Boyle J, Sidhu B. Unexplained decrease in measured oxygen saturation by pulse oximetry following injection of Lymphazurin 1% (isosulfan blue) during a lymphatic mapping procedure. J Surg Oncol. 1999;70:126–9.
84. Larsen VH, Freudendal A, Fogh-Andersen N. The influence of patent blue V on pulse oxymetry and haemoximetry. Acta Anaesthesiol Scand Suppl. 1995;107:53–5.
85. Scheller J, Unger RJ, Kelner MJ. Effects of intravenously administered dyes on pulse oximetry readings. Anesthesiology. 1986;65:550–2.
86. Kessler MR, Eide T, Humayun B, Poppers PJ. Spurious pulse oximeter desaturation with methylene blue injection. Anesthesiology. 1986;65:435–6.
87. Hirche C, Mohr Z, Kneif S, et al. Ultrastaging of colon cancer by sentinel node biopsy using fluorescence navigation with indocyanine green. Int J Colorectal Dis. 2012;27:319–24.
88. van der Pas MH, Ankersmit M, Stockmann HB, et al. Laparoscopic sentinel lymph node identification in patients with colon carcinoma using a near-infrared dye: description of a new technique and feasibility study. J Laparoendosc Adv Surg Tech A. 2013;23:367–71.
89. Merrie A, van Rij A, Phillips L, Rossaak JI, Yun K, Mccall JL. Diagnostic use of the sentinel node in colon cancer. Dis Colon Rectum. 2001;44:410–7.
90. Joosten J, Strobbe L, Wauters C, Pruszczynski M, Wobbes T, Ruers TJ. Intraoperative lymphatic mapping in colorectal carcinoma. Br J Surg. 1999;86:482–6.
91. Wood TF, Saha S, Morton DL, et al. Validation of lymphatic mapping in colorectal cancer: in-vivo, ex-vivo, and laparoscopic techniques. Ann Surg Oncol. 2001;8:150–7.
92. Saha S, Dan AG, Bilchik AJ, Kitagawa Y, Schochet E, Choudhri S, Saha LT, Wiese D, Morton D, Kitajima M. Historical review of lymphatic mapping in gastrointestinal malignancies. Ann Surg Oncol. 2004;11(3 Suppl):245S–9. Review.
93. Nastro P, Sodo M, Dodaro CA, Gargiulo S, Acampa W, Bracale U, Renda A. Intraoperative radiochromo-guided mapping of sentinel lymph node in colon cancer. Tumori. 2002;88(4):352–3.
94. de Haas RJ, Wicherts DA, Hobbelink MG, et al. Sentinel lymph node mapping in colon cancer using radiocolloid as a single tracer: a feasibility study. Nucl Med Commun. 2012;33:832–7.
95. Kitagawa Y, Fujii H, Mukai M, Ando N, Kubota T, Ikeda T, Ohgami M, Watanabe M, Otani Y, Ozawa S, Hasegawa H, Furukawa T, Nakahara T, Kubo A, Kumai K, Kitajima M. The validity of the sentinel node concept in gastrointestinal cancers. Nippon Geka Gakkai Zasshi. 2000;101(3):315–9.
96. Trocha SD, Nora DT, Saha SS, Morton DL, Wiese D, Bilchik AJ. Combination probe and dye-directed lymphatic mapping detects micrometastases in early colorectal cancer. J Gastrointest Surg. 2003;7(3): 340–5; discussion 345–6.
97. Patten LC, Berger DH, Rodriguez-Bigas M, et al. A prospective evaluation of radiocolloid and immunohistochemical staining in colon carcinoma lymphatic mapping. Cancer. 2004;100:2104–9.
98. Povovski SP, Neff RL, Mojzisik CM, et al. A comprehensive overview of radioguided surgery using gamma detection probe technology. World J Surg Oncol. 2009;7:11.
99. Kitagawa Y, Fujii H, Mukai M, Kubota T, Ando N, Watanabe M, Ohgami M, Otani Y, Ozawa S, Hasegawa H, Furukawa T, Kumai K, Ikeda T, Nakahara T, Kubo A, Kitajima M. The role of the sentinel lymph node in gastrointestinal cancer. Surg Clin North Am. 2000;80:1799–809.
100. Bembenek A, Rau B, Moesta T, Markwardt J, Ulmer C, Gretschel S, Schneider U, Slisow W, Schlag PM. Sentinel lymph node biopsy in rectal cancer – Not yet ready for routine clinical use. Surgery. 2004;135:498–505.
101. Aikou T, Kitagawa Y, Kitajima M, et al. Sentinel lymph node mapping with GI cancer. Cancer Metastasis Rev. 2006;25:269–77.
102. Baton O, Lasser P, Sabourin JC, Boige V, Duvillard P, Elias D, Malka D, Ducreux M, Pocard M. Ex vivo sentinel lymph node study for rectal adenocarcinoma: preliminary study. World J Surg. 2005;29:1166–70.
103. Braat AE, Oosterhuis JWA, Moll FCP, de Vries JE, Wiggers T. Sentinel node detection after preoperative short-course radiotherapy in rectal carcinoma is not reliable. Br J Surg. 2005;92:1533–8.

104. Yagci G, Unlu A, Kurt B, Can MF, Kaymakcioglu N, Cetiner S, Tufan T, Sen D. Detection of micrometastases and skip metastases with ex vivo sentinel node mapping in carcinoma of the colon and rectum. Int J Colorectal Dis. 2007;22:167–73.
105. Bobin JY, Gérard JP, Chapet O, Romestaing P, Isaac S. Lymphatic mapping and inguinal sentinel lymph node biopsy in anal canal cancers to avoid prophylactic inguinal irradiation. Cancer Radiother. 2003;7(Suppl 1):85s–90s.
106. Damin DC, Rosito MA, Gus P, Spiro BL, Amaral BB, Meurer L, Cartel A, Schwartsmann G. Sentinel lymph node procedure in patients with epidermoid carcinoma of the anal canal: early experience. Dis Colon Rectum. 2003;46:1032–7.
107. Gretschel S, Warnick P, Bembenek A, Dresel S, Koswig S, String A, Hünerbein M, Schlag PM. Lymphatic mapping and sentinel lymph node biopsy in epidermoid carcinoma of the anal canal. Eur J Surg Oncol. 2008;34:890–4.
108. Perera D, Pathma-Nathan N, Rabbitt P, Hewett P, Rieger N. Sentinel node biopsy for squamous-cell carcinoma of the anus and anal margin. Dis Colon Rectum. 2003;46:1027–9.
109. Ulmer C, Bembenek A, Gretschel S, Markwardt J, Koswig S, Schneider U, Schlag PM. Refined staging by sentinel lymph node biopsy to individualize therapy in anal cancer. Ann Surg Oncol. 2004;11(3 Suppl):259S–62.
110. Mistrangelo M, Bellò M, Mobiglia A, Beltramo G, Cassoni P, Milanesi E, Cornaglia S, Pelosi E, Giunta F, Sandrucci S, Mussa A. Feasibility of the sentinel node biopsy in anal cancer. Q J Nucl Med Mol Imaging. 2009;53:3–8.

19 Radioguided Surgery for Gastroenteropancreatic Neuroendocrine Tumors

Nathan C. Hall, Christina Bluemel, Sergi Vidal-Sicart, and Stephen P. Povoski

Contents

Portions of the contents of this chapter are adapted from 1 prior article:
(1) Hall et al.: Intraoperative utilization of a portable large field of view gamma camera and handheld gamma detection probe for radioguided localization and prediction of complete surgical resection of gastrinoma: Proof of concept. *J Am Coll Surg*. 2015;221(2):300–308. doi: http://dx.doi.org/10.1016/j.jamcollsurg.2015.03.047

N.C. Hall, MD, PhD (✉)
Department of Radiology, University of Pennsylvania, Philadelphia, PA 19104, USA
e-mail: nathan.hall@uphs.upenn.edu

C. Bluemel, MD
Department of Nuclear Medicine, University Hospital of Würzburg, Würzburg, Germany
e-mail: Bluemel_C@ukw.de

S. Vidal-Sicart, MD, PhD
Department of Nuclear Medicine, Hospital Clinic-Barcelona, Barcelona, Spain
e-mail: svidalclinic@ub.es

Abstract

Gastroenteropancreatic (GEP) neuroendocrine tumors (NETs) are rare neoplasms, but the incidence is rising. Surgery plays a central role in its management, as it is the only potentially curative treatment option for limited primary and recurrent disease and is critical in the surgical debulking and cytoreduction of advanced recurrent and metastatic disease. For preoperative detection of disease, gamma-emitting radiopharmaceuticals are available which can also be intraoperatively used for radioguided surgery. Most experience exists

S.P. Povoski, MD
Division of Surgical Oncology, Department of Surgery, Arthur G. James Cancer Hospital and Richard J. Solove Research Institute and Comprehensive Cancer Center, The Ohio State University, Columbus, OH 43210, USA
e-mail: stephen.povoski@osumc.edu

K. Herrmann et al. (eds.), *Radioguided Surgery: Current Applications and Innovative Directions in Clinical Practice*, DOI 10.1007/978-3-319-26051-8_19

for ^{111}In-octreotide, a radiopharmaceutical targeting agent specifically binding to somatostatin receptors expressed on the tumor cell surface. In comparison to traditional intraoperative inspection and palpation techniques, intraoperative localization using ^{111}In-octreotide has demonstrated high sensitivity and detection rates. Recently, first promising results have been reported for utilization of intraoperative scintigraphic imaging in GEP-NETs in addition to more commonplace gamma probe localization.

19.1 The Role of Surgery in the Treatment of Gastroenteropancreatic Tumors

Gastroenteropancreatic (GEP) neuroendocrine tumors (NETs) represent a heterogeneous subset of functioning or nonfunctioning tumors arising from the neuroendocrine system. GEP-NETs have the potential of producing, storing, and secreting a variety of peptide hormones and biogenic amines which can lead to distinct clinical syndromes which can have significant symptoms. Based on this, GEP-NETs are broadly subdivided into "functional" or "nonfunctional" tumors (with or without a clinical syndrome attributable to biochemical hypersecretion, respectively) [1]. These tumors have historically been relatively rare but are increasing in incidence [2–5]. GEP-NETs can involve a variety of morphologic structures including the stomach, small intestine, colon, rectum, pancreas, appendix, and liver [1, 6–8].

In general, GEP-NETs are relatively slow-growing tumors and have longer survival statistics than their adenocarcinoma counterparts affecting the same organs [8]. The symptoms of these tumors range from asymptomatic nonfunctioning tumors to carcinoid syndrome or carcinoid crisis arising from functioning tumors that can secrete a variety of hormones and peptides [9]. Nonfunctioning GEP-NETs typically become large and/or widely metastatic before becoming symptomatic and subsequently diagnosed [8, 10].

Independent of the functionality and/or anatomic origin, one attribute most of the GEP-NETs share in common is that the only curative therapeutic option is complete surgical resection in patients with limited disease [1, 6, 8, 10–13]. Radical oncologic surgical resection is generally indicated unless the tumors are small carcinoids (<2 cm) of the stomach, small intestine, appendix, rectum, or insulinomas [14–20]. In these cases, conservative surgical or endoscopic resections may be appropriate as these usually have low malignant potential. Surgical resection has also proven useful for debulking and cytoreduction of advanced or metastatic disease and remains integral in the management of recurrent disease [6, 8].

Before surgery, the detection and localization of disease manifestations are crucial. The introduction of ^{123}I-Metaiodobenzylguanidine (MIBG) and ^{111}In-DTPA-D-Phe^{1}-octreotide/^{123}I-Tyr^{3}-octreotide, binding to somatostatin receptors expressed on neuroendocrine tumor cells, specifically addresses this issue [21]. High detection rates for MIBG or somatostatin-directed imaging were shown, exceeding magnetic resonance imaging (MRI) or computed tomography (CT) and also revised staging and management in patients [21–24].

For planning a radioguided surgery approach to GEP-NETs, a whole-body scintigraphy must be performed and, if possible, a single photon emission computed tomography (SPECT) or SPECT/CT to fully evaluate all sites of disease that are planned to be surgically removed. SPECT/CT helps to plan the surgical approach and contributes to the success of radioguided surgery. In addition, subsequent to preoperative radiotracer injection and prior to surgical intervention, scintigraphic imaging is recommended to verify adequate uptake of the radiotracer by all lesions planned for surgical removal [25, 26].

Despite improvements in preoperative imaging technologies, intraoperative localization of small tumor lesions remains challenging. Therefore, various intraoperative localization techniques have been investigated [6, 27].

Many groups have reported improved success of intraoperative GEP-NET detection using a handheld gamma detection probe (HGDP) during surgery in conjunction with preoperatively administration of various radiotracers [28–38]. When an

HGDP is used to assist the surgeon in identification of small tumors within the abdominal surgical field, a high degree of technical proficiency is required by the surgeon [39–41]. Successful use of the HGDP to identify all sites of disease requires: (1) appropriate preoperative diagnostic imaging to map the general locations of the sites of disease, (2) obtaining adequate surgical exposure, and (3) the performance of a methodical and systematic HGDP survey of the abdominal surgical field. Despite improvements demonstrated by utilization of the HGDP in combination with preoperative diagnostic imaging for verification of the general locations of the sites of disease, incorporation of the preoperative imaging data into useful real-time information for localization of tumor with the HGDP is limited. Real-time intraoperative images during the radioguided resection procedure could be very beneficial for verifying resection of all sites of disease, a technique which is described in detail later in this chapter.

19.2 Historical Use of Gamma-Ray-Emitting Radiotracers for Intraoperative Localization of GEP-NET during Radioguided Surgery

There are a variety of specific and nonspecific radiotracers and radionuclides that target multiple cellular components used in the diagnosis and intraoperative localization of GEP-NETs during radioguided surgery. It has been demonstrated by a number of research groups that an improvement in intraoperative detectability of GEP-NETs can result from combining preoperative GEP-NET-targeted radiotracer scintigraphy with real-time intraoperative localization assistance using an HGDP.

19.2.1 ^{111}In-Pentetreotide (OctreoScan)

^{111}In-pentetreotide is widely used in scintigraphic imaging of NETs and also used in radioguided surgery. Fortunately, most GEP-NETs express somatostatin (SS) receptors, specifically subtypes 2 and 5. As a result, long-acting somatostatin analogues, such as octreotide, have been developed to target these receptors [42, 43]. By labeling octreotide with radionuclides, those GEP-NETs expressing somatostatin receptors, specifically subtypes 2 and 5, can be successfully identified [32, 44, 45].

The most frequently used radiotracer is ^{111}In-pentetreotide. ^{111}In-pentetreotide is a radiolabeled eight-peptide protein segment of somatostatin binding well to the SS2 and SS5 receptors [46]. Somatostatin has a relatively short half-life with respect to its usefulness in imaging ($\approx$2 min), whereas ^{111}In-pentetreotide has a longer biological half-life (1 h) and is, therefore, more useful for diagnostic imaging as the radiotracer requires time to reach and bind to the tumor receptors after injection and prior to imaging. ^{111}In-pentetreotide is commonly used in diagnosis and staging of a variety of NETs, including the GEP-NETs. The detection rate of somatostatin receptor scintigraphy with ^{111}In-pentetreotide was reported between 80 and 100 % in different studies. Somatostatin receptor scintigraphy also provides information about somatostatin receptor expression that might indicate efficacy of treatment with octreotide or other somatostatin analogues.

The injected activity reported in literature ranges from 120 to 220 MBq (3.2–5.9 mCi). The recommended activity to obtain good image quality is about 200 MBq (5.4 mCi). However, activities lower than 200 MBq can be administered without loss of imaging quality by adjusting the acquisition parameters accordingly. The amount of injected ^{111}In-pentreotide for radioguided surgery ranged between 111 and 275 MBq [35, 47–49]. Injection was mainly performed 24–48 h prior to surgery [35, 47, 48], but radiotracer injection up to 7 days prior to surgery is suitable [49].

Planar images (anterior and posterior of the head, neck, chest, abdomen, pelvis, and lower extremities; 15 min per view in a gamma camera fitted with a medium-energy, parallel-hole collimator) should be acquired at 4 and 24 h or 24 and 48 h post-injection. Four-hour images benefit from a minimal bowel activity. At least one SPECT or SPECT/CT should be acquired in order to more precisely localize disease and assist in preoperative planning for resection. Spot views may be repeated at 48, 72, and/or 96 h to reduce interfering bowel radioactivity. Laxatives can be administered between 24 and 48 h as well for minimizing bowel activity [50]. Imaging prior to surgery depends on results of previous scintigraphic imaging and the time point of surgery post-injection.

As such, the use of ^{111}In-pentetreotide has significantly improved the success of radioguided surgery in the treatment of GEP-NETs [51, 52].

At least 90 % success rate has been demonstrated using preoperative ^{111}In-pentetreotide scintigraphy for diagnostic and staging information along with real-time intraoperative HGDP in the operating room [35, 47, 49]. The improved efficacy of using intraoperative radioguided detection of GEP-NETs with ^{111}In-pentetreotide for lesions difficult to localize on preoperative scintigraphy was demonstrated [35, 47]. Adams et al. demonstrated the incremental benefit of radioguided intraoperative lesion detection in comparison to preoperative scintigraphic imaging and intraoperative palpation only. They investigated 12 patients with GEP-NETs. Intraoperative lesion localization using HGDP identified 70 lesions, whereas preoperative scintigraphic imaging identified only 74 % and intraoperative palpation only 44 % of the 70 identified lesions. Tumor-to-nontumor ratios with count rates (counts per second) of at least 2:1, but in most cases 4:1, resulted in no resection of false-positive lesions [47]. Ohrvall et al. investigated 21 patients with pancreatic or midgut NETs. They also reported a reduced sensitivity of preoperative SPECT (34 of 60 lesions identified). The resected specimens were measured using a scintillation well counter, and ten specimens including 35 carcinoid tumors were placed under the gamma camera. Only 68 % of the tumor lesions were identified using the gamma camera [53].

The high intraoperative detection rate can be explained by the finding that HGDPs are more sensitive at detecting small lesions (≥5 mm) compared to SPECT scintigraphy alone and surgeon's hands (typically more useful for tumor deposits ≥1 cm) [35, 47, 48].

In addition to assisting the surgeon in finding all areas of somatostatin receptor-positive tissue during the operation to ensure highest likelihood of complete extirpation of disease, the HGDP, in conjunction with preoperative injection of ^{111}In-pentetreotide, has also proven useful in assisting with planned cytoreduction surgery with only palliative intent [54, 55]. Hellman et al. demonstrated a survival benefit in removing the primary midgut tumor as well as resecting all mesenteric lymph nodes even in patients with known metastatic disease to the liver [54]. Wang et al. demonstrated that utilization of the gamma probe during cytoreduction surgery can decrease operative time, minimize unnecessary dissection, and assist in differentiation of benign versus malignant tissue. To achieve these results, they consider an injection of 222 MBq (6 mCi) ^{111}In-pentreotide 7 days prior to surgery as optimal, because get rid of then the tumor-to-background ratio is still high enough and the scattering effect from physiological uptake in the kidney and liver at a minimum. This group also demonstrated that use of the gamma probe during re-intervention surgical resection proved useful in 97 % of the 30 cases studied [55].

19.2.2 ^{125}I-Labeled Somatostatin Analogues

^{125}I-labeled octreotide has some disadvantages. Due to the long physical half-life (60 days), radiation exposure is relatively high, and because of the hepatobiliary excretion, high intestinal background activity reduces the image quality [41]. ^{125}I-Tyr3-octreotide was replaced by ^{111}In-pentetreotide because of the advantages provided: easy preparation, availability, appropriate half-life, and less interference from physiological activity in the upper abdomen due to its predominantly urinary excretion [21, 37, 46].

19.2.3 ^{99m}Tc-Labeled Somatostatin Analogues

Less common and more scarcely available radiotracers have been used to assist surgeons with intraoperative localization of NETs with varying degrees of success. Gabriel et al. demonstrated that ^{99m}Tc-EDDA/HYNIC-TOC had an overall sensitivity of 80 %, specificity of 94.4 %, and precision of 82.9 % in 88 patients with GEP-NET tumors [56]. In all patients, whole-body imaging and SPECT 4-h post-injection of 400 MBq ^{99m}Tc-EDDA/HYNIC-TOC were performed. In 68 patients, additional early whole-body images were obtained 2 h post-injection. The authors concluded that despite rapid background clearance, single imaging protocol leads to false-positive results. They recommend a dual-time imaging protocol including SPECT [56]. With regard to radioguided surgery, the energy of ^{99m}Tc is more adequate than that of ^{111}In for detection with HGDP, because it allows the use of a greater amount of administered activity due to its short half-life, and shows less renal uptake [57]. A ^{99m}Tc-labeled somatostatin analogue, ^{99m}Tc-EDDA/HYNIC-octreotate has also been used in radioguided surgery of occult GEP-NETs [58]. ^{99m}Tc-EDDA/HYNIC-octreotate is intravenously administered using an activity of 600–740 MBq [57, 58]. Hubalewska-Dydejczyk et al. successfully localized primary tumors (≥8 mm in diameter) and lymph node metastases during surgery with the assistance for the HGDP. In one case, the radioguided procedure identified additional lymph node metastases, which were not found in preoperative imaging. The authors conclude that ^{99m}Tc-EDDA/HYNIC-TOC-guided surgery "… is a promising technique to improve both the rate of detection of GEP-NET and the treatment efficacy…" [58].

19.2.4 ^{123}I-MIBG

MIBG scintigraphy is used to image tumors of neuroendocrine origin particularly those of the neuroectodermal (sympathoadrenal) origin (pheochromocytomas, paragangliomas, and neuroblastomas) [59]. In addition, other neuroendocrine tumors (e.g., carcinoids, medullary thyroid carcinoma) can also be visualized by MIBG, which can be labeled with either ^{131}I or ^{123}I. The 159 keV gamma energy of ^{123}I is more suitable for imaging (especially when using SPECT) than the 360 keV photons of ^{131}I, and the difference in terms of radiation burden permits higher activities of ^{123}I-MIBG to be injected. Furthermore, results with ^{123}I-MIBG are usually available within 24 h, whereas with ^{131}I-MIBG delayed images are required for optimal target to background ratios [60]. To obtain high image quality, patients have to be prepared prior to radiotracer injection (e.g., discontinuing inferring drugs, hydration, blocking thyroid uptake of free radioiodine by stable iodine or potassium perchlorate).

The activities administered to adults should be 40–80 MBq (1.2–2.2 mCi) for^{131}I-MIBG and 400 MBq (10.8 mCi) for ^{123}I-mIBG. The activity administered to children has to be adapted [61]. The administered activity for radioguided surgery ranged from 18.5 MBq (0.5 mCi) to 370 MBq (10 mCi) [55]. Scanning time points for preoperative diagnostic imaging are related to the radiotracer used (^{131}I-MIBG scan 1 and 2 days post-injection vs. ^{123}I-MIBG scan 20 and 24 h post-injection). Selected delayed images may be useful in equivocal findings. Whole-body imaging; limited field images, especially in pediatric patients; and SPECT or SPECT/CT are recommended. Anterior and posterior (>150 kcounts for ^{131}I and >500 kcounts for ^{123}I) views of the head, neck, chest, abdomen, pelvis, and upper and lower extremities are encouraged to be acquired [61]. Imaging protocols prior to radioguided surgery have to be planned according to the injected radiotracer (^{131}MIBG vs. ^{123}MIBG) and the time point of surgery post-injection.

Radioiodine-labeled MIBG has also been used for radioguided surgery, mainly in pheochromocytoma, but also in GEP-NETs [53, 55, 62]. In a previously referenced work by Wang et al., 6 patients with NETs (5 of the small bowel and 1 pancreatic) presenting with low scintigraphic uptake of ^{111}In-penetreotide, ^{123}I-MIBG was used in the radioguided surgery and was only found to be useful in 1 of the patients [55]. The authors assumed this to be due to the short interval between injection and the surgery. In a review of 20 studies on the role of ^{123}I-MIBG in radioguided surgery of NETs, van Hulsteijn et al. concluded that this radiotracer has less sensitivity than the radiolabeled somatostain analogues to detect metastatic lesions of carcinoid tumors [53, 62].

19.2.5 ^{68}Ga-Somatostatin Analogues

Besides gamma-emitting radiotracers (preoperative), staging and restaging is also performed with positron emission radiotracers like ^{18}F-fluorodeoxyglucose (^{18}F-FDG) in highly aggressive GEP-NETs [63]. positron emission tomography (PET) with ^{68}Ga-DOTATATE or ^{68}Ga-DOTATOC, both with a high affinity to the somatostatin receptor subtype 2, enables diagnosis of well-differentiated NETs with a very high sensitivity [33].

Intraoperative HGDP-guided techniques for resecting GET-NETs have included the use of ^{68}Ga-somatostatin analogue [64]. Kaemmerer et al. studied nine patients with primary or recurrent GEP tumors. Whole-body PET/CT was performed 2–4 weeks prior to surgery. Another PET/CT scan of the region of interest was performed 1.5–2 h before the intraoperative intervention using an injection of 180 MBq of ^{68}Ga DOTA-NOC (DOTA-1-Na1^{3}-octreotide) or DOTA-TATE (DOTA-D-Phe^{1}-Tyr^{3}-Thr^{8}-octreotide) [64]. HGDP detected 94 % of all histologically quantified lesions, whereas palpation and preoperative PET/CT identified only 50 % and 69 %, respectively [64]. These analogues are therefore also an interesting option for real-time detection of primary tumors and small metastases.

19.3 Intraoperative Imaging for Localization and Verification of Resection of GEP-NETs: Illustration of This Approach Using Real-Time, Large Field-of-View, Portable Gamma Camera Imaging during Radioguided Surgery in Patients with Zollinger-Ellison Syndrome

Although many investigators and clinicians have utilized targeted radiopharmaceuticals to assist with radioguided surgical intervention using the HGDP, there has been very limited use of intraoperative scintigraphic imaging techniques to assist in these interventions in real-time. Preoperative collection of imaging data has been used as a road map to guide surgeons on where to search for areas of tumor using an HGDP. Intraoperative real-time scintigraphic imaging to assist with localization and verification of resection of tumor is only at its early stages of utilization despite the fact that such technology has been available for decades [65–76]. An example of utilization of real-time intraoperative scintigraphic imaging during GEP-NET-radioguided surgery has very recently been published by Hall et al. [77]. In this study, a large field-of-view gamma camera (LFOVGC) was used to assist with the radioguided surgical treatment of patients with Zollinger-Ellison syndrome (ZES).

ZES is a rare cause of severe peptic ulcer disease by gastrin-secreting NETs of the gastrointestinal tract (60–90 % of gastrinomas are considered malignant), which are located predominately in the duodenum and pancreas [30, 78]. Due to the vague and nonspecific symptoms associated with ZES, diagnosis from symptom onset is typically delayed by approximately 6 years [30]. Despite the increasing prevalence of utilizing H2-antagonist and proton pump inhibitor medications to medically manage symptoms of ZES, surgical management, in appropriately selected patients, affords the only chance for cure [30, 79]. Surgical treatment for gastrinoma focuses on eradication of primary disease, treating refractory disease, and prolonging survival, with postoperative cure rates of 60 % and 34 % at 5 and 10 years, respectively [80–82].

Gastrinoma tumors and their metastatic foci are commonly very small, multiple in number, and found in variable locations, making them difficult to identify by visual examination and palpation and, therefore, difficult to completely remove during surgery. Because of this, surgical management frequently fails to accomplish a sustainable cure of disease. The successful surgical management of ZES requires that all gastrinoma lesions be localized and extirpated, which is best done at the time of the first operation. However, over the past several decades, apart from the previously noted improvement in the available technology for the preoperative scintigraphic localization of sites of disease in patients with GET-NETs, including ZES patients, very few significant advances have occurred in the surgical management of ZES. The incorporation of real-time, intraoperative, portable LFOVGC imaging during radioguided surgery with an HGDP represents an example of a potentially significant advancement in the surgical management of ZES. The combined use of intraoperative scintigraphic imaging and the HGDP, as applied to both the patient and the resected surgical specimens, can resultantly provide the surgeon with instantaneous, real-time navigational feedback for optimizing the identification and complete surgical resection of all possible sites of disease.

In a recent report by Hall et al. [77], they addressed the utility of the combined use of intraoperative scintigraphic imaging and the HGDP in the radioguided surgical management of ZES patients. In their report, they used a portable LFOVGC (Ergo™, Digirad Corporation, Poway, CA, 15.6 × 12.2 in. field of view), capable of detecting gamma photon emissions in the 50–350 keV range and providing real-time intraoperative imaging and navigational assistance. Five patients with ZES and previously characterized ^{111}In-pentetreotide-positive lesions on prior diagnostic ^{111}In-pentetreotide imaging were included in this prospective feasibility study. The overarching goal was complete resection and extirpation of all areas of disease with intraoperative real-time confirmation. Each patient received an intravenous dose of ^{111}In-pentetreotide (mean dose, 229.6 ± 15.2 MBq/6.2 ± 0.4 mCi) on the day before surgery, and for which this was followed by whole-body planar and/or SPECT/CT imaging at 4–6 h and/or 20–24 h post-injection to localize the lesions. Patients underwent surgical exploration approximately 24 h after ^{111}In-pentetreotide administration. In the operating room and just prior to the surgical incision, reconfirmation of the previously detected ^{111}In-pentetreotide-avid lesions was accomplished with the portable LFOVGC (Fig. 19.1). An HGDP was used to systemically survey the exposed abdominal surgical field for sites of disease. The HGDP threshold for positivity in lesion detection was based on the signaling setting for three-sigma criteria, a method developed and used successfully for radioimmunoguided surgery [83, 84]. Intraoperatively, static planar

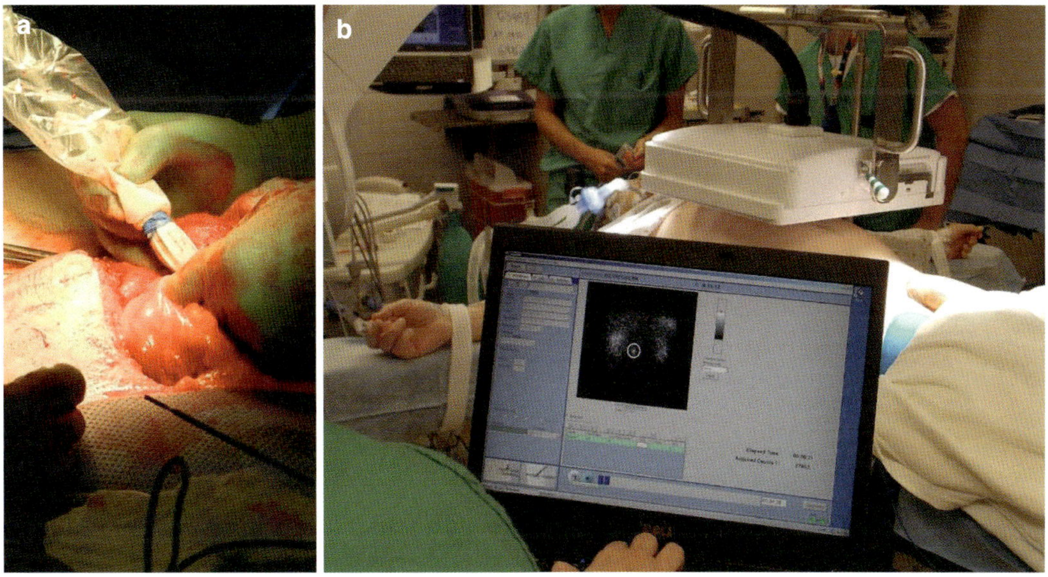

Fig. 19.1 (**a**) Digital photograph of HGDP use during ^{111}In-pentetreotide radioguided surgery to assist in localization of tumors. (**b**) Intraoperative image acquisition with the LFOVGC for real-time intraoperative evaluation of the surgical bed; image displayed on computer monitor (Reproduced from Hall et al. [77]

images obtained with the LFOVGC were used to guide the surgeon's use of the HGDP to identify and resect sites of disease. Quality readable imaging can be obtained within five minutes of the start time of image acquisition for the patient scans and one minute for the specimen scans, which is easily viewable to the surgeon on a laptop workstation, providing immediate real-time navigational feedback using the LFOVGC [77, 85]. The portable LFOVGC allowed the detection of radiotracers within the operating room in a manner which was manipulated by the surgeon without interfering with work flow or surgical field sterility. The complete surgical resection of all sites of disease was then confirmed using LFOVGC imaging of the post-resection surgical field.

In these 5 ZES patients, 15 surgical specimens were resected during a total of 6 separate radioguided surgical procedures. These surgical specimens were classified as either benign (5 specimens) or involved with NET (10 specimens). Standard surgical techniques of visual and palpable cues failed to detect 3 of the 10 NET-

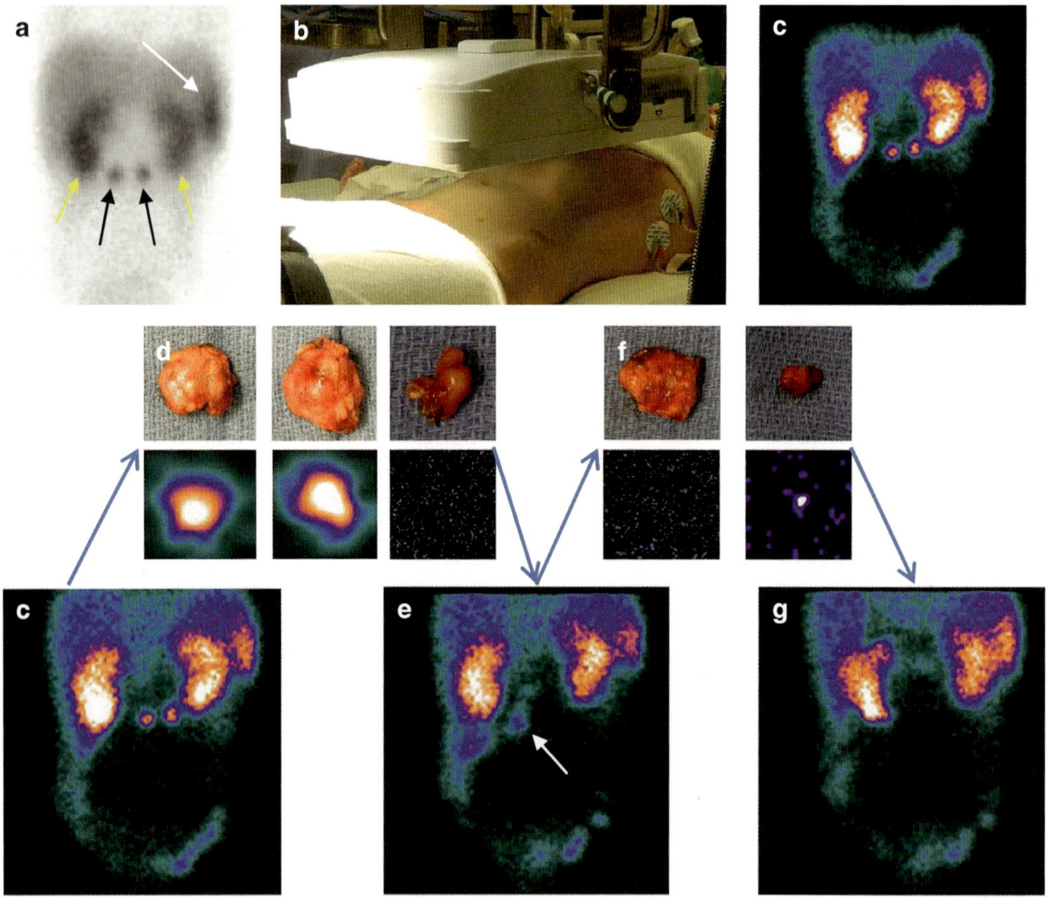

Fig. 19.2 (**a**) Preoperative ^{111}In-pentetreotide imaging identifying two tumors (*black arrows*), kidneys (*yellow arrows*), and the spleen (*white arrow*). (**b**) Pre-incision LFOVGC imaging setup and (**c**) associated image identifying same structures. (**d**) Digital photos of three initially excised specimens and paired LFOVGC images. The left and middle specimens had ^{111}In-pentetreotide activity, while the third specimen (*right*) did not. (**e**) Initial post-resection LFOVGC image showing residual activity (*white arrow*). (**f**) Digital photo and LFOVGC image of two additionally excised tissue specimens, having no and a small amount of ^{111}In-pentetreotide activity on the left and right pictures, respectively. (**g**) Final post-resection LFOVGC image indicating no further activity and verifying completeness of resection, with activity remaining in the right kidneys and spleen (Reproduced from Hall et al. [77]

positive specimens (30 %), even the use of the HGDP did not delineate the benign status of the remaining 5 specimens. Intraoperative LFOVGC imaging detected all 10 NET-positive specimens also positive for radiolabeled activity (Fig. 19.2) and all 5 benign specimens negative for activity. There were no false positives with specimen or patient imaging. The discordance between detection and differentiation of benign versus malignant tissue by histopathologic assessment with radiolabeling imaging techniques versus detection and differentiation using standard operative techniques was statistically significant ($P<0.03$).

Of note, one of the patients in this study required two separate operations secondary to residual tumor unintentionally left at the initial operation. In this particular patient, the investigators noted, in retrospect, that there was a mild focus of activity in the left upper quadrant, not convincing to the surgeon to represent tumor and which could not be found with standard surgical techniques or with the HGDP, at the time of the initial operative procedure (Fig. 19.3). Aside from this patient's first operation, intraoperative post-resection LFOVGC imaging of the abdomen confirmed complete excision of all detectable ^{111}In-pentetreotide-avid lesions prior to closure.

Overall, in this study by Hall et al. [77], utilization of the HGDP along with LFOVGC imaging aided the surgeon in localizing the gastrinoma tumors. Effectively, use of ^{111}In-pentetreotide with intraoperative LFOVGC imaging changed management in 3 of the 6 radioguided surgical cases. Use of combined intraoperative HGDP detection techniques and LFOVGC imaging subjectively improved efficiency and confidence management in all 6 cases and enhanced tumor identification and resection of all sites of disease.

19.4 Concluding Remarks

The management of GEP-NETs remains challenging. The surgical management of these tumors offers the best possibility for cure and has a significant impact on survival. Various radiotracers are available for pre- and intraoperative detection of GEP-NETs. The combined intraoperative utilization of the HGDP in concert with using real-time portable imaging devices for attempted tumor localization during radioguided surgery provides the surgeon with instantaneous navigational feedback for optimizing the precise identification of all possible sites of disease, for

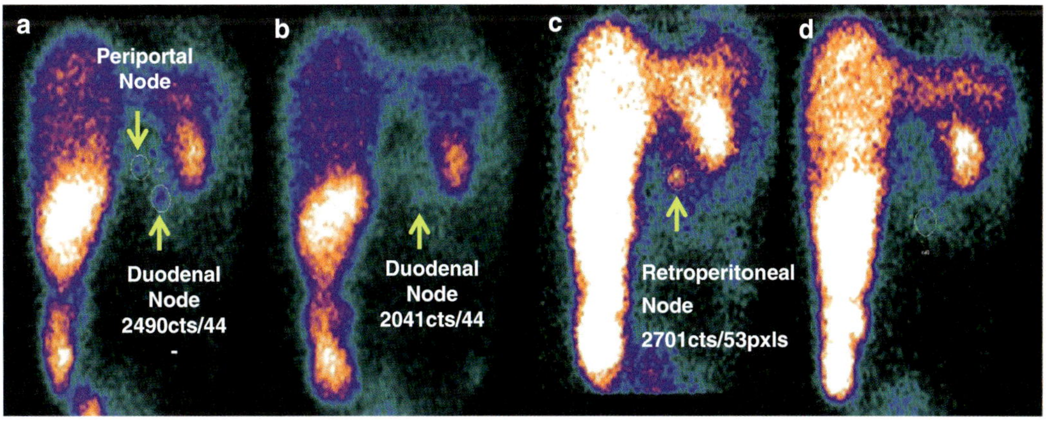

Fig. 19.3 Patient 2, first surgical procedure, pre-incision LFOVGC image (**a**) indicating two foci of activity with associated quantitative counts. The corresponding post-resection image (**b**) indicates decreased but persistent activity (thought to be artifactual at time of surgery). Same patient, second surgical procedure, pre-incision LFOVGC image (**c**) indicating focus of increased activity in the same location as on image **b**, with interval growth of the lesion between operations. Corresponding post-resection image (**d**) indicating no further activity and complete resection of detectable ^{111}In-pentetreotide-avid lesions (Reproduced from Hall et al. [77]

minimizing the unnecessary destruction and removal of uninvolved adjacent tissues, and for ultimately potentially impacting favorably on long-term patient outcomes.

References

1. Diez M, Teule A, Salazar R. Gastroenteropancreatic neuroendocrine tumors: diagnosis and treatment. Ann Gastroenterol. 2013;26:29–36.
2. Fraenkel M, Kim MK, Faggiano A, Valk GD. Epidemiology of gastroenteropancreatic neuroendocrine tumours. Best Pract Res Clin Gastroenterol. 2012;26:691–703. doi:10.1016/j.bpg.2013.01.006.
3. Hallet J, Law CH, Cukier M, Saskin R, Liu N, Singh S. Exploring the rising incidence of neuroendocrine tumors: a population-based analysis of epidemiology, metastatic presentation, and outcomes. Cancer. 2015;121:589–97. doi:10.1002/cncr.29099.
4. Lawrence B, Gustafsson BI, Chan A, Svejda B, Kidd M, Modlin IM. The epidemiology of gastroenteropancreatic neuroendocrine tumors. Endocrinol Metab Clin North Am. 2011;40:1–18, vii. doi:10.1016/j.ecl.2010.12.005.
5. Yao JC, Hassan M, Phan A, Dagohoy C, Leary C, Mares JE, et al. One hundred years after "carcinoid": epidemiology of and prognostic factors for neuroendocrine tumors in 35,825 cases in the United States. J Clin oncol. 2008;26:3063–72. doi:10.1200/JCO.2007.15.4377.
6. Modlin IM, Oberg K, Chung DC, Jensen RT, de Herder WW, Thakker RV, et al. Gastroenteropancreatic neuroendocrine tumours. Lancet Oncol. 2008;9:61–72. doi:10.1016/S1470-2045(07)70410-2.
7. Plockinger U, Rindi G, Arnold R, Eriksson B, Krenning EP, de Herder WW, et al. Guidelines for the diagnosis and treatment of neuroendocrine gastrointestinal tumours. A consensus statement on behalf of the European Neuroendocrine Tumour Society (ENETS). Neuroendocrinology. 2004;80:394–424. doi:10.1159/000085237.
8. Ramage JK, Ahmed A, Ardill J, Bax N, Breen DJ, Caplin ME, et al. Guidelines for the management of gastroenteropancreatic neuroendocrine (including carcinoid) tumours (NETs). Gut. 2012;61:6–32. doi:10.1136/gutjnl-2011-300831.
9. Bendelow J, Apps E, Jones LE, Poston GJ. Carcinoid syndrome. Eur J Surg Oncol. 2008;34:289–96. doi:10.1016/j.ejso.2007.07.202.
10. Boudreaux JP. Surgery for gastroenteropancreatic neuroendocrine tumors (GEPNETS). Endocrinol Metab Clin North Am. 2011;40:163–71, ix. doi:10.1016/j.ecl.2010.12.004.
11. Knigge U, Hansen CP. Surgery for GEP-NETs. Best Pract Res Clin Gastroenterol. 2012;26:819–31. doi:10.1016/j.bpg.2012.12.005.
12. Partelli S, Maurizi A, Tamburrino D, Baldoni A, Polenta V, Crippa S, et al. GEP-NETS update: a review on surgery of gastro-entero-pancreatic neuroendocrine tumors. Eur J Endocrinol. 2014;171:R153–62. doi:10.1530/EJE-14-0173.
13. Plockinger U, Gustafsson B, Ivan D, Szpak W, Davar J. ENETS consensus guidelines for the standards of care in neuroendocrine tumors: echocardiography. Neuroendocrinology. 2009;90:190–3. doi:10.1159/000225947.
14. Delle Fave G, Capurso G, Milione M, Panzuto F. Endocrine tumours of the stomach. Best Pract Res Clin Gastroenterol. 2005;19:659–73. doi:10.1016/j.bpg.2005.05.002.
15. Hill JS, McPhee JT, McDade TP, Zhou Z, Sullivan ME, Whalen GF, et al. Pancreatic neuroendocrine tumors: the impact of surgical resection on survival. Cancer. 2009;115:741–51. doi:10.1002/cncr.24065.
16. Eriksson B, Orlefors H, Oberg K, Sundin A, Bergstrom M, Langstrom B. Developments in PET for the detection of endocrine tumours. Best Pract Res Clin Endocrinol Metab. 2005;19:311–24. doi:10.1016/j.beem.2004.11.001.
17. Pape UF, Perren A, Niederle B, Gross D, Gress T, Costa F, et al. ENETS consensus guidelines for the management of patients with neuroendocrine neoplasms from the jejuno-ileum and the appendix including goblet cell carcinomas. Neuroendocrinology. 2012;95:135–56. doi:10.1159/000335629.
18. Plockinger U, Couvelard A, Falconi M, Sundin A, Salazar R, Christ E, et al. Consensus guidelines for the management of patients with digestive neuroendocrine tumours: well-differentiated tumour/carcinoma of the appendix and goblet cell carcinoma. Neuroendocrinology. 2008;87:20–30. doi:10.1159/000109876.
19. Ramage JK, Goretzki PE, Manfredi R, Komminoth P, Ferone D, Hyrdel R, et al. Consensus guidelines for the management of patients with digestive neuroendocrine tumours: well-differentiated colon and rectum tumour/carcinoma. Neuroendocrinology. 2008;87:31–9. doi:10.1159/000111036.
20. Jensen RT, Rindi G, Arnold R, Lopes JM, Brandi ML, Bechstein WO, et al. Well-differentiated duodenal tumor/carcinoma (excluding gastrinomas). Neuroendocrinology. 2006;84:165–72. doi:10.1159/000098008.
21. Krenning EP, Kwekkeboom DJ, Bakker WH, Breeman WA, Kooij PP, Oei HY, et al. Somatostatin receptor scintigraphy with [111In-DTPA-D-Phe1]- and [123I-Tyr3]-octreotide: the Rotterdam experience with more than 1000 patients. Eur J Nucl Med. 1993;20:716–31.
22. Lamberts SW, Bakker WH, Reubi JC, Krenning EP. Somatostatin-receptor imaging in the localization of endocrine tumors. N Engl J Med. 1990;323:1246–9. doi:10.1056/NEJM199011013231805.
23. Kaltsas G, Korbonits M, Heintz E, Mukherjee JJ, Jenkins PJ, Chew SL, et al. Comparison of somatosta-

tin analog and meta-iodobenzylguanidine radionuclides in the diagnosis and localization of advanced neuroendocrine tumors. J Clin Endocrinol Metab. 2001;86:895–902. doi:10.1210/jcem.86.2.7194.
24. Kvols LK, Brown ML, O'Connor MK, Hung JC, Hayostek RJ, Reubi JC, et al. Evaluation of a radiolabeled somatostatin analog (I-123 octreotide) in the detection and localization of carcinoid and islet cell tumors. Radiology. 1993;187:129–33. doi:10.1148/radiology.187.1.8383865.
25. Ober K, Akerstrom G, Rindi G, Jelic S. Neuroendocrine gastroenteropancreatic tumours: ESMO Clinical practice guidelines for diagnosis, treatment and follow up. Ann Oncol. 2010;21 Suppl 5:v223–7.
26. Gulec SA, Baum R. Radio-guided surgery in neuroendocrine tumors. J Surg Oncol. 2007;96:309–15. doi:10.1002/jso.20868.
27. Norton JA. Intraoperative methods to stage and localize pancreatic and duodenal tumors. Ann Oncol. 1999;10 Suppl 4:182–4.
28. Albertario S, Forti P, Bianchi C, Morone G, Tinozzi FP, Moglia P, et al. Radioguided surgery for gastrinoma: a case report. Tumori. 2002;88:S41–3.
29. Benevento A, Dominioni L, Carcano G, Dionigi R. Intraoperative localization of gut endocrine tumors with radiolabeled somatostatin analogs and a gamma-detecting probe. Semin Surg Oncol. 1998;15:239–44.
30. Ellison EC, Johnson JA. The Zollinger-Ellison syndrome: a comprehensive review of historical, scientific, and clinical considerations. Curr Probl Surg. 2009;46:13–106. doi:10.1067/j.cpsurg.2008.09.001.
31. Hosoya Y, Satoh K, Hironaka M, Nokubi M, Kurashina K, Shibayama C, et al. Multiple gastric carcinoids associated with parietal cell hyperplasia: intraoperative detection with a radiolabeled somatostatin analog. Gastric cancer. 2008;11:123–6. doi:10.1007/s10120-008-0457-8.
32. Gibril F, Reynolds JC, Doppman JL, Chen CC, Venzon DJ, Termanini B, et al. Somatostatin receptor scintigraphy: its sensitivity compared with that of other imaging methods in detecting primary and metastatic gastrinomas. A prospective study. Ann Intern Med. 1996;125:26–34.
33. Koukouraki S, Strauss LG, Georgoulias V, Schuhmacher J, Haberkorn U, Karkavitsas N, et al. Evaluation of the pharmacokinetics of 68Ga-DOTATOC in patients with metastatic neuroendocrine tumours scheduled for 90Y-DOTATOC therapy. Eur J Nucl Med Mol Imaging. 2006;33:460–6. doi:10.1007/s00259-005-0006-1.
34. Modlin IM, Cornelius E, Lawton GP. Use of an isotopic somatostatin receptor probe to image gut endocrine tumors. Arch Surg. 1995;130:367–73; discussion 73–4.
35. Ohrvall U, Westlin JE, Nilsson S, Juhlin C, Rastad J, Lundqvist H, et al. Intraoperative gamma detection reveals abdominal endocrine tumors more efficiently than somatostatin receptor scintigraphy. Cancer. 1997;80:2490–4.
36. Ohrvall U, Westlin JE, Kjellberg F, Nilsson S, Juhlin C, Rastad J, et al. A gamma detector probe with ex vivo detection of carcinoid tumors superior to intraoperative palpation. Cancer. 1997;80:2495–500.
37. Schirmer WJ, O'Dorisio TM, Schirmer TP, Mojzisik CM, Hinkle GH, Martin EW. Intraoperative localization of neuroendocrine tumors with 125I-TYR(3)-octreotide and a hand-held gamma-detecting probe. Surgery. 1993;114:745–51; discussion 51–2.
38. Woltering EA, Barrie R, O'Dorisio TM, O'Dorisio MS, Nance R, Cook DM. Detection of occult gastrinomas with iodine 125-labeled lanreotide and intraoperative gamma detection. Surgery. 1994;116:1139–46; discussion 46–7.
39. Hall NC, Povoski SP, Murrey DA, Knopp MV, Martin EW. Bringing advanced medical imaging into the operative arena could revolutionize the surgical care of cancer patients. Expert Rev Med Devices. 2008;5:663–7. doi:10.1586/17434440.5.6.663.
40. Hall NC, Povoski SP, Zhang J, Knopp MV, Martin Jr EW. Use of intraoperative nuclear medicine imaging technology: strategy for improved patient management. Expert Rev Med Devices. 2013;10:149–52. doi:10.1586/erd.13.2.
41. Povoski SP, Neff RL, Mojzisik CM, O'Malley DM, Hinkle GH, Hall NC, et al. A comprehensive overview of radioguided surgery using gamma detection probe technology. World J Surg Oncol. 2009;7:11. doi:10.1186/1477-7819-7-11.
42. Ellison EC, Gower WR, Elkhammas E, Woltering EA, Sparks J, O'Dorisio TM, et al. Characterization of the in vivo and in vitro inhibition of gastrin secretion from gastrinoma by a somatostatin analogue (SMS 201–995). Am J Med. 1986;81:56–64.
43. Geelhoed GW, Bass BL, Mertz SL, Becker KL. Somatostatin analog: effects on hypergastrinemia and hypercalcitoninemia. Surgery. 1986;100:962–70.
44. Carnaille B, Nocaudie M, Pattou F, Huglo D, Deveaux M, Marchandise X, et al. Scintiscans and carcinoid tumors. Surgery. 1994;116:1118–21; discussion 21–2.
45. Krenning EP, Kwekkeboom DJ, Oei HY, de Jong RJ, Dop FJ, de Herder WW, et al. Somatostatin receptor scintigraphy in carcinoids, gastrinomas and Cushing's syndrome. Digestion. 1994;55 Suppl 3:54–9.
46. Krenning EP, Bakker WH, Kooij PP, Breeman WA, Oei HY, de Jong M, et al. Somatostatin receptor scintigraphy with indium-111-DTPA-D-Phe-1-octreotide in man: metabolism, dosimetry and comparison with iodine-123-Tyr-3-octreotide. J Nuc Med. 1992;33:652–8.
47. Adams S, Baum RP, Hertel A, Wenisch HJ, Staib-Sebler E, Herrmann G, et al. Intraoperative gamma probe detection of neuroendocrine tumors. J Nuc Med. 1998;39:1155–60.
48. Banzo J, Vidal-Sicat S, Prats E, Galofre G, Razola P, Mane S, et al. In-111 DTPA octreotide scintigraphy and intraoperative gamma probe detection in the diagnosis and treatment of residual lymph node metastases of a rectal carcinoid tumor. Clin Nucl Med. 2005;30:308–11.
49. Benjegard SA, Forssell-Aronsson E, Wangberg B, Skanberg J, Nilsson O, Ahlman H. Intraoperative

tumour detection using 111In-DTPA-D-Phe1-octreotide and a scintillation detector. Eur J Nucl Med. 2001;28:1456–62. doi:10.1007/s002590100600.
50. Bombardieri E, Ambrosini V, Aktolun C, Baum RP, Bishof-Delaloye A, Del Vecchio S, et al. 111In-pentetreotide scintigraphy: procedure guidelines for tumour imaging. Eur J Nucl Med Mol Imaging. 2010;37:1441–8. doi:10.1007/s00259-010-1473-6.
51. Serrano Vicente J, Dominguez Grande ML, Infante De La Torre JR, Duran Barquero C, Garcia Bernardo L, Rayo Madrid JI, et al. Radioguided surgery of intestinal carcinoid tumor relapse. Role of SPECT-CT. Revista espanola de medicina nuclear. 2010;29:177–80. doi:10.1016/j.remn.2010.02.011.
52. Wong KK, Cahill JM, Frey KA, Avram AM. Incremental value of 111-in pentetreotide SPECT/CT fusion imaging of neuroendocrine tumors. Acad Radiol. 2010;17:291–7. doi:10.1016/j.acra.2009.08.015.
53. van Hulsteijn LT, Corssmit EP, van der Hiel B, Smit JW, Stokkel MP. Is there a role for radioguided surgery with iodine-labeled metaiodobenzylguanidine in resection of neuroendocrine tumors? Clin Nucl Med. 2012;37:1083–8. doi:10.1097/RLU.0b013e318266cb3d.
54. Hellman P, Ladjevardi S, Skogseid B, Akerstrom G, Elvin A. Radiofrequency tissue ablation using cooled tip for liver metastases of endocrine tumors. World J Surg. 2002;26:1052–6. doi:10.1007/s00268-002-6663-3.
55. Wang YZ, Diebold A, Woltering E, King H, Boudreaux JP, Anthony LB, et al. Radioguided exploration facilitates surgical cytoreduction of neuroendocrine tumors. J Gastrointest Surg. 2012;16:635–40. doi:10.1007/s11605-011-1767-4.
56. Gabriel M, Muehllechner P, Decristoforo C, von Guggenberg E, Kendler D, Prommegger R, et al. 99mTc-EDDA/HYNIC-Tyr(3)-octreotide for staging and follow-up of patients with neuroendocrine gastro-entero-pancreatic tumors. Q J Nucl Med Mol Imaging. 2005;49:237–44.
57. Fettich J, Pepse S, Snoj M, Zitko-Krhin M, Markovic M. 99mTc-EDDA/HAYNIC-TOC is suitable radiopharmaceutical for radioguided surgery of neuroendocrine tumours. In: Trends in radiopharmaceuticals (ISTR-2005), vol. 1. Vienna: IAEA; 2007. p. 183–4.
58. Hubalewska-Dydejczyk A, Fross-Baron K, Mikolajczak R, Maecke HR, Huszno B, Pach D, et al. 99mTc-EDDA/HYNIC-octreotate scintigraphy, an efficient method for the detection and staging of carcinoid tumours: results of 3 years' experience. Eur J Nucl Med Mol Imaging. 2006;33:1123–33. doi:10.1007/s00259-006-0113-7.
59. Taieb D, Timmers HJ, Hindie E, Guillet BA, Neumann HP, Walz MK, et al. EANM 2012 guidelines for radionuclide imaging of phaeochromocytoma and paraganglioma. Eur J Nucl Med Mol Imaging. 2012;39:1977–95. doi:10.1007/s00259-012-2215-8.
60. Meyer-Rochow GY, Schembri GP, Benn DE, Sywak MS, Delbridge LW, Robinson BG, et al. The utility of metaiodobenzylguanidine single photon emission computed tomography/computed tomography (MIBG SPECT/CT) for the diagnosis of pheochromocytoma. Ann Surg Oncol. 2010;17:392–400. doi:10.1245/s10434-009-0850-5.
61. Bombardieri E, Giammarile F, Aktolun C, Baum RP, Bischof Delaloye A, Maffioli L, et al. 131I/123I-metaiodobenzylguanidine (mIBG) scintigraphy: procedure guidelines for tumour imaging. Eur J Nucl Med Mol Imaging. 2010;37:2436–46. doi:10.1007/s00259-010-1545-7.
62. van Hulsteijn LT, van der Hiel B, Smit JW, Stokkel MP, Corssmit EP. Intraoperative detection of ganglioneuromas with 123I-MIBG. Clin Nucl Med. 2012;37:768–71. doi:10.1097/RLU.0b013e31825add9b.
63. Adams S, Baum R, Rink T, Schumm-Drager PM, Usadel KH, Hor G. Limited value of fluorine-18 fluorodeoxyglucose positron emission tomography for the imaging of neuroendocrine tumours. Eur J Nucl Med. 1998;25:79–83.
64. Kaemmerer D, Prasad V, Daffner W, Haugvik SP, Senftleben S, Baum RP, et al. Radioguided surgery in neuroendocrine tumors using Ga-68-labeled somatostatin analogs: a pilot study. Clin Nucl Med. 2012;37:142–7. doi:10.1097/RLU.0b013e3182291de8.
65. Aitken DR, Thurston MO, Hinkle Jr GH, Martin DT, Haagensen Jr DE, Houchens D, et al. Portable gamma probe for radioimmune localization of experimental colon tumor xenografts. J Surg Res. 1984;36:480–9.
66. Aitken DR, Hinkle GH, Thurston MO, Tuttle SE, Martin DT, Olsen J, et al. A gamma-detecting probe for radioimmune detection of CEA-producing tumors. Successful experimental use and clinical case report. Dis Colon Rectum. 1984;27:279–82.
67. Desai B, Elatre W, Quinn DI, Jadvar H. FDG PET/CT demonstration of pancreatic metastasis from prostate cancer. Clin Nucl Med. 2011;36:961–2. doi:10.1097/RLU.0b013e3182291d1a.
68. Desai DC, Arnold M, Saha S, Hinkle G, Soble D, Fry J, et al. Correlative whole-body FDG-PET and intraoperative gamma detection of FDG distribution in colorectal cancer. Clin Positron Iimaging. 2000;3:189–96.
69. Hall NC, Povoski SP, Murrey DA, Knopp MV, Martin Jr EW. Combined approach of perioperative 18F-FDG PET/CT imaging and intraoperative 18F-FDG handheld gamma probe detection for tumor localization and verification of complete tumor resection in breast cancer. World J Surg Oncol. 2007;5:143. doi:10.1186/1477-7819-5-143.
70. Martinez DA, King DR, Romshe C, Lozano RA, Morris JD, O'Dorisio MS, et al. Intraoperative identification of parathyroid gland pathology: a new approach. J Pediatr Surg. 1995;30:1306–9.
71. Povoski SP, Hall NC, Martin Jr EW, Walker MJ. Multimodality approach of perioperative 18F-FDG PET/CT imaging, intraoperative 18F-FDG handheld gamma probe detection, and intraoperative ultrasound for tumor localization and verification of

resection of all sites of hypermetabolic activity in a case of occult recurrent metastatic melanoma. World J Surg Oncol. 2008;6:1. doi:10.1186/1477-7819-6-1.
72. Povoski SP, Hall NC, Murrey Jr DA, Chow AZ, Gaglani JR, Bahnson EE, et al. Multimodal imaging and detection approach to 18F-FDG-directed surgery for patients with known or suspected malignancies: a comprehensive description of the specific methodology utilized in a single-institution cumulative retrospective experience. World J Surg Oncol. 2011;9:152. doi:10.1186/1477-7819-9-152.
73. Povoski SP, Chapman GJ, Murrey Jr DA, Lee R, Martin Jr EW, Hall NC. Intraoperative detection of (1)(8)F-FDG-avid tissue sites using the increased probe counting efficiency of the K-alpha probe design and variance-based statistical analysis with the three-sigma criteria. BMC Cancer. 2013;13:98. doi:10.1186/1471-2407-13-98.
74. Povoski SP, Hall NC, Murrey Jr DA, Sharp DS, Hitchcock CL, Mojzisik CM, et al. Multimodal imaging and detection strategy with 124 I-labeled chimeric monoclonal antibody cG250 for accurate localization and confirmation of extent of disease during laparoscopic and open surgical resection of clear cell renal cell carcinoma. Surg Innov. 2013;20:59–69. doi:10.1177/1553350612438416.
75. Povoski SP, Murrey Jr DA, Smith SM, Martin Jr EW, Hall NC. 18F-FDG PET/CT oncologic imaging at extended injection-to-scan acquisition time intervals derived from a single-institution 18F-FDG-directed surgery experience: feasibility and quantification of 18F-FDG accumulation within 18F-FDG-avid lesions and background tissues. BMC Cancer. 2014;14:453. doi:10.1186/1471-2407-14-453.
76. Sickle-Santanello BJ, O'Dwyer PJ, Mojzisik C, Tuttle SE, Hinkle GH, Rousseau M, et al. Radioimmunoguided surgery using the monoclonal antibody B72.3 in colorectal tumors. Dis Colon Rectum. 1987;30:761–4.
77. Hall NC, Nichols SD, Povoski SP, James IA, Wright CL, Harris R, et al. Intraoperative Use of a portable large field of view gamma camera and handheld gamma detection probe for radioguided localization and prediction of complete surgical resection of gastrinoma: proof of concept. J Am Coll Surg. 2015;221:300–8. doi:10.1016/j.jamcollsurg.2015.03.047.
78. Zollinger RM, Ellison EH. Primary peptic ulcerations of the jejunum associated with islet cell tumors of the pancreas. Ann Surg. 1955;142:709–23; discussion 24–8.
79. McCarthy DM, Hyman PE. Effect of isopropamide on response to oral cimetidine in patients with Zollinger--Ellison syndrome. Dig Dis Sci. 1982;27:353–9.
80. Norton JA, Fraker DL, Alexander HR, Venzon DJ, Doppman JL, Serrano J, et al. Surgery to cure the Zollinger-Ellison syndrome. N Engl J Med. 1999;341:635–44.doi:10.1056/NEJM199908263410902.
81. Norton JA, Jensen RT. Role of surgery in Zollinger-Ellison syndrome. J Am Coll Surg. 2007;205:S34–7. doi:10.1016/j.jamcollsurg.2007.06.320.
82. Norton JA, Fraker DL, Alexander HR, Gibril F, Liewehr DJ, Venzon DJ, et al. Surgery increases survival in patients with gastrinoma. Ann Surg. 2006;244:410–9. doi:10.1097/01.sla.0000234802.44320.a5.
83. Chapman GJ, Povoski SP, Hall NC, Murrey Jr DA, Lee R, Martin Jr EW. Comparison of two threshold detection criteria methodologies for determination of probe positivity for intraoperative in situ identification of presumed abnormal 18F-FDG-avid tissue sites during radioguided oncologic surgery. BMC Cancer. 2014;14:667. doi:10.1186/1471-2407-14-667.
84. Thurston MO. Development of the gamma detecting probe for radioimmunoguided surgery. In: Martin EW, editor. Radioimmunoguided Surgery (RIGS) in the detection and treatment of colorectal cancer, 1st ed. Austin: R.G. Landes Company; 1994. p. 41–65.
85. Siman W, Kappadath SC. Performance characteristics of a new pixelated portable gamma camera. Med Phys. 2012;39:3435–44. doi:10.1118/1.4718874.

Part IX

Clinical Application: Thoracic

Radioguided Sentinel Lymph Node Mapping and Biopsy in Non-small Cell Lung Cancer (NSCLC)

20

Leili Zarifmahmoudi, David N. Krag, Ramin Sadeghi, Reza Bagheri, and Susan Shafiee

Contents

L. Zarifmahmoudi, PhD • R. Sadeghi, MD
S. Shafiee, MD
Nuclear Medicine Research Center, Mashhad University of Medical Sciences, Mashhad, Iran

D.N. Krag, MD (✉)
Division of Surgical Oncology, Department of Surgery, College of Medicine, University of Vermont Given Building, Rm E309, 89 Beaumont Ave, Burlington, VT 05405, USA
e-mail: david.krag@uvm.edu

R. Bagheri, MD
Endoscopic & Minimal Invasive Surgery Research Center, Mashhad University of Medical Sciences, Mashhad, Iran

Abstract

Mediastinal lymph node dissection is an integral part of non-small cell lung cancer (NSCLC) surgical treatment. However, mediastinal lymph nodes are involved in less than 30 % of clinically stage I patients. Sentinel lymph node (SLN) mapping and biopsy has been proposed as an alternative to mediastinal lymph node dissection in NSCLC since 1999. Most studies thus far have used radiotracers for lymphatic mapping in NSCLC. Successful SLN mapping and biopsy needs careful selection of patients (only cN0 patients without history of chemotherapy) and proper administration route of the radiotracer (peri-tumoral is preferred over intra-tumoral injections). Alternative methods such as magnetic particles and fluorescent dyes seem to be very promising and need further validation studies in the future.

K. Herrmann et al. (eds.), *Radioguided Surgery: Current Applications and Innovative Directions in Clinical Practice*, DOI 10.1007/978-3-319-26051-8_20

20.1 Clinical Value and Relevance in Clinical Practice

Non-small cell lung cancer (NSCLC) accounts for almost 85 % of all types of lung cancers and is one of the major causes of cancer-related death. Mediastinal lymph node metastasis is one powerful and significant prognostic factor which leads to the considerable decrease in the 5-year survival rate and increase in disease recurrence possibility. Mediastinal lymph node dissection is an integral part of NSCLC surgical treatment which is associated with improved staging and survival. However, mediastinal lymph nodes may not be pathologically involved in the majority of patients with NSCLC (less than 30 % of clinically stage I patients) [1]. This is why less invasive methods for evaluating mediastinal lymph nodes are actively sought including CT scan, MRI, 18-F-FDG PET, mediastinoscopy, and SLN mapping.

SLN mapping and biopsy was used for NSCLC in 1999 by Little et al. [2] for the first time. However, Little et al. only used blue dye for this purpose. The first true radioguided SLN mapping and biopsy for NSCLC was done by Liptay et al. in 2000 [3], and since then numerous groups have published their experience in this regard [4]. Table 20.1 shows the characteristics of available studies on SLN mapping and biopsy in NSCLC in the medical literature [2, 5–50]. In case of duplicate reports, only the most recent one is summarized in Table 20.1.

20.1.1 Indications for SLN Mapping and Biopsy

Patients with cN0 NSCLC tumors are the best candidates for SLN mapping and biopsy. Very large necrotic tumors (>5 cm in diameter) and history of previous chemotherapy can also decrease the accuracy of lymphatic mapping in NSCLC. Liptay reported that reasons of detection failure were hilar and/or mediastinal adenopathy in eight patients, nine patients had tumors greater than 5 cm, and two patients underwent preoperative chemoradiation [13]. Melfi et al. in a study on 26 NSCLC patients reported only one SLN detection failure which was in a patient with a very large tumor [16]. In another study Faries et al. reported only one false-negative SLN result in 28 NSCLC patients, and this false-negative case had a history of chemotherapy [7]. The reason is straightforward: patients with large tumors and clinical (or radiological) large lymph nodes are more likely to have their SLNs completely replaced by tumor cells with resulting detection failure and false negativity.

Histological type and location of NSCLC and gender of the patients do not seem to be related to the success or accuracy of SLN mapping and biopsy in NSCLC [4].

20.2 Lymphatic Mapping Using Radiotracers

Most of the studies thus far have used radiotracers for lymphatic mapping in NSCLC. Tc-99 m-labeled HSA (human serum albumin), filtered or non-filtered SC (sulfur colloid), NC (nanocolloid), phytate, tin colloid, rhenium colloid, and antimony sulfide colloid have all been used for SLN mapping in NSCLC with very high detection rate and sensitivity. Type of the radiotracer does not seem to change the success or accuracy of SLN mapping and biopsy in NSCLC [4].

In a study by Rzyman et al., four radiotracers (Tc-99 m SC, Tc-99 m NC, Tc-99 m tin colloid, and Tc-99 m rhenium colloid) were compared for SLN mapping in 110 NSCLC patients, and no difference between the tracers was observed [36].

It should be noted that not all groups agree with our conclusion on the type of the radiotracer. Most importantly, Nomori et al. compared Tc-99 m phytate and Tc-99 m tin colloid for SLN mapping and biopsy of 147 patients. They reported that Tc-99 m phytate could identify SLNs more readily than Tc-99 m tin colloid, even in patients with a low FEV1 [24]. These results need to be validated in further trials; overall all radiotracers thus far seem to be reliable enough for SLN mapping and biopsy in NSCLC.

20.2.1 Route of Administration

Two injection locations have been used thus far for lymphatic mapping in NSCLC: peri-tumoral and intra-tumoral. Most studies thus far used

Table 20.1 Characteristics of the studies on SLN mapping and biopsy in NSCLC

First author	Country of origin	Publication year	Number of patients	Number of patients with detected SLN	Number of patients with positive lymph nodes	Number of patients with positive SLN	Radiotracer	Dose/volume (mCi/mL)	Blue dye	Volume (mL)	Other methods	Time from injection to surgery	Injection site	Time of injection	Type of surgery
Little et al.	Las Vegas, USA	1999	36	17	8	8	N/A	N/A	Isosulfan blue	5	N/A	N/A	Peri-tumoral	Intraoperative	Open
Klein et al.	The Czech Republic, Olomouc	2001	16	13	5	5	N/A	N/A	Patent blue V	4	N/A	10 min	Peri-tumoral	Intraoperative	Open
Schmidt et al.	Louisiana, USA	2002	31	25	3	3	Filtered Tc-99 m SC	0.5/1	Isosulfan blue	1	N/A	N/A	Peri-tumoral	Intraoperative 28; through bronchoscope 3	Open
Jedlicka et al.	The Czech Republic, Brno	2003	33	28	12	7	N/A	N/A	Patent blue V	5	N/A	N/A	Peri-tumoral	Intraoperative	Open
Melfi et al. (2003 study)	Pisa, Italy	2003	26	25	7	7	Tc-99 m nanocolloid	1	N/A	N/A	N/A	1 h (50–70 min)	Peri-tumoral	Intraoperative [10] and preoperative [16]	Open
Nakagawa et al.	Japan, Akita	2003	38	31	7	6	N/A	N/A	N/A	N/A	Ferumoxide 5 mL	15 min	Peri-tumoral	Intraoperative	Open
Sugi et al. (indocyanine green group)	Japan, Yamaguchi	2003	16	1	0	0	N/A	N/A	Indocyanine green	3	N/A	N/A	Peri-tumoral	Intraoperative	Open
Sugi et al. (isosulfan blue group)	Japan, Yamaguchi	2003	18	9	5	4	N/A	N/A	Isosulfan blue	3	N/A	N/A	Peri-tumoral	Intraoperative	Open
Sugi et al. (radiotracer group)	Japan, Yamaguchi	2003	14	9	2	2	Tc-99 m tin colloid	1/1.5	N/A	N/A	N/A	135 ± 55 (78–300) min	Peri-tumoral	Preoperative CT-guided	Open

(continued)

Table 20.1 (continued)

First author	Country of origin	Publication year	Number of patients	Number of patients with detected SLN	Number of patients with positive lymph nodes	Number of patients with positive SLN	Radiotracer	Dose/volume (mCi/mL)	Blue dye	Volume (mL)	Other methods	Time from injection to surgery	Injection site	Time of injection	Type of surgery
Lardinois et al.	Switzerland, Zürich	2003	20	19	10	9	Tc-99 m nanocolloid	2/1	N/A	N/A	N/A	1.4 h (1–3 h)	Peri-tumoral	Preoperative using bronchoscope	Open
Faries et al.	California, USA	2004	28	28	11	10	Tc-99 m HSA or Tc-99 m SC	1 or 0.5	Isosulfan blue (7 patients only blue dye, the rest both methods)	0.5–2	N/A	10–15 min	Peri-tumoral	Intraoperative	Open
Ni et al.	China	2004	12	12	7	6	Tc-99 m SC	2/2	N/A	N/A	N/A	N/A	Peri-tumoral	Intraoperative	Open
Liptay	Illinois, USA	2004	148	104	30	21	Filtered Tc-99 m SC	0.25–2	N/A	N/A	N/A	10–15 min	Intra-tumoral	Intraoperative	Open
Forte et al.	Rome, Italy	2004	11	6	2	2	N/A	N/A	Patent blue V	2–5	N/A	N/A	Peri-tumoral	Intraoperative	Open
Nomori et al. (2004 study)	Japan, Tokyo	2004	104	84	15	13	Tc-99 m tin colloid	8/1–1.5	N/A	N/A	N/A	18 h	Peri-tumoral	Preoperative CT-guided	N/A
Ito et al.	Japan, Tottori	2004	38	7	2	2	N/A	N/A	Indocyanine green AND hyaluronidase	5	N/A	N/A	Peri-tumoral	Intraoperative	Open
Ueda et al.	Japan, Yamaguchi	2004	9	8	0	0	N/A	N/A	N/A	N/A	Iopamidol 1.5–2 mL	N/A	Peri-tumoral	Preoperative	N/A
Bohanes et al.	The Czech Republic, Olomouc	2004	48	40	17	14	N/A	N/A	Patent blue V	2–4	N/A	5–10 min	Peri-tumoral	Intraoperative	Open
Zhu et al.	China	2005	50	33	15	11	N/A	N/A	Isosulfan blue	4	N/A	N/A	Peri-tumoral	Intraoperative	Open

Tiffet et al.	France, the UK	2005	24	13	6	5	Tc-99 m NC or Tc-99 m SC (one patient had only tracer injection)	1.6	Patent blue V (first two patients only had blue dye)	2	N/A	18.5 min (5–30 min)	Peri-tumoral	Intraoperative	Open
Sugi et al. (2005 study)	Japan, Yamaguchi	2005	15	14	3	3	N/A	N/A	N/A	N/A	Iohexol 1 mL	N/A	Peri-tumoral	Preoperative (percutaneous)	Open
Pulte et al.	New York, USA	2005	15	13	11	10	N/A	N/A	Isosulfan blue	0.5–2	N/A	5–21 min	Peri-tumoral	Intraoperative	Open
Atinkaya et al.	Turkey	2005	28	26	7	7	Filtered Tc-99 m SC	0.25	N/A	N/A	N/A	45 min (30–60 min)	Peri-tumoral	Intraoperative	Open
Ma et al.	China	2006	60	55	N/A	N/A	N/A	N/A	Methylene blue	4	N/A	N/A	Peri-tumoral	Intraoperative	Open
Minamiya et al.	Japan, Akita	2006	20	16	4	4	N/A	N/A	N/A	N/A	Ferumoxide 5 mL	28.4	Peri-tumoral	Intraoperative	Open
Rzyman et al.	Norway, Poland	2006	110	110	35	30	Tc-99 m nanocolloid OR Tc-99 m rhenium colloid OR Tc-99 m tin colloid OR Tc-99 m filtered SC	0.5/2	Patent blue V 42; methylene blue 68	4	N/A	15–100 min (median 50 min)	Peri-tumoral	Intraoperative	Open
Di Lieto et al. (dye group)	Napoli	2007	24	12	4	4	N/A	N/A	Isosulfan blue	2.5	N/A	N/A	Peri-tumoral	Intraoperative	Open
Di Lieto et al. (radiotracer group)	Napoli	2007	29	29	12	12	Tc-99 m HSA	1 (30 MBq)	N/A	N/A	N/A	N/A	Peri-tumoral	Intraoperative	Open
Minamiya et al. (peri-tumoral group)	Japan, Akita	2007	49	41	10	7	N/A	N/A	N/A	N/A	Ferucarbotran 1.6 mL	15 min	Peri-tumoral	Intraoperative	Open

(continued)

Table 20.1 (continued)

First author	Country of origin	Publication year	Number of patients	Number of patients with detected SLN	Number of patients with positive lymph nodes	Number of patients with positive SLN	Radiotracer	Dose/ volume (mCi/mL)	Blue dye	Volume (mL)	Other methods	Time from injection to surgery	Injection site	Time of injection	Type of surgery
Minamiya et al. (peri-tumoral and subpleural group)	Japan, Akita	2007	27	22	3	3	N/A	N/A	N/A	N/A	Ferucarbotran 1.6 mL	15 min	Peri-tumoral + subpleural	Intraoperative	Open
Meyer et al.	Switzerland, Lausanne	2007	10	0	N/A	N/A	Tc-99 m nanocolloid	0.4	Patent blue V	2	Fluorescein 10 % (1 mL)	Every 10 min till 60 min	Peri-tumoral	Intraoperative	Open
Bustos et al.	Brazil	2008	32	15	5	4	N/A	N/A	Patent blue V	2	N/A	15–30 min (in 12.5 % more than 30 min)	Peri-tumoral	Intraoperative	Open
Melfi et al. (2008 study)	Pisa, Italy	2008	19	16	8	8	Tc-99 m NC	1	N/A	N/A	N/A	1 h (50–70 min)	Peri-tumoral	Preoperative (by bronchoscopy or CT-guided)	Open; 2 VATS
Sugi et al. (2008 study)	Japan, Yamaguchi	2008	170	133	32	32	Tc-99 m tin colloid	2–8	N/A	N/A	N/A	1 day	Peri-tumoral	Preoperative CT-guided	Open
Liu et al.	China	2009	30	27	9	8	N/A	N/A	Methylene blue	4	N/A	N/A	Peri-tumoral	Intraoperative	Open
Liptay et al.	Illinois, USA	2009	39	24	6	2	Filtered Tc-99 m SC	0.25	N/A	N/A	N/A	N/A	Intra-tumoral	Intraoperative	Open
Ono et al.	Japan, Akita	2009	51	41	4	3	N/A	N/A	N/A	N/A	Ferucarbotran 1.6 mL	15 min	Peri-tumoral	Intraoperative	Open 25; VATS 26

Nomori et al. (tin colloid group)	Japan, Tokyo	2009	73	54	5	5	Tc-99 m tin colloid	6–8/1–1.5	N/A	N/A	N/A	18 h	Peri-tumoral	Preoperative CT-guided	Open 58; VATS 15
Nomori et al. (phytate group)	Japan, Tokyo	2009	74	66	6	6	Tc-99 m phytate	6–8/1–1.5	N/A	N/A	N/A	18 h	Peri-tumoral	Preoperative CT-guided	Open 58; VATS 15
Ichinose et al.	Japan, Tokyo	2009	20	20	8	7	N/A	N/A	N/A	N/A	Indocyanine green fluorescence 2–5 mL	N/A	Peri-tumoral	Intraoperative	Open
Matsuoka et al.	Japan, Tokushima	2009	12	8	2	2	N/A	N/A	N/A	N/A	Indocyanine green fluorescence 0.25 mL	5	Peri-tumoral	Intraoperative	Open
Barcelo-Galindez et al.	Spain	2009	37	35	7	5	Tc-99 m albumin	0.25	N/A	N/A	N/A	5 min	Peri-tumoral	Intraoperative	Open
Jiang-Peng et al.	China	2010	15	11	7	6	N/A	N/A	N/A	N/A	carbon nanoparticles suspension	N/A	Peri-tumoral	Intraoperative	Open
Yamashita et al.	Japan, Oita	2011	61	49	2	1	N/A	N/A	N/A	N/A	Indocyanine green fluorescence	10 min	Peri-tumoral	Intraoperative	VATS
Takizawa et al.	Japan, Tokushima	2012	13	12	2	2	N/A	N/A	N/A	N/A	Iopamidol 3 mL	N/A	Peri-tumoral	Preoperative (by bronchoscopy)	VATS
Kim et al. (preoperative group)	South Korea	2012	48	46	11	11	Tc-99 m MSA	1/0.2	N/A	N/A	N/A	1–2 h	Peri-tumoral	Preoperative CT-guided	VATS in 40
Kim et al. (intraoperative group)	South Korea	2012	34	33	6	6	Tc-99 m MSA	1/0.2	N/A	N/A	N/A	5 min	Peri-tumoral	Intraoperative	VATS in 26
Karamustafaoglu et al.	Turkey	2013	25	23	11	6	Tc-99 m nanocolloid	0.25	N/A	N/A	N/A	1 h	Peri-tumoral	Intraoperative	Open

(continued)

Table 20.1 (continued)

First author	Country of origin	Publication year	Number of patients	Number of patients with detected SLN	Number of patients with positive lymph nodes	Number of patients with positive SLN	Radiotracer	Dose/ volume (mCi/mL)	Blue dye	Volume (mL)	Other methods	Time from injection to surgery	Injection site	Time of injection	Type of surgery
Gilmore et al.	Boston, USA	2013	38	15 (success rate increased with increasing dose of the mapping material)	6	6	N/A	N/A	N/A	N/A	Indocyanine green fluorescence	5 min	Peri-tumoral	Intraoperative	Open [18], Thoracoscopic [20]
Hong et al.	China	2014	61	59	14	13	Tc-99 m SC	N/A	Methylene blue	N/A	N/A	30 min	Peri-tumoral	Intraoperative	Open
Zeybek et al.	Turkey	2014	12	10	1	1	Tc-99 m SC	5/5	N/A	N/A	N/A	96 min	Peri-tumoral	Intraoperative	Open
Galbis Caravajal et al.	Spain	2014	29	29	N/A	N/A	Tc-99 m nanocolloid	2/0.3	N/A	N/A	N/A	59 min	Peri-tumoral	Intraoperative	Open
Eo et al.	South Korea	2015	34	34	8	8	N/A	N/A	N/A	N/A	Ga-68-MSA for PET/CT imaging	1–3 h	Peri-tumoral	Pre operative CT-guided	Open

peri-tumoral injection of the tracer for SLN mapping and biopsy with excellent results [4, 51]. On the other hand, intra-tumoral injection was used in two studies by Liptay et al. with lower detection rate and sensitivity [13, 14]. The latter study *(CALGB 140203 multicenter phase II trial)* was terminated due to disappointing accuracy of the technique [14]. In another study by Melfi et al., the reason of three SLN detection failures was reported to be intratumoral injection of the radiotracer [17]. It seems that intra-tumoral injection of the tracer should be avoided and only peritumoral injection should be used.

20.2.2 Intraoperative vs. Preoperative Injection

The time of radiotracer injection in relation to the surgery is a matter of debate. Rationale of preoperative CT-guided or bronchoscopy-guided injection is to let the time pass enough for the radiotracer to reach the SLNs in the lymphatic system. Several studies used preoperative injection of the tracer with excellent detection rate and sensitivity. Taghizadeh et al. in a systematic review showed pooled detection rate and sensitivity of 82.1 % [75.4–87.3 %] and 97 % [90–99 %], respectively [4].

However, experience of SLN mapping and biopsy in breast cancer showed that radiotracer movement in the lymphatic system is very rapid, and there is no need for a long time interval between injection and surgery [52–55]. Experience on NSCLC also showed the same findings (Fig. 20.1), and intraoperative injection of the radiotracer showed comparable detection rate and sensitivity as the preoperative injection technique. Mean time of injection to SLN detection by a gamma detection probe was 10 min. Taghizadeh et al. showed pooled detection rate and sensitivity of 88.5 % [75.4–95.17 %] and 92 % [72–98 %], respectively, for intraoperative injection technique.

Overall, it seems that intraoperative radiotracer injection is as accurate and as successful as preoperative injection without any need for CT for

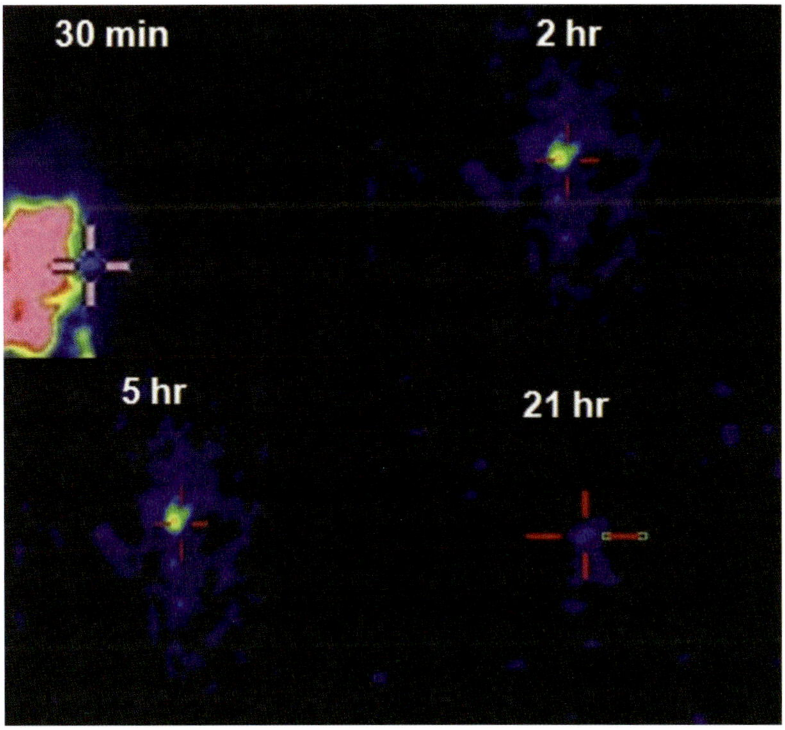

Fig. 20.1 Time course of sentinel lymph node visualization after preoperative injection of the radiotracer. The sentinel node could be easily identified as early as 30 min to 21 h postinjection (Reproduced with permission (10.1016/j.ejcts.2010.01.012))

bronchoscopy guidance. Time to wait after intraoperative injection does not need to be very long and 10–15 min is enough for successful SLN detection.

The radiotracer should be injected carefully to not penetrate the airways as leakage into the airways can make intraoperative SLN mapping and biopsy difficult (Tiffet et al. reported four detection failures due to airway injection in their study) [12]. Figure 20.2 shows planar lymphoscintigraphy images with radiotracer leakage into the airways. This does not seem to be of concern in preoperative injections as radiotracer would wash away the airways with time [56, 57].

20.2.3 Dose and Volume of the Injected Radiotracer

The dose of the radiotracer is highly dependent on the time of injection in relation to the surgery. For intraoperative injection usually 1–2 mCi divided into four aliquots is used, and for preoperative injection, 6–8 mCi divided into four aliquots [58]. Volume of injection is totally 1–1.5 mL which is divided into four samples for injection.

20.2.4 Role of Preoperative Lymphoscintigraphy and SPECT/CT

The prerequisite of preoperative lymphoscintigraphy imaging is preoperative CT- or bronchoscopy-guided injection of the radiotracer. There is not enough information in the literature regarding preoperative lymphoscintigraphy and SPECT/CT. However few reports showed that preoperative imaging especially SPECT/CT can identify the location of SLNs before surgery which can guide the surgeons intraoperatively.

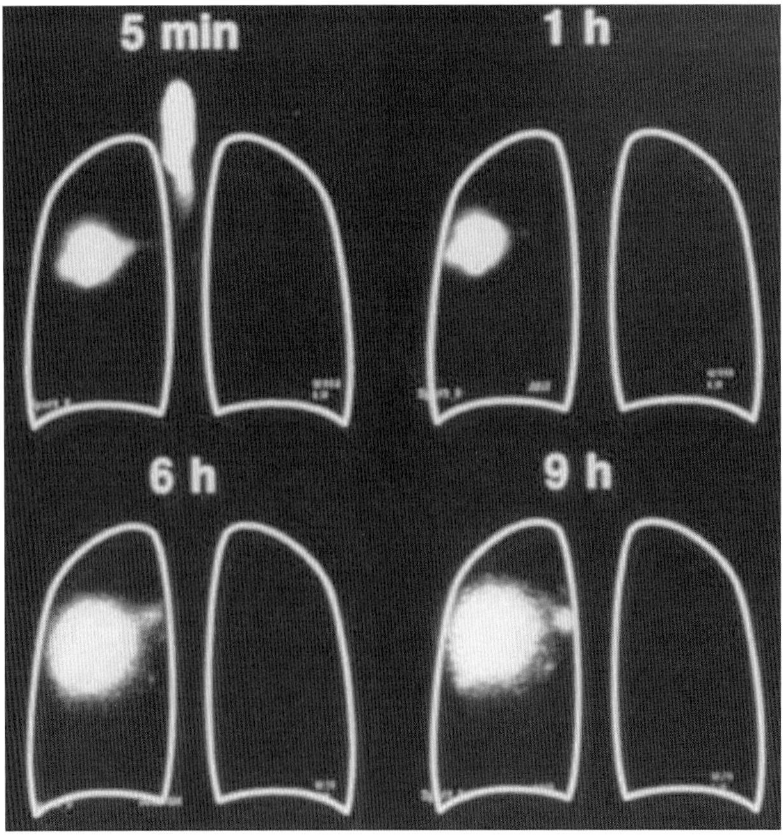

Fig. 20.2 Planar lymphoscintigraphy images of an NSCLC patient. Note airway leakage of the radiotracer on the early image (5 min image) which disappeared on the delayed images and the sentinel lymph node which is apparent on the 6 h image (Reproduced with permission (10.1067/mtc.2002.124496))

Unusual location of the SLNs can also be easily identified which otherwise would be neglected by the surgeons. By better preoperative localization, SPECT/CT findings may decrease operating time, decrease patient morbidity, and improve the accuracy of pathological examination. Injection problems such as leakage of the radiotracer into the airways and pleural space could also be identified readily by SPECT/CT imaging [59, 60]. Figures 20.3, 20.4, 20.5, and 20.6 show examples of SPECT/CT findings in NSCLC SLN mapping and biopsy.

However, compared to the other solid tumors such as genitourinary cancers, breast cancer, and melanoma, the utility of SPECT/CT in NSCLC SLN mapping and biopsy seems to be limited. In the Abele et al. study, SLNs were identified only in 50 % of the patients on SPECT/CT imaging [60]. Another study by Nomori et al. showed that SPECT/CT could identify SLNs in the hila especially in segmental and lobar lymph node areas, but not in the mediastinum. This can be an advantage for SPECT/CT imaging as intraoperative SLN localization by gamma probes can be hard in the hilar and segmental areas [61] (Figure 20.7). Figure 20.6 shows an example of a patient with hilar SLN on SPECT/CT images.

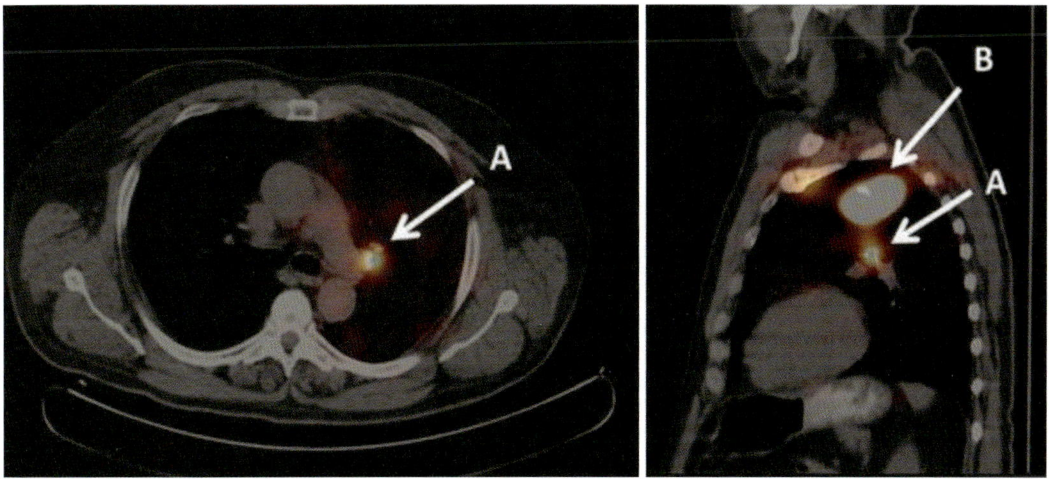

Fig. 20.3 Transverse and sagittal fused SPECT/CT images of an NSCLC in the LUL. *A* is a sentinel lymph node in the left suprahilar area and *B* is the injection site (Reproduced with permission (10.1007/s12149-014-0821-1))

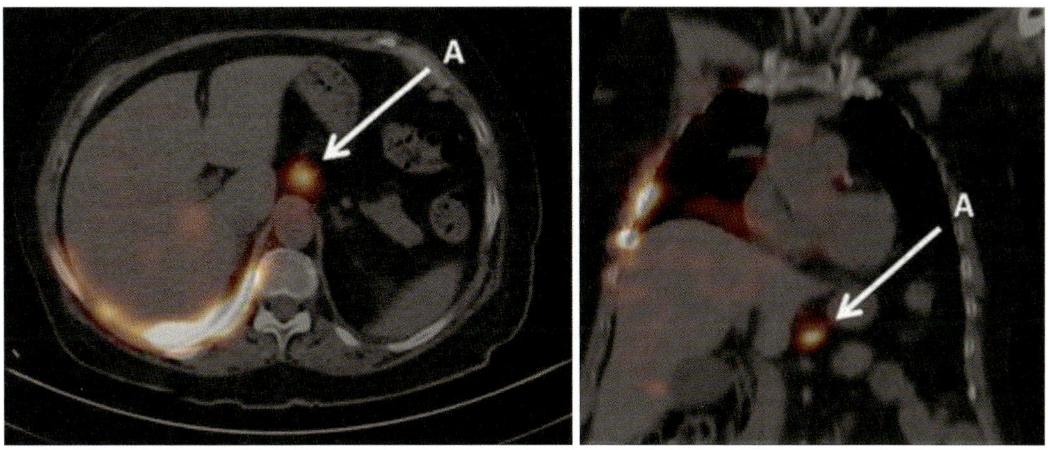

Fig. 20.4 Transverse and coronal fused SPECT/CT images of an NSCLC in the RUL. *A* is a sentinel lymph node in the gastrohepatic area (Reproduced with permission (10.1007/s12149-014-0821-1))

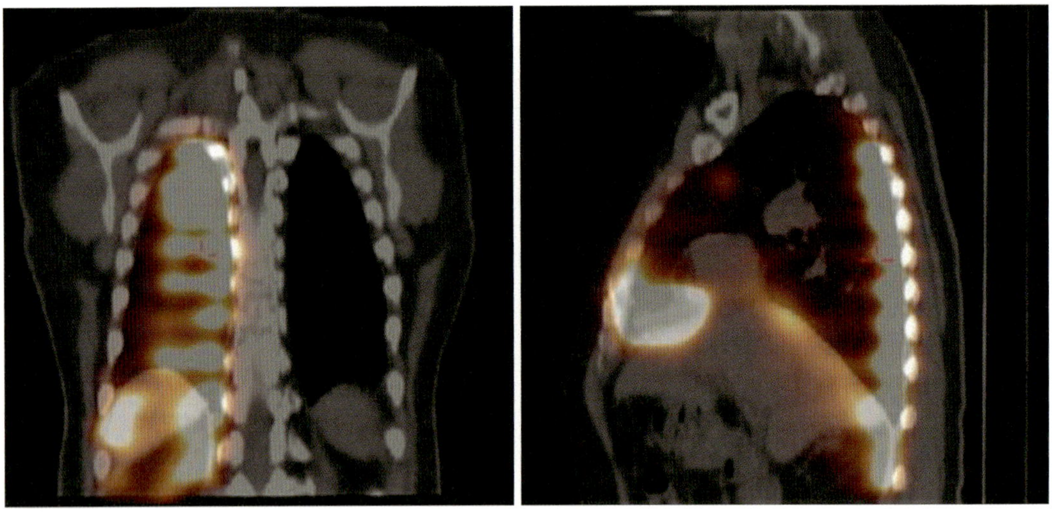

Fig. 20.5 Coronal and sagittal fused SPECT/CT images of an NSCLC in the RLL. Diffuse activity in the pleural space is due to radiotracer pleural space leakage (Reproduced with permission (10.1007/s12149-014-0821-1))

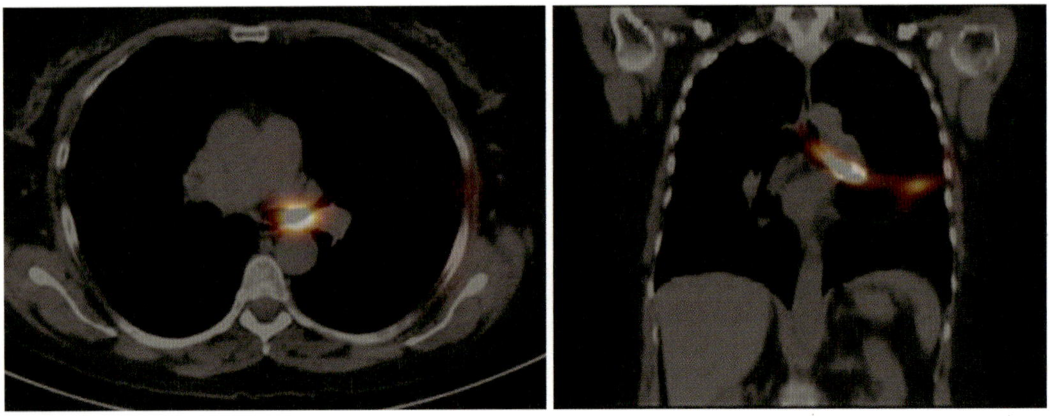

Fig. 20.6 Transverse and coronal fused SPECT/CT images of an NSCLC in the LUL. Note airway leakage of the radiotracer into the left mainstem bronchus (Reproduced with permission (10.1007/s12149-014-0821-1))

20.3 Alternative Approaches to SLN Mapping and Biopsy in NSCLC

20.3.1 Blue Dyes

SLN mapping and biopsy using a dye-only method is not as successful as other solid tumors. A systematic review by Taghizadeh Kermani et al. showed only 64.4 % which is pretty low as compared to the radiotracer method [4].

Lower detection rate by dye alone is related to black discoloration of the mediastinal lymph nodes in most patients (anthracosis) which makes it difficult to find dye-stained SLNs in the mediastinum [58]. Among the dye methods, indocyanine green had the worst detection rate as indocyanine green (although bright under fluorescent light) is not readily visible by the unaided eye [32].

Due to possible occurrence of some allergic and nonallergic complications including hypersensitivity (even anaphylactic) reaction in the form of pulmonary edema, blue discoloration of the skin or body fluids, and skin necrosis [62, 63] and very low detection rate by dye techniques,

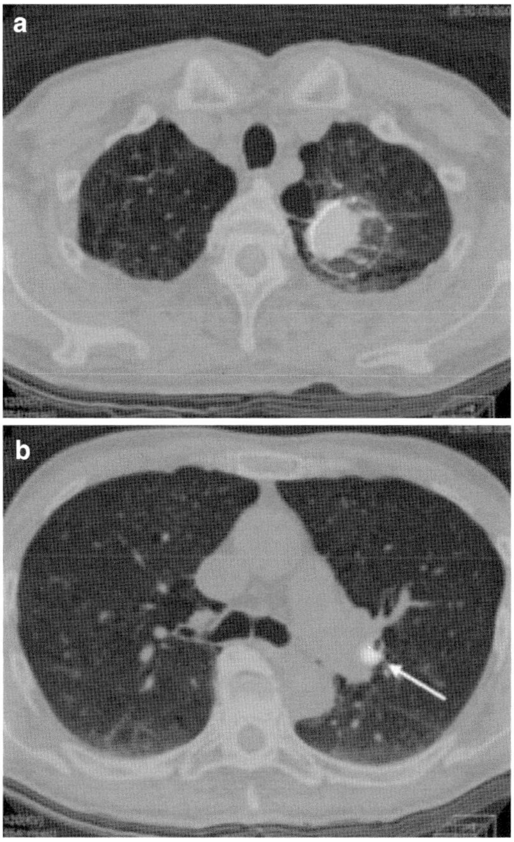

Fig. 20.7 Fused SPECT/CT images in an NSCLC of the LUL. (**a**) is the injection site and (**b**) is a segmental sentinel lymph node (*white arrow*) (Reproduced with permission (10.1016/j.jtcvs.2007.02.013))

using blue dye (alone or in combination) in NSCLC SLN mapping and biopsy is not justified.

20.3.2 PET Radiotracers

Thus far, only one group reported application of PET radiotracers for SLN mapping and biopsy in NSCLC. Eo et al. used Ga-68-labeled mannosylated human serum albumin (Ga-68-MSA) for SLN mapping and biopsy in NSCLC (Figure 20.8). They enrolled 34 patients of clinically stage I NSCLC. The radiotracer was injected peri-tumorally under CT guidance 1–3 h before surgery, and PET imaging was started 15–30 min postinjection. They had 100 % detection rate and no false-negative results [50].

Despite being a promising alternative to the conventional radiotracers, PET tracers are limited by their cost.

20.3.3 Magnetic Particles

Ferumoxides (a colloidal superparamagnetic iron oxide of nonstoichiometric magnetite), which are used as a contrasting agent for MRI, have been recently applied for SLN mapping and biopsy in NSCLC patients. The magnetic particles are injected peri-tumorally and the magnetic force within SLNs is detected by handheld magnetometer [19, 64]. Intraoperative application of mentioned magnetic particle for SLN mapping and biopsy of NSCLC patients resulted in the detection, accuracy, sensitivity, and false-negative rates of 81.6 %, 96.8 %, 85.7 %, and 14.3 %, respectively [19]. Similar outcomes have been obtained by using ferucarbotran (clinically approved superparamagnetic iron oxide) for SLN mapping and biopsy of patients with NSCLC [21].

It is suggested that applying magnetic particles for SLN mapping and biopsy is associated with high sensitivity, detection rate, and accuracy without any radiation burden to the patients and surgical staff. Larger studies are still needed to validate the abovementioned findings.

20.3.4 Fluorescent Dyes

Near-infrared (NIR) fluorescent lymphatic imaging is a novel method for SLN mapping and biopsy in solid tumors and also has been used for SLN mapping and biopsy in NSCLC.

Although indocyanine green (ICG) was difficult to visualize using regular room light with the unaided eye because it was masked by the black appearance of the SLNs, its ability of absorbing infrared rays (as an NIR lymphatic fluorophore) during in vivo binding with serum proteins appeared to be advantageous for SLN mapping and biopsy of NSCLC.

The clinical efficacy of this new technique for NSCLC has been investigated by several

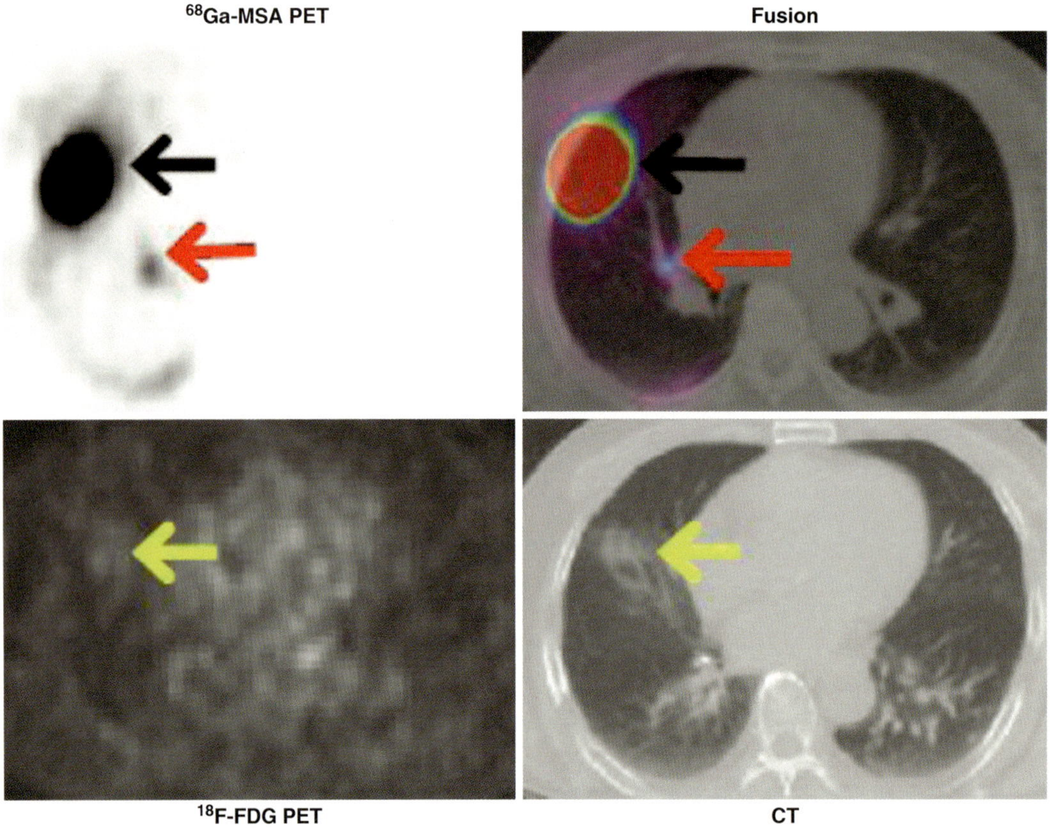

Fig. 20.8 Sentinel lymph node imaging by 68Ga-MSA PET/CT. *Black arrow* shows the injection site, and *red arrow* shows the sentinel node activity. *Yellow arrow* shows tumor activity (Reproduced with permission (10.1245/s10434-014-3986-x))

research groups. In 2012, Yamashita et al. reported the results of fluorescent imaging for SLN mapping and biopsy in 61 NSCLC patients with 80.3 % detection rate and 2.1 % false-negative rate [65]. Ichinose et al. also reported excellent results by NIR imaging in 12 patients with 91.6 % detection rate and no false-negative case [25]. However, Matsuoka et al. showed less satisfactory results on 12 NSCLC patients with 66.6 % detection rate [27].

The advantages of this new technique over radioisotopes are lower radioactivity exposure and no shine-through effect. The technique may also reveal deeply located SLNs in the lung parenchyma or mediastinal fat tissue; however identification of SLNs should begin as soon as possible because dye may pass through to the non-SLNs as time passes [65].

Further studies are needed to increase the validity of ICG fluorescence imaging-guided lung surgery and to be used for SLN mapping and biopsy in NSCLC. Dose, imaging time and method, and many other variables should be optimized before routine clinical imaging [46].

20.3.5 Carbon Nanoparticles Suspension

In a single report, Jiang-Peng et al. studied the efficacy of carbon nanoparticles for SLN mapping and biopsy in 15 NSCLC patients with 73.3 % detection rate and 85.7 % sensitivity [10]. However, carbon nanoparticles do not seem to be a viable alternative for radiotracers as they share the same shortcoming as the blue dyes.

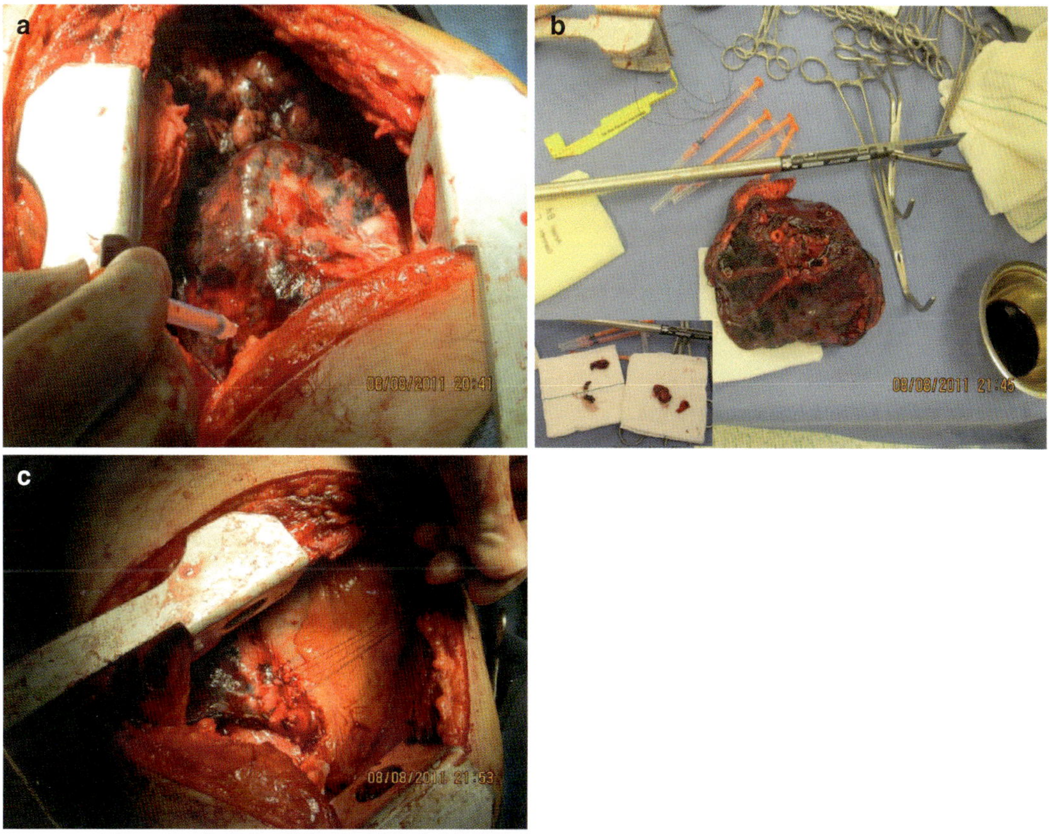

Fig. 20.9 (**a**) NSCLC after exposure of the lung and injection of the tracer in the peri-tumoral area. (**b**) Resected tumor and harvested lymph nodes. (**c**) Tumoral bed after resection of the tumor and lymph node dissection

20.4 Intraoperative Detection and Resection of SLNs

For intraoperative SLN detection, an acoustic gamma detection probe is used to guide the surgeons to the location of SLNs.

As mentioned above, the success rate (surgical detection rate) for radiotracer-guided SLN biopsy in NSCLC is high and comparable to other solid tumors such as breast cancer and melanoma. Pooled surgical detection rate was highest for studies using radiotracer intraoperatively and peri-tumorally: 95.3 % [89.9–97.9 %] [4, 58].

Acoustic gamma detection probes are very reliable for SLN localization in NSCLC; even laparoscopic gamma detection probes for video-assisted thoracoscopic surgery (VATS) work very well with very high surgical detection rate [58]. Preoperative CT- or bronchoscopy-guided radiotracer injection can provide the opportunity for preoperative lymphoscintigraphy and SPECT/CT which can guide the surgeons to the correct position of the intrathoracic SLNs. However, intraoperative injection also works well as shown by multiple studies. Figure 20.9 shows intraoperative SLN mapping and biopsy in an NSCLC.

However, detection of SLNs near the injection site can be very hard due to obscured uptake in the nearby SLNs. Learning curve effect also can be a problem in utilizing acoustic gamma detection probes. Thus far, two studies have reported possible learning curve effect when performing SLN mapping and biopsy in NSCLC patients using radiotracers and fluorescent imaging [14, 65]. This learning curve effect can compromise the performance of the thoracic surgeon early on in the process of gaining experience with this technique.

20.4.1 Role of Portable Gamma Cameras and 3D Systems (fhSPECT)

Thus far, no study has reported the application of intraoperating portable gamma cameras and freehand SPECT devices for SLN mapping and biopsy in NSCLC. Due to the complex anatomy of the thorax, these novel technologies could potentially be of real help in NSCLC, and this future studies should be considered using these devices.

Conclusion

SLN mapping and biopsy is an accurate method for mediastinal lymph node staging in NSCLC patients. Successful SLN mapping and biopsy needs careful selection of patients (only cN0 patients without history of chemotherapy) and proper administration route of the radiotracer (peri-tumoral injection is preferred over intra-tumoral injection). Alternative methods, such as magnetic particles and fluorescent dyes, seem to be very promising and need further validation studies in the future.

References

1. Zhong W, Yang X, Bai J, Yang J, Manegold C, Wu Y. Complete mediastinal lymphadenectomy: the core component of the multidisciplinary therapy in resectable non-small cell lung cancer. Eur J Cardiothorac Surg. 2008;34(1):187–95. Epub 2008/05/07.
2. Little AG, DeHoyos A, Kirgan DM, Arcomano TR, Murray KD. Intraoperative lymphatic mapping for non-small cell lung cancer: the sentinel node technique. J Thorac Cardiovasc Surg. 1999;117(2):220–4. Epub 1999/01/27.
3. Liptay MJ, Masters GA, Winchester DJ, Edelman BL, Garrido BJ, Hirschtritt TR, et al. Intraoperative radioisotope sentinel lymph node mapping in non-small cell lung cancer. Ann Thorac Surg. 2000;70(2):384–9. discussion 9–90. Epub 2000/09/02.
4. Taghizadeh Kermani A, Bagheri R, Tehranian S, Shojaee P, Sadeghi R. D NK. Accuracy of sentinel node biopsy in the staging of non-small cell lung carcinomas: systematic review and meta-analysis of the literature. Lung Cancer. 2013;80(1):5–14. Epub 2013/01/29.
5. Bustos ME, Camargo JJ, Resin Geyer G, Feijo AC. Intraoperative detection of sentinel lymph nodes using Patent Blue V in non-small cell lung cancer. Minerva Chir. 2008;63(1):29–36. Epub 2008/01/24.
6. Jedlicka V, Capov I, Pestal A, Stasek T, Wechsler J. Sentinel node detection and its importance in the surgical treatment of non-small cell lung carcinoma--review. Rozhl Chir. 2003;82(5)):273–7. Epub 2003/08/23. Detekce sentinelove uzliny a jeji vyznam v chirurgicke lecbe nemalobunecneho karcinomu plic--prehled.
7. Faries MB, Bleicher RJ, Ye X, Essner R, Morton DL. Lymphatic mapping and sentinel lymphadenectomy for primary and metastatic pulmonary malignant neoplasms. Arch Surg. 2004;139(8):870–6. discussion 6–7. Epub 2004/08/11.
8. Liu P, Wang H. Non-small cell lung cancer sentinel lymph node biopsy in clinical research. Contemp Chin Med. 2009;20:187–8.
9. Ma L, Zhou W, Wu S, Chen Z, Ye M. Intraoperative sentinel lymph node mapping for non-small cell lung cancer. Chin J Prim Med Pharm. 2006;13(1):173–5.
10. Jian-Peng Z, Zou W, Wang K, Liu F, Ma G, Cao L. Intraoperative detection of sentinel lymph nodes using carbon nanoparticles suspension injection in non-small cell lung cancer. Chin J Surg Oncol. 2010;2(2):74–7.
11. Zhu ZH, Li BJ, Zhang SY, Rong TH, Zeng CG, Yu H, et al. Predictive value of detection of sentinel lymph nodes on lymphatic metastasis of non-small cell lung cancer. Ai Zheng. 2005;24(3):341–4. Epub 2005/03/11.
12. Tiffet O, Nicholson AG, Khaddage A, Prevot N, Ladas G, Dubois F, et al. Feasibility of the detection of the sentinel lymph node in peripheral non-small cell lung cancer with radio isotopic and blue dye techniques. Chest. 2005;127(2):443–8. Epub 2005/02/12.
13. Liptay MJ. Sentinel node mapping in lung cancer. Ann Surg Oncol. 2004;11(3 Suppl):271S–4. Epub 2004/03/17.
14. Liptay MJ, D'Amico TA, Nwogu C, Demmy TL, Wang XF, Gu L, et al. Intraoperative sentinel node mapping with technitium-99 in lung cancer: results of CALGB 140203 multicenter phase II trial. J Thorac Oncol. 2009;4(2):198–202. Epub 2009/01/31.
15. Di Lieto E, Gallo G, Scarpati VD, Di Tommaso P, Carpenito A, Perrone A. Lymph node sentinel detection in lung resection for non small cell lung cancer: our experience. Recenti Prog Med. 2007;98(6):327–8. Epub 2007/06/22. Tecnica del linfonodo sentinella nella resezione polmonare per cancro polmonare non a piccole cellule: nostra esperienza.
16. Melfi FM, Chella A, Menconi GF, Givigliano F, Boni G, Mariani G, et al. Intraoperative radioguided sentinel lymph node biopsy in non-small cell lung cancer. Eur J Cardiothorac Surg. 2003;23(2):214–20. Epub 2003/02/01.

17. Melfi FM, Lucchi M, Davini F, Viti A, Fontanini G, Boldrini L, et al. Intraoperative sentinel lymph node mapping in stage I non-small cell lung cancer: detection of micrometastases by polymerase chain reaction. Eur J Cardiothorac Surg. 2008;34(1):181–6. Epub 2008/05/27.
18. Forte A, D'Urso A, Urbano V, Lo Russo R, Gallinaro LS, Petrozza V, et al. Intraoperative limphonodal mapping in gastric, pulmonary and large bowel tumors. The sentinel limphonode technique. G Chir. 2004;25(3):101–4. Epub 2004/06/29. Mappatura linfonodale intraoperatoria in tumori gastrici, polmonari e del grosso intestino. La tecnica del linfonodo sentinella.
19. Nakagawa T, Minamiya Y, Katayose Y, Saito H, Taguchi K, Imano H, et al. A novel method for sentinel lymph node mapping using magnetite in patients with non-small cell lung cancer. J Thorac Cardiovasc Surg. 2003;126(2):563–7. Epub 2003/08/21.
20. Minamiya Y, Ito M, Katayose Y, Saito H, Imai K, Sato Y, et al. Intraoperative sentinel lymph node mapping using a new sterilizable magnetometer in patients with nonsmall cell lung cancer. Ann Thorac Surg. 2006;81(1):327–30. Epub 2005/12/22.
21. Ono T, Minamiya Y, Ito M, Saito H, Motoyama S, Nanjo H, et al. Sentinel node mapping and micrometastasis in patients with clinical stage IA non-small cell lung cancer. Interact Cardiovasc Thorac Surg. 2009;9(4):659–61. Epub 2009/08/01.
22. Minamiya Y, Ito M, Hosono Y, Kawai H, Saito H, Katayose Y, et al. Subpleural injection of tracer improves detection of mediastinal sentinel lymph nodes in non-small cell lung cancer. Eur J Cardiothorac Surg. 2007;32(5):770–5. Epub 2007/09/04.
23. Nomori H, Watanabe K, Ohtsuka T, Naruke T, Suemasu K. In vivo identification of sentinel lymph nodes for clinical stage I non-small cell lung cancer for abbreviation of mediastinal lymph node dissection. Lung Cancer. 2004;46(1):49–55. Epub 2004/09/15.
24. Nomori H, Ohba Y, Yoshimoto K, Shibata H, Mori T, Shiraishi S, et al. Difference of sentinel lymph node identification between tin colloid and phytate in patients with non-small cell lung cancer. Ann Thorac Surg. 2009;87(3):906–10. Epub 2009/02/24.
25. Ichinose S, Usuda J, Maehara S, Ohtani K, Ishizumi T, Ohira T, et al. Sentinel node navigation surgery (SNNS) using indocyanine green (ICG) and near infrared spectroscopy in lung cancer. J Thorac Oncol. 2009;4(9):S563–S.
26. Yamashita SI, Tokuishi K, Miyawaki M, Anami K, Moroga T, Takeno S, et al. Sentinel Node Navigation Surgery by Thoracoscopic Fluorescence Imaging System and Molecular Examination in Non-Small Cell Lung Cancer. Ann Surg Oncol. 2011;19(3):728–33. Epub 2011/11/22.
27. Matsuoka H, Kondo K, Takizawa H, Uyama K, Hiroaki T, Koichiro K, et al. Sentinel lymph nodes detection using indocyanine green in patients with lung cancer. J Thorac Oncol. 2009;4(9):S562–3.
28. Takizawa H, Kondo K, Toba H, Kajiura K, Takashima M, Uyama K, et al. Computed Tomography Lymphography by Transbronchial Injection of a Water-Soluble Extracellular Ct Contrast Agent to Identify the Sentinel Lymph Nodes in Preoperative Nsclc Patients. J Thorac Oncol. 2011;6(6):S1335–6.
29. Ito N, Fukuta M, Tokushima T, Nakai K, Ohgi S. Sentinel node navigation surgery using indocyanine green in patients with lung cancer. Surg Today. 2004;34(7):581–5. Epub 2004/06/29.
30. Sugi K, Kitada K, Yoshino M, Hirazawa K, Matsuda E, Azuma T, et al. New method of visualizing lymphatics in lung cancer patients by multidetector computed tomography. J Comput Assist Tomogr. 2005;29(2):210–4. Epub 2005/03/18.
31. Ueda K, Suga K, Kaneda Y, Li TS, Hamano K. Preoperative imaging of the lung sentinel lymphatic basin with computed tomographic lymphography: a preliminary study. Ann Thorac Surg. 2004;77(3):1033–7. discussion 7–8. Epub 2004/03/03.
32. Sugi K, Fukuda M, Nakamura H, Kaneda Y. Comparison of three tracers for detecting sentinel lymph nodes in patients with clinical N0 lung cancer. Lung Cancer. 2003;39(1):37–40. Epub 2002/12/25.
33. Sugi K, Kobayashi S, Yagi R, Matsuoka T. Usefulness of sentinel lymph node biopsy for the detection of lymph node micrometastasis in early lung cancer. Interact Cardiovasc Thorac Surg. 2008;7(5):913–5. Epub 2008/06/07.
34. Schmidt FE, Woltering EA, Webb WR, Garcia OM, Cohen JE, Rozans MH. Sentinel nodal assessment in patients with carcinoma of the lung. Ann Thorac Surg. 2002;74(3):870–4. discussion 4–5. Epub 2002/09/20.
35. Pulte D, Li E, Crawford BK, Newman E, Alexander A, Mustalish DC, et al. Sentinel lymph node mapping and molecular staging in nonsmall cell lung carcinoma. Cancer. 2005;104(7):1453–61. Epub 2005/09/01.
36. Rzyman W, Hagen OM, Dziadziuszko R, Kobierska-Gulida G, Karmolinski A, Lothe IM, et al. Intraoperative, radio-guided sentinel lymph node mapping in 110 nonsmall cell lung cancer patients. Ann Thorac Surg. 2006;82(1):237–42. Epub 2006/06/27.
37. Klein J, Bohanes T, Kral V, Neoral C, Tichy T, Skarda J, et al. Technical details of sentinel node detection during lung cancer resection. Klin Onkol. 2001;14(5):170–3.
38. Bohanes T, Klein J, Kral V, Neoral C, Tichy T. Detection of the sentinel lymph nodes in lung carcinoma cases using patent blue and its clinical significance. Rozhl Chir. 2004;83(6):210–6. Epub 2004/09/24. Detekce sentinelove uzliny u plicniho karcinomu pomoci patentni modri a jeji klinicky vyznam.
39. Barcelo-Galindez R, Uribe-Etxebarria N, Viteri A, Genolla J, Jimenez-Maestre U, Lorenzo-Martin M, et al. Feasibility and safety of detection of sentinel node in lung cancer. J Clin Oncol. 2009;27(15):7587.

40. Kim HK, Kim S, Sung HK, Lee YS, Jeong JM, Choi YH. Comparison between preoperative versus intraoperative injection of technetium-99 m neomannosyl human serum albumin for sentinel lymph node identification in early stage lung cancer. Ann Surg Oncol. 2011. Epub 2011/12/07.
41. Meyer A, Cheng C, Antonescu C, Pezzetta E, Bischof-Delaloye A, Ris HB. Successful migration of three tracers without identification of sentinel nodes during intraoperative lymphatic mapping for non-small cell lung cancer. Interact Cardiovasc Thorac Surg. 2007;6(2):214–8. Epub 2007/08/03.
42. Lardinois D, Brack T, Gaspert A, Spahr T, Schneiter D, Steinert HC, et al. Bronchoscopic radioisotope injection for sentinel lymph-node mapping in potentially resectable non-small-cell lung cancer. Eur J Cardiothorac Surg. 2003;23(5):824–7. Epub 2003/05/20.
43. Atinkaya C, Ozlem Kucuk N, Koparal H, Aras G, Sak SD, Ozdemir N. Mediastinal intraoperative radioisotope sentinel lymph node mapping in non-small-cell lung cancer. Nucl Med Commun. 2005;26(8):717–20. Epub 2005/07/08.
44. Ni X, Wang Q, Tan L, Jiang W, Yong F, Pang X, et al. Clinical research on the technique of sentinel lymph node biopsy in patients with NSCLC. Clin J Chin Med. 2004;11(5):730–1.
45. Karamustafaoglu YA, Yoruk Y, Yanik F, Sarikaya A. Sentinel lymph node mapping in patients with operable non-small cell lung cancer. J thorac dis. 2013;5(3):317–20. Epub 2013/07/05.
46. Gilmore DM, Khullar OV, Jaklitsch MT, Chirieac LR, Frangioni JV, Colson YL. Identification of metastatic nodal disease in a phase 1 dose-escalation trial of intraoperative sentinel lymph node mapping in non-small cell lung cancer using near-infrared imaging. J Thorac Cardiovasc Surg. 2013;146(3):562–70. discussion 9–70. Epub 2013/06/25.
47. Hong B, Shen X, Chen J. Intraoperative methylene blue and (99m)Tc-sulfur colloid isotope tracing for sentinel node mapping in early-stage non-small cell lung cancer. Nan Fang Yi Ke Da Xue Xue Bao. 2014;34(7):1053–6. Epub 2014/07/25.
48. Zeybek A, Sarper A, Erdogan A, Dertsiz L, Demircan A. Determination of sentinel lymph node by Tc(99m) in small-cell lung cancer. Tuberk Toraks. 2014;62(1):45–50. Epub 2014/05/13. Kucuk hucreli disi akciger kanserlerinde Tc(99m) ile sentinel lenf nodunun saptanmasi.
49. Galbis Caravajal JM, Mira AC, Cabrera AZ, Guerrero ME, Ferrairo AT, Martinez Hernandez NJ, et al. Sentinel lymph node in pulmonary carcinoma. Molecular study after radioisotope detection. Cir Esp. 2014;92(1):11–5. Epub 2014/03/04. El ganglio centinela en el carcinoma pulmonar. Estudio molecular tras deteccion con radioisotopo.
50. Eo JS, Kim HK, Kim S, Lee YS, Jeong JM, Choi YH. Gallium-68 neomannosylated human serum albumin-based PET/CT lymphoscintigraphy for sentinel lymph node mapping in non-small cell lung cancer. Ann Surg Oncol. 2015;22(2):636–41. Epub 2014/08/27.
51. Shersher DD, Liptay MJ. Status of sentinel lymph node mapping in non-small cell lung cancer. Cancer J. 2015;21(1):17–20. Epub 2015/01/23.
52. Sadeghi R, Forghani MN, Memar B, Rajabi Mashhadi MT, Dabbagh Kakhki VR, Abdollahi A, et al. How long the lymphoscintigraphy imaging should be continued for sentinel lymph node mapping? Ann Nucl Med. 2009;23(6):507–10. Epub 2009/07/10.
53. Abdollahi A, Jangjoo A, Dabbagh Kakhki VR, Rasoul Zakavi S, Memar B, Naser Forghani M, et al. Factors affecting sentinel lymph node detection failure in breast cancer patients using intradermal injection of the tracer. Rev Esp Med Nucl. 2010;29(2):73–7. Epub 2009/11/26.
54. Jangjoo A, Forghani MN, Mehrabibahar M, Rezapanah A, Kakhki VR, Zakavi SR, et al. Comparison of early and delayed lymphoscintigraphy images of early breast cancer patients undergoing sentinel node mapping. Nucl Med Commun. 2010;31(6):521–5. Epub 2010/04/30.
55. Aliakbarian M, Memar B, Jangjoo A, Zakavi SR, Reza Dabbagh Kakhki V, Aryana K, et al. Factors influencing the time of sentinel node visualization in breast cancer patients using intradermal injection of the radiotracer. Am J Surg. 2011;202(2):199–202. Epub 2011/08/04.
56. Nomori H. Sentinel node mapping in lung cancer: the Japanese experience. Semin Thorac Cardiovasc Surg. 2009;21(4):316–22. Epub 2009/01/01.
57. Nomori H, Horio H, Naruke T, Orikasa H, Yamazaki K, Suemasu K. Use of technetium-99m tin colloid for sentinel lymph node identification in non-small cell lung cancer. J Thorac Cardiovasc Surg. 2002;124(3):486–92. Epub 2002/08/31.
58. Shafiei S, Bagheri R, Sadri K, Jafarian AH, Attaran D, Mohammadzadeh Lari S, et al. Sentinel node mapping for intra-thoracic malignancies: systematic review of the best available evidence. Rev Clin Med. 2015;2(2):52–7.
59. Kim S, Kim HK, Kang DY, Jeong JM, Choi YH. Intraoperative sentinel lymph node identification using a novel receptor-binding agent (technetium-99m neomannosyl human serum albumin, 99mTc-MSA) in stage I non-small cell lung cancer. Eur J Cardiothorac Surg. 2010;37(6):1450–6. Epub 2010/04/01.
60. Abele JT, Allred K, Clare T, Bedard EL. Lymphoscintigraphy in early-stage non-small cell lung cancer with technetium-99m nanocolloids and hybrid SPECT/CT: a pilot project. Ann Nucl Med. 2014;28(5):477–83. Epub 2014/02/22.
61. Nomori H, Ikeda K, Mori T, Shiraishi S, Kobayashi H, Iwatani K, et al. Sentinel node identification in clinical stage Ia non-small cell lung cancer by a combined single photon emission computed tomography/computed tomography system. J Thorac Cardiovasc Surg. 2007;134(1):182–7. Epub 2007/06/30.
62. Teknos D, Ramcharan A, Oluwole SF. Pulmonary edema associated with methylene blue dye

administration during sentinel lymph node biopsy. J Natl Med Assoc. 2008;100(12):1483–4. Epub 2008/12/30.

63. Jangjoo A, Forghani MN, Mehrabibahar M, Sadeghi R. Anaphylaxis reaction of a breast cancer patient to methylene blue during breast surgery with sentinel node mapping. Acta Oncol. 2010;49(6):877–8. Epub 2010/05/01.

64. Minamiya Y, Ito M, Katayose Y, Katayose Y, Saito H, Imai K, Sato Y, Ogawa JI, et al. Intraoperative sentinel lymph node mapping using a new sterilizable magnetometer in patients with nonsmall cell lung cancer. Ann Thorac Surg. 2006;81(1):327–30.

65. Yamashita S, Tokuishi K, Miyawaki M, Anami K, Moroga T, Takeno S, et al. Sentinel node navigation surgery by thoracoscopic fluorescence imaging system and molecular examination in non-small cell lung cancer. Ann Surg Oncol. 2012;19(3):728–33. Epub 2011/11/22.

Radioguided Surgery of Small Pulmonary Nodules

21

Amelia W. Maiga and Eric L. Grogan

Contents

Dr. Maiga is supported by the Office of Academic Affiliations, Department of Veterans Affairs (VA) National Quality Scholars Program. Dr. Grogan is a recipient of the Department of Veterans Affairs, Veterans Health Administration, Health Services Research and Development Service Career Development Award (10-024). The views expressed in this chapter are those of the authors and do not necessarily represent the views of the Department of Veterans Affairs.

A.W. Maiga, MD, MPH
Department of Surgery, Vanderbilt University Medical Center, Nashville, TN, USA

Department of Surgery, Veterans Affairs Tennessee Valley Healthcare System, Nashville, TN, USA

E.L. Grogan, MD, MPH, FACS (✉)
Department of Thoracic Surgery, Veterans Affairs Tennessee Valley Healthcare System, Nashville, TN, USA

Department of Thoracic Surgery, Vanderbilt University Medical Center, 609 Oxford House, 1313 21st Ave. South, Nashville, TN 37232, USA
e-mail: eric.grogan@vanderbilt.edu

Abstract

The incidence of pulmonary nodules discovered by imaging is increasing. These pulmonary nodules may be discovered incidentally or through a computed tomography (CT) scan screening program. Small lesions suspicious for lung cancer may require tissue, and surgical resection may be necessary to rule out malignancy. Due to the small size of these lesions, intraoperative localization with minimally invasive surgical techniques may be challenging and require lesion localization prior to resection. Radioguided surgery using a radiotracer and a handheld gamma probe technology facilitates real-time pulmonary

K. Herrmann et al. (eds.), *Radioguided Surgery: Current Applications and Innovative Directions in Clinical Practice*, DOI 10.1007/978-3-319-26051-8_21

nodule localization and surgical resection. Most commonly, this involves two steps. First, a radiotracer (usually injectable technetium-99m) is preoperatively and percutaneously delivered into or immediately deep to the pulmonary nodule under CT guidance. Second, a handheld gamma probe is used to localize the pulmonary nodule for thoracoscopic resection. Alternatively, a radiotracer can be given intravenously, such as radiolabeled monoclonal antibodies, ^{18}F-fluorodeoxyglucose (FDG), bleomycin derivatives, or DOTATATE (i.e., a highly selective somatostatin analog). These other techniques remain experimental. Radioguidance with transthoracic technetium-99m injection and intraoperative gamma probe detection offers several advantages over CT-guided hookwires or markers, locally administered radiopaque contrast and blue dyes, and thoracoscopic ultrasound. These techniques may be employed alone or in combination with radioguidance. Precise localization of small pulmonary nodules will become more pressing as national lung cancer CT screening guidelines are implemented.

21.1 Background

In 2011, the National Lung Screening Trial (NLST) reported a 20 % reduction in lung cancer-specific mortality with low-dose chest CT screening in a population at high risk, namely, older male smokers [1]. In December 2013, the US Preventive Service Task Force (USPSTF) began recommending annual screening for lung cancer with low-dose CT scans in adults aged 55–80 years with a recent 30 pack-year smoking history [2]. In light of these recommendations and the eight million Americans at risk, more than three million lung abnormalities are projected to be identified in the first three years of a national CT screening program [3]. This will create an unprecedented number of pulmonary nodules to manage appropriately.

Whereas some pulmonary nodules can be sampled noninvasively, most commonly with bronchoscopy or CT-guided fine needle aspiration (FNA), surgical biopsy of such pulmonary nodules is often necessary for definitive diagnosis, to be followed by an immediate or staged formal resection in the event malignancy is confirmed. The success rates of nonoperative diagnostic modalities are inversely related to pulmonary nodule size, resulting in unacceptably high false-negative rates [4, 5]. In particular, subcentimeter pulmonary nodules cannot be reliably biopsied percutaneously [6, 7]. Positron emission tomography (PET) also has low sensitivity in screening for subcentimeter lesions, particularly those 7 mm or smaller [8, 9]. For this reason, both the American College of Chest Physicians (ACCP) and the American Association of Thoracic Surgery (AATS) recommend obtaining a tissue diagnosis via surgical excision of subcentimeter pulmonary nodules with suspicious changes in size and appearance [10, 11].

21.1.1 Need for Surgical Localization Adjuncts for Small Pulmonary Nodules

Unfortunately, small indeterminate pulmonary nodules identified on high-resolution CT images as candidates for excisional biopsy can be challenging to identify thoracoscopically via the traditional combination of direct visualization, instrument palpation, and digital palpation [12]. This is particularly true with pulmonary nodules located deep in the lung parenchyma and with so-called ground glass pulmonary nodules that are less solid to the touch and difficult to palpate thoracoscopically. Preoperative marking for subcentimeter pulmonary nodules has been recommended to facilitate a successful minimally invasive approach [13]. Various perioperative adjuncts have been developed to facilitate video-assisted thoracoscopic surgery (VATS) excision of small pulmonary nodules and thereby avoid the morbidity of a thoracotomy. These include radioguided surgery and its alternatives, which will be reviewed below.

21.2 Radioguided Surgery: Percutaneous Delivery Techniques

A radioguided surgical approach to pulmonary nodules involves either percutaneous transthoracic or intravenous delivery of a radiotracer, followed by intraoperative gamma detection, typically with a handheld gamma probe. Percutaneous transthoracic delivery of the radiotracer is by far the most common, typically relying on CT guidance for precise placement of the radiotracer into or deep to the pulmonary nodule of interest. Advantages of this approach include better differential uptake of the radiotracer in the relevant area and the resultant superior spatial resolution and selectivity. Disadvantages include those inherent to introducing a needle into the pleural space and lung parenchyma, namely, pneumothorax, hemothorax, and parenchymal bleeding, as well as the additional time and coordination of services needed between radiology, surgery, and operating room staff. Bronchoscopic delivery of a radiotracer, still experimental and highly specialized with a steep learning curve, may avoid some of the disadvantages of the percutaneous transthoracic route while maintaining the advantages of a localized approach.

21.2.1 Percutaneous Transthoracic Injection of Technetium-99m

Most of the published experience with CT-guided injection of a radiotracer for pulmonary nodule localization and excisional biopsy has relied on technetium-99m (Tc-99m), a commonly used medical radioisotope. This approach dates back to 2000, when Chella et al. first described CT-guided percutaneous transthoracic injection of Tc-99m-labeled human serum microspheres into or near a target pulmonary nodule to guide subsequent thoracoscopic excisional biopsy [14]. They successfully localized and excised pulmonary nodules with a mean size of 8.3 mm in 39 of 39 patients, with surgery performed 2 h after intralesional injection. The specific radiotracer they used is unavailable in the United States (US). A variety of radiotracers have subsequently been used for this indication. Burdine et al. used Tc-99m sulfur colloid, the standard tracer in melanoma and breast cancer sentinel lymph node dissections, for a similar radiotracer localization technique in 17 patients [15]. Although they successfully resected all lesions, one caveat they identified was the radiotracer's rapid diffusion away from the pulmonary nodule. Sugi et al. used Tc-99m tin colloid and Tc-99m phytate in Japan and also reported good success with locating and resecting 25 pulmonary nodules averaging 13.8 mm in size [16]. Neither of these radiolabeled Tc-99m compounds is available in the US, however, and both require special handling due to radioactivity.

The radiotracer now most commonly employed for pulmonary nodule radioguided surgery in the US is Tc-99m macroaggregated albumin (MAA). This radiotracer was first developed for this purpose by a group at the University of Virginia [17]. Daniel et al. tested a variety of Tc-99m solutions in an animal model, including Tc-99m sulfur colloid, Tc-99m MAA, and Tc-99m pertechnetate (TcO4). They determined that Tc-99m MAA provided the most precise and sustained localization, up to 8 h, likely due to its larger particle size, thus preventing diffusion away from the pulmonary nodule through the lung parenchyma. They then successfully piloted the Tc-99m MAA radiotracer injection in lesions in 13 of 13 humans with thoracoscopic biopsy [12, 17, 18].

On the basis of this work, in 2008, the same group at the University of Virginia published their results of the successful identification and excision of 77 of 81 indeterminate pulmonary nodules (95 %), with 71 of the 77 (92 %) removed thoracoscopically [19]. The mean size of the pulmonary nodules was 9.8 mm. Under CT guidance on the day of surgery, these 81 pulmonary nodules were injected with 0.1 mL Tc-99m MAA (approximately 0.3 mCi) just deep to the lesion to ensure adequate incorporation of the lesion. The corresponding pulmonary nodule was then identified and confirmed as frequently as needed intraoperatively using a special angled gamma detection probe. Of note, the four patients in whom the lesion was not identified and successfully excised had accidental spillage of the radiotracer, either into the pleural space or the soft tissues of the chest wall. This occurred early in the series. The team subsequently modified their protocol to include an immediate preoperative scintigraphy, in order to confirm an intraparenchymal location of the injected radiotracer for the remaining patients, and with 100 % success with localization and excision thereafter (77 of 77). This additional step adds 10–15 min to the procedure. An unknown number of patients required a second CT-guided radiotracer injection based on the findings of preoperative scintigraphy.

The radiotracer injection itself was performed under conscious sedation and was well tolerated. A total 8 of 81 patients (10 %) developed pneumothoraces requiring pigtail catheter placement into the intrathoracic pleural space in the radiology suite. This is comparable to the 6 patients with asymptomatic pneumothoraces of the 39 (15 %) in the original series by Chella et al. [14]. Most patients underwent surgery the same day as radiotracer injection, but the team also successfully performed excision the following morning with an increased radiotracer dose (0.3–0.4 mL of Tc-99m MAA rather than the standard 0.1 mL). This in vivo radiotracer longevity facilitates practical incorporation of this technology given the often unpredictable nature of surgical schedules and operating room case start times. This technique is described in detail below. The University of Virginia provides some additional educational information at the following website: http://www.med-ed.virginia.edu/courses/rad/rsnanucs/.

21.2.2 Technique in Detail

21.2.2.1 CT-Guided Radiotracer Injection

On the morning of or day prior to the operation, the patient undergoes placement of the radiotracer as follows (Fig. 21.1). Conscious sedation is administered. A limited CT scan confirms the nodule's position. The surgeon and interventional radiologist agree on the optimal approach angle, avoiding the pleural surface of major fissures. Local anesthesia is administered. The radiologist positions a 20-gauge coaxial needle along the intended track with the tip ending just proximal to the pleural cavity. Under CT fluoroscopy, a 22-gauge needle is then advanced through this needle into or just deep to the pulmonary nodule. Between 0.1 and 0.3 mL (~0.3–0.9 mCi) of Tc-99m MAA is injected. An immediate post-procedural scintigram confirms intraparenchymal location of radiotracer. If unsuccessful, the procedure is repeated as needed.

21.2.2.2 Radioguided VATS Surgery

Later that day or the following morning, the patient is brought to the operating room (Fig. 21.2). General anesthesia with single-lung ventilation is induced. The patient is placed in the left lateral decubitus position and prepped and draped in the standard fashion. A sterile handheld angled gamma detection probe is used to identify the area of maximum signal on the external chest wall. Three standard VATS incisions are made, one 5-mm port for the thoracoscopic grasper and two 10-mm ports for the thoracoscope and the gamma detection probe alternating with the endostapler, respectively. Inside the chest cavity, the gamma detection probe is again used to identify the site of maximum counts per second signal on the surface of the lung parenchyma.

The area of interest is grasped and elevated with an endoscopic grasper. The lung parenchyma is scanned with the angled probe to confirm the signal from multiple angles and to determine the depth of the lesion. The lesion is then wedged out with one or more fires of an endostapler, taking care to incorporate the entire lesion distal to the staple line. The specimen is removed in an Endobag. After excision, the specimen is probed ex vivo with the gamma detection probe to confirm the presence of radiotracer activity within the excised specimen and then opened on the operative field and/or sent directly to pathology for frozen sectioning. The gamma detection probe is then reintroduced into the thoracic cavity to scan the adjacent lung parenchyma and ensure removal of all areas of radiotracer

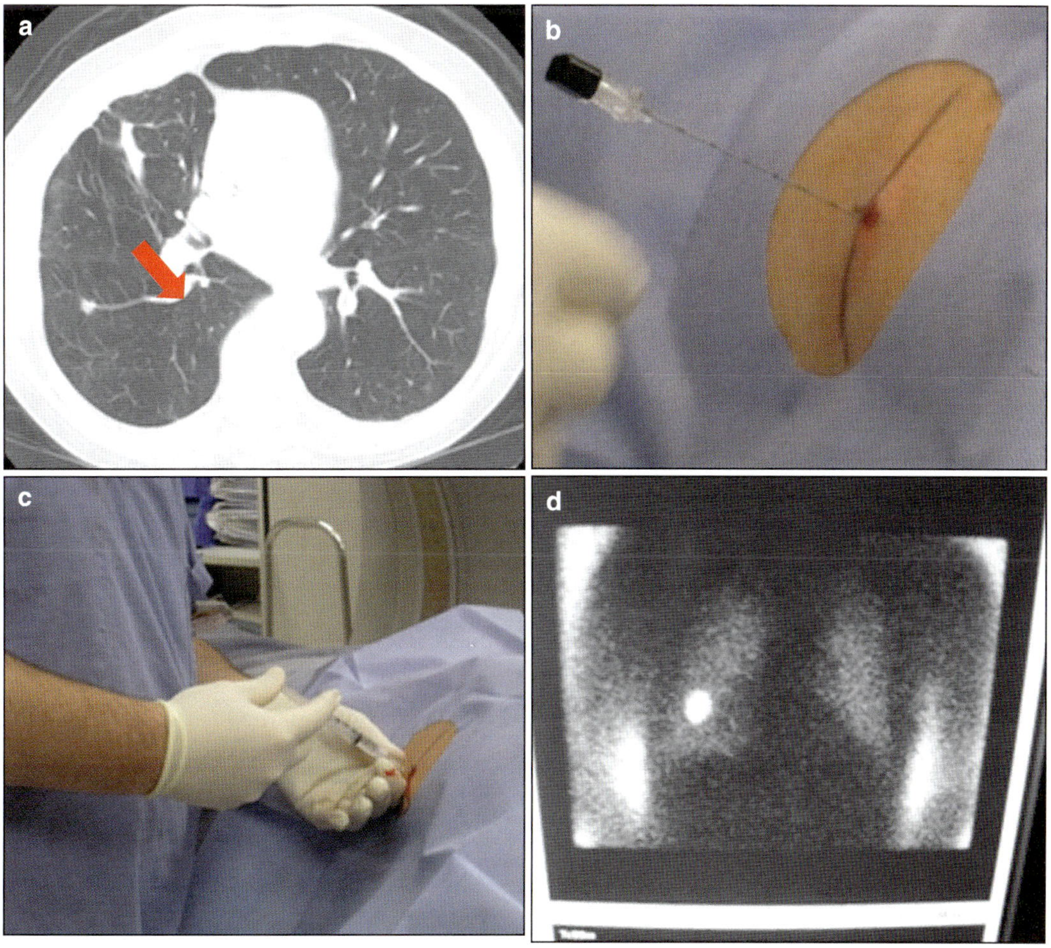

Fig. 21.1 CT-guided injection of Tc-99m. (**a**) A 77-year-old smoker was referred to the thoracic surgery service with a 0.7×0.9 cm right lower lobe nodule, greater than 2 cm from the pleura. The pulmonary nodule was noted incidentally 6 months prior and had increased in size from 0.5×0.6 cm at that time. His preoperative FEV1 was 49 %. (**b**) Under CT guidance, the interventional radiologist positions the needle with the tip just deep to the pulmonary nodule. (**c**) The radiologist injects 0.1–0.3 mL of technetium-99m-labeled albumin at the site of interest. (**d**) Post-procedural scintigram confirms precise intraparenchymal radiotracer uptake

activity. As needed, additional lung parenchyma is removed and the process repeated. Based on frozen section results, a formal lung resection may or may not be required.

21.2.3 Co-localization with Radiotracer and Another Modality

A number of researchers have also combined Tc-99m radiotracer localization with other common localization adjuncts, including radiopaque contrast injection, hookwire placement, and methylene blue injection. Radiopaque contrast media has been the most common adjunct reported in the literature [20–22]. For example, Bellomi et al. used Tc-99m MAA mixed with nonionic iodinated contrast medium to successfully localize and resect 47 indeterminate pulmonary nodules (mean 11 mm size and 11 mm depth) in 44 patients [20]. A post-procedural CT scan was performed to define the distribution of the contrast media and rule out an iatrogenic pneumothorax, followed by a confirmatory scintigram and then surgery within 24 h, typically on

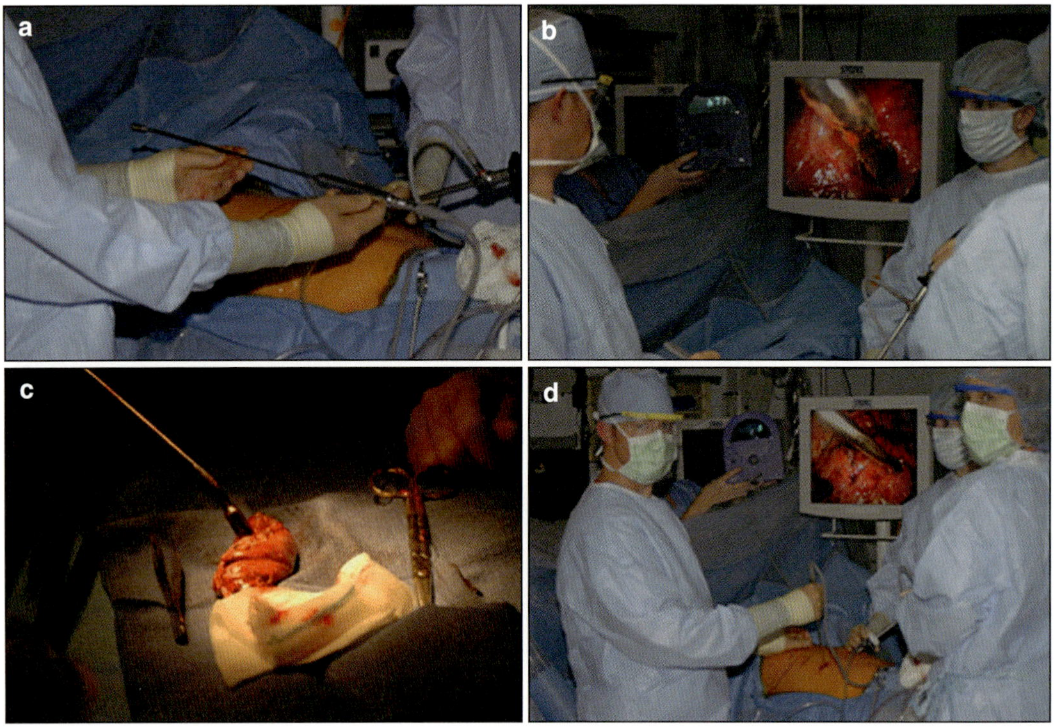

Fig. 21.2 Localization of lung nodule using gamma probe during VATS excisional biopsy. (**a**) A sterile gamma radioprobe is introduced into one of the thoracoscopic port sites. (**b**) The lung parenchyma is scanned with the radioprobe to identify the area of maximum radioactive signal, rotating to confirm the depth of the pulmonary nodule. Note the Navigator™ displaying the radioactivity counts per second. (**c**) After wedge excision, the lesion is examined ex vivo with the gamma detection probe to confirm focal radioactivity. (**d**) The staple line and adjacent lung parenchyma are scanned to ensure there is no significant residual radioactivity

the following day. Thirteen patients (30 %) had asymptomatic pneumothoraces on CT imaging, none requiring drainage. Similarly, Bertolaccini et al. used Tc-99m MAA diluted with iodized contrast medium in a prospective series of 19 patients with pulmonary nodules <15 mm located 20–40 mm from the pleural surface and also reported good success with minimal complications [21]. In the largest series, Ambrogi et al., a group from Italy, reported success in 208 of 211 cases (99 %), again with the Tc-99m MAA/contrast co-localization method [22]. A total of 10.4 % developed pneumothoraces, none requiring drainage.

Local injection of simple blue dyes, typically methylene blue, is a long-standing localization adjunct for small pulmonary nodules. Wang et al. reported using both Tc-99m sulfur colloid and methylene blue to locate and resect pulmonary nodules in a small case series of three patients [23]. They deposited both the Tc-99m and blue dye in two locations, one in the subcutaneous fat in line with the target and then within or just deep to the lesion, hypothesizing that this would better highlight the "linear projecting tract" for intraoperative localization and ex vivo confirmation.

The hookwire localization technique is described in the "Alternatives to Radioguidance" section later in this chapter. One group has reported a dual-localization technique using both a percutaneous transthoracic hookwire and Tc 99m phytate for 36 pulmonary nodules in 34 patients [24]. Of note, 7 hookwires (19 %) dislodged prior to surgery, although these pulmonary nodules were all successfully excised secondary to detection of the radiotracer.

21.2.4 Iodine-125 (I-125) Seeds

Whereas Tc-99m is the most commonly used radiotracer, iodine-125 (I-125) seeds have been employed in radioguided surgery for pulmonary nodules in a limited fashion. In 2013, Gobardhan et al. from the Netherlands reported using CT-guided percutaneous transthoracic placement of I-125 seeds, one per pulmonary nodule, for 28 patients with suspicious pulmonary nodules, followed by VATS wedge resection guided by a handheld gamma probe [25]. Downsides of this technique include the possibility for I-125 seed dislodgement with subpleural placement (occurring in 5 of 28 patients in this study), the need to ensure removal of the radioactive seeds in accordance with local and national guidelines, and the increased risk of hematoma and pneumothorax given the larger 18-gauge needle that is required to implant I-125 seeds. There have been no subsequent reports in the literature of using I-125 seed placement in pulmonary nodule surgery. However, in contrast to using the I-125 seed localization approach for radioguided surgery for pulmonary nodules, the I-125 seed localization approach is much more commonplace for radioguided surgery for non-palpable breast lesions (see Chap. 8).

21.3 Radioguided Surgery: Intravenous Delivery Techniques

The intravenous administration of a radiotracer to guide resection of pulmonary nodules remains experimental. Nevertheless, the attraction of the intravenous route is clear. Intravenous injection avoids the innate morbidity and mortality of any percutaneous transthoracic procedure and obviates the need to coordinate services between radiology and surgery during the perioperative time frame [26]. The primary challenge remains ensuring adequate radiotracer uptake at the site of interest to allow for sufficient contrast to that of the background lung parenchyma.

21.3.1 Radioimmunoguided Surgery

Limited work has been published on the application of radioimmunoguided surgery (RIGS) to the identification and resection of pulmonary nodules [27–29]. In 1998, Grazia et al. described intravenously injecting 10 patients with I-125-labeled monoclonal antibodies at an average of 20 days prior to surgery and then employed a handheld gamma probe for intraoperative detection [27]. Despite the higher background radioactivity in the thorax, specific binding (i.e., RIGS positivity) to histologically confirmed sites of adenocarcinoma in the lung parenchyma was confirmed in 9 of 10 cases, with the one RIGS-negative lesion demonstrating benign histology. Another Italian group reported less promising results with monoclonal antibodies (MAb) radiolabeled with either I-125 or Tc-99m, with binding occurring in a minority of primary non-small cell lung cancers, and no in situ selective localization of I-125- or Tc-99m-tagged MAb within the area of the primary lung tumor cells during RIGS but in situ selective localization of Tc-99m-MAb to a small lymph node metastasis previously unidentified on preoperative imaging [28]. Resected neoplastic tissue had an ex vivo 2:1 tumor to background ratio, but this differential was not sufficient for in vivo identification. In 2000, Wang et al. reported on a pilot animal study of a RIGS technique using biotinylated monoclonal antibodies in mice to identify adenocarcinoma lung micrometastases, with a reported sensitivity, specificity, and accuracy of 96 %, 98 %, and 97 %, respectively [29]. However, this technique reported by Wang et al. has not been subsequently replicated in humans. Therefore, overall, RIGS appears to potentially be most relevant to pulmonary nodules suspected to be adenocarcinoma, but for which further clinical research would be necessary for more conclusive validation.

21.3.2 ^{18}F-FDG-Guided Surgery

When administered intravenously, ^{18}F-fluorodeoxyglucose (^{18}F-FDG) accumulates within pulmonary nodules and thoracic lymph nodes harboring metastatic cancer, lighting up as hypermetabolic lesions on positron emission tomography (PET) imaging [30]. Gamma radiation should also be detectable intraoperatively with a handheld gamma probe, facilitating the identification and localization of any sites of cancer. Nwogu et al. describe using intravenous injection of ^{18}F-FDG in a series of 10 patients on the day of surgery to guide resection, specifically of intrathoracic lymph nodes with suspected micrometastases [31]. All resected primary tumor sites and true-positive lymph nodes were ^{18}F-FDG avid when measured ex vivo, but in vivo avidity was less reliable due to cardiac background activity, despite appropriate shielding. Moffatt-Bruce et al. also published a single case report of using radioguided localization of ^{18}F-FDG-avid tissue after an intravenous injection of ^{18}F-FDG approximately 98 min prior to surgery [32]. Notably, they relied on a triad of preoperative patient PET/CT, specimen PET/CT, and postoperative patient PET/CT, as well as intraoperative gamma probe detection. This technology is likely most applicable to lymph node "ultrastaging" rather than to the localization and resection of suspicious pulmonary nodules or primary lung cancers themselves.

21.3.3 Bleomycin Derivatives

Bleomycin is a chemotherapeutic agent produced by the *Streptomyces* bacterium as an antiviral drug. It is known to localize to the lung and when given in high doses for systemic chemotherapy can thus cause pulmonary fibrosis. The first use of a gamma detection probe in lung cancer actually relied on cobalt-57 (^{57}Co) bleomycin as a localization compound. In 1984, Woolfenden et al. reported intravenously injecting 34 patients with bleomycin and then used a sodium iodine crystal attached to the tip of a bronchoscope to attempt to detect and localize tumors [33]. Although these results were intriguing, the long physical half-life of the ^{57}Co radionuclide (i.e., 271.8 days) renders it impractical for radioguided surgery.

Although the same lines, in 2003 a Chinese group described administering an intravenous injection of peplomycin, a bleomycin derivative, linked to Tc-99m as a "tumor tracer" to not only identify pulmonary nodules in 37 patients but also to differentiate malignant versus benign lesions intraoperatively as based upon the tumor radioactivity relative to normal lung parenchyma as calculated by a handheld gamma detection probe [34]. They reported a sensitivity, specificity, and accuracy of 90 %, 88 %, and 89 %, respectively. This work remains experimental.

21.3.4 DOTATATE

Somatostatin receptor scintigraphy is a proven means to visualize many malignancies, including lung cancer [35]. Investigators have demonstrated the utility of scintigraphy with older somatostatin analogs, such as depreotide, in localizing lung neoplasms, other neoplasms, and inflammatory nodules such as active granulomas [36–40]. The somatostatin analog, 4,7,10-tricarboxymethyl-1,4,7,10-tetraaza-cyclododecan-1-yl-acetyl-D-Phe-Cys-Tyr-D-Trp-Lys-Thr-Cys-Thr-OH (DOTATATE), is a highly selective SSTR2 agonist with greater affinity for SSTR2 than older somatostatin analogs [41]. Some data support DOTATATE PET/CT in the routine diagnosis of suspected neuroendocrine tumors [42]. In particular, bronchial carcinoids have been shown to have avid, selective uptake of DOTATATE over that of ^{18}F-FDG [43].

Early experimental data suggest that DOTATATE, when labeled with indium-111 (^{111}In), could serve to localize small pulmonary nodules not only for imaging but also for intraoperative detection with a handheld gamma probe and wedge resection. The low normal background uptake of DOTATATE in the lung parenchyma should facilitate localization of lung lesions with an adequate lesion/background ratio. Furthermore, the 2.8-day ^{111}In physical half-life would also allow intravenous administration 1–2 days prior to surgery. Our research team has begun preliminary research into this area.

Ongoing challenges include determining the optimal injected activity of ^{111}In-DOTATATE and the optimal time interval between intravenous injection and lesion resection in order to maximize the signal to noise ratio for pulmonary nodule detection. Furthermore, improved gamma detection probe performance or shielding is needed to reduce background noise and enhance lesion localization.

21.4 Alternatives to Radioguidance

In addition to the radioguidance techniques summarized in this chapter, multiple other localization adjuncts are available and have been described in the literature. These will be reviewed briefly in this section of this chapter. A comparison chart of localization techniques for surgical resection of pulmonary nodules is provided in Table 21.1. After a comprehensive review, the British Thoracic Society concluded in their 2015 guidelines for the investigation and management of pulmonary nodules that surgeons should "use localisation techniques depending on local availability and expertise to facilitate limited resection of pulmonary nodules" [44].

21.4.1 CT-Guided Hookwire

The use of CT-guided percutaneous transthoracic placement of hookwires to guide intraoperative identification and resection of small indeterminate pulmonary nodules has been described by a number of authors and has perhaps been the most commonly used preoperative marking strategy [45–52]. It is greater than 85 % effective but carries a risk of pneumothorax ranging from 3 to 50 %, depending on the series, as well as a risk of pulmonary hemorrhage upward of 30 %. The main technical disadvantage of this approach is the tendency of the hookwire tip to dislodge from its target over time. To address this problem, Partik and others have more recently described using a helical tip wire specially designed to hold lung parenchyma [53, 54]. However, any wire may cross a fissure in transit to the pulmonary nodule, and intraoperatively it can be difficult to track down from the external wire to the lesion unless the thoracoscope is in the exact plane as the wire.

Comparative studies are limited. Gonfiotti et al. conducted a small prospective, randomized trial comparing the hookwire technique and radioguided surgery with Tc-99m human albumin microspheres [55]. Fifty patients were divided into two groups well matched for size (mean 1.1 cm) and depth (2.5 cm) of pulmonary lung nodules. Pulmonary nodule localization was 84 % successful (21 of 25) in the hookwire group compared to 96 % (24 of 25) in the radioguided group.

21.4.2 CT-Guided Coil or Marker Placement

Alternatively, Powell and others have described using platinum microcoil markers for pulmonary nodule localization [56–58]. This technique is similar to hookwire implantation, but no external wire is left in place. Rather than following the wire down to the pulmonary nodule, surgeons rely on intraoperative fluoroscopy to visualize the implanted marker, adding to operating room time and introducing awkwardness given the lateral decubitus positioning of the patient. Other caveats exist. In one study, the coil was displaced in one of the 12 patients due to atelectasis [56]. Moon et al. used a similar technique of CT-guided microcoil placement with fluoroscopic-guided VATS resection for 32 pulmonary nodules in 30 patients, with 2 cases of intrathoracic displacement of the coils [58].

Koyama et al. have also described their experience with a 5-mm point marker with an attached 30-cm-long nylon suture and introducer system, with low morbidity and good success [59]. In theory, this suture obviates the need for fluoroscopy while avoiding some disadvantages of the classic hookwire technique. All CT-guided localization procedures employing hooks and wires carry a risk of pneumothorax, as well as a rare but catastrophic risk of air embolism [47, 60].

Table 21.1 Case series reporting localization techniques for surgical resection of pulmonary nodules

Authors/ Reference	Localization technique	Patient population	Efficacy	Complications
Dendo et al. [49]	CT-guided hookwire	150 Patients undergoing VATS resection of 168 nodules	97.6 % hookwire placed successfully	32.1 % pneumothorax (chest tube in 1.2 %) 14.9 % pulmonary hemorrhage
Ciriaco et al. [50]	CT-guided hookwire	53 patients undergoing VATS nodule resection	92.5 % hookwire remained in situ facilitating VATS in 58 %	7.5 % pneumothorax
Saito et al. [46]	CT-guided hookwire	61 patients undergoing VATS nodule resection	85 % hookwire facilitated VATS	None reported
Miyoshi et al. [51]	CT-guided hookwire	108 patients undergoing VATS nodule resection	93.6 % successful resection 4 % nodule not in resection specimen, 2.4 % hookwire left in situ	3.7 % of patients, chest drain for pneumothorax
Yoshida et al. [52]	CT-guided hookwire	57 patients undergoing VATS nodule resection	One hookwire dislodged by time of surgery. Successful surgery for all cases	49.1 % pneumothorax (no chest drain) 29.8 % pulmonary hemorrhage 7 % pain
Koyama et al. [59]	CT-guided point marker system	52 patients undergoing VATS nodule resection	Successful placement in 98 % cases (one dislodged) and resection	19 % asymptomatic pneumothorax 10 % pulmonary hemorrhage
Mayo et al. [57]	CT-guided microcoil wire	69 patients undergoing VATS resection of 75 nodules	Successful placement in all cases but dislodged in 3 %. 97 % of nodules removed	3 % pneumothorax requiring drain 1 % asymptomatic hemothorax
Watanabe et al. [64]	Lipiodol marking	150 patients undergoing VATS nodule resection	All nodules successfully resected	11 % pain requiring analgesia 17 % pneumothorax (6 % drain) 0.6 % hemopneumothorax (emergency operation)
Kawanaka et al. [84]	Lipiodol marking	65 patients undergoing VATS resection of 107 nodules	All nodules successfully marked and resected	31 % pneumothorax (5 % drain) 15 % pulmonary hemorrhage
Kim et al. [63]	Lipiodol marking	67 patients undergoing VATS resection of 68 nodules	Marking successful in 98 %	29 % pneumothorax 7 % pulmonary hemorrhage
Vandoni et al. [67]	Methylene blue marking	51 patients undergoing VATS resection of 54 nodules	Successful thoracoscopic resection in 91 % of patients	25.4 % pneumothorax (no drain)

Table 21.1 (continued)

Authors/ Reference	Localization technique	Patient population	Efficacy	Complications
Grogan et al. [19]	Radiotracer injection	81 patients undergoing VATS nodule resection	Successful localization and excision in 95.1 % of cases	10 % pneumothorax with drain
Ambrogi et al. [22]	Radiotracer injection	211 patients undergoing VATS nodule resection	Successful localization and resection in 99 % of cases	10.4 % pneumothorax no drain
Mattioli et al. [75]	Transthoracic ultrasound	54 patients undergoing VATS resection of 65 nodules	Successful identification of 15/16 non-visible or palpable nodules (94 %)	None
Gonfiotti et al. [55]	Hookwire vs. radiotracer	50 patients randomized to each procedure for VATS resection	Successful localization: 84 % hookwire 96 % for radiotracer (not significant)	24 % pneumothorax no drain hookwire 4 % pneumothorax radiotracer 4 % ($n = 1$) hookwire displacement

Reproduced with permission from Callister et al. [44]
VATS video-assisted thoracoscopic surgery

21.4.3 Radiopaque Dyes

After hookwires, the next most commonly employed technique is CT-guided injection of a radiopaque marker such as lipiodol, an iodized oil, or barium sulfate, followed by intraoperative fluoroscopy for real-time detection [61–63]. Watanabe et al. reported their experience with CT-guided lipiodol injection followed by intraoperative fluoroscopic detection in 174 patients, reporting 100 % success but complications including a 17 % incidence of pneumothorax, with 11 patients requiring drainage and one patient requiring an emergent operation for hemopneumothorax [64]. This technique does allow for a delay of a day or more between injection and surgery. Additional theoretical risk is systemic embolization of the contrast media. Interestingly, Okumura et al. describes bronchoscopic rather than CT-guided injection of the barium marker [65]. While innovative, it requires sophisticated bronchoscopic skill available at few institutions. Ultimately, the need for intraoperative fluoroscopy limits the utility and appeal of all of these techniques.

21.4.4 Methylene Blue

The oldest marking technique relies on the simple injection of methylene blue in the vicinity of the pulmonary nodule, enhancing its intraoperative visibility [66–68]. For example, Vandoni et al. describe successful resection in 91 % of 51 patients undergoing VATS resection of 54 pulmonary nodules, with a 25 % pneumothorax rate [67]. Recent data suggest that this approach is safe and feasible in children as well [68]. However, simple dye injection is less successful with pulmonary nodules located deep in the lung parenchyma, and the blue dye does diffuse away from the injection site over time.

Methylene blue can also be delivered via bronchoscopy. Navigational bronchoscopy has recently been developed as a method for transbronchial biopsy or, alternatively, the delivery of fiducial markers, to facilitate either pulmonary nodule resection or radiation [69, 70]. Bolton et al. describe using intraoperative navigational bronchoscopy in a series of 19 patients to locate the lesion, obtain one or two transbronchial needle biopsy specimens, and then inject methylene blue dye as a local marker to guide immediate surgical excision [71]. If the biopsy specimens returned as positive for malignancy, a formal lobectomy and lymph node dissection was performed. If the biopsy was negative or inconclusive, a robotic-assisted wedge resection was performed, using the parenchyma dyed blue to guide the resection.

In cases where CT-guided percutaneous marking or injection is not feasible or is high risk, simple noninvasive use of dyes can provide some benefit. For example, Okuda et al. describe using crystal violet to intraoperatively mark the visceral pleura adjacent to the pulmonary nodule using the preoperative CT scan as a guide [72].

21.4.5 Ultrasound

Intraoperative thoracoscopic ultrasonography is another adjunct to pulmonary nodule localization that can be employed as needed across the entire pleural surface. A few authors have reported successful identification of small, firm pulmonary nodules with this technique [73–77]. Sortini et al. reported a small nonrandomized study comparing intrathoracoscopic ultrasound to radioguided occult lesion localization with Tc-99m human serum albumin microspheres, demonstrating 96 % success with ultrasound (24 of 25) and 80 % success with radioguidance (20 of 25) [78, 79]. However, thoracoscopic ultrasonography has a steep learning curve and relies on complete atelectasis, as visualization is limited by intraparenchymal air causing reverberating artifacts.

21.4.6 Experimental Techniques

Several experimental pulmonary nodule localization techniques have been described in the literature, including local injection of acrylates, bronchoscopic delivery of radiofrequency identification (RFID) tags, and the use of near-infrared (NIR) technology.

21.4.6.1 Acrylates

Yoshida et al. have described CT-guided injection of a cyanoacrylate agent to aid in both intraoperative visualization and palpation [80]. Although effective, the hardness of the polymer interferes with pathologic sectioning, and there is a risk of systemic embolization, rendering the technique less useful.

21.4.6.2 RFID Tags

A Japanese group has recently described a canine model of employing radiofrequency identification (RFID) technology as a wireless marker for subcentimeter pulmonary nodules [81]. The 1-mm RFID tags are delivered bronchoscopically, and the detection system is accurate down to the millimeter for pinpoint pulmonary nodule localization. Although the RFID tags have been approved for use in humans, this proof-of-concept study remains to be replicated in humans. More work also needs to be done to improve the current effective communication range of 7 mm between the RFID tag and the detector probe (which powers the RFID tag remotely to permit detection).

21.4.6.3 NIR Technology

Okusanya et al. have described administering systemic indocyanine green and using near-infrared technology to successfully identify and resect pulmonary nodules 24 h later in 14 of the 18 (78 %) patients [82]. Of note, all patients had intentional thoracotomies to correlate finger palpation with the NIR findings. Five additional pulmonary nodules were identified by NIR that were not visualized on preoperative CT scans, and these were also resected. This technique remains experimental.

21.5 Summary

Radioguided surgery of small pulmonary nodules provides critical real-time guidance to surgeons regarding pulmonary nodule identification and adequacy of surgical resection margins. This is typically accomplished via the CT-guided transthoracic injection of Tc-99m MAA and intraoperative detection with a handheld gamma probe. A variety of other percutaneous transthoracic and intravenous delivery techniques have been described, many of which remain experimental. Management of subcentimeter pulmonary nodules is a critical and timely topic, especially given the encouraging results of the NLST and the USPSTF's recommendations to adopt annual screening chest CT scans for high-risk individuals.

Radiotracer-guided thoracoscopic surgery for small pulmonary nodules has been shown to be more cost-effective than thoracotomy for the management of indeterminate subcentimeter pulmonary nodules [83]. It also avoids the higher morbidity and mortality of diagnostic thoracotomy. A variety of localization alternatives to radioguidance exist, including hookwires and markers, simple and radiopaque dyes, thoracoscopic ultrasound, and more experimental techniques like bronchoscopic delivery of RFID tags and near-infrared technology. Regardless of other techniques in use and in development, radioguided surgery is likely to play an increasingly important role in the management of indeterminate pulmonary nodules.

References

1. TNLSTR Team. Reduced lung-cancer mortality with Low-dose computed tomographic screening. N Engl J Med. 2011;365(5):395–409.
2. Force USPST. Lung Cancer: Screening 2013 [7/17/2015]. Available from: http://www.uspreventiveservicestaskforce.org/Page/Document/UpdateSummaryFinal/lung-cancer-screening.
3. Bureau UDoCC. National Cancer Institute-sponsored Tobacco Use Supplement to the Current Population Survey (2010–11): http://appliedresearch.cancer.gov/tus-cps/. 2012.
4. Wallace JM, Deutsch AL. Flexible fiberoptic bronchoscopy and percutaneous needle lung aspiration for evaluating the solitary pulmonary nodule. Chest. 1982;81(6):665–71.
5. Levine MS, Weiss JM, Harrell JH, Cameron TJ, Moser KM. Transthoracic needle aspiration biopsy following negative fiberoptic bronchoscopy in solitary pulmonary nodules. Chest. 1988;93(6):1152–5.
6. Ohno Y, Hatabu H, Takenaka D, Higashino T, Watanabe H, Ohbayashi C, et al. CT-guided transthoracic needle aspiration biopsy of small (≤20 mm) solitary pulmonary nodules. Am J Roentgenol. 2003;180(6):1665–9.
7. Tsukada H, Satou T, Iwashima A, Souma T. Diagnostic accuracy of CT-guided automated needle biopsy of lung nodules. Am J Roentgenol. 2000;175(1):239–43.
8. Coleman RE, Laymon CM, Turkington TG. FDG imaging of lung nodules: a phantom study comparing SPECT, camera-based PET, and dedicated PET. Radiology. 1999;210(3):823–8.
9. Bunyaviroch T, Coleman RE. PET evaluation of lung cancer. J Nucl Med. 2006;47(3):451–69.
10. Gould MK, Fletcher J, Iannettoni MD, Lynch WR, Midthun DE, Naidich DP, et al. Evaluation of patients with pulmonary nodules: when is it lung cancer?: ACCP evidence-based clinical practice guidelines (2nd edition). Chest. 2007;132(3 Suppl):108S–30.
11. Jaklitsch MT, Jacobson FL, Austin JHM, Field JK, Jett JR, Keshavjee S, et al. The American association for thoracic surgery guidelines for lung cancer screening using low-dose computed tomography scans for lung cancer survivors and other high-risk groups. J Thorac Cardiovasc Surg. 2012;144(1):33–8.
12. Daniel TM. A proposed diagnostic approach to the patient with the subcentimeter pulmonary nodule: techniques that facilitate video-assisted thoracic surgery excision. Semin Thorac Cardiovasc Surg. 2005;17(2):115–22.
13. Suzuki K, Nagai K, Yoshida J, Ohmatsu H, Takahashi K, Nishimura M, et al. Video-assisted thoracoscopic surgery for small indeterminate pulmonary nodules*: Indications for preoperative marking. Chest. 1999;115(2):563–8.
14. Chella A, Lucchi M, Ambrogi MC, Menconi G, Melfi FMA, Gonfiotti A, et al. A pilot study of the role of TC-99 radionuclide in localization of pulmonary nodular lesions for thoracoscopic resection. Eur J Cardiothorac Surg. 2000;18(1):17–21.
15. Burdine J, Joyce LD, Plunkett MB, Inampudi S, Kaye MG, Dunn DH. Feasibility and value of video-assisted thoracoscopic surgery wedge excision of small pulmonary nodules in patients with malignancy*. Chest. 2002;122(4):1467–70.
16. Sugi K, Kaneda Y, Hirasawa K, Kunitani N. Radioisotope marking under ct guidance and localization using a handheld gamma probe for small or indistinct pulmonary lesions*. Chest. 2003;124(1):155–8.
17. Daniel TM, Altes TA, Rehm PK, Williams MB, Jones DR, Stolin AV, et al. A novel technique for localization and excisional biopsy of small or Ill-defined pulmonary lesions. Ann Thorac Surg. 2004;77(5):1756–62.
18. Stiles BM, Altes TA, Jones DR, Shen KR, Ailawadi G, Gay SB, et al. Clinical experience with radiotracer-guided thoracoscopic biopsy of small, indeterminate lung nodules. Ann Thorac Surg. 2006;82(4):1191–7.
19. Grogan EL, Jones DR, Kozower BD, Simmons WD, Daniel TM. Identification of small lung nodules: technique of radiotracer-guided thoracoscopic biopsy. Ann Thorac Surg. 2008;85(2):S772–7.
20. Bellomi M, Veronesi G, Trifirò G, Brambilla S, Bonello L, Preda L, et al. Computed tomography-guided preoperative radiotracer localization of

nonpalpable lung nodules. Ann Thorac Surg. 2010;90(6):1759–64.
21. Bertolaccini L, Terzi A, Spada E, Acchiardi F, Ghirardo D. Not palpable? Role of radio-guided video-assisted thoracic surgery for nonpalpable solitary pulmonary nodules. Gen Thorac Cardiovasc Surg. 2012;60(5):280–4.
22. Ambrogi M, Melfi F, Zirafa C, Lucchi M, De Liperi A, Mariani G, et al. Radio-guided thoracoscopic surgery (RGTS) of small pulmonary nodules. Surg Endosc. 2012;26(4):914–9.
23. Wang Y-Z, Boudreaux JP, Dowling A, Woltering EA. Percutaneous localisation of pulmonary nodules prior to video-assisted thoracoscopic surgery using methylene blue and TC-99. Eur J Cardiothorac Surg. 2010;37(1):237–8.
24. Doo K, Yong H, Kim H, Kim S, Kang E-Y, Choi Y. Needlescopic resection of small and superficial pulmonary nodule after computed tomographic fluoroscopy-guided dual localization with radiotracer and hookwire. Ann Surg Oncol. 2015;22(1): 331–7.
25. Gobardhan PD, Djamin RS, Romme PJHJ, de Wit PEJ, de Groot HGW, Adriaensen T, et al. The use of iodine seed (I-125) as a marker for the localisation of lung nodules in minimal invasive pulmonary surgery. Eur J Surg Oncol (EJSO). 2013;39(9):945–50.
26. Povoski S, Neff R, Mojzisik C, O'Malley D, Hinkle G, Hall N, et al. A comprehensive overview of radioguided surgery using gamma detection probe technology. World J Surg Oncol. 2009;7(1):11.
27. Grazia M, Bini A, Stella F, Pagani D, Bazzocchi R. Radioimmunoguided surgery and intraoperative lung cancer staging. Semin Surg Oncol. 1998;15(4):215–9.
28. Mansi L, Di Lieto E, Rambaldi PF, Bergaminelli C, Fallanca F, Vicidomini G, et al. Preliminary experience with radioimmuno-guided surgery of primary neoplasms of the lung. Minerva Chir. 1998;53(5): 369–72.
29. Wang Y, Sun Y, Gao A. The experimental study of radioimmunoguided surgery for lung cancer. Zhongguo Fei Ai Za Zhi. 2000;3(1):46–9.
30. Kelloff GJ, Hoffman JM, Johnson B, Scher HI, Siegel BA, Cheng EY, et al. Progress and promise of FDG-PET imaging for cancer patient management and oncologic drug development. Clin Cancer Res. 2005;11(8):2785–808.
31. Nwogu C, Fischer G, Tan D, Glinianski M, Lamonica D, Demmy T. Radioguided detection of lymph node metastasis in Non-small cell lung cancer. Ann Thorac Surg. 2006;82(5):1815–20.
32. Moffatt-Bruce SD, Povoski SP, Sharif S, Hall NC, Ross Jr P, Johnson MA, et al. A novel approach to positron emission tomography in lung cancer. Ann Thorac Surg. 2008;86(4):1355–7.
33. Woolfenden JM, Nevin WS, Barber HB, Donahue DJ. Lung cancer detection using a miniature sodium iodide detector and cobalt-57 bleomycin. Chest. 1984; 85(1):84–8.
34. Wang YQ, Sun YE, Zhang JM, Liu X. Clinical practice of 99mTc-peplimycin imaging and radio guided surgery for lung neoplasms. Ai Zheng. 2003;22(7): 749–52.
35. Reubi JC, Laissue J, Krenning E, Lamberts SW. Somatostatin receptors in human cancer: incidence, characteristics, functional correlates and clinical implications. J Steroid Biochem Mol Biol. 1992;43(1–3):27–35.
36. Blum J, Handmaker H, Lister-James J, Rinne N. A multicenter trial with a somatostatin analog (99m)Tc depreotide in the evaluation of solitary pulmonary nodules. Chest. 2000;117(5):1232–8.
37. Grewal RK, Dadparvar S, Yu JQ, Babaria CJ, Cavanaugh T, Sherman M, et al. Efficacy of Tc-99m depreotide scintigraphy in the evaluation of solitary pulmonary nodules. Cancer J. 2002;8(5):400–4.
38. Miliziano JS, Bradley YC. Soft tissue metastases and lung cancer recurrence detected by Tc-99m depreotide scintigraphy. Clin Nucl Med. 2002;27(6):410–2.
39. Menda Y, Kahn D. Somatostatin receptor imaging of non-small cell lung cancer with 99mTc depreotide. Semin Nucl Med. 2002;32(2):92–6.
40. Kahn D, Menda Y, Kernstine K, Bushnell D, McLaughlin K, Miller S, et al. The utility of 99mTc depreotide compared with F-18 fluorodeoxyglucose positron emission tomography and surgical staging in patients with suspected non-small cell lung cancer. Chest. 2004;125(2):494–501.
41. Reubi JC, Schar JC, Waser B, Wenger S, Heppeler A, Schmitt JS, et al. Affinity profiles for human somatostatin receptor subtypes SST1-SST5 of somatostatin radiotracers selected for scintigraphic and radiotherapeutic use. Eur J Nucl Med. 2000;27(3):273–82.
42. Haug AR, Cindea-Drimus R, Auernhammer CJ, Reincke M, Wängler B, Uebleis C, et al. The role of 68Ga-DOTATATE PET/CT in suspected neuroendocrine tumors. J Nucl Med. 2012;53(11):1686–92.
43. Kayani I, Conry BG, Groves AM, Win T, Dickson J, Caplin M, et al. A comparison of 68Ga-DOTATATE and 18F-FDG PET/CT in pulmonary neuroendocrine tumors. J Nucl Med. 2009;50(12):1927–32.
44. Callister MEJ, Baldwin DR, Akram AR, Barnard S, Cane P, Draffan J, et al. British thoracic society guidelines for the investigation and management of pulmonary nodules. Thorax. 2015;70 Suppl 2:ii1–54.
45. Paci M, Annessi V, Giovanardi F, Ferrari G, De Franco S, Casali C, et al. Preoperative localization of indeterminate pulmonary nodules before videothoracoscopic resection. Surg Endosc. 2002;16(3):509–11.
46. Saito H, Minamiya Y, Matsuzaki I, Tozawa K, Taguchi K, Nakagawa T, et al. Indication for preoperative localization of small peripheral pulmonary nodules in thoracoscopic surgery. J Thorac Cardiovasc Surg. 2002;124(6):1198–202.
47. Suzuki K, Shimohira M, Hashizume T, Ozawa Y, Sobue R, Mimura M, et al. Usefulness of CT-guided hookwire marking before video-assisted thoracoscopic surgery for small pulmonary lesions. J Med Imaging Radiat Oncol. 2014;58(6):657–62.

48. Huang W, Ye H, Wu Y, Xu W, Tang X, Liang Y, et al. Hook wire localization of pulmonary pure ground-glass opacities for video-assisted thoracoscopic surgery. Thorac Cardiovasc Surg. 2014;62(02):174–8.
49. Dendo S, Kanazawa S, Ando A, Hyodo T, Kouno Y, Yasui K, et al. Preoperative localization of small pulmonary lesions with a short hook wire and suture system: experience with 168 procedures. Radiology. 2002;225(2):511–8.
50. Ciriaco P, Negri G, Puglisi A, Nicoletti R, Del Maschio A, Zannini P. Video-assisted thoracoscopic surgery for pulmonary nodules: rationale for preoperative computed tomography-guided hookwire localization. Eur J Cardiothorac Surg. 2004;25(3):429–33.
51. Miyoshi K, Toyooka S, Gobara H, Oto T, Mimura H, Sano Y, et al. Clinical outcomes of short hook wire and suture marking system in thoracoscopic resection for pulmonary nodules. Eur J Cardiothorac Surg. 2009;36(2):378–82.
52. Yoshida Y, Inoh S, Murakawa T, Ota S, Fukayama M, Nakajima J. Preoperative localization of small peripheral pulmonary nodules by percutaneous marking under computed tomography guidance. Interact Cardiovasc Thorac Surg. 2011;13(1):25–8.
53. Partik BL, Leung AN, Müller MR, Breitenseher M, Eckersberger F, Dekan G, et al. Using a dedicated lung-marker system for localization of pulmonary nodules before thoracoscopic surgery. Am J Roentgenol. 2003;180(3):805–9.
54. Eichfeld U, Dietrich A, Ott R, Kloeppel R. Video-assisted thoracoscopic surgery for pulmonary nodules after computed tomography-guided marking with a spiral wire. Ann Thorac Surg. 2005;79(1):313–6.
55. Gonfiotti A, Davini F, Vaggelli L, De Francisci A, Caldarella A, Gigli PM, et al. Thoracoscopic localization techniques for patients with solitary pulmonary nodule: hookwire versus radio-guided surgery. Eur J Cardiothorac Surg. 2007;32(6):843–7.
56. Powell TI, Jangra D, Clifton JC, Lara-Guerra H, Church N, English J, et al. Peripheral lung nodules: fluoroscopically guided video-assisted thoracoscopic resection after computed tomography-guided localization using platinum microcoils. · Ann Surg. 2004;240(3):481–9.
57. Mayo JR, Clifton JC, Powell TI, English JC, Evans KG, Yee J, et al. Lung nodules: CT-guided placement of microcoils to direct video-assisted thoracoscopic surgical resection. Radiology. 2009;250(2):576–85.
58. Moon SW, Cho DG, Do Cho K, Kang CU, Seop Jo M, Park HJ. Fluoroscopy-assisted thoracoscopic resection for small intrapulmonary lesions after preoperative computed tomography-guided localization using fragmented platinum microcoils. Thorac Cardiovasc Surg. 2012;60(06):413–8.
59. Koyama H, Noma S, Tamaki Y, Goto K, Kitamura E, Maeda T, et al. CT localisation of small pulmonary nodules prior to thorascopic resection: evaluation of a point marker system. Eur J Radiol. 2008;65(3):468–72.
60. Horan TA, Pinheiro PM, Araújo LM, Santiago FF, Rodrigues MR. Massive gas embolism during pulmonary nodule hook wire localization. Ann Thorac Surg. 2002;73(5):1647–9.
61. Moon S-W, Wang Y-P, Jo K-H, Kwack M-S, Kim S-W, Kwon O-K, et al. Fluoroscopy-aided thoracoscopic resection of pulmonary nodule localized with contrast media. Ann Thorac Surg. 1999;68(5):1815–20.
62. Nomori H, Horio H, Naruke T, Suemasu K. Fluoroscopy-assisted thoracoscopic resection of lung nodules marked with lipiodol. Ann Thorac Surg. 2002;74(1):170–3.
63. Kim YD, Jeong YJ, Hoseok I, Cho JS, Lee JW, Kim HJ, et al. Localization of pulmonary nodules with lipiodol prior to thoracoscopic surgery. Acta Radiol. 2011;52(1):64–9.
64. Watanabe K, Nomori H, Ohtsuka T, Kaji M, Naruke T, Suemasu K. Usefulness and complications of computed tomography-guided lipiodol marking for fluoroscopy-assisted thoracoscopic resection of small pulmonary nodules: Experience with 174 nodules. J Thorac Cardiovasc Surg. 2006;132(2):320–4.
65. Okumura T, Kondo H, Suzuki K, Asamura H, Kobayashi T, Kaneko M, et al. Fluoroscopy-assisted thoracoscopic surgery after computed tomography-guided bronchoscopic barium marking. Ann Thorac Surg. 2001;71(2):439–42.
66. Partrick DA, Bensard DD, Teitelbaum DH, Geiger JD, Strouse P, Harned RK. Successful thoracoscopic lung biopsy in children utilizing preoperative CT-guided localization. J Pediatr Surg. 2002;37(7): 970–3.
67. Vandoni RE, Cuttat J-F, Wicky S, Suter M. CT-guided methylene-blue labelling before thoracoscopic resection of pulmonary nodules. Eur J Cardiothorac Surg. 1998;14(3):265–70.
68. Lenglinger FX, Schwarz CD, Artmann W. Localization of pulmonary nodules before thoracoscopic surgery: value of percutaneous staining with methylene blue. Am J Roentgenol. 1994;163(2): 297–300.
69. Bolton WD, Richey J, Ben-Or S, Hale AL, Ewing JA, Stephenson JE. Electromagnetic navigational bronchoscopy: a safe and effective method for fiducial marker placement in lung cancer patients. Am Surg. 2015;81(7):659–62.
70. Weiser TS, Hyman K, Yun J, Litle V, Chin C, Swanson SJ. Electromagnetic navigational bronchoscopy: a Surgeon's perspective. Ann Thorac Surg. 2008; 85(2):S797–801.
71. Bolton WD, Howe Iii H, Stephenson JE. The utility of electromagnetic navigational bronchoscopy as a localization tool for robotic resection of small pulmonary nodules. Ann Thorac Surg. 2014;98(2):471–6.
72. Okuda K, Yano M, Sasaki H, Moriyama S, Hikosaka Y, Shitara M, et al. A safe method for marking small pulmonary nodules with crystal violet. Surg Today. 2015;45(7):871–5.
73. Santambrogio R, Montorsi M, Bianchi P, Mantovani A, Ghelma F, Mezzetti M. Intraoperative ultrasound during thoracoscopic procedures for solitary pulmonary nodules. Ann Thorac Surg. 1999;68(1):218–22.

74. Sortini A, Carrella G, Sortini D, Pozza E. Single pulmonary nodules: localization with intrathoracoscopic ultrasound — a prospective study. Eur J Cardiothorac Surg. 2002;22(3):440–2.
75. Mattioli S, D'Ovidio F, Daddi N, Ferruzzi L, Pilotti V, Ruffato A, et al. Transthoracic endosonography for the intraoperative localization of lung nodules. Ann Thorac Surg. 2004;79(2):443–9.
76. Kondo R, Yoshida K, Hamanaka K, Hashizume M, Ushiyama T, Hyogotani A, et al. Intraoperative ultrasonographic localization of pulmonary ground-glass opacities. J Thorac Cardiovasc Surg. 2009;138(4):837–42.
77. Gow KW, Saad DF, Koontz C, Wulkan ML. Minimally invasive thoracoscopic ultrasound for localization of pulmonary nodules in children. J Pediatr Surg. 2008;43(12):2315–22.
78. Sortini D, Feo CV, Carrella G, Bergossi L, Soliani G, Carcoforo P, et al. Thoracoscopic localization techniques for patients with a single pulmonary nodule and positive oncological anamnesis: a prospective study. J Laparoendosc Adv Surg Tech. 2003;13(6):371–5.
79. Sortini D, Feo CV, Carcoforo P, Carrella G, Pozza E, Liboni A, et al. Thoracoscopic localization techniques for patients with solitary pulmonary nodule and history of malignancy. Ann Thorac Surg. 2005;79(1):258–62.
80. Yoshida J, Nagai K, Nishimura M, Takahashi K. Computed tomography-fluoroscopy guided injection of cyanoacrylate to mark a pulmonary nodule for thoracoscopic resection. Jpn J Thorac Caridovasc Surg. 1999;47(5):210–3.
81. Kojima F, Sato T, Takahata H, Okada M, Sugiura T, Oshiro O, et al. A novel surgical marking system for small peripheral lung nodules based on radio frequency identification technology: feasibility study in a canine model. J Thorac Cardiovasc Surg. 2014;147(4):1384–9.
82. Okusanya OT, Holt D, Heitjan D, Deshpande C, Venegas O, Jiang J, et al. Intraoperative near-infrared imaging can identify pulmonary nodules. Ann Thorac Surg. 2014;98(4):1223–30.
83. Grogan EL, Stukenborg GJ, Nagji AS, Simmons W, Kozower BD, Jones DR, et al. Radiotracer-guided thoracoscopic resection is a cost-effective technique for the evaluation of subcentimeter pulmonary nodules. Ann Thorac Surg. 2008;86(3):934–40.
84. Kawanaka K, Nomori H, Mori T, Ikeda K, Ikeda O, Tomiguchi S, Yamashita Y. Marking of small pulmonary nodules before thoracoscopic resection: injection of lipiodol under CT-fluoroscopic guidance. Acad Radiol. 2009;16(1):39–45.

Part X
Miscellaneous

Radioguided Localization of Bone Lesions

22

Erik M. Von Meyenfeldt and Karel W.E. Hulsewé

Contents

Abstract

Nuclear medicine techniques are used increasingly in primary staging and follow-up of several malignancies and imaging of benign bone diseases.

Bone scans using Technetium-99m (^{99m}Tc) are highly sensitive in detecting bone lesions, but due to low specificity, false-positive lesions are detected frequently. Although SPECT and PET techniques have improved diagnostic imaging accuracy, histological diagnosis of suspected metastatic lesions is often needed to be able to make important treatment decisions. When radiological biopsy is not successful or feasible due to absence of a radiologically detectable target, radionuclide-guided surgical bone biopsy is a highly accurate and well-tolerated technique to obtain histological diagnosis. When benign lesions are not amenable to less invasive treatment options, radioguided surgery can limit the extent and increase the success rate of surgical resection.

E.M. Von Meyenfeldt (✉)
Department of Surgery, Albert Schweitzer Hospital, Dordrecht, The Netherlands
e-mail: e.m.von.meyenfeldt@asz.nl

K.W.E. Hulsewé
Departments of Surgery, Zuyderland Hospital, Sittard/Heerlen, The Netherlands
e-mail: k.hulsewe@orbisconcern.nl

22.1 Clinical Value and Relevance in Clinical Practice

Nuclear medicine imaging techniques are used increasingly during analysis of primary tumours or follow-up after their curative treatment. Depending on primary tumour histology, bone metastases occur in up to 70 % of patients [1]. Skeletal scintigraphy with Technetium-99m (^{99m}Tc)-labeled agents has been the mainstay of imaging of osteoblastic bone metastases, but has limited sensitivity (86.0 %) and especially limited specificity

K. Herrmann et al. (eds.), *Radioguided Surgery: Current Applications and Innovative Directions in Clinical Practice*, DOI 10.1007/978-3-319-26051-8_22

(81.4 %), leading to false-positive scintigraphy results [2]. Addition of single-photon emission computed tomography (SPECT) and SPECT/CT techniques has increased especially specificity (92.8 %) of ^{99m}Tc-based imaging [2–4].

The increased use of highly sensitive (93.7 %) and specific (97.4 %) ^{18}F-fluorodeoxyglucose (^{18}F-FDG) – positron emission tomography (PET)/CT imaging, which relies on glucose metabolism of the tumour itself rather than the osteoblastic activity caused by the tumour, has improved detection rate of bone metastases as well as extra-skeletal metastases [2]. Improved PET technique and PET availability have revived interest in ^{18}F-fluoride as a specific bone tracer. ^{18}F-Fluoride accumulates in both osteoblastic and osteolytic lesions, has highly specific bone uptake and has rapid clearance from the blood pool; these characteristics combined with CT imaging result in improved detection and characterisation of bone lesions, compared to ^{99m}Tc bone imaging [5].

Despite the use of these more sensitive and specific imaging modalities, confirmation of the histology of a bone lesion is still essential to determine the appropriate treatment plan in many cases.

Confirmation of synchronous bone metastases during primary analysis will often preclude curative treatment and warrant a change in treatment strategy. Proving a bone lesion, detected during follow-up, to be benign, rather than cancer recurrence, will reassure the patient and prevent overtreatment.

When radiological abnormalities are present, percutaneous biopsy by the radiologist is the preferred, least invasive, technique. In radio-occult lesions, or when the percutaneous biopsy result is inconclusive, radioguided surgical biopsy is a highly reliable, well-tolerated technique to obtain histological diagnosis [6–8].

Radioguided (i.e., gamma probe-guided) bone biopsy is generally reported to have a specificity of approximately 100 % and a sensitivity in the 97 %–100 % range [6–8], and with anywhere between 30 %–70 % of radioguided biopsied bone lesions proving to be malignant. An illustrated case description of radioguided rib biopsy is included in Chapter 29 of this book.

Radioguided surgery for benign bone lesions, like enchondroma and especially osteoid osteoma, results in excellent symptom relief with more limited dissection, more complete resection of the nidus and less extensive resection of healthy bone tissue, as compared to conventional open resection [9–12]. Radioguided resection therefore provides a valuable alternative, when other minimally invasive techniques, like radiofrequency ablation (RFA), are not feasible [10, 11]. Reports on the added value of radioguided surgery in infectious disease have been published as well, but have not been consistently reproduced [13].

22.2 Preoperative Localization

Most early and small bone lesions are asymptomatic and are discovered with whole-body imaging techniques, performed during work up or follow-up in oncological patient care. These lesions do not always show on conventional radiological imaging, which would take around 50 % bone destruction to be visible [7]. Especially in osteoblastic bone lesions, limited bone destruction of 5–10 % can be visualised on skeletal scintigraphy [7]. As mentioned in 22.1, detection, characterisation and localization of bone lesions can be enhanced by adding 3-D imaging technique (i.e., SPECT, PET, SPECT/CT, PET/CT) and by using other radiotracers (i.e., ^{18}F-FDG or ^{18}F-fluoride).

Lesions detected primarily with PET/CT will often be detected by skeletal scintigraphy as well. Considering the wide availability of 140 keV gamma probes for use in sentinel node biopsy procedures in breast cancer and melanoma (as opposed to 511 keV PET probes needed to detect ^{18}F-FDG or ^{18}F-fluoride), performing a ^{99m}Tc skeletal scintigraphy to confirm uptake in the suspected lesion will improve the detection rate during 140 keV probe-guided surgery using ^{99m}Tc-labeled radiotracers.

22.2.1 Tracers Usually Used and Route of Administration

Intravenously administered ^{99m}Tc-labeled diphosphonates (hydroxy diphosphonate (HDP) or methylene diphosphonate (MDP)) are the most commonly used agents for skeletal scintigraphy.

For radioguided bone biopsies, doses between 15–30 mCi (550–1110 MBq) have been described, injected 2–12 h preoperatively [6–8, 14].

Even though ^{18}F-labeled agents have increased sensitivity and specificity in nuclear medicine, skeletal imaging and 511 keV probe-guided surgery have been demonstrated to be feasible; however, no series of PET probe-guided bone biopsies have been published [15].

In osteoid osteoma, comparable doses of intravenously administered ^{99m}Tc-labeled diphosphonates or oxidronate were used [10–12, 16].

22.2.2 Preoperative Imaging

One to four hours after injection, preoperative scintigraphic images can be obtained, but this is not described in all series [6–12]. When deemed necessary by the nuclear medicine specialist, SPECT or SPECT/CT images can be obtained to aid precise localization and marking on the skin. In many surgical cases, skeletal scintigraphy, SPECT scan or SPECT/CT images will already be available from the original diagnostic evaluation of the bone lesion. In addition to intraoperative use of a140 keV gamma probe, skin marking of the site of shortest distance between the skin and the bone lesion by the nuclear medicine specialist remains helpful to the surgeon.

22.3 Alternatives to Radioguided Surgery or Combination of Techniques

Radioguided surgery for bone lesions is indicated when less invasive techniques, like percutaneous radiological biopsy or RFA for osteoid osteoma, is not possible or proves unsuccessful.

For standard radiological biopsy, sufficient bone destruction is needed to provide a target on CT scan. In addition to standard radiologically guided biopsy, reports on the value of PET/CT-guided percutaneous biopsy have been published recently with a high rate of adequate biopsies (94.3 %) and up to 100 % sensitivity in detecting malignant bone lesions [17–19].

22.4 Radioguided Localization, Biopsy, and Possible Resection of Bone Lesions

Radioguide surgery is planned 4–12 h after intravenous injection of the ^{99m}Tc-labeled agent. After anaesthesia and positioning on the operating table, the handheld 140 keV gamma probe can be used to check the activity at the skin mark and confirm localization of the bone lesion. After preparation and draping of the operative field, the handheld gamma probe is put in a sterile plastic sleeve for intraoperative use. Since most bone lesions targeted with radioguided surgery are located in superficially located bones (ribs/sternum), a 3–5 cm incision directly over the lesion is sufficient to expose the bone [6–8]. Depending on the site of the bone lesion, indication (biopsy or complete excision) and build of the patient (muscular or obese) exposure might be more extensive.

The target area (i.e., bone lesion) is identified with the handheld gamma probe; the activity of the target is generally 1.6–10 times higher than background activity of the adjacent bone tissue [6–8, 11, 12].

Several artefacts might occur during gamma probe-guided surgery:

1. Use of electrical appliances, like the electrocautery, can distort the gamma probe signal. Simultaneous use of these appliances and the gamma probe is problematic.
2. Areas of increased concentration of the ^{99m}Tc-labeled agent close to the bone lesion can hinder localization. Orientation of the gamma probe in the direction of the bladder and bony growth plates should be avoided.
3. Abrupt movement of the gamma probe with regard to the bone surface can result in artefactual alterations of the counts per second. Slow and even movements with the gamma probe are advised [12].

Depending on the indication for gamma probe-guided surgery, the outer cortex of the rib or sternum can be opened and biopsied with a rongeur as well as the medulla. This leaves the inner cortex intact, reducing the chance of a pneumothorax. If complete resection is required, the extent of rib resection can be determined, as based on the detected activity. The same applies to osteoid osteoma resection. Guided by the measured activity, the cortex is opened over the nidus, enabling excision or curettage with very limited exploration and loss of normal bone tissue. When, in vertebral osteoid osteoma, en bloc resection is not possible, high-speed intra-lesional drill excision can be monitored with the gamma probe as well [16].

The immediate decrease of activity at the target area and activity in the specimen indicates an adequate biopsy of the bone lesion, or complete removal in case of osteoid osteoma [6, 8, 11, 12, 16]. Limited experience with detection of high-uptake bone lesions with portable gamma camera imaging devices has been described in osteoid osteoma and in diabetic foot problems. For bone lesions, this experience has remained limited [13, 20].

22.4.1 Previously Used and/or Alternative Techniques

Preoperative marking on the skin, using a cobalt marker overlying the focus of increased uptake, gives surgeons a general direction for the surgical biopsy that needed to be performed. Based on imaging and skin markings alone, generous biopsies of grossly normal looking bone were still needed to increase the chance of an adequate sample [21].

In addition to skin markings, percutaneous marking of the bone lesion with methylene blue by the nuclear medicine specialist has been described as well. This serves as an adjunct to direct the surgeon more precisely to the bone lesion with increased uptake [22]. This technique, however, is more time consuming and cumbersome for the patient. The availability of 140 keV gamma probes and the rate of successful localizations have made methylene blue dye skin marking obsolete.

22.4.2 Success Rates of 1D Gamma Probes for Intraoperative Detection

Using the readily available handheld 1D 140 keV gamma probes, radioguided surgery for suspected metastatic skeletal lesions has a sensitivity of 97–100 % and a specificity of 100 % in the largest published series [6–8]. Although 3D techniques (freehand SPECT) should be feasible in intraoperative localization of bone lesions, no series have been published [23]. Since the technique with handheld 1D 140 KeV gamma probes is highly accurate, the added value of intraoperative 3D localization might be limited and of no significant added value.

Apart from postoperative pain, no significant procedure-related complications are reported. Chest tube drainage during 24 h after opening the pleural cavity during rib resection is reported in 2/10 procedures [7]. When only the outer cortex and medulla of the rib are biopsied, no pneumothoraxes occurred [6].

Conclusion

A bone lesion on nuclear medicine imaging in a patient with a known malignancy does not necessarily implicate metastatic disease. Since the presence of a metastasis will significantly change the prognosis and treatment strategy in most patients, histological proof is often highly important. If the bone lesion is radio-occult and not amenable to radiologic, or PET-guided percutaneous biopsy, then radioguided localization is a highly accurate and well-tolerated technique to aid a minimally invasive surgical biopsy of a bone lesion.

In benign bone lesions, like osteoid osteoma, nonsurgical treatment is often preferred. If less invasive treatment is not feasible, radioguided bone lesion resection can facilitate minimally invasive resection of these lesions.

Radioguided surgery for bone lesions requires the same equipment and infrastructure that is readily available in most hospitals performing radioguided sentinel lymph node biopsies and is relatively easy to learn. Since the result of this very reliable procedure is often of great consequence to the patient and his or her treatment plan, radioguided surgery for bone lesions belongs in the armamentarium of any surgical and nuclear medicine department (Figs. 22.1, 22.2, 22.3, and 22.4).

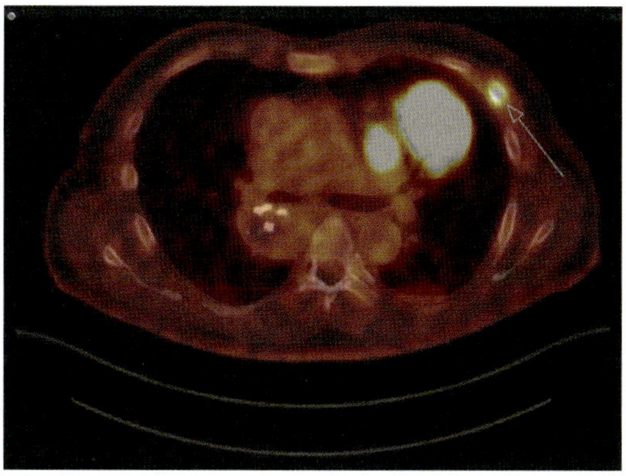

Fig. 22.1 PET/CT scan image with the large FDG-avid primary tumor in the left upper lobe and the bone lesion (white arrow)

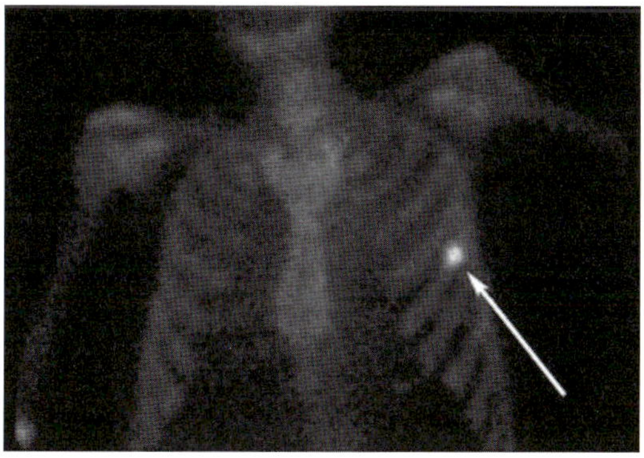

Fig. 22.2 99mTc-bone scan image with high uptake in the bone lesion (white arrow)

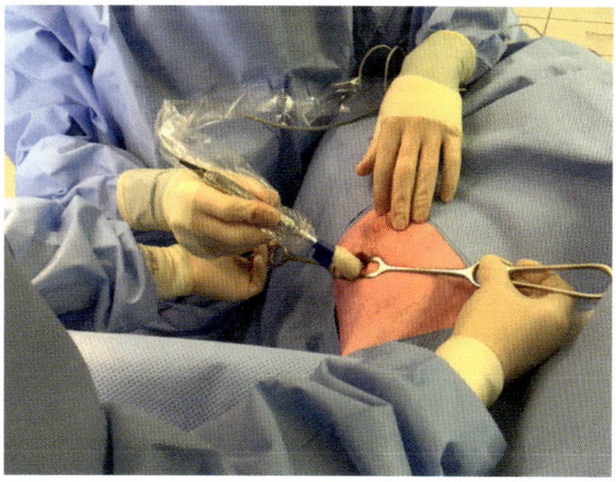

Fig. 22.3 140keV hand-held probe localization of the left 5th rib area with the Highest uptake

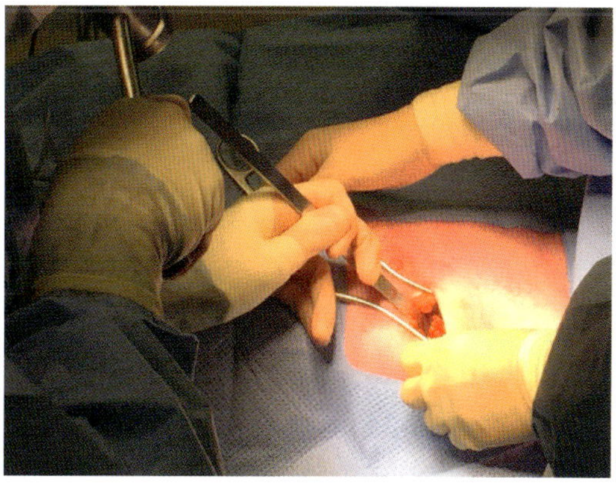

Fig. 22.4 Opening of the outer cortex of the left 5th rib with chisel

References

1. Heindel W, Gübitz R, Weckesser M, et al. The diagnostic imaging of bone metastases. Deutches Ärtzeblatt Int. 2014;111:741–7.
2. Yang HL, Liu T, Wang XM, et al. Diagnosis of bone metastases: a meta-analysis comparing 18FDG PET, CT, MRI and bone scintigraphy. Eur Radiol. 2011;21:2604–17.
3. Helyar V, Mohan HK, Barwick T, et al. The added value of multislice SPECT/CT in patients with equivocal bony metastasis from carcinoma of the prostate. Eur J Nucl Med Mol Imaging. 2010;37:706–13.
4. Römer W, Nömayr A, Uder M, et al. SPECT-guided CT for evaluating foci of increased bone metabolism classified as indeterminate on SPECT in cancer patients. J Nucl Med. 2006;47:1102–6.
5. Grant FD, Fahey FH, Packard AB, et al. Skeletal PET with 18F-fluoride: applying New technology to an Old tracer. J Nucl Med. 2008;49:68–78.
6. von Meyenfeldt EM, Siebenga J, van der Pol HAG, et al. Radionuclide-guided biopsy of bone lesions in cancer patients; a reliable, well-tolerated technique. EJSO. 2014;40:193–6.
7. Robinson LA, Preksto D, Muro-Cacho C, et al. Intraoperative gamma probe-directed biopsy of asymptomatic suspected bone metastases. Ann Thorac Surg. 1998;65:1426–32.
8. Andrade RS, Blondet JJ, Kast T, et al. Evaluation of isolated Rib lesions with radionuclide-guided biopsy. Ann Thorac Surg. 2008;86:1111–5.
9. Harvey WC, Lancaster JL. Technical and clinical characteristics of a surgical biopsy probe. J Nucl Med. 1981;22:184–6.

10. Pratali R, Zuiani G, Inada G, et al. Open resection of osteoid osteoma guided by a gamma-probe. Int Orthop. 2009;33:219–23.
11. Hempfing A, Hoffend J, Bitsch RG, et al. The indication for gamma probe-guided surgery of spinal osteoid osteomas. Eur Spine J. 2007;16:1668–72.
12. Wioland M, Sergent-Alaoui A. Didactic review of 175 radionuclide-guided excisions of osteoid osteomas. Eur J Nucl Med. 1996;23:1003–11.
13. Soluri A, Massari R, Trotta C, et al. High resolution mini-gammacamera and 99mTc [HMPAO] – leukocytes for diagnosis of infection and radioguided surgery in diabetic foot. G Chir. 2005;26:246–50.
14. Povoski SP, Neff RL, Mojzisik CM, et al. A comprehensive review of radioguided surgery using gamma detection probe technology. World J Surg Oncol. 2009;7:11. doi:10.1186/1477-7819-7-11.
15. Gulec SA. PET pobe-guided surgery. J Surg Oncol. 2007;96:353–7.
16. Van Royen BJ, Baayen JC, Pijpers R, et al. Osteoid osteoma of the spine: a novel technique using combined computer-assisted and gamma probe-guided high-speed intralesional drill excision. Spine. 2005;30:369–73.
17. Purandare NC, Kulkarni AV, Kulkarni SS, et al. 18F-FDG PET/CT-directed biopsy: does it offer incremental benefit? Nucl Med Commun. 2013;34: 203–10.
18. Cornelis F, Silk M, Schoder H. Performance of intra-procedural 18-fluorodeoxyglucose PET/CT-guided biopsies for lesions suspected of malignancy but poorly visualized with other modalities. Eur J Nucl Med Mol Imaging. 2014;41:2265–72.
19. Klaeser B, Wiskirchen J, Wartenberg J, et al. PET/CT-guided biopsies of metabolically active bone lesions: applications and clinical impact. Eur J Nucl Med Mol Imaging. 2010;37:2027–36.
20. D'Errico G, Rosa MA, Soluri A, et al. Radioguided biopsy of osteoid osteoma: usefulness of imaging probe. Tumori. 2002;88:S30–2.
21. Shih WJ, DeLand FH, Domstad PA, et al. Open rib biopsy guided by radionuclide technique. Ann Thorac Surg. 1984;38:59–62.
22. Little AG, DeMeester TR, Kirchner PT, et al. Guided biopsies of abnormalities on nuclear bone scans technique and indications. J Thorac Cardiovasc Surg. 1983;85:396–403.
23. Vetter C, Lasser T, Okur A, et al. 1D-3D registration for intra-operative nuclear imaging in radio-guided surgery. IEEE Trans Med Imaging. 2015;34: 608–17.

Radioguided Monitoring of Systemic Leakage During Isolated Limb Perfusion for Melanoma

23

Sergi Vidal-Sicart, Ramon Rull, Clemente Barriuso, and Omgo E. Nieweg

Contents

Abstract

Isolated perfusion is a treatment option when metastases are located on a limb and they are too numerous or when they recur too frequently for excision, even in the presence of distant metastases. Isolated limb perfusion enables treatment of an entire extremity with drugs without exposing the rest of the body to the medication. In the isolated limb, drug concentrations of up to 20 times the level that would be tolerated in the rest of the body may be reached. Perfusion provides the opportunity to treat not only the lesions that are evident but also occult lesions that could become evident later. Continuous monitoring can detect systemic leakage at an early stage. This is needed in situations when systemic leakage is known to occur and when tumor necrosis factor is administered. The detection of systemic leakage was classically performed by measurement of radiotracer concentrations in blood samples from the perfusate and systemic circulation. Radioguided monitoring of potential systemic leakage has been accomplished by using a precordial scintillation detector, a handheld gamma ray probe, or a mobile small field-of-view gamma camera in the operating room.

S. Vidal-Sicart (✉)
Melanoma Unit, Nuclear Medicine Department, Hospital Clínic Barcelona, Barcelona, Spain
e-mail: SVIDAL@clinic.ub.es

R. Rull
Melanoma Unit, Surgery Department, Hospital Clínic Barcelona, Barcelona, Spain

C. Barriuso
Melanoma Unit, Cardiovascular Surgery Department, Hospital Clínic Barcelona, Barcelona, Spain

O.E. Nieweg
Surgery Department, Melanoma Institute Australia, North Sydney, NSW, Australia
e-mail: omgo.nieweg@melanoma.org.au

23.1 Introduction

The biology of melanoma has particular features that are not found in other types of cancer. Satellite and in-transit dissemination are typical of this disease and occur in a small percentage of the patients. These metastases originate from tumor

K. Herrmann et al. (eds.), *Radioguided Surgery: Current Applications and Innovative Directions in Clinical Practice*, DOI 10.1007/978-3-319-26051-8_23

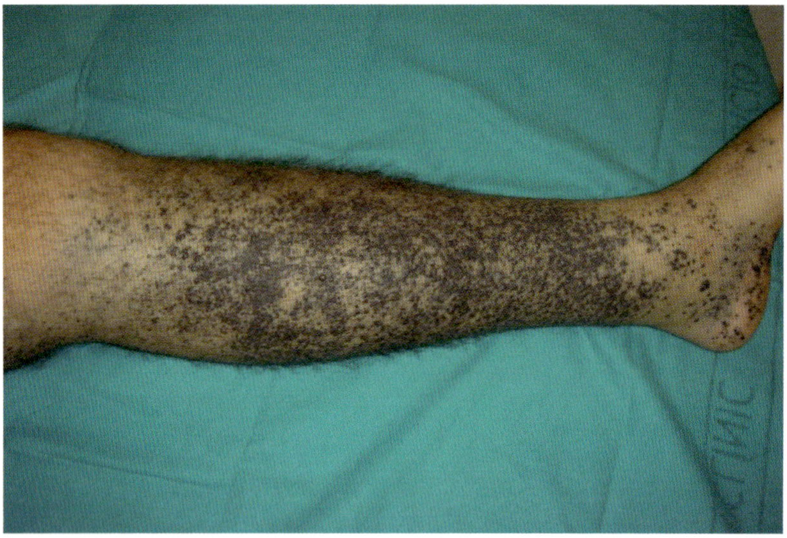

Fig. 23.1 Multiple in-transit cutaneous metastases in a left lower limb of a patient who had a primary melanoma located on left heel

cells that are caught in lymph vessels in the skin or in the subcutaneous tissues. Such metastases are typically excised, but they often recur in larger numbers (Fig. 23.1). Isolated perfusion is a well-established treatment option when such metastases are located on a limb and they are too numerous or when they recur too frequently for excision, even in the presence of distant metastases. A range of other options is available for inoperable in-transit disease, like intralesional injection with BCG, Rose Bengal, or T-VEC. Options for cutaneous lesions are topical application of dinitrochlorobenzene, diphencyprone, or monobenzone and imiquimod. Other options are diathermy, cryotherapy, carbon dioxide laser ablation, electrochemotherapy, and radiotherapy. New effective systemic drugs may provide another option. With all these alternatives available, amputation is rarely performed these days in patients with locally or regionally advanced melanoma [1, 2].

23.2 Definitions and Prognosis

The nomenclature used for recurrences in melanoma can be confusing because terms such as locoregional recurrence, satellitosis, and in-transit disease have all been used with varying definitions and intentions. Local recurrence is preferably defined as the regrowth of the primary melanoma in the excision scar or graft [3, 4].

The most recent American Joint Committee on Cancer (AJCC) and Union International Contre le Cancer (UICC) staging system for melanoma define in-transit metastases as any skin or subcutaneous metastases that are more than 2 cm from the primary lesion but are not beyond the regional nodal basin. Satellite metastases are defined as cutaneous or subcutaneous metastases occurring within 2 cm of the primary melanoma. The staging classification does not differentiate between in-transit lesions and satellitosis in the assignment of stage, both being designated as N2 disease, or N3 if regional nodes are also involved [5, 6].

Satellites and in-transit metastases are associated with a 5-year survival rate of 69 % and a 10-year survival rate of 52 %. These numbers are somewhat better than the 59 % 5-year and 43 % 10-year survival for stage IIIB patients overall [7].

23.3 Isolated Limb Perfusion

Isolated limb perfusion enables treatment of an entire extremity with systemic drugs without exposing the rest of the body to the medication.

Isolating the limb from the main circulation and creating a separate blood circuit accomplish this goal. The rationale is that melanoma is sensitive to chemotherapy, but requires a higher dose than is customary in other types of cancer. In the isolated limb, drug concentrations of up to 20 times the level that would be tolerated in the rest of the body may be reached. Perfusion provides the opportunity to treat not only the lesions that are evident but also occult lesions that could become evident later.

An 80 % response rate is accomplished with perfusion with a complete response rate of 54 % [8]. Approximately half of the patients with a complete response recur in the perfused limb after a median interval of 6 months. In 70 % of these patients, such recurrences can be managed by simple local treatment modalities like excision, or laser ablation, or radiotherapy. The 10-year survival rate in patients with a complete response is 49 % [9]. Repeat perfusion can be considered for patients who recur following an initial response and is often effective [10]. Long-term survivors have a better quality of life than comparable control individuals [11, 12].

Melphalan is the standard drug for isolated limb perfusion. The addition of tumor necrosis factor (TNF)-α to the perfusate results in tumor vasculature destruction, increased cytotoxicity, and modulation of the immune response. TNF-α augments the response rate, but can cause serious morbidity when substantial leakage occurs [13–15].

Systemic toxicity can be avoided by adequate isolation of the limb. For this purpose, a tourniquet around the base of the limb is used and is combined with ligation of collateral vessels. Systemic leakage can be limited by avoiding a high flow rate of perfusion and limiting the venous pressure. Continuous monitoring can detect systemic leakage at an early stage. This is needed in situations when systemic leakage is known to occur and when high dose TNF-α is administered.

The aim of this chapter is to describe the current options for intraoperative radioguided monitoring of systemic leakage during isolated limb perfusion.

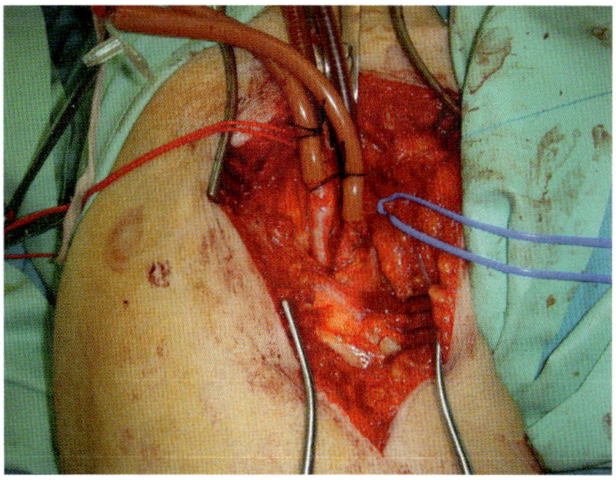

Fig. 23.2 Both common femoral vessels are cannulated and connected to perfusion pump

23.4 Description of Perfusion Technique

Isolated limb perfusion requires a multidisciplinary effort by the surgeon, the perfusionist, the nuclear medicine physician, and the operating room team. A detailed description of the technique can be found elsewhere [16]. There is variation in the perfusion technique between institutions. A summary of our protocol at Hospital Clinic of Barcelona is described here.

General anesthesia is used. Perfusion can be performed in the lower limb at the level of the external iliac vessels, at the femoral level, or the popliteal level and in the upper limb at the axillary or brachial level. A tourniquet, for subsequent compression, is placed at the base of the limb under sterile conditions. After disinfection of the entire limb, an arterial line is inserted in the dorsal pedal (or radial) artery to assess the mean arterial pressure, reflecting the perfusion pressure. Subsequently, the main artery and vein are dissected at the base of the limb. Collateral vessels are ligated to prevent leakage to and from the systemic circulation. Arteriotomy and venotomy are performed and cannulae are inserted and connected to the perfusion circuit lines (Fig. 23.2). The blood draining from the venous cannula is propelled by a pump through an oxygenator and a heat exchanger and reintroduced via the arterial cannula, with a pressure lower than the mean systemic arterial pressure.

Isolation of the limb is finalized by wrapping a rubber bandage or inflatable tourniquet around its root to compress the smaller vessels in the muscles and subcutaneous tissue. Thermal probes are inserted into the subcutaneous tissue and a muscle compartment to monitor the temperature.

For leakage monitoring, a small dose of a radiopharmaceutical like ^{99m}Tc-labeled serum human albumin (i.e., Vasculocis ®) is added to the perfusion circuit. Leakage of this tracer into the systemic circulation is continuously monitored by a gamma ray detector (gamma camera) placed over the heart. After establishing the absence of venous blood leakage to the main circulation, the perfusion of cytostatic drugs (melphalan 1.50 mg/kg – TNF-alpha 3 mg for the arm and 4 mg/kg for the leg) is initiated. At the end of the perfusion, the limb is washed out with 1 l (arm) to 4 l (iliac perfusion) of physiological saline solution, the tourniquet is released, and all the blood from the venous line is drained. Subsequently, all vascular cannulae are removed and the arteriotomy and venotomy are closed with vascular suture material.

23.5 Systemic Leakage Monitoring

Originally, the detection of systemic leakage was performed by measurement of radiotracer concentrations in blood samples from the perfusate and systemic circulation with intervals of several minutes. The different volumes involved in the procedure of extracorporeal perfusion are total blood volume (Vt) as the sum of systemic blood volume (Vs) and the blood volume of the perfused extremity (Ve).

For extracorporeal circulation (Vc), the overall volume consists of Ve plus the volume of the pump oxygenator with the connecting tubes (Vo).

Usually, the value for Vo is known. Vt can be extracted from medical tables and Ve values are estimated to be 5 % of the Vt for the upper limbs and 10 % for the lower limbs. For a more exact determination of Vt, Ve, or Vc, it is important to do a dilution analysis. Thus, a known quantity of a blood pool tracer in a known volume must be injected into an unknown volume. After a mixing period, a blood sample is drawn from the unknown volume and the concentration is measured.

Human serum albumin (HSA) tagged with a radioactive tracer is one of the radiopharmaceuticals that can be administered to measure this potential leakage. HSA labeled with ^{125}I or ^{131}I (half-life 60 and 8 days, respectively) was used for this purpose in the past. Thyroid uptake of the radioiodine released after HSA catabolism should be prevented with potassium iodide or sodium perchlorate given 1 or 2 days before the procedure, and these should be continued for 1 or 2 weeks. HSA is also available for labeling with ^{99m}Tc-pertechnetate and this isotope is currently used. The labeling efficiency should be greater than 90 %.

When radioactive blood pool indicators are used, their presence is expressed in counts per minute (cpm). The count rate is proportional to the concentration of the indicator. Thus, systemic leakage is calculated as the quotient of the difference between tracer concentration in the systemic circulation at the beginning and at the end of one perfusion time frame and the total amount of tracer in the perfusion circulation at the beginning of that interval.

23.6 Radioguided Monitoring

Intraoperative radioguided monitoring of systemic leakage during isolated limb perfusion surgery is well described in the literature [17–28], and can be performed using a precordial scintillation detector, a handheld gamma ray probe, or a mobile small field-of-view gamma camera in the operating room. During perfusion, this device is positioned in the precordial region to acquire the background count rate from the blood pool within the heart. A small amount of radiopharmaceutical is injected into systemic circulation to calibrate the system before monitoring. Subsequently, a larger dose (usually ten times greater) of the same tracer is added to the perfusion circuit. The background count rate over the heart is nearly proportional to the activity in the systemic circulation, and the latter can thus be monitored continuously. A rapid calculation of leakage is possible at any time.

• The basic principles of this radioguided technique were described by Stehlin et al. using a single, large, overhead-mounted scintillation detector that displayed continuous tracing results in cpm, on a rectilinear recorder for detecting ^{131}I-HSA [17]. This same principle using a more modern handheld gamma detection probe system was later described by Sardi et al. [18]. The system described by Sardi et al. [18] consisted of two handheld gamma ray detectors, one positioned over the precordial area and one positioned over the distal aspect of the thigh. Each patient received nearly 30 MBq of ^{99m}Tc-pentetate through the volume of perfusion pump. The percentage of leakage was calculated by a simultaneous reading of the two gamma ray detection probes at 1-min intervals. Identical percentages of leakage were detected when this approach was compared to a method of intermittent simultaneous blood sampling from the perfusate and systemic circulations at intervals of several minutes. In contrast to the intermittent (i.e., every 15 min) blood sampling from the perfusate and systemic circulations, the minute-by-minute monitoring of the two handheld gamma probe system allowed for a real-time indication of any fluctuations in the percentage of leakage.

Since then, variations of the radioguided systemic leakage monitoring technique have been described [19–28]. For example, Manner et al. described the use of a two-probe system (precordial region and thigh) with 18.5 MBq of ^{111}In-labeled red blood cells added to the perfusate [19]. Sprenger et al. used a three-probe system (precordial, thigh, and perfusate circuit) with low dose (0.15 MBq) of ^{111}In-labeled red blood cells injected into the systemic circulation to establish a minimum baseline reference activity within the systemic circulation. A subsequent high dose (12 MBq) of ^{111}In-labeled red blood cells was injected into the perfusate [20]. Barker et al. used a one-probe precordial system with a low dose (0.74 MBq) of ^{131}I-labeled human serum albumin injected into the systemic circulation and a subsequent tenfold higher dose (7.4 MBq) of ^{131}I-HSA injected into the perfusate circulation [21]. Van Ginkel et al. described the use of a precordial one-probe system and a combination of two radionuclides. They administered a low dose (0.5 MBq) of ^{131}I-HSA and 10 MBq of ^{99m}Tc-HSA into the systemic circulation and a subsequent tenfold higher dose (5 MBq) of ^{131}I-HSA injected into the perfusion circuit [22].

All these classic real-time leakage determination methods displayed continuous tracing results on a rectilinear recorder. The percentage of leakage was manually calculated every minute, making this procedure tedious and increasing the possibility of mistakes. Also, the intraoperative equipment (detector + recorder) used to perform this procedure was bulky (Fig. 23.3). In order to overcome some drawbacks associated with the properties of ^{131}I, a procedure based on HSA labeled with ^{99m}Tc in combination with a handheld gamma ray detection probe was developed. Sandrock et al. used a portable gamma probe with digital display and investigated the physical properties in a phantom study simulating blood pool activity at different angles of the probe to the surface and at different distances. In twenty patients, the limb circulation was surgically separated from the systemic blood circulation, and the limb was then selectively perfused for 1 h. Initially, 15 MBq ^{99m}Tc-labeled autologous red blood cells were injected into the limb circulation, and an equal amount was kept as a standard. Every 10 min, blood samples were drawn from the body circulation and count rates were simultaneously measured using the probe system in the precordial area. All blood samples were counted for calculation of leakage in terms of percent of the injected dose, and the results were compared with the intraoperative count rates of the probe system. They found a high correlation between the two techniques ($r = 0.92$) [23].

Lately, Casara et al. advocated a precordial one-probe system following well-defined steps. Firstly, 48–72 h before perfusion, a ^{99m}Tc-HSA dose corresponding to 10 % of the dose calculated for perfusion (i.e., 0.05 MBq/kg body weight) was administered to the patient. The maximum count-rate zone detected on the precordial area was marked on patient's skin. During the perfusion

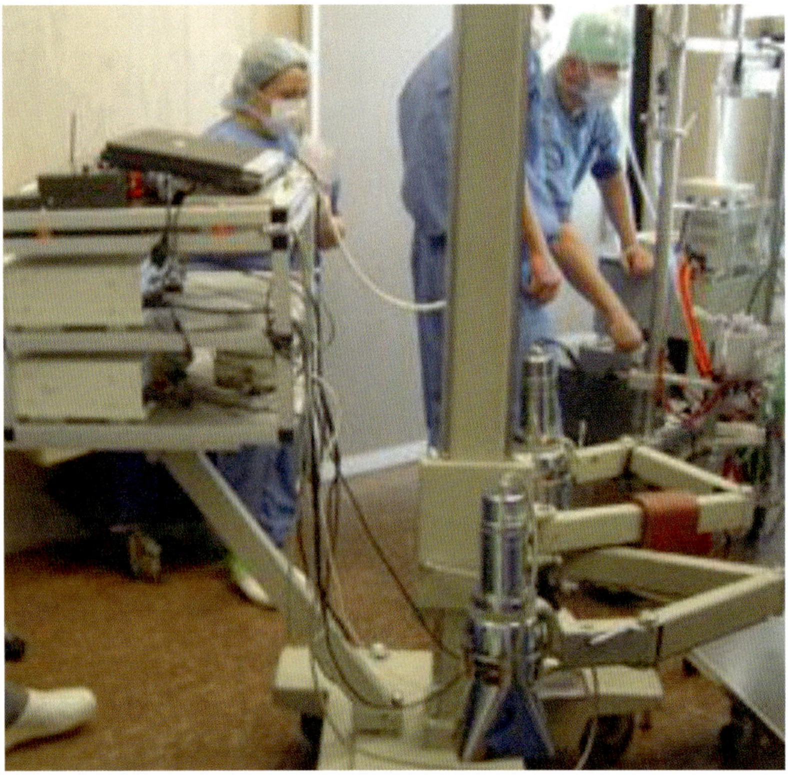

Fig. 23.3 Bulky external detectors used for systemic leakage monitoring during perfusion

procedure, a ^{99m}Tc-HSA dose of 0.5 MBq/kg body weight was injected into the perfusion circuit before TNF-α administration. A handheld gamma probe, usually employed in sentinel lymph node procedure, was placed over the precordial area in the zone premarked during the simulation test. A 60-min time-activity curve corresponding to the circulating ^{99m}Tc-HSA radioactivity effective decay was calculated to compensate for the leakage systemic counting observed during perfusion.

A good correlation was found ($R^2=0.965$, $P<0.01$) when the results of handheld gamma probe monitoring were compared with the results of patient blood and perfusion circuit samples taken simultaneously every 5 min. So, this approach appeared to be technically simple and accurate enough for the real-time monitoring of perfusion leakage [24, 25].

Orero et al. developed a method using a portable gamma camera (Sentinella S102 (ONCOVISION, Valencia, Spain)), specially designed for intraoperative use [26]. This device is a compact scintillation camera with a CsI (Na) crystal optically coupled to a flat panel-type position-sensitive photomultiplier tube [27]. A USB port connects the camera to a computer. The gamma camera is mounted on a lightweight support to facilitate transport to the operating theater (Fig. 23.4). A parallel multi-hole collimator was developed because monitoring of tracer activity requires a higher sensitivity than can be provided by a pinhole collimator (Fig. 23.5). Software to acquire the data needed to detect leakage from the perfusion limb to the systemic circulation was designed. This program measures activity data in the precordial region at 30-s intervals throughout the procedure. The basal activity in this region is measured after the radiotracer measurements in both circuits have reached a steady state and before the drug is administered. Knowing the injected activity in the body A_b, in the isolated extremity A_e, and the measured basal counts B, a detection increase Δ corresponds to a certain leakage L. An approximate value for the leakage, L_a, can be obtained by using the formula:

$$L_a(\%) = 100 \cdot \frac{A_b}{A_e} \cdot \frac{\Delta}{B}$$

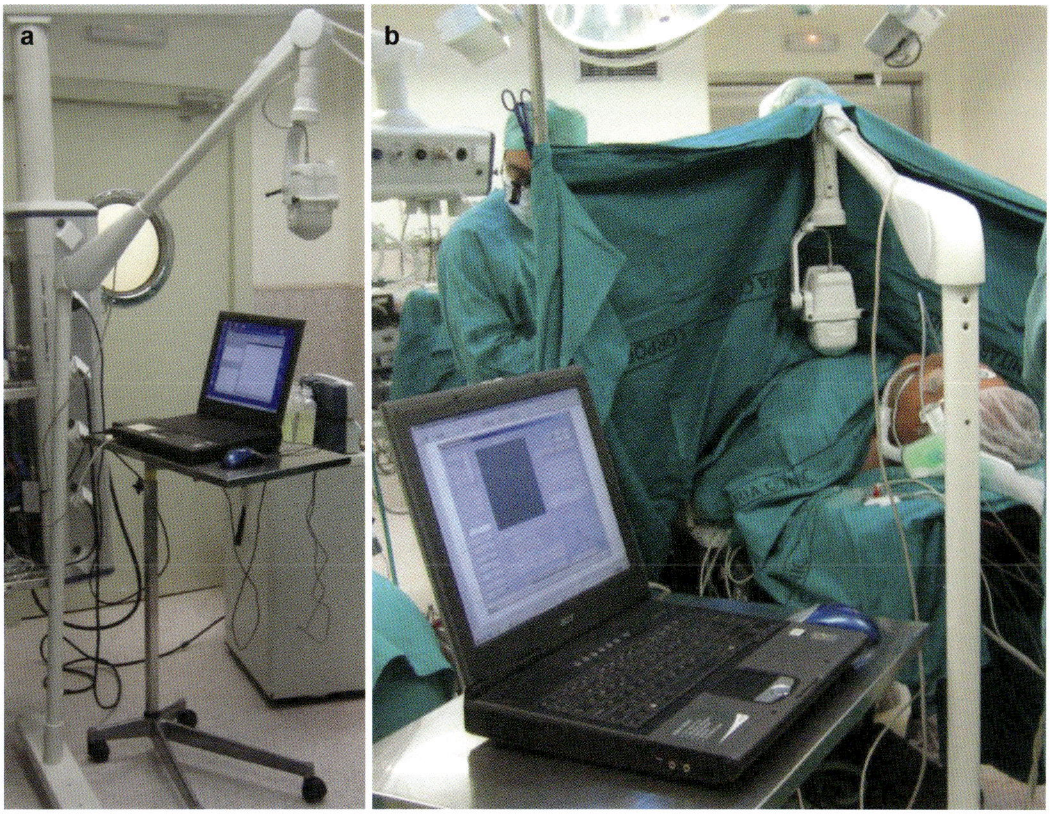

Fig. 23.4 First device used for radioguided monitoring of systemic leakage in our center. The portable gamma camera mounted on an articulated arm connected to a laptop (**a**). The gamma camera is placed over precordial area of patient for continuously radiotracer activity reading (**b**)

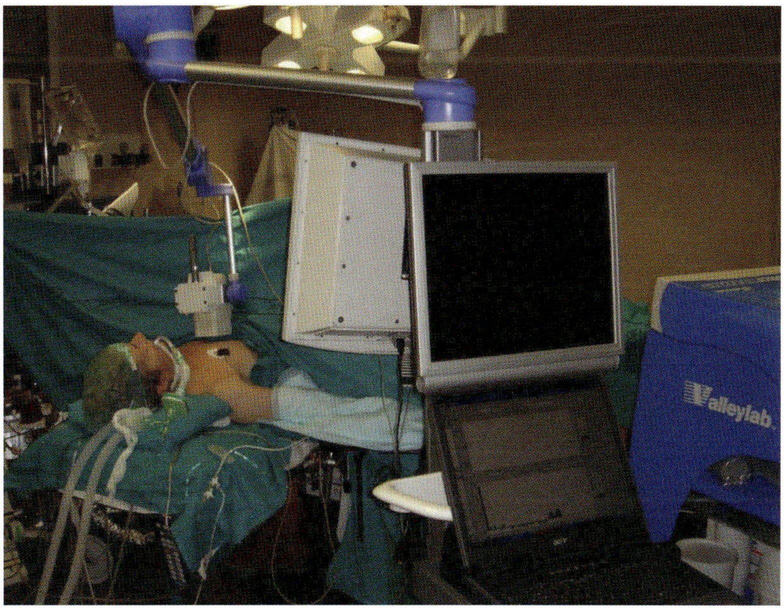

Fig. 23.5 Current device used for ILP. The supporting arm belongs to the new design of portable gamma camera (Sentinella S102). The collimator used is a self-built parallel multi-hole collimator

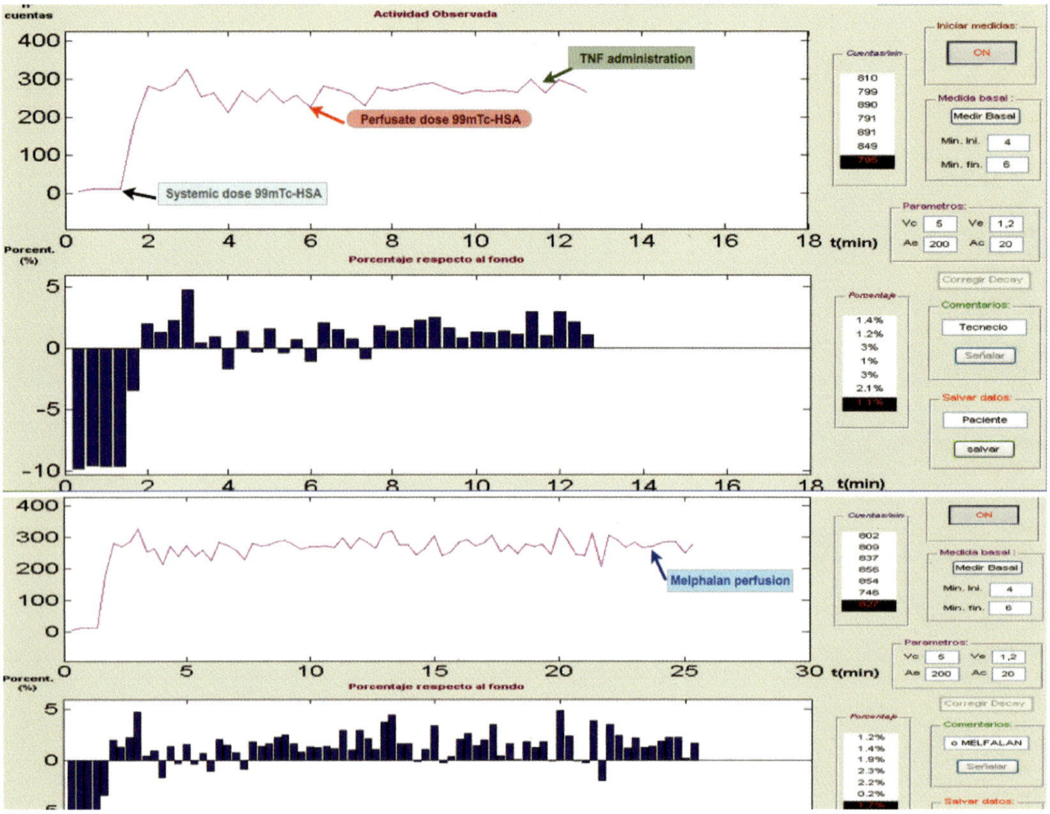

Fig. 23.6 Example of software developed for monitoring systemic leakage. The *upper row* shows tracer activity (in counts). The *lower row* depicts the percentage of systemic activity variation from the baseline readings as histograms. This example is of a patient with a stable count rate during radiotracer injection (TNF-alpha administration and melphalan perfusion)

Orero et al. [27] concluded from their pilot work that the monitoring system could give reliable values for the leakage. Using this approach, the percentage of blood leakage to the systemic vascular territory is calculated and displayed on the computer screen for the duration of the procedure (Figs. 23.6, 23.7, and 23.8). The initial experience was obtained in sixteen melanoma patients in whom the percentage of leakage ranged from 0.5 to 8 % (mean = 3.1 %).

Our group has performed 45 perfusions with this radioguided system. The median leakage percentage demonstrated was 3.5 % (range 0–10 %). During the immediate postoperative period (1–7 days after the operation), there were two vascular complications. Fourteen patients presented bone marrow toxicity (eight leukopenia and six thrombocytopenia) that was successfully managed using colony-stimulating factor. Complete regional response was achieved in 50 % of cases, with a nearly 30 % of the remaining patients showing partial response (unpublished data, Ramon Rull, 2014).

23.7 Concluding Remarks

Despite a plethora of innovative therapeutic options, isolated limb perfusion remains a reasonable option for patients with extensive or bulky disease in a limb. The complete response rate is 54 % and the response is durable in half of them. Given the nature and dose of the drugs that are used in the perfusion circuit, monitoring of systemic leakage is of utmost importance. Throughout the years, different approaches have been used for this purpose. The current standard technique involves radiotracers and continuous

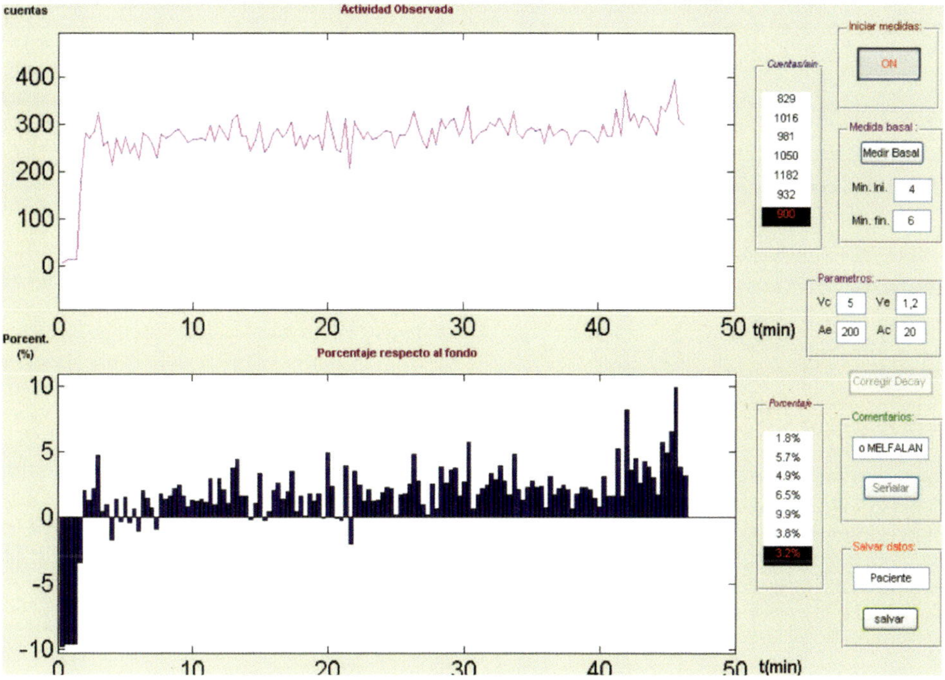

Fig. 23.7 Same patient as in Fig. 23.6 with a more prolonged monitoring (after 30 min of melphalan perfusion). Systemic leakage was maintained below 5 % with minimal peaks of systemic leakage higher than this value

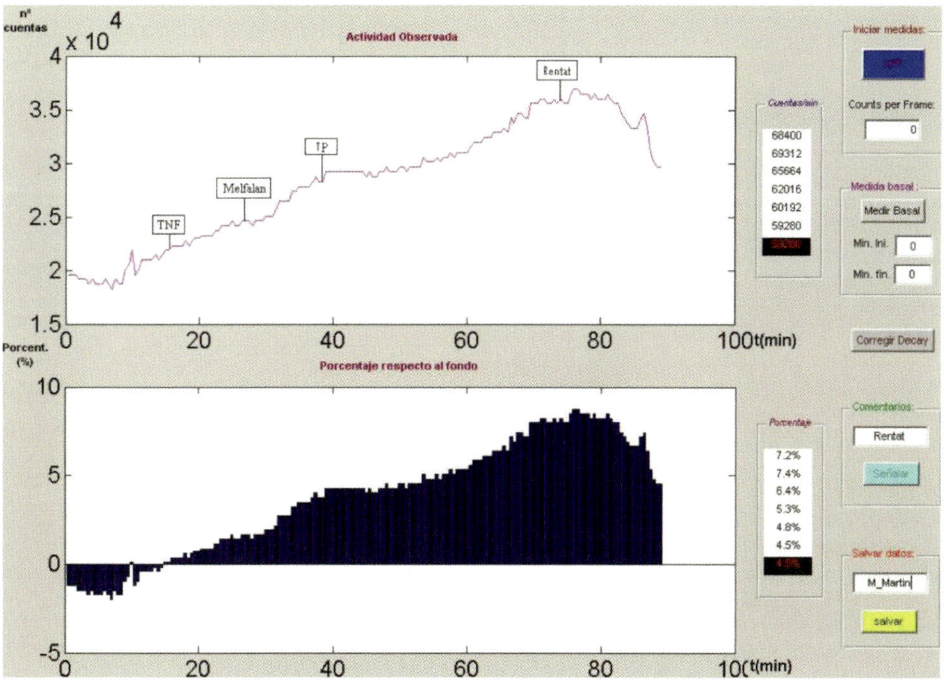

Fig. 23.8 Example of a progressive and maintained systemic leakage (<10 %) during the entire perfusion procedure. The surgical team did not terminate the perfusion prematurely. No serious systemic complications were noted. A partial response of her regional illness was subsequently achieved

monitoring. The new detection devices used in other fields of radioguided surgery (e.g., sentinel lymph node localization) have replaced traditional approaches based on blood samples or bulky detectors. Within this framework, several technical variations all appear to have good results.

References

1. Kapma MR, Vrouenraets BC, Nieweg OE, van Geel AN, Noorda EM, Eggermont AMM, et al. Major amputation for intractable extremity melanoma after failure of isolated limb perfusion. Eur J Surg Oncol. 2005;31:95–9.
2. Read RL, Haydu L, Saw RPM, Quinn MJ, Shannon K, Spillane AJ, et al. In-transit melanoma metastases: incidence, prognosis, and the role of lymphadenectomy. Ann Surg Oncol. 2015;22:475–81.
3. Pawlik TM, Ross MI, Johnson MM, Schacherer CW, McClain DM, Mansfield PF, et al. Predictors and natural history of in-transit melanoma after sentinel lymphadenectomy. Ann Surg Oncol. 2005;12:587–96.
4. Meier F, Will S, Ellwanger U, Schlagenhauff B, Schittek B, Rassner G, et al. Metastatic pathways and time courses in the orderly progression of cutaneous melanoma. Br J Dermatol. 2002;147:62–70.
5. Balch CM. Melanoma of the skin. In: Edge, S. B., Byrd, D. R., Compton, C. C., Fritz, A. G., Greene, F. L., Trotti, A. (Eds). American Joint Committee on cancer staging manual. 7th ed. New York: Springer; 2010. p. 325.
6. Balch CM, Gershenwald JE, Soong SJ, Thompson JF, Atkins MB, Byrd DR, et al. Final version of 2009 AJCC melanoma staging and classification. J Clin Oncol. 2009;27:6199–206.
7. Edge SB, Compton CC. The American Joint Committee on Cancer: the 7th edition of the AJCC cancer staging manual and the future of TNM. Ann Surg Oncol. 2010;17:1471–4.
8. Nieweg OE, Kroon BBR. Isolated limb perfusion with melphalan for melanoma. J Surg Oncol. 2014;109:132–7.
9. Sanki A, Kam PC, Thompson JF. Long-term results of hyperthermic, isolated limb perfusion for melanoma: a reflection of tumor biology. Ann Surg. 2007;245:591–6.
10. Klop WM, Vrouenraets BC, van Geel BN, Eggermont AMM, Klaase JM, Nieweg OE, et al. Repeat isolated limb perfusion with melphalan for recurrent melanoma of the limbs. J Am Coll Surg. 1996;182:467–72.
11. Noorda EM, van Kreij RH, Vrouenraets BC, Nieweg OE, Muller M, Kroon BBR, et al. The health-related quality of life of long-term survivors of melanoma treated with isolated limb perfusion. Eur J Surg Oncol. 2007;33:776–82.
12. Raymond AK, Beasley GM, Broadwater G, Augustine CK, Padussis JC, Turley R, et al. Current trends in regional therapy for melanoma: lessons learned from 225 regional chemotherapy treatments between 1995 and 2010 at a single institution. J Am Coll Surg. 2011;213:306–18.
13. Lienard D, Ewalenko P, Delmotte JJ, Renard N, Lejeune FJ. High-dose recombinant tumor necrosis factor alpha in combination with interferon gamma and melphalan in isolation perfusion of the limbs for melanoma and sarcoma. J Clin Oncol. 1992;10:52–60.
14. Fraker DL, Alexander HR, Andrich M, Rosenberg SA. Treatment of patients with melanoma of the extremity using hyperthermic isolated limb perfusion with melphalan, tumor necrosis factor, and interferon gamma: results of a tumor necrosis factor dose-escalation study. J Clin Oncol. 1996;14:479–89.
15. Zwaveling JH, Maring JK, Clarke FL, van Ginkel RJ, Limburg PC, Hoekstra HJ, et al. High plasma tumor necrosis factor (TNF)-alpha concentrations and a sepsis-like syndrome in patients undergoing hyperthermic isolated limb perfusion with recombinant TNF-alpha, interferon-gamma, and melphalan. Crit Care Med. 1996;24:765–70.
16. Nieweg OE, Imhof O, Kroon BBR. Isolated limb perfusion. In: Mulholland MW, Hawn MT, Hughes SJ, Albo D, Sabel MS, Dalman RL, editors. Operative techniques in surgery. Riverwoods: Wolters Kluwer; 2014. p. 1647–55.
17. Stehlin Jr JS, Clark Jr RL, Dewey WC. Continuous monitoring of leakage during regional perfusion. Arch Surg. 1961;83:943–9.
18. Sardi A, Minton JP, Mojzisik C, Nieroda CA, Ferrara PJ, Hinkle GH, et al. The use of a hand-held gamma detector improves the safety of isolated limb perfusion. J Surg Oncol. 1989;41:172–6.
19. Manner M, Sinn H, Bubeck H, Kettelhack C, Schlag P. Improved intraoperative leak control in cytostatic drug isolation perfusion of tumors of the extremities. Langenbecks Arch Chir. 1990;375:208–13.
20. Sprenger HJ, Markwardt J, Schlag PM. Quantitative radionuclide leakage control during isolated limb perfusion. Nuklearmedizin. 1994;33:248–53.
21. Barker WC, Andrich MP, Alexander HR, Fraker DL. Continuous intraoperative external monitoring of perfusate leak using iodine-131 human serum albumin during isolated perfusion of the liver and limbs. Eur J Nucl Med. 1995;22:1242–8.
22. van Ginkel RJ, Limburg PC, Piers DA, Koops HS, Hoekstra HJ. Value of continuous leakage monitoring with radioactive iodine-131-labeled human serum albumin during hyperthermic isolated limb perfusion with tumor necrosis factor-alpha and melphalan. Ann Surg Oncol. 2002;9:355–63.
23. Sandrock D, Horst F, Gatzemeier W, Ghorbani M, Rauschecker H, Munz DL, et al. Leakage measurement during selective limb perfusion using a gamma probe. Eur J Nucl Med. 1996;23:534–8.

24. Casara D, Rubello D, Pilati PL, Scalerta R, Foletto M, Rossi CR. A simplified procedure for continuous intraoperative external monitoring of systemic leakage during isolated limb perfusion. Tumori. 2002;88:S61–3.
25. Casara D, Rubello D, Pilati P, Scalerta R, Foletto M, Rossi CR. Optimized procedure of real-time systemic leakage monitoring during isolated limb perfusion using a hand held gamma probe and 99mTc-HSA. Nucl Med Commun. 2004;25:61–6.
26. Orero A, Vidal-Sicart S, Roé N, Muxí A, Rubí S, Duch J, et al. Monitoring system for isolated limb perfusion based on a portable gamma camera. Nuklearmedizin. 2009;48:166–72.
27. Sánchez F, Fernández MM, Giménez M, Benlloch JM, Rodríguez-Alvarez MJ, García de Quirós F, et al. Performance tests of two portable mini gamma cameras for medical applications. Med Phys. 2006;33:4210–20.
28. Povoski SP, Neff RL, Mojzisik CM, O'Malley DM, Hinkle GH, Hall NC, Murrey Jr DA, Knopp MV, Martin Jr EW. A comprehensive overview of radioguided surgery using gamma detection probe technology. World J Surg Oncol. 2009;7:11.

Radioimmunoguided Surgery: Intraoperative Radioimmunodetection for the Radioguided Localization and Resection of Tumors

24

Stephen P. Povoski, Cathy M. Mojzisik, and Brandon J. Sullivan

Contents

Portions of the contents of this chapter are adapted from the prior Open Access review article:

S.P. Povoski, MD (✉) • C.M. Mojzisik, RN, BSN, MS
Division of Surgical Oncology, Department of Surgery, Arthur G. James Cancer Hospital and Richard J. Solove Research Institute and Comprehensive Cancer Center, The Ohio State University, Columbus, OH 43210, USA
e-mail: stephen.povoski@osumc.edu; cathymojzisik@gmail.com

B.J. Sullivan, PhD
Department of Chemistry and Biochemistry, The Ohio State University, Columbus, OH 43210, USA
e-mail: sullivan.272@osu.edu

K. Herrmann et al. (eds.), *Radioguided Surgery: Current Applications and Innovative Directions in Clinical Practice*, DOI 10.1007/978-3-319-26051-8_24

Abstract
Radioimmunoguided surgery is a specific application of radioguided surgery which involves intraoperative radioimmunodetection, using a handheld radiation detection device within the operating room in a real-time fashion, for the identification of a radiolabeled antibody or antibody fragment/derivative that has been administered to a patient prior to the time of attempted intraoperative detection and for the sole purpose of guiding the successful performance of the surgical procedure. This chapter discusses (1) the history and development of radioimmunoguided surgery, (2) tumor-associated antigens, (3) monoclonal antibodies, (4) clinical applications of radioimmunoguided surgery, and (5) the future clinical relevance of radioimmunoguided surgery in cancer diagnostics and cancer therapeutics (i.e., oncologic theranostics) as a potential powerful form of antigen-directed cancer surgery.

24.1 Background

Radioimmunoguided surgery is a specific application of radioguided surgery which involves intraoperative radioimmunodetection, using a handheld radiation detection device within the operating room in a real-time fashion, for the identification of a radiolabeled antibody or antibody fragment/derivative that has been administered to a patient prior to the time of attempted intraoperative detection and for the sole purpose of guiding the successful performance of the surgical procedure [1].

Intraoperative radioimmunodetection using a handheld radiation detection device during radioimmunoguided surgery has its own origin from the work of Tarun Ghose and Philip Belitsky at the Dalhousie University Medical School and the Victoria General Hospital (Halifax, Nova Scotia, Canada), which focused upon diagnostic radioimmunodetection using external gamma scintillation imaging [2–5]. In 1975, Ghose et al. [2, 3] reported localization of iodine-131 (^{131}I)-labeled antitumor antibodies on external gamma scintillation imaging within sites of metastatic disease in 2 cancer patients (i.e., metastatic renal adenocarcinoma and metastatic squamous cell of the lung) injected with ^{131}I-labeled goat globulin produced against their own tumors. Then, in 1978, Belitsky et al. [4, 5] reported localization of ^{131}I-labeled antitumor antibodies (consisting of goat-derived antibody generated against pooled homogenate of renal cell carcinomas from 2 patients) on external gamma scintillation imaging in 6 of 6 patients with metastatic renal carcinoma [4] and in 6 of 7 patients with primary renal carcinoma [5]. In that same year, Goldenberg et al. [6] from the University of Kentucky (Lexington, Kentucky, USA) similarly reported localization of ^{131}I-labeled antitumor antibodies (consisting of goat-derived IgG antibody directed against carcinoembryonic antigen (CEA)) on external gamma scintillation imaging in 18 cancer patients, including 3 with colon cancer, 1 with rectal cancer, 4 with ovarian cancer, 5 with cervical cancer, 1 with endometrial cancer, 1 with breast cancer, 1 with lymphoma, 1 with lung cancer, and 1 with bile duct cancer. In the frequently cited work of Goldenberg et al. [6], localization of ^{131}I-labeled antitumor antibodies on external gamma scintillation imaging was seen in 15 of 18 (83 %) cancer patients, excluding 1 case of cervical cancer, 1 case of lymphoma, and 1 case of lung cancer.

24.2 The Genesis of the Concept of Radioimmunoguided Surgery

As previously discussed in Chap. 1, the year 1984 marked the inauguration of the radioguided surgical concept of radioimmunoguided surgery

[1]. The idea of utilizing antibodies directed against cancer-specific antigens for intraoperative radioimmunodetection, localization, and resection of tumors was pioneered at The Ohio State University (Columbus, Ohio, USA) by a surgical oncologist, Dr. Edward W. Martin, Jr., and a professor emeritus of electrical engineering, Dr. Marlin O. Thurston [1], as based upon a collaborative effort that they first established in August 1979 [7] [Personal communication: Cathy M. Mojzisik, Formerly from The Ohio State University, Columbus, OH, USA, cathymojzisik@gmail.com, January 11, 2015]. Their initial findings regarding both experimental animal model testing and the clinical application of intraoperative radioimmunodetection were subsequently first published in 1984 [1, 8, 9] and were predominantly directed toward the surgical management of adenocarcinomas of the colon and rectum. The overriding concept of radioimmunoguided surgery was driven by Dr. Martin's everlasting belief that oncologic surgery should be based upon "more science and less emotion" [Personal communication: Cathy M. Mojzisik, Formerly from The Ohio State University, Columbus, OH, USA, cathymojzisik@gmail.com, January 11, 2015].

In their initial experimental animal model testing, Aitken et al. [1, 8, 9] at The Ohio State University (Columbus, Ohio, USA) grow CEA-producing human colonic adenocarcinoma cells (CX-1) as subcutaneous tumor implants xenografted on the flank in Swiss nude mice. They demonstrated the feasibility of gamma probe detection of ^{131}I-labeled baboon anti-CEA polyclonal antibody within such subcutaneous tumor implants and demonstrated the greater sensitivity of the gamma detection probe as compared to gamma camera imaging for small tumor implants. In addition to these initial animal model experiments, they also published the first clinical application of intraoperative radioimmunodetection in a single patient case report study of a 59-year-old male with a rectal carcinoma located 6 cm above the anal verge [1, 9]. The patient was intravenously injected with 1.9 mCi (70.3 MBq) of ^{131}I-labeled baboon anti-CEA polyclonal antibody at a time of 3 days prior to the planned surgical procedure. They utilized a prototype handheld gamma detection probe system, consisting of a single CdTe semiconductor crystal housed within a 16 mm diameter lead collimator with a 4 mm aperture and connected to a preamplifier and an amplifier with a digital display counter for radioactive count recording. The prototype handheld gamma detection probe intraoperatively detected an increased level of the ^{131}I-labeled baboon anti-CEA polyclonal antibody in the rectal tumor (135 counts/min) as compared to normal sigmoid colon (111 counts/min), ileum (57 counts/min), abdominal wall (105 counts/min), and anal verge (66 counts/min).

Shortly thereafter in 1985, Martin et al. [1, 10] at The Ohio State University (Columbus, Ohio, USA) reported the results of the first radioimmunoguided surgery clinical feasibility study, consisting of a series of 28 patients with colorectal cancer, including 12 patients with primary colorectal cancer and 16 patient with recurrent disease. The patients were intravenously injected with 2.2 mCi (81.4 MBq) of ^{131}I baboon anti-CEA polyclonal antibody at approximately 48–72 h prior to surgery. There were 23 of the 28 patients who underwent preoperative whole-body scintillation imaging. All 28 patients underwent intraoperative gamma counting of gross tumor and adjacent tissues using the same previously described prototype handheld gamma detection probe system. Preoperative whole-body scintillation imaging correctly localized tumor in only 33 % of the patients with primary colorectal cancer and only 64 % of patients with recurrent colorectal cancer. In contrast, intraoperative radioimmunodetection with the prototype handheld gamma detection probe system was successful in all 28 patients, with a mean tumor-to-background ratios of 3.97-to-1 in primary lesions and 4.18-to-1 in recurrent lesions. The author concluded that this clinical feasibility study demonstrated the ability of radioimmunoguided surgery technology to provide immediate intraoperative information regarding the assessment of colorectal cancer.

For all subsequent radioimmunoguided surgery clinical studies conducted at The Ohio State

University (Columbus, Ohio, USA), a variety of prototype handheld gamma detection probe systems were utilized up until 1987, and for which thereafter, a commercially available gamma detection probe system (Neoprobe® 1000; formerly Neoprobe Corporation, Dublin, Ohio, USA) was standardly employed [1, 11] [Personal communication: Cathy M. Mojzisik, Formerly from The Ohio State University, Columbus, OH, USA, cathymojzisik@gmail.com, January 11, 2015]. In this regard, the timing of the eventual radioimmunoguided surgery procedure was determined by serially accessing external precordial counts on each patient with the gamma detection probe, with surgery proceeding forward when external precordial counts reached ≤10 counts per second. Likewise, for all subsequent radioimmunoguided surgery clinical studies conducted at The Ohio State University (Columbus, Ohio, USA) in the 1980s and 1990s, iodine-125 (^{125}I) was selected to replace ^{131}I [1, 11–13]. ^{125}I, a radionuclide gamma emitter with a physical half-life of 60.1 days, as selected as the radionuclide of choice for all subsequent radioimmunoguided surgery since the design of the gamma detection probe utilized at that time was much more efficient at detecting ^{125}I than ^{131}I, predominantly as a result of the lower energy level of the primary gamma photon emitter of ^{125}I as compared to ^{131}I (35 keV vs. 364 keV, respectively) [1, 13–15]. The lower energy gamma photons emitted by ^{125}I were much more likely to be detected by the gamma detection probe system secondary to the fact that the resultant gamma photon emissions were less likely to pass through the small-sized detector crystal within the head of the gamma detection probe without being counted. Similarly, as demonstrated in tumor-bearing mice studies, higher tumor-to-background ratios could be achieved with ^{125}I-labeled antibodies as opposed to ^{131}I-labeled antibodies [1, 14]. This observation of an improved tumor-to-background ratio was a function of the lower energy gamma photon emission of ^{125}I leading to less tissue scatter and greater tissue attenuation [1, 13, 15]. Finally, for all subsequent radioimmunoguided surgery clinical studies conducted at The Ohio State University (Columbus, Ohio, USA) in the 1980s and 1990s using ^{125}I-labeled antibodies, patients were routinely pretreated with an oral saturated solution of potassium iodide (10 drops, twice daily, beginning 2 days prior to injection and continued for approximately 3 weeks after injection of the ^{125}I-labeled antibody or until the day or surgery), in order to block thyroid uptake of ^{125}I [16].

24.3 The History of the Development of Monoclonal Antibody Technology

The specific application of antibodies precisely targeted against tumor-associated antigens represents the basic foundation and groundwork behind the successful implementation of radioimmunoguided surgery and diagnostic radioimmunodetection strategies [1, 17–19]. Antibodies used in these various radioimmunoguided strategies can be targeted against antigens expressed on the surface of tumor cells or targeted against antigens expressed within the extracellular environment around tumor cells. Such antibodies can exist in the form of whole antibody molecules or as various antibody fragments/derivatives. When an antibody is radiolabeled with one of any of a variety of radionuclides, the resultant radiolabeled conjugates can potentially be utilized for (1) diagnostic nuclear medicine imaging, (2) integrated technologies involving handheld radiation detection devices and advanced nuclear medicine imaging for guidance and optimization of the intraoperative detection and resection of tumors, and (3) cancer radiotherapeutics [1].

Over the years, there has been an ongoing evolution in the techniques for the production of antibodies [20] utilized in various radioimmunoguided strategies. Early radioimmunoguided strategies utilized antibodies of polyclonal origin, while later radioimmunoguided strategies took advantage of antibodies of monoclonal origin. The general schema for the production of polyclonal and monoclonal antibodies is shown in Fig. 24.1. Polyclonal antibodies are easily produced by immunization and harvesting from mammalian nonhuman species (i.e., murine, rat,

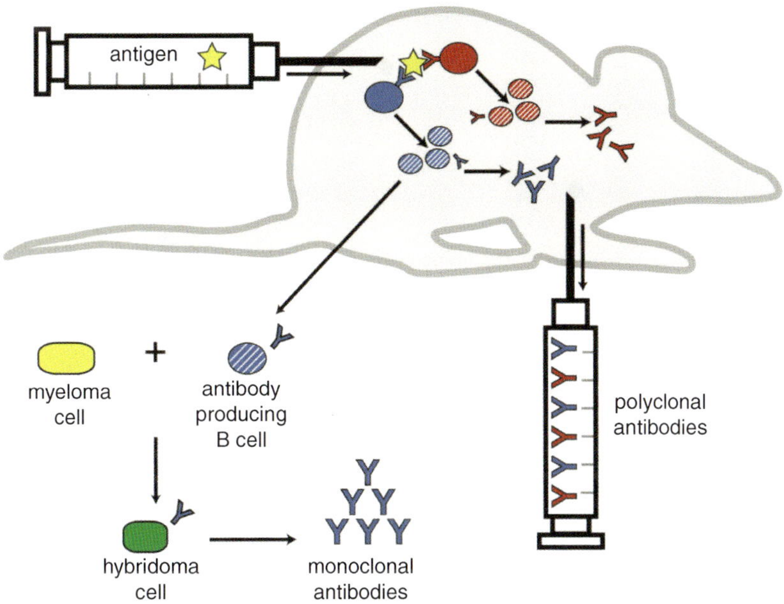

Fig. 24.1 Production of polyclonal and monoclonal antibodies. Here, a host animal (i.e., mouse) is injected with a tumor-associated antigen (i.e., presenting antigen) that elicits an immune response. Immunoglobulin receptors on multiple B-cell lymphocyte clones (depicted as single blue cell and single red cell) bind the antigen, each at distinct epitopes, leading to activation, proliferation, and secretion of antibody from the resultant antibody-producing cell lines (depicted as group of blue-hashed cells and group of red-hashed cells). These resultant antibodies (i.e., antibodies that each recognize distinct epitopes on a single presenting antigen) are designated as polyclonal antibodies and may be collectively harvested from the host animal for broad applications. Alternatively, a single antibody-producing B-cell clone may be harvested from the spleen and fused with myeloma cells to create immortalized hybridoma cells. These hybrid cells produce monoclonal antibodies (i.e., antibodies that recognize a single epitope on the presenting antigen) and may be grown in cell culture in a manner independent from the original host animal

guinea pig, rabbit, sheep, goat, and baboon) but represent a heterogeneous population of immunoglobulins that may target different epitopes on the same presenting antigen. While easier to produce, the resultant polyclonal antibodies may have drastically different and diverse binding and physical properties, resulting in the potential for significant batch-to-batch variability. In order to avoid the pitfalls of polyclonal antibodies, antibody engineers sought new technologies for generating antibodies with improve homogeneity and consistency. Although far more complex to produce, these resultant homogeneous antibodies, designated as monoclonal antibodies (MAbs), allow for enhanced performance and reliability when applied to radioimmunoguided strategies.

The production of MAbs from mouse hybridoma cells by way of a technique called hybridoma fusion technology has its origins in the early 1970s [1, 21–23]. This technology was first reported in 1973/1974 by Jerold Schwaber and Edward Cohen from the University of Chicago (Chicago, Illinois, USA) [21, 22] and was later popularized in 1975 by Georges Köhler and César Milstein from the MCR Laboratory of Molecular Biology (Cambridge, United Kingdom) [23], and for which Köhler and Milstein subsequently received and shared the Nobel Prize in Physiology or Medicine in 1984 with Niels K. Jerne. Simply stated, hybridoma fusion technology represents a process in which a B-cell lymphocyte (which recognized a single particular epitope on a presenting antigen and subsequently produced a single antibody targeting that particular epitope) and a myeloma cell are fused together to create a hybridoma cell (Fig. 24.1). This immortalized hybridoma cell has the ability to be tissue cultured and grown independently of the original host animal. Each stable hybridoma cell culture can produce a large amount of a single antibody, thus representing the resultant monoclonal antibody (MAb).

Homogeneous antibody production has not been the only challenge facing researchers for creating antibody products with enhanced performance and reliability that can be utilized in clinical medicine, including in various radioimmunoguided strategies. Most notably, MAbs have been shown to elicit a human anti-mouse antibody (HAMA) response in patients, especially with repeated administrations of murine antibodies [24]. In the years that followed the Köhler and Milstein accomplishment, several recombinant strategies were developed to engineer less immunogenic MAbs (Fig. 24.2). In 1984, Sherie Morrison (Columbia University, New York, New York, USA), Jacqueline Johnson and Leonard Herzenberg (Stanford University School of Medicine, Stanford, California, USA), and Vernon Oi (Becton-Dickinson Monoclonal Center, Mountain View, California, USA) engineered the first chimeric MAbs [25]. Specifically, they genetically fused the variable domain genes of a mouse antibody-producing myeloma cell line to the human immunoglobulin constant domain genes. This recombinant gene yielded a chimeric antibody that was approximately 67 % human in amino acid composition and retained its ability to bind antigen. Unfortunately, the two remaining murine domains (i.e., variable heavy and variable light domains) each had some potential for eliciting a HAMA response. This immunogenicity issue was further addressed in 1988 by Greg Winter and colleagues from the MCR Laboratory of Molecular Biology (Cambridge, United Kingdom) by the development of grafting techniques for humanization of MAbs [26]. Here, only the complementary determining regions (CDRs) from a rat antibody directed against human lymphocytes were grafted into a human IgG antibody framework. Immunoglobulins that were recombinantly produced in this fashion were approximately 90–95 % humanized. Later on, the degree of humanization for MAbs was further increased by Jeffrey Schlom and his colleagues from the National Cancer Institute (Bethesda, Maryland, USA) [27]. Here, they empirically determined the minimal set of murine residues within the CDRs required for antibody binding to an anti-

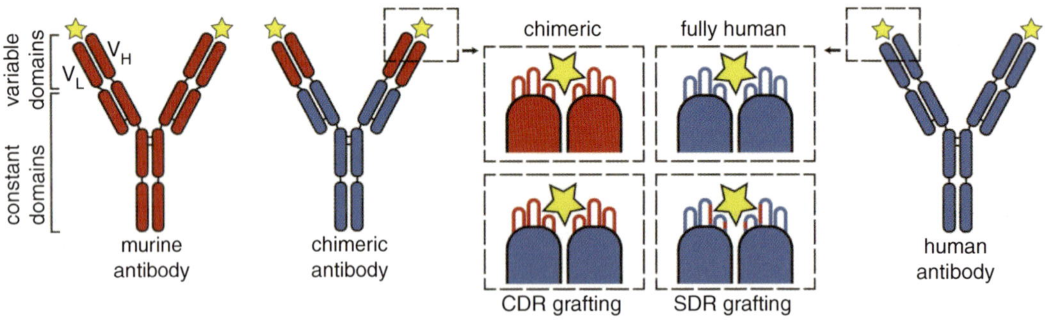

Fig. 24.2 Humanization of IgG monoclonal antibodies. Monoclonal antibodies developed from nonhuman species may elicit an undesired immune response when administered to a patient (i.e., HAMA – human anti-mouse antibodies response). Several recombinant strategies have been developed to humanize these antibody molecules. Here, murine domains and amino acid residues are depicted in red, human domains and amino acid residues are depicted in blue, antigen is shown as yellow stars, and CDR (complementary determining region) loops are shown as lines interacting with antigen within the inset *dashed-lined boxes*. Chimeric antibodies are gene fusions between the variable domains (*VL* variable light, *VH* variable heavy) of nonhuman antigen-binding antibodies to human constant domains. CDR grafting replaces the variable loops of human antibodies with the nonhuman loops of an antibody that recognizes the antigen of interest. Finally, SDR (site determining region) grafting replaces only the nonhuman loop residues essential for antigen binding in a human antibody scaffold. Grafting strategies yield monoclonal antibodies that retain the desirable property (i.e., binding) of the nonhuman monoclonal antibody but are significantly humanized (approximately 90–95 %), thus reducing the potential for HAMA response in patients

gen of interest. In this specific case, 5 amino acid residues within the 6 CDRs were identified as essential for binding to antigen. These investigators recombinantly engineered those 5 murine amino acid residues into a homologous human antibody. This designed antibody retained binding and did not react with the anti-variable region antibodies within stored patient serum samples being tested.

The techniques described within the previous paragraph represent strategies for converting mammalian nonhuman MAbs (i.e., those isolated from murine, rat, guinea pig, rabbit, sheep, goat, or baboon) into immunoglobulins that more closely resemble those that are circulating in human sera (i.e., humanization), in order to prevent any undesired immune responses such as HAMA. These techniques can be especially useful for pre-existing mammalian nonhuman MAbs that recognize known tumor-associated antigens and other antigenic targets of interests that have established applications in clinical medicine. While many talented researchers have developed these methods for humanizing MAbs, other investigators have sought techniques to directly produce human antibodies that are directed against antigenic targets of interest. One such strategy enables human MAbs to be obtained through transgenic mice that express the human antibody repertoire [28, 29] followed by traditional hybridoma techniques. After immunization, B cells from the spleens of these transgenic mice are isolated and immortalized via hybridoma technologies. Subsequent tissue cultures produce fully human MAbs. Another strategy enables human MAbs to be obtained through recombinant techniques paired with *in vitro* selection strategies [30–32]. Once Greg Winter and John McCafferty from the MCR Laboratory of Molecular Biology (Cambridge, United Kingdom) showed that antibody fragments could be displayed on filamentous phage and selected for antigen binding [30], the *in vitro* technology was aimed at selecting and engineering human antibodies that bypassed immunization and hybridoma operations [31, 32]. In this recombinant MAb process, antibody domain genes were first recovered from the human source cell type, and these antibody genes were then amplified and cloned into an appropriate vector (generally derived from plasmids or viruses) for phage display and selected in vitro for antigen binding. Subsequently, phage carrying genes that encoded binding activity were isolated, subcloned into expression vectors, and introduced into a host (such as a bacteria, yeast, filamentous fungi, and mammalian cell) for which expression of adequate amounts of the resultant functional antibody was ultimately achieved. MAbs produced in these manners were fully human, were easily produced, and did not elicit any HAMA response.

All of these pioneering studies to produce homogenous (i.e., MAbs) and nonimmunogenic (i.e., humanized and fully human) antibodies have set the stage for further development and engineering of MAbs with ideal properties for various radioimmunoguided strategies, including radioimmunoguided surgery.

24.4 The Ideal Monoclonal Antibody and Radiolabeling

There are several important features which are considered essential for designing the ideal MAb [1, 13, 15, 17, 33–35]. These features include (1) a high association constant for the antigen of interest ($K_a = k_{on}/k_{off}$, where k_{on} is the rate of association and k_{off} is the rate of dissociation), (2) rapid penetration into the tumor tissue environment, (3) specificity for the antigen of interest, (4) rapid clearance of unbound MAb from the systemic circulation, (5) minimal accumulation of MAb within normal tissues, (6) the absence of a HAMA response, and (7) favorable biophysical properties, including ease of manufacturing, homogeneity, low aggregation propensity, serum stability, and thermodynamic stability.

The particular structural form of the MAb utilized for radioimmunodetection (i.e., whether it is a whole MAb or a MAb fragment/derivative) can affect the degree and success of tumor localization [1, 17]. MAb fragments/derivatives have smaller molecular weights, more rapid tumor penetration, and faster clearance from the systemic circulation. As a result, the use of radiolabeled MAb fragments/derivatives can lead to lower background activity within normal tissues and sera and an increased tumor-to-background ratio, thus improving overall tumor detection. However, if the retention time of the MAb fragment/derivative by the tumor is too short and the clearance rate from the systemic circulation is too rapid, the resultant window of time for radioimmunodetection may be too brief to make its use clinically efficacious. Likewise, since MAb fragments/derivatives tend to accumulate more rapidly within the kidneys and urinary system, radioimmunodetection of the tumors within or around the regions of the kidneys, ureters, and bladder can be significantly impaired. For all of these reasons, it is critically important to understand the pharmacokinetic and biodistribution properties of each molecule.

Whole MAbs and their fragments/derivatives require radiolabeling for their application to various radioimmunoguided strategies, including radioimmunoguided surgery. The MAb radiolabeling process can be impactful on the efficacy of a radionuclide-MAb conjugate [1, 13, 17]. The conjugation of a radionuclide to a MAb may potentially change the specific target antigen-binding properties of a given MAb. If the specific target antigen-binding properties of the MAb are significantly altered, the resultant radiolabeled MAb may be left with significantly reduced affinity (i.e., binding) for the intended target antigen, thus ultimately rendering the radionuclide-MAb conjugate clinically ineffective. However, it is worth noting that in most instances the radiolabeling of whole MAbs and MAb fragments/derivatives has little effect on affinity (i.e., binding) of the resultant radionuclide-MAb conjugate for the intended target antigen.

Two of the most significant challenges faced when utilizing radiolabeled MAb in radioimmunodetection are related to the radioactivity ratio of the radiolabeled MAb between tumor and normal surrounding tissues (i.e., tumor-to-background ratio) and the time interval between the initial administration of the radiolabeled MAb and the performance of radioimmunodetection (i.e., diagnostic nuclear medicine imaging or radioimmunoguided surgery) [1]. In an attempt to increase the radioactivity ratio between tumor and normal surrounding tissues and to decrease the time interval between the initial administration of the radiolabeled MAb and the performance of radioimmunodetection, pretargeting strategies for MAbs and radionuclides have been investigated [36–39].

One such pretargeting strategy utilizes the principle of the avidin-biotin binding system [1, 36, 37]. In this avidin-biotin binding system, the MAb is labeled with biotin, and the radionuclide is labeled with avidin, thus permitting complete temporal separation of the systemic delivery of the MAb from the systemic delivery of the radionuclide and ultimately leading to a reduction of nonspecific binding of the radiolabeled MAb. The biotin-labeled MAb is first administered, allowing binding of the biotin-labeled MAb to the tumor and thus allowing the nonspecific uptake of the biotin-labeled MAb to be cleared. Subsequently, the avidin-labeled radionuclide is then administered, with resultant localization to the tumor secondary to the high affinity and specificity of the avidin-labeled radionuclide for the biotin-labeled MAb.

Another such pretargeting strategy utilizes an unradiolabeled bispecific antibody and radiolabeled bivalent hapten system for cooperative binding to target cells [1, 37–39]. This strategy is analogous to the avidin-biotin binding system. However, in this pretargeting approach, a bispecific antibody is used to link the tumor-associated antigen to a radiolabeled hapten. The bispecific antibody generally contains two distinct recognition arms, one arm responsible for tumor-associated antigen binding and a second arm that associates with the radiolabeled hapten that is administered to the patient after the bispecific antibody has associated with sites of tumor and has fully cleared from the systemic circulation.

While further pretargeting strategies are currently in active development, most radioimmunoguided applications continue to rely upon non-pretargeting strategies which simply involve the direct conjugation of the radionuclide to the MAb prior to its systemic administration.

24.5 Tumor-Associated Antigens and Their Specific Monoclonal Antibodies Used in Radioimmunoguided Surgery

A variety of MAbs have been developed against numerous tumor-associated antigens and have been evaluated regarding their clinical application to radioimmunodetection and radioimmunoguided surgery [1, 17, 19]. The most intensely investigated and clinically evaluated MAbs, which have been utilized in radioimmunoguided surgery, have been those directed against tumor-associated glycoprotein-72 (TAG-72), carcinoembryonic antigen (CEA), tumor-associated antigen 17-1A, and carbonic anhydrase IX (CAIX).

24.5.1 Tumor-Associated Glycoprotein-72 (TAG-72)

TAG-72 is a tumor-associated glycoprotein, which is comprised of approximately 80 % carbohydrate moieties and which has a molecular weight of greater than 10 million daltons [1, 40, 41]. It has mucin-like biochemical and biophysical properties which are similar to that of colonic, small intestine, and gastric mucins and is believed to be specifically secreted by epithelial-derived tissues. The TAG-72 antigen is predominantly found within extracellular mucin pools of the tumor environment and is to a lesser degree located on adenocarcinoma cell surfaces. Numerous human adenocarcinomas are known to overexpress the TAG-72 antigen, including colorectal, gastric, esophageal, pancreatic, endometrial, ovarian, lung, prostate, and breast [1, 40–47], with TAG-72 overexpression reported in over 90 % of the colorectal, gastric, and ovarian adenocarcinomas and in approximately 70 % of breast adenocarcinomas [1, 42, 44–47]. While TAG-72 is rarely expressed in normal human adult tissues or in benign disease processes, it is known to be expressed in some normal human fetal tissues, including normal fetal intestine [1, 48]. It should be acknowledged that nearly all of the pioneering work done on the TAG-72 antigen and subsequently on the development of anti-TAG-72 MAbs was conducted by Jeffrey Schlom and his colleagues from the National Cancer Institute (Bethesda, Maryland, USA) [1, 17, 40, 41, 43–54].

The first generation of anti-TAG-72 MAb was the B72.3 murine MAb [1, 17]. From a factual standpoint, it is most interesting and somewhat ironic that B72.3 was originally derived from human mammary tumor cells [1, 49], rather than from human colorectal cancer cells. B72.3 murine MAb is known to be reactive with a variety of human adenocarcinomas, including colorectal (94 %), breast (84 % of invasive ductal carcinomas of the breast), ovarian (100 % of common epithelial ovarian tumors), as well as the majority of gastric, pancreatic, endometrial, and lung adenocarcinomas [1, 17, 42, 44, 46–48, 50]. For the most part, B72.3 murine MAb is only very weakly reactive or nonreactive to most normal adult human tissues [1, 17]. The only exception being that normal postovulatory (secretory phase) endometrium demonstrates reactivity to B72.3 murine MAb, whereas normal preovulatory (proliferative phase) endometrium is nonreactive [1, 17, 50].

The second generation of anti-TAG-72 MAbs was murine CC49 and murine CC83 [1, 17, 41, 51–53]. The CC49 murine MAb and CC83 murine MAb are known to recognize overlapping but distinctly different epitopes on the TAG-72 antigen as opposed to the B72.3 murine MAb. Both of these second generations of anti-TAG-72 MAbs have only minimal reactivity to a variety of normal human tissues, in a fashion similar to that of B72.3 murine MAb. However, from a comparative standpoint, CC49 murine MAb and CC83 murine MAb demonstrated higher association constants (K_a 16.2 × 10^9 M^{-1} and K_a 27.7 × 10^9 M^{-1}, respectively) as compared to B72.3 murine MAb (K_a 2.5 × 10^9 M^{-1}), exhibiting higher reactivity to a wide range of human adenocarcinomas, including colorectal, breast, ovarian, and lung adenocarcinomas, as compared to B72.3 murine MAb [1, 17, 51–53].

It is well documented in the literature that a majority of patients receiving murine MAbs develop some degree of a HAMA response [1, 17, 24, 43, 54, 55]. Despite the fact that this resultant HAMA response has been well studied and thoroughly reported within the literature, its actual clinical relevancy and impact on cancer patients, whether deleterious or beneficial, has never been well borne out, as it generally represents a subclinical event [1, 56, 57]. Nonetheless, in an effort to eliminate this HAMA response, a third-generation anti-TAG-72 MAb, humanized CC49 MAb (HuCC49 MAb), was genetically engineered in the mid-1990s [1, 58]. This intact HuCC49 MAb demonstrates equivalent tumor targeting for human colon carcinoma xenografts but exhibits the trade-off of having a slightly less relative affinity to the TAG-72 antigen as compared to CC49 murine MAb and CC49 chimeric MAb. In contrast to CC49 murine MAb and CC49 chimeric MAb, the intact HuCC49 MAb was shown to not produce a HAMA response [1, 59]. Further refinements were engineered into the intact HuCC49 MAb by the development of a higher affinity HuCC49 MAb molecule possessing a C_H2 domain deletion (i.e., HuCC49ΔC_H2 MAb) [1, 60]. This HuCC49ΔC_H2 MAb exhibited more rapid clearance from the systemic circulation, higher association constant (K_a 5.1 × 10^{-9} M^{-1} versus K_a 2.1 × 10^{-9} M^{-1}), and significantly lower percent of the injected dose in normal background tissues as compared to intact HuCC49 MAb, thus representing factors thought to be more desirable for diagnostic and therapeutic clinical applications. Furthermore, a population pharmacokinetic modeling analysis performed on precordial count data from 21 patients receiving intravenous injection of ^{125}I-HuCC49ΔC_H2 MAb and 34 patients receiving intravenous injection of ^{125}I-CC49 murine MAb demonstrated that HuCC49ΔC_H2 MAb had a more rapid clearance (65 % increase) from the systemic circulation and a resulting shorter "residence time" (24 % shorter) than that of CC49 murine MAb [1, 61].

By the later half of the 2000s, a fourth-generation anti-TAG-72 MAb was engineered, with the hope of creating an adenocarcinoma targeting agent that could be applied toward future-integrated radioimmunodetection and therapeutic strategies [62, 63]. This fourth-generation anti-TAG-72 MAb was a new humanized version of CC49 murine MAb. This humanized version of CC49 murine MAb was constructed by grafting only the specificity-determining residues (SDRs) within the complementarity-determining regions (CDRs) onto homologous human immunoglobulin (IgG) germ line segments while retaining two mouse heavy chain framework amino acid residues that supported the conformation of the CDRs [62]. The resultant humanized antibody (AKA) demonstrated only a twofold lower association constant (K_a) compared with the original murine CC49 and a 27-fold lower reactivity to patient serum compared with HuCC49 that was constructed by CDR grafting. The affinity of this parental AKA was improved by random mutagenesis of 5 SDR residues in the heavy chain CDR3 (HCDR3). The highest affinity variant (i.e., 3E8) showed 22-fold higher association constant (K_a) compared with the parental AKA and retained the original epitope specificity. In a subsequent separate study [63], the light chain of the parental AKA was modified using a phage display chain shuffling approach to create a completely humanized light chain against the TAG-72 antigen, which contained no residual mouse-derived amino acid residues. In this approach, the heavy chain variable region of the parental AKA was used to guide the selection of a human TAG-72-specific light chain variable region from a human light chain variable region repertoire constructed from human peripheral blood lymphocytes. This phage display chain shuffling procedure yielded a fully humanized light chain that bound the TAG-72 antigen with higher affinity than the parental AKA. The authors suggested that the fully humanized light chain produced in this study could be used to guide the complete humanization of the matching heavy chain via further phage display shuffling. A molecule of this design would represent the complete humanization of an immunoglobulin from its murine origin.

The Thomas Magliery Laboratory (The Ohio State University, Columbus, Ohio, USA; https://chemistry.osu.edu/~magliery/) has continued to engineer the 3E8 MAb for enhanced performance in radioimmunoguided imaging and radioimmunoguided surgery applications by reducing the size to single-chain variable fragments (scFvs) and other small oligomers (such as diabody and tetrabody molecules) with maintained higher avidity. These various antibody fragments of 3E8 retain antigen binding to TAG-72 and are as thermally stable as the full-length IgG form of the 3E8 MAb [Personal communications: Thomas J. Magliery, The Ohio State University, Columbus, Ohio, USA, magliery.1@osu.edu, February 5, 2015; and Brandon J. Sullivan, The Ohio State University, Columbus, Ohio, USA, sullivan.272@osu.edu, February 5, 2015].

24.5.2 Carcinoembryonic Antigen (CEA)

Carcinoembryonic antigen (CEA) is a tumor-associated glycoprotein with a molecular weight of approximately 200,000 daltons [1, 17, 64, 65]. CEA is well known to be highly expressed on the cell surface of both embryonic colonic mucosa and a variety of human adenocarcinomas, including colorectal, gastric, pancreatic, ovarian, endometrial, lung, and breast [1, 17, 64–66]. As it specifically pertains to colorectal adenocarcinomas, it is well documented that anywhere from 66 to 100 % of colorectal adenocarcinomas express CEA.

Various murine MAbs have been developed to specifically target CEA, including COL-1, A_5B_7, IMMU-4, and CL58 [1, 17, 64, 67–72]. These anti-CEA murine MAbs have a very high affinity to CEA and have been shown to have a high reactivity to a significant percentage of colon, lung, and breast adenocarcinomas. Their high reactivity to CEA-producing human adenocarcinomas have made these anti-CEA murine MAbs the subject of prior intense investigation into their clinical utility for diagnostic radioimmunodetection imaging, as well as for possible radioimmunoguided surgery applications.

24.5.3 Tumor-Associated Antigen 17-1A

Tumor-associated antigen 17-1A (also referred to as EpCAM) is a tumor-associated glycoprotein which has a molecular weight of approximately 30,000–40,000 daltons and is believed to represent a surface, epithelial cell-to-cell adhesion-type molecule [1, 73–77]. The existence of 17-1A was first characterized on a human colorectal adenocarcinoma cell line SW1083. 17-1A is widely expressed on the cell surface of various normal human epithelial tissues and in a variety of human adenocarcinomas, including colorectal, gastric, and breast.

Murine MAbs against 17-1A were originally developed in the hybridoma SW1083-17-1A [1, 18, 78, 79]. The localization and clearance properties of the 17-1A whole murine MAb and its MAb fragment were previously assessed in a mouse xenograft model by Martin et al. [1, 12, 18], and for which they demonstrated high tumor-to-normal tissue ratios, with the highest tumor-to-normal tissue ratios seen at 72 and 24 h for the 17-1A whole murine MAb and MAb fragment, respectively.

24.5.4 Carbonic Anhydrase IX (CAIX)

The carbonic anhydrase IX (CAIX) antigen is a cytosolic transmembrane glycoprotein [80–84]. The CAIX antigen represents one of the many carbonic anhydrase enzymes that are involved in catalyzing the reaction $CO_2 + H_2O \leftrightarrow HCO_3^- + H^+$, a process ultimately important in the regulation of cellular proton flux and pH regulation. It is well established that the CAIX antigen is constitutively expressed by up to 97–98 % of all clear cell renal cell carcinomas [80–88], including both primary tumors and sites of metastatic disease. Yet it is absent from normal kidney tissues (including normal adult proximal tubular epithelial cells and fetal kidney tissue) and is minimally expressed or absent in other much less common renal epithelial neoplasms, including papillary renal cell carcinomas, chromophobe renal cell carcinomas, and oncocytoma.

The MAb G250 recognizes the CAIX antigen [1, 82–84]. In 1986, the IgG murine MAb Grawitz 250 (G250) was first described in the literature by Egbert Oosterwijk and his colleagues at the University of Leiden (Leiden, The Netherlands)

[82, 84, 85, 89, 90]. Later on, for attempting to minimize the occurrence of HAMA response, a chimerized version of the murine MAb G250 was developed (chimeric MAb cG250) with the same affinity and binding characteristics as murine MAb G250 [84, 90, 91]. All forms of G250 MAb are well known to bind to clear cell renal cell carcinomas with relatively high specificity [1, 89–93]. The use of G250 MAbs for clear cell renal cell carcinoma applications related to radioimmunoimaging and various radioimmunotherapy strategies has long been recognized by Oosterwijk [82–85, 89–92].

24.6 Clinical Applications of Radioimmunoguided Surgery

24.6.1 Colorectal Cancer

24.6.1.1 Radioimmunoguided Surgery Using 17-1A Murine Monoclonal Antibody

Early on, it was the availability of MAb antibody and antibody fragment against the tumor-associated antigen 17-1A which allowed investigators at The Ohio State University (Columbus, Ohio, USA) to conduct initial radioimmunoguided surgery clinical studies for exploring the utility of ^{125}I-labled MAbs and for allowing the development and refinement of various prototype handheld gamma detection probe system designs which could discriminate between tumor-bearing tissues and normal background tissues [1, 12, 94].

In 1986, O'Dwyer et al. [1, 94] at The Ohio State University (Columbus, Ohio, USA) reported on intraoperative radioimmunodetection of ^{125}I-17-1A murine MAbs using a prototype handheld gamma detection probe system in a total of 16 evaluable colorectal cancer patients (with 2 patients excluded secondary to intraoperative malfunctioning of the prototype handheld gamma detection probe system). Patients were intravenously injected with 1–4 mCi (37–148 MBq) of either ^{125}I-17-1A whole murine MAb at approximately 3–6 days prior to surgery or ^{125}I-labeled murine MAb fragment F(ab')$_2$ at approximately 2–3 days prior to surgery. A total of 20 potential tumor sites were evaluated in the 16 evaluable patients with the prototype handheld gamma detection probe. Overall tumor localization of ^{125}I-17-1A murine MAbs was confirmed with the prototype handheld gamma detection probe in 15 of 20 (75 %) potential tumor sites examined, with higher tumor-to-background ratios detected in ^{125}I-17-1A whole murine MAb patients (3.4-to-1.0) as compared to ^{125}I-labeled murine MAb fragment F(ab')$_2$ patients (2.3-to-1.0). From the 16 evaluable patients, histologically confirmed occult or subclinical disease was identified in 18 % of these patients that was not otherwise clinically detectable by traditional intraoperative inspection and palpation techniques. This initial study demonstrated the clinical feasibility of ^{125}I-labeled MAb radioimmunoguided surgery and provided useful information on issues related to optimization of the timing between ^{125}I-labeled MAb injection and surgery for enhancing intraoperative radioimmunodetection in all subsequent ^{125}I-labeled MAb clinical investigations.

In 1991, Petty et al. [1, 95] at The Ohio State University (Columbus, Ohio, USA) reported on intraoperative radioimmunodetection of ^{125}I-17-1A murine MAb using a commercially available gamma detection probe system in 13 colorectal cancer patients, including 6 primary colorectal cancer patients and 7 recurrent colorectal cancer patients. Patients were intravenously injected with 2 mCi (74 MBq) of ^{125}I-17-1A murine MAb. In this clinical study, radioimmunodetection accomplished by a commercially available gamma detection probe system that incorporated a microprocessor into the control unit (Neoprobe® 1000 gamma detection probe; formerly Neoprobe Corporation, Dublin, Ohio, USA), and for which the control unit maintained a running average of the count rate and produced an audible siren sound when the count rate of an area of increased radioactivity exceeds the background count rate by a statistically significant amount using the three-sigma statistical threshold for probe positivity [1, 15]. The feasibility of predicting ^{125}I-17-1A murine MAb blood clearance was reproducible utilizing the external precordial count method (i.e., when external precordial counts reached ≤10 counts per second), with 11 of 13 (85 %) patients demonstrating adequate clearance by 10 days after the ^{125}I-17-1A murine MAb injection. Overall tumor localization of ^{125}I-17-1A murine MAb by radioimmunoguided surgery was confirmed in 8 of 13 (62 %) patients, with successful localization demonstrated in 2 of 6 (33 %) primary colorectal cancer patients and 6 of 7 (86 %) recurrent colorectal cancer patients [1, 95]. There was localization of ^{125}I-17-1A murine MAb at radioimmunoguided surgery in 12 of 18 (67 %) suspected sites of disease. Of the 12 sites of tumor localization of ^{125}I-17-1A murine MAb, histologic confirmation of malignant cells by hematoxylin and eosin (H&E) staining was demonstrated in 8 of 12 sites (67 %), and additional histologic evaluation with immunohistochemical staining and autoradiography identified malignant cells in all 12 sites of tumor localization of ^{125}I-17-1A murine MAb. Radioimmunoguided surgery identified occult disease in 3 of 7 (43 %) of the recurrent colorectal cancer patients which was not identified by traditional intraoperative inspection and palpation techniques. In comparison to the prior initial clinical report by O'Dwyer et al. [1, 94], a higher occult disease detection rate was seen by Petty et al. [1, 95], and for which this was thought to be a reflection of lower blood-pool background levels of ^{125}I-17-1A murine MAb at the time of surgery and secondary to technical design improvements to the gamma detection probe system.

24.6.1.2 Radioimmunoguided Surgery Using B72.3 Murine Monoclonal Antibody

Radioimmunoguided surgery specifically directed against the TAG-72 antigen has its origins in preclinical investigations on a human colon carcinoma xenograft mouse model in athymic mice using B72.3 murine MAb, the first-generation anti-TAG-72 MAb [1, 96]. In these preclinical investigations, it was determined that significant specific uptake of ^{131}I-B72.3 murine MAb within subcutaneous tumor implants occurred within the first 48 h after the intravenous injection of ^{131}I-B72.3 murine MAb. It was shown that subcutaneous tumor implant uptake of ^{131}I-B72.3 murine MAb subsequently remained stable over a 19-day study period, while blood-pool background and the normal tissue background levels continued to clear over time, thus yielding continued increasing tumor-to-background ratios over the 19-day study period. This high degree of specific tumor targeting and associated prolonged retention of the radiolabeled B72.3 murine MAb that was demonstrated in this preclinical work was important in the decision-making to utilize the B72.3 murine MAb for subsequent radioimmunoguided surgery clinical trials involving colorectal cancer patients [1, 96–115].

In 1987, Sickle-Santanello et al. [1, 97] at The Ohio State University (Columbus, Ohio, USA) reported their first human clinical trial utilizing ^{125}I-B72.3 murine MAb and a prototype handheld gamma detection probe system in 37 colorectal cancer patients, including 6 patients with primary colorectal cancer and 31 with recurrent disease. Patients were injected intravenously with approximately 4 mCi (148 MBq) of ^{125}I-B72.3 murine MAb at a time of 5–34 days (mean 16.4 days) prior to surgery. The ^{125}I-B72.3 murine MAb localized in 8 of 9 (89 %) sites in the 6 primary colorectal cancer patients, including in 5 of 6 primary tumors and in 3 of 3 metastatic sites. The ^{125}I-B72.3 murine MAb localized in 47 of 57 (82 %) suspected sites of disease in the 31 recurrent colorectal cancer patients, with a resultant modification of the planned surgical procedure in 8 of 31 (26 %) of those recurrent colorectal cancer patients.

Subsequently, in 1988, Martin et al. [1, 98, 99] at The Ohio State University (Columbus, Ohio, USA) reported on the utilization of ^{125}I-B72.3 murine MAb and a prototype handheld gamma detection probe system in a total of 66 patients with various types of adenocarcinoma, including 45 colorectal cancer patients (6 primary colorectal cancer patients and 39 patients with recurrent disease). All colorectal cancer patients were injected intravenously with approximately

4–5 mCi (148–185 MBq) of ^{125}I-B72.3 murine MAb at a time of 7–22 days (mean 15 days) prior to surgery for the primary colorectal cancer patients and at a time of 5–42 days (mean 19 days) prior to surgery for patients with recurrent disease. Tumor localization of ^{125}I-B72.3 MAb was observed in 5 of 6 (83 %) patients with primary colorectal cancer and in 31 of 39 (79 %) patients with recurrent colorectal cancer. There was an observed correlation between the length of the injection-to-surgery interval and the adequacy of clearance of the blood-pool background, yielding greater tumor-to-normal tissue count ratios of localized ^{125}I-B72.3 murine MAb at longer injection-to-surgery intervals. Likewise, there was an observed improvement in the counting rate by a factor of approximately 2.5 when the diameter of the probe detector crystal was increased and the crystal mounting and preamplifier were modified.

In 1990, Nieroda et al. [1, 100] at The Ohio State University (Columbus, Ohio, USA) further demonstrated the prolonged retention of ^{125}I-B72.3 murine MAb and adequate clearance of the blood-pool background at the time of radioimmunoguided surgery in primary colon cancer patients. A total of 30 patients with primary colon cancer were intravenously injected with 1–5 mCi (37–185 MBq) of ^{125}I-B72.3 murine MAb, as part of a dose-range study, at a time of 22.3 days (range from 8 to 34 days) prior to surgery. Intraoperative radioimmunodetection of ^{125}I-B72.3 murine MAb was undertaken using a commercially available gamma detection probe system. The ^{125}I-B72.3 murine MAb localized in histologically confirmed tumor among 23 of 30 (77 %) of patients. Of the 23 localized patients, 7 (30 %) patients had occult disease within either the liver, lymph nodes, and/or invasion in adjacent tissues that was identified by the gamma detection probe but which was not identified by traditional intraoperative inspection and palpation techniques. The finding of occult disease led to a major alteration of the surgical plan in 6 of 23 (26 %) localized patients and a change in postoperative adjuvant therapy in 4 of 23 (17 %) localized patients. Additionally, the use of radioimmunoguided surgery provided pertinent and accurate intraoperative confirmatory information (i.e., gamma detection probe counts comparable to background) regarding tumor margin assessment and confirmation of histologically proven benign lesions of the liver and ovaries.

In 1991, Martin and Carey [1, 101] at The Ohio State University (Columbus, Ohio, USA) and The University of South Florida (Tampa, Florida, USA) reported on the ability of radioimmunoguided surgery using ^{125}I-B72.3 murine MAb to accurately determine resectability in patients with recurrent colorectal cancer undergoing a second-look surgery procedure. A total of 86 patients received a preoperative intravenous injection of 2 mCi (74 MBq) of ^{125}I-B72.3 murine MAb at approximately 24 days (range from 21 to 28 days) prior to surgery. The abdomen and pelvis were first explored by using traditional intraoperative inspection and palpation techniques. Prior to the use of the gamma detection probe, sites of tumor identified by traditional intraoperative inspection and palpation techniques were documented, and the surgeon indicated a surgical plan as based upon the findings noted by traditional intraoperative inspection and palpation techniques. The surgical field was then systematically re-explored using a commercially available gamma detection probe system, in order to attempt to identify areas of increased radioactivity compared to normal adjacent tissues and to determine whether the findings would alter the previously declared planned surgical procedure. Fifty-three patients of the 86 patients (62 %) were initially deemed resectable by traditional intraoperative inspection and palpation techniques. However, in contrast, only 40 patients of the 86 patients (47 %) were subsequently determined to be resectable by the application of radioimmunoguided surgical techniques. The survival data were reported for 3 classifications of patients: (1) radioimmunoguided surgery determined resectable patients ($n=40$), (2) traditional intraoperative inspection and palpation determined nonresectable patients ($n=33$), and (3) radioimmunoguided surgery determined nonresectable patients ($n=13$). Overall survival rate for the radioimmunoguided surgery determined resectable group was 83 % versus 21 % and 31 %

for the traditional intraoperative inspection and palpation determined nonresectable and radioimmunoguided surgery determined nonresectable groups, respectively. Significant differences in survival were observed in the radioimmunoguided surgery determined resectable versus traditional nonresectable groups ($p<0.0001$) and in the radioimmunoguided surgery determined resectable versus radioimmunoguided surgery determined nonresectable groups ($p<0.0008$). No significant differences were noted in the traditional intraoperative inspection and palpation determined nonresectable versus radioimmunoguided surgery determined nonresectable groups ($p=0.24$). The 2-year, 3-year, and 5-year survival rates were 95 %, 83 %, and 60 % for the radioimmunoguided surgery determined resectable group; 36 %, 7 %, and 0 % for the traditional intraoperative inspection and palpation determined nonresectable group; and 57 %, 37 %, and 0 % for the radioimmunoguided surgery determined nonresectable group, respectively.

In 1991, the safety and efficacy of ^{125}I-B72.3 murine MAb for tumor localization and occult disease detection was evaluated in a multicenter radioimmunoguided surgery clinical trial of 104 patients with primary ($n=26$) or known/suspected recurrent colorectal cancer ($n=78$; of which 72 were ultimately found to have histologic confirmation of recurrent disease) [1, 102]. This multicenter clinical trial was conducted at Memorial Sloan-Kettering Cancer Center (New York, New York, USA), The Ohio State University (Columbus, Ohio, USA), University of Pennsylvania (Philadelphia, Pennsylvania, USA), Ochsner Clinic (New Orleans, Louisiana, USA), University of Florida (Gainesville, Florida, USA), Cleveland Clinic Foundation (Cleveland, Ohio, USA), and Loma Linda University Medical Center (Loma Linda, CA, USA). All patients received a preoperative intravenous injection of 2 mCi (74 MBq) of ^{125}I-B72.3 murine MAb at approximately 24 days prior to surgery. At the time of surgery, traditional intraoperative inspection and palpation techniques were performed to the surgical field, followed by a systematically re-exploration of the surgical field using a commercially available gamma detection probe system. Tumor localization was identified with the gamma detection probe system in 78 % of the patients. This included 24 (75 %) of 32 sites in patients with primary tumor and 126 (63 %) of 199 sites in patients with recurrent disease. A total of 30 occult tumor sites of disease (not identified on prior clinical exam, preoperative diagnostic imaging, or were identified by traditional intraoperative inspection and palpation techniques) were identified with the gamma detection probe system alone in a total of 26 patients. Of all histologically confirmed tumor sites, 9.2 % represented clinically occult sites of disease identified only by the gamma detection probe system. The location of occult sites of disease in primary tumor patients included the liver ($n=4$), retroperitoneum ($n=2$), pelvis ($n=1$), and periportal region ($n=1$). Of the 72 patients with recurrent disease, 37 patients were deemed unresectable, with 10 of those patients (27 %) deemed unresectable by the gamma detection probe system alone. Additionally, of the 35 patients with recurrent disease who were deemed resectable, 8 of those patients (23 %) deemed resectable underwent a more extended surgical resection based upon the findings by the gamma detection probe system alone. Based upon serial serum samples taken from the time of injection of ^{125}I-B72.3 MAb and through the postoperative time frame, it was documented that 40 % of the patients injected with ^{125}I-B72.3 murine MAb ultimately developed HAMA; yet this was not felt to be negatively impactful on overall tumor localization with ^{125}I-B72.3 murine MAb. This multicenter radioimmunoguided surgery clinical trial using ^{125}I-B72.3 murine MAb confirmed a relatively low toxicity profile for ^{125}I-B72.3 murine MAb and demonstrated its utility in identifying occult sites of disease based upon the findings by the gamma detection probe system alone and its impact on altering the surgical management of patients with primary and recurrent colorectal cancer.

Further investigations regarding the clinical utility of radioimmunoguided surgery with ^{125}I-B72.3 murine MAb in colorectal cancer patients continued to be reported throughout the 1990s [1, 103–113].

From 1991 to 1995, Di Carlo et al. [103–108] from University of Milan (Milan, Italy) reported on radioimmunoguided surgery using ^{125}I-B72.3 murine MAb in a cumulative series of 66 colorectal cancer patients, including 36 primary colorectal cancer patients and 30 recurrent colorectal cancer patients. Patients were intravenously injected with 2 mCi (74 MBq) of ^{125}I-B72.3 murine MAb at an interval of approximately 21 days prior to surgery. This included 7 of 66 patients who were intravenously injected with ^{125}I-biotinylated B72.3 murine MAb, followed by 2 sequential intravenous injections of avidin for promoting more rapid clearance of the MAb from the blood-pool circulation prior to surgery. Intraoperative tumor localization with a gamma detection probe was successful in 18 of 36 (50 %) primary colorectal cancer patients and in 24 of 30 (80 %) recurrent colorectal cancer patients. The intraoperative gamma detection probe findings were instrumental in modifying the surgical approach in 9 of 66 (14 %) of patients, including 2 of 36 (6 %) primary colorectal cancer patients and 7 of 30 (23 %) recurrent colorectal cancer patients and thus leading to removal of occult sites of disease that would have otherwise gone unrecognized by traditional intraoperative inspection and palpation techniques alone.

In 1998, Bertoglio et al. [1, 109, 110] from University of Genoa (Genoa, Italy) evaluated radioimmunoguided surgery using ^{125}I-B72.3 murine MAb in 16 asymptomatic patients with a history of previously treated primary colorectal cancer who were suspected of having recurrent disease as based upon rising CEA levels. Patients were intravenously injected with a nonspecified dose of ^{125}I-B72.3 murine MAb at a nonspecified time prior to surgery. They found recurrent disease in only 9 of 16 patients (56 %) by traditional intraoperative inspection and palpation techniques alone at the time of surgical exploration but in 14 of 16 patients (88 %) using a combined approach of traditional intraoperative inspection and palpation techniques and systematic re-exploration of the surgical field using a commercially available gamma detection probe system, thus demonstrating additional occult sites of disease 5 of 16 patients (31.3 %) based upon the findings by the gamma detection probe alone. There were 9 of 16 patients (56 %) who were resected for cure as based upon additional findings with the gamma detection probe, whereas only 4 of 16 patients (25 %) would have been resected for cure as based upon the findings by traditional intraoperative inspection and palpation techniques.

In 1998, Percivale et al. [1, 109–111] from University of Genoa (Genoa, Italy) evaluated radioimmunoguided surgery with ^{125}I-B72.3 murine MAb in a group of 30 patients with recurrent or metastatic colorectal cancer using a commercially available gamma detection probe system. Patients were intravenously injected with 2 mCi (74 MBq) of ^{125}I-B72.3 murine MAb at a mean of 22.7 ± 3.1 days prior to surgery. A total of 46 histologically confirmed tumor sites were identified by traditional surgical exploration and radioimmunoguided surgery. Intraoperative gamma detection probe assessment identified 39 sites of ^{125}I-B72.3 murine MAb uptake. Radioimmunoguided surgery correctly identified tumor in 37 of 46 (80 %) histologically confirmed tumor sites, with only 2 of 39 (5 %) false-negative results. Based upon the findings of intraoperative gamma detection probe assessment alone, radioimmunoguided surgery identified additional occult sites of disease in 7 of 30 patients (23 %) which was not detected by traditional surgical exploration alone. The authors concluded that radioimmunoguided surgery with ^{125}I-B72.3 murine MAb provided essential information in selected cases for patients with recurrent or metastatic colorectal cancer.

In 1998, Renda et al. [1, 112] from University of Naples Federico II (Naples, Italy) reported on the detection of ^{125}I-B72.3 murine MAb by radioimmunoguided surgery in 23 patients with colorectal cancer. Patients were intravenously injected with a nonspecified dose of ^{125}I-B72.3 murine MAb at approximately 12–28 days prior to surgery. Radioimmunoguided surgery successfully identified tumor in 18 of 23 (78 %) ^{125}I-B72.3 murine MAb patients. The authors were unable to draw any significant conclusions from their radioimmunoguided surgery experience and recommended the evaluation of newer MAbs.

In 1999, Veroux et al. [113] from University of Catania (Catania, Italy) evaluated 25 colorectal cancer patients (including 20 primary colorectal cancer patients and 5 recurrent colorectal cancer patients) who were intravenously injected with 1.5–3 mCi (54–111 MBq) of ^{125}I-B72.3 murine MAb at approximately 16–19 days prior to surgery. Radioimmunoguided surgery successfully identified tumor in 18 of 25 patients (72 %), including 15 of 20 (75 %) primary colorectal cancer patients and 3 of 5 (60 %) recurrent colorectal cancer patients [Personal communication: Massimiliano Veroux, University Hospital of Catania, Catania, Italy, veroux@unict.it, January 8, 2015].

The utilization of ^{111}In-B72.3 murine MAb in radioimmunoguided surgery for colorectal cancer has been previously investigated in a somewhat limited fashion [1, 112, 114–116]. However, a common obstacle faced when using ^{111}In-B72.3 murine MAb in radioimmunodetection of colorectal cancer was the nonspecific accumulation of any given ^{111}In-B72.3 murine MAb conjugate within the liver, thus making it difficult to identify liver metastases and limiting its usefulness to the identification of only extrahepatic disease [117].

In 1992, Krag et al. [114] from University of California at Davis (Sacramento, California, USA) and University of Vermont (Burlington, Vermont, USA) investigated the detection of ^{111}In-CYT-103, an immunoconjugate of the B72.3 murine MAb, evaluated both by radioimmunoscintigraphy and radioimmunoguided surgery, in 8 patients with colorectal cancer, including 7 primary colorectal cancer patients and 1 patient with hepatic metastases. Patients were intravenously injected with approximately 5 mCi (185 MBq) of ^{111}In-CYT-103 at a time of 2–4 days prior to radioimmunoscintigraphy and 4–15 days prior to undergoing radioimmunoguided surgery. At the time of surgery, patients underwent surgical exploration by traditional inspection and palpation, followed by a systematically re-exploration of the surgical field using a commercially available gamma detection probe system. However, the authors did not perform a subgroup analysis of their data for the 8 patients with colorectal cancer as compared to the other 5 included patients with suspected recurrent ovarian cancer, thus making it impossible to gleam any information regarding their radioimmunoscintigraphy and radioimmunoguided surgery experience as it specifically related to colorectal cancer.

In 1998, Renda et al. [1, 112] from University of Naples Federico II (Naples, Italy) reported on the detection of ^{111}In-B72.3 murine MAb by radioimmunoguided surgery in 8 patients with colorectal cancer. Patients were intravenously injected with a nonspecified dose of ^{111}In-B72.3 murine MAb at approximately 5–8 days prior to surgery. Radioimmunoguided surgery successfully identified tumor in 5 of 8 (63 %) ^{111}In-B72.3 murine MAb patients. The authors were unable to draw any significant conclusions from their radioimmunoguided surgery experience and recommended the evaluation of newer MAbs.

In 1999, Muxi et al. [1, 115] from University of Barcelona (Barcelona, Spain) evaluated the detection of ^{111}In-CYT-103 by both radioimmunoscintigraphy and radioimmunoguided surgery in 28 patients with colorectal cancer, including 18 primary colorectal cancer patients and 10 patients with suspicion for recurrent disease. Patients were intravenously injected with 4–5 mCi (148–185 MBq) of ^{111}In-CYT-103 at approximately 72–96 h prior to surgery. Radioimmunoscintigraphy was performed 48–72 h after the injection of ^{111}In-CYT-103. At surgery, attempts were made to identified all possible sites of tumor by traditional intraoperative inspection and palpation techniques, and subsequently the surgical field was then systematically re-explored using a commercially available gamma detection probe, and a target-to-background ratio of greater than 1.5 was used as the cutoff for successful tumor localization. The overall sensitivity for radioimmunoscintigraphy was 71 %, consisting of successful tumor localization in 10 of 18 (56 %) primary tumors and in 10 of 10 (100 %) cases of recurrent disease. The overall sensitivity for radioimmunoguided surgery was 82 %, consisting of successful tumor localization in 15 of 18 (83 %) primary tumors and in 8 of 10 (80 %) cases of recurrent disease. There were 5 primary tumors of the rectum identified at radioimmunoguided surgery that were not detected on preoperative radioimmunoscintigraphy. Radioimmunoguided surgery changed the surgical management in 2 cases, including finding a small primary rectal cancer in one case and finding a small pelvic recurrence in another case, with both representing small-volume disease which was not identifiable by traditional intraoperative inspection and palpation techniques. The authors concluded that radioimmunoguided surgery complemented radioimmunoscintigraphy and was useful in the identification of small-volume disease that was difficult to identify by traditional surgical exploration.

In 2001, Hladik et al. [1, 116] from Charles University/Faculty of Medicine in Hradec Králové (Hradec Králové, Czech Republic) evaluated the detection of ^{111}In-CYT-103 by preoperative radioimmunoscintigraphy, radioimmunoguided surgery, and histology (H&E and immunohistochemistry) in 56 patients with either primary or recurrent colorectal cancer. Patients were intravenously injected with 4.3–5.0 mCi (160–185 MBq) of ^{111}In-CYT-103 at a time of approximately 5–7 days prior to surgery. Preoperative radioimmunoscintigraphy identified primary or recurrent tumor in 52 of 56 (93 %) patients. They determined that preoperative radioimmunoscintigraphy using ^{111}In-CYT-103 led to a sensitivity and accuracy for the detection of primary tumor or local recurrence of 93 % and 93 %, for the detection of hepatic metastases of 79 % and 95 %, and for the detection of extrahepatic metastases of 50 % and 66 %, respectively. Intraoperative gamma detection probe assessment identified radioimmunoguided surgery-positive lymph nodes in 32 of 56 (57 %) patients. Of the 32 radioimmunoguided surgery-positive lymph node patients, 24 (75 %) were confirmed positive for lymph node involvement by histology, including histologic confirmation recognized by immunohistochemistry alone in 6 of 24 (25 %) histologically confirmed lymph node-positive patients. The authors concluded that radioimmunoguided surgery was potentially useful in the surgical management of primary colorectal patients by improving the intraoperative assessment of the extent of disease and staging of disease as a result of more accurately identifying occult lymph node disease.

The utilization of ^{131}I-B72.3 murine MAb in radioimmunoguided surgery for colorectal cancer has been limited to only one report [112]. In 1998, Renda et al. [1, 112] from University of Naples Federico II (Naples, Italy) reported on the detection of ^{131}I-B72.3 murine MAb plus beta-interferon by radioimmunoguided surgery in 7 patients with colorectal cancer. Patients were intravenously injected with a nonspecified dose of ^{131}I-B72.3 murine MAb plus beta-interferon at approximately 7–10 days prior to surgery. Radioimmunoguided surgery successfully identified tumor in 4 of 7 (57 %) ^{131}I-B72.3 murine MAb plus beta-interferon patients. The authors were unable to draw any significant conclusions from their radioimmunoguided surgery experience and recommended the evaluation of newer MAbs.

24.6.1.3 Radioimmunoguided Surgery Using CC49 Murine Monoclonal Antibody and CC83 Murine Monoclonal Antibody

The most widely clinically investigated second generation of radiolabeled anti-TAG-72 MAb in radioimmunoguided surgery was the CC49 murine MAb [1]. Clinical investigations using ^{125}I-CC49 murine MAb in colorectal cancer were numerous during the 1990s [1, 118–130]. From a clinical perspective, CC49 murine MAb was shown to be superior to B72.3 murine MAb for tumor detection during radioimmunoguided surgery for colorectal cancer.

In 1992, Arnold et al. [1, 118] at The Ohio State University (Columbus, Ohio, USA) evaluated the efficiency of ^{125}I-CC49 murine MAb and its impact on radioimmunoguided surgery in a clinical trial of 54 colorectal cancer patients, including 24 patients with primary colorectal cancer and 30 patients with recurrent disease. All patients received an intravenous injection of 2 mCi (74 MBq) of ^{125}I-CC49 murine MAb at approximately 14–21 days prior to surgery. At the time of surgery, traditional intraoperative inspection and palpation techniques were performed to the surgical field, followed by a systematic re-exploration of the surgical field using a commercially available gamma detection probe system. At surgery, all radioimmunoguided surgery-positive tissue was considered malignant and was excised whenever possible. Tumor localization of the ^{125}I-CC49 murine MAb was successful in 86 % of primary colorectal cancer patients and in 97 % of patients with recurrent disease. In comparison to prior clinical trials using ^{125}I-B72.3 murine MAb, the tumor localization rates for ^{125}I-CC49 murine MAb were superior for targeting both primary colorectal cancer lesions and sites of recurrent disease. The intraoperative findings at the time of radioimmunoguided surgery altered the planned surgical procedure in 50 % of primary colorectal cancer patients and in 47 % of patients with recurrent disease, with the intraoperative identification of extrahepatic occult disease by the gamma detection probe resulting in the abandonment of hepatic resections in 3 patients. In this study, tissue specimens were categorized into 4 tissue specimen types, as based upon whether they were detected by radioimmunoguided surgery and by the presence or absence of histologically confirmed carcinoma by H&E staining. The 4 tissue specimen classifications were type I (radioimmunoguided surgery negative and histologic negative), type II (radioimmunoguided surgery negative and histologic positive), type III (radioimmunoguided surgery positive and histologic negative), and type IV (radioimmunoguided surgery positive and histologic positive). Arnold et al. [1, 118] were particularly interested in the type III lymph nodes and believed that the intraoperative detection of type III lymph nodes by radioimmunoguided surgery was a function of the presence of the TAG-72 within the extracellular environment. Type III lymph nodes were detected in both primary colorectal cancer cases ($n = 40$ specimens) and recurrent colorectal cancer cases ($n = 16$ specimens). The authors felt strongly that the intraoperative detection of type III lymph nodes by radioimmunoguided surgery was a reflection of greater disease burden than could be assess by standard histologic evaluation alone and therefore was important for the intraoperative assessment of the extent of disease and for predicting long-term patient outcomes. Along similar lines, Quinlan et al. [1, 131] evaluated excised lymph nodes from colorectal cancer patients and demonstrated a direct correlation between the immunohistochemical staining of the germinal centers of excised lymph nodes with CC49 murine MAb and poorer patient prognosis.

In 1995, Burak et al. [132] from The Ohio State University (Columbus, Ohio, USA) evaluated radioimmunoguided surgery in 17 patients with suspected recurrent colorectal cancer using ^{125}I-CC83 murine MAb. Patients were intravenously injected with 2 mCi (74 MBq) of ^{125}I-CC83 murine MAb at a time of 13–35 days (mean 26.6 days) prior to surgery. All patients underwent surgical exploration using traditional inspection and palpation, followed by a systematic re-exploration of the surgical field using a commercially available gamma detection probe system. There were 15 of 17 patients who were found to have histologically confirmed recurrent colorectal cancer. All 15 patients with histologically confirmed recurrent colorectal cancer demonstrated tumor localization of ^{125}I-CC83 murine MAb, whereas the 2 patients with no evidence of histologically confirmed recurrent colorectal cancer demonstrated no localization of ^{125}I-CC83 murine MAb. Traditional surgical exploration identified 32 sites as suspicious for tumor, and of which 23 (72 %) suspicious sites were histologically confirmed to contain carcinoma. Radioimmunoguided surgery identified 27 sites as suspicious for tumor, and of which all 27 (100 %) suspicious sites were histologically confirmed to contain carcinoma. Radioimmunoguided surgery identified occult disease that was histologically confirmed to contain carcinoma in 4 of 15 (27 %) patients, but which was not identified during surgical exploration using traditional inspection and palpation. There was a change in the surgical plan as a result of the occult findings at radioimmunoguided surgery in 3 of 15 (20 %) patients.

In 1995, Arnold et al. [1, 120] at The Ohio State University (Columbus, Ohio, USA) investigated the role of radioimmunoguided surgery as an intraoperative prognostic indicator of survival in primary colorectal cancer patients. All patients were intravenously injected with 2 mCi (74 MBq) of ^{125}I- CC49 murine MAb at approximately 21 days prior to the time of surgery. A total of 31 primary colorectal cancer patients with ^{125}I-CC49 murine MAb localization were assessed for the presence or absence of residual radioimmunoguided surgery-positive tissue detected in surgical field at the completion of the operative procedure. Patients were classified as radioimmunoguided surgery positive (i.e., residual radioimmunoguided surgery-positive tissue detected in surgical field at the completion of the operative procedure) or radioimmunoguided surgery negative (i.e., no residual radioimmunoguided surgery-positive tissue detected in surgical field at the completion of the operative procedure). A total of 109 extra-regional sites of radioimmunoguided surgery positivity were identified with the gamma detection probe, including the gastrohepatic ligament, celiac axis, pelvis, retroperitoneum, liver, omentum, small bowel and its mesentery, abdominal wall, and diaphragm. At the conclusion of the surgical procedure, there were 17 and 14 patients, respectively, who were assessed as radioimmunoguided surgery positive and radioimmunoguided surgery negative. For a patient follow-up duration that ranged from 30 to 54 months, only 2 of 17 patients (12 %) with residual radioimmunoguided surgery-positive tissue were still alive, while all 14 patients (100 %) with no residual radioimmunoguided surgery-positive tissue were still alive at last follow-up ($p<0.0001$). The authors concluded that the presence or absence of residual radioimmunoguided surgery-positive tissue provided immediate and accurate prognostic information regarding the behavior of the tumor and patient outcomes in primary colorectal cancer patients, with radioimmunoguided surgery-negative patients having improved overall survival.

In 1995, Bertsch et al. [1, 121] at The Ohio State University (Columbus, Ohio, USA) similarly investigated the role of radioimmunoguided surgery as an intraoperative prognostic indicator of survival in recurrent colorectal cancer patients. A total of 131 patients with recurrent colorectal cancer were injected with 2 mCi (74 MBq) of ^{125}I-B72.3 murine MAb ($n=86$) or 1 mCi (37 MBq) of ^{125}I-CC49 murine MAb ($n=45$) and underwent surgical exploration using traditional inspection and palpation, followed by a systematic re-exploration of the surgical field using a commercially available gamma detection probe system. Of the 49 patients judged as successfully resected at the end of their surgical procedure (i.e., radioimmunoguided surgery-negative patients with successful removal of all traditionally evident disease and all radioimmunoguided surgery-positive tissue), 55 % (27 patients) were alive at 2–8 years following surgery, with a minimal patient follow-up duration of 28 months. In contrast, of the 82 patients judged as unresectable or incompletely resected at the end of their surgical procedure (including by radioimmunoguided surgery), only 2.4 % (2 patients) were still alive at the end of the same analyzed patient follow-up duration. Likewise, none of the patients deemed to be surgically resectable by traditional intraoperative inspection and palpation techniques but unresectable by radioimmunoguided surgery were still alive. A significant improvement in survival ($p<0.0001$) was observed among patients with recurrent colorectal cancer undergoing a resection of all disease found by a combination of both traditional intraoperative inspection and palpation techniques and by radioimmunoguided surgery. The authors concluded that radioimmunoguided surgery provided useful immediate information regarding extent of disease and resectability, and provided accurate prognostic information regarding long-term patient outcome for recurrent colorectal cancer patients.

In 1998, Arnold et al. [1, 124] at The Ohio State University (Columbus, Ohio, USA) published a survival analysis of a longer follow-up duration on a group of 97 primary colorectal cancer patients who received a second-generation ^{125}I-labeled anti-TAG-72 MAb, consisting of either ^{125}I-CC49 murine MAb or ^{125}I-CC83 murine MAb, but for which the number of patients receiving ^{125}I-CC49 murine MAb versus ^{125}I-CC83 murine MAb was not specified. Survival was assessed using standard TNM staging (based upon histologic confirmation of disease) and using the presence or absence of radioimmunoguided surgery-positive tissue at the end of the surgical procedure. There were 38 patients deemed nonevaluable, secondary to the presence of nonresectable, stage IV disease ($n=26$), failure of tumor localization of ^{125}I-labeled murine MAb ($n=10$), and no postoperative histologic evidence of malignancy ($n=2$). The mean follow-up among the 59 evaluable patients was 62 months (range 34–89 months). Based on standard TNM staging, 13, 18, and 28 patients were classified as stage I, stage II, and stage III, respectively. Of the 59 evaluable patients, 24 patients (41 %) were deemed radioimmunoguided surgery negative, and 35 patients (59 %) were deemed radioimmunoguided surgery positive at the end of the surgical procedure. Due to the small sample size of each stage of disease within the evaluable group, no significant differences could be observed in survival by stage using standard TNM staging ($p=0.12$) or in survival by stage using radioimmunoguided surgery status ($p=0.73$). However, a significant difference in survival was observed by analyzing the radioimmunoguided surgery status alone ($p<0.0002$), with 87 % (21/24) of radioimmunoguided surgery-negative patients alive and only 40 % (14/35) of radioimmunoguided surgery-positive patients alive at a mean follow-up duration of 62 months. The authors concluded that radioimmunoguided surgery provided pertinent intraoperative information, thus functioning as an intraoperative prognostic tool for predicting long-term patient outcome and for helping to individualize and optimize therapeutic strategies of each colorectal cancer patient.

Since that time, there have been several subsequent longer duration survival analyses published by the group at The Ohio State University (Columbus, Ohio, USA) on primary colorectal cancer patients receiving ^{125}I-labeled murine anti-TAG-72 MAb and who underwent radioimmunoguided surgery [1, 19, 133]. Most recently, in 2012, Povoski et al. [133] performed a comprehensive survival analysis of primary colorectal cancer patients with a minimum 15-year duration of patient follow-up after radioimmunoguided surgery, in order to assess the impact of complete surgical resection of all detectable ^{125}I-labeled anti-TAG-72 murine MAb (i.e., detectable TAG-72 antigen) on long-term patient outcome. Between July 1990 and August 1995, 102 primary colorectal cancer patients were intravenously injected with a ^{125}I-labeled anti-TAG-72 murine MAb (98 patients with ^{125}I-CC49 murine MAb and 4 patients with ^{125}I-CC83 murine MAb). At surgery, 92 patients (90.2 %) demonstrated tumor localization of ^{125}I-labeled anti-TAG-72 murine MAb (88 patients with ^{125}I-CC49 murine MAb and 4 patients with ^{125}I-CC83 murine MAb). The 92 patients demonstrating tumor localization at surgery were defined as the study group and were compared with 546 control group patients, consisting of all other colorectal cancer patients (both biopsy-proven primary carcinomas and villous adenomas suspected of containing carcinoma) who were seen at The Ohio State University (Columbus, Ohio, USA) during the same time interval. There was no difference in the time-dependent survival analysis performed at 5-, 10-, and 15-year intervals between the study group and the control group, signifying that the study group was representative of all primary colorectal cancer patients evaluated during the same time frame. The 92 patient study group was then used to assess the correlation between TAG-72 antigen status at the completion of surgery and long-term patient outcome. Of the 92 patients in the study group, 33 patients (35.9 %) had no evidence of detectable TAG-72 antigen-bearing tissues (i.e., TAG-72-negative group) upon completion of the operation, whereas 59 patients (64.1 %) had evidence of persistent detectable TAG-72 antigen-bearing tissues (i.e., TAG-72-positive group) upon completion of the operation. For all stages of disease (stage 0, I, II, III, and IV), the TAG-72-negative group had a significantly improved median survival as compared to the TAG-72-positive group (8.8 years vs. 2.5 years, $p=0.005$), with no significant survival difference at the first 5-year interval between the two TAG-72 groups (69.7 % vs. 32.2 %, $p=0.27$) but with improved survival for the TAG-72-negative group as compared to the TAG-72-positive group at the subsequent 10- and 15-year intervals (45.4 % vs. 22.0 % at 10 years; $p=0.002$, and 39.4 % vs. 20.3 % at 15 years; $p=0.003$). For early-stage disease (stages 0, I, and II), there were no significant differences in the median survival or time-dependent survival analysis at the 5-, 10-, and 15-year intervals between the two TAG-72 groups. For advanced-stage disease (stage III and IV), the TAG-72-negative group had a significantly improved median survival (6.2 years vs. 1.6 years, $p<0.001$), and time-dependent survival analysis revealed that although survival was not significantly different at the first 5-year interval (57.9 % vs. 18.4 %, $p=0.13$), the TAG-72-negative group had significantly improved survival as compared to the TAG-72-positive group at the subsequent 10- and 15-year intervals (42.1 % vs. 7.9 % at both 10 years and 15 years; $p=0.03$). Finally, time-dependent multivariate Cox proportional hazards regression analysis was carried out and demonstrated that pathologic stage of disease and TAG-72 positivity were both significantly associated with long-term mortality at both the 10-year interval (with a 57 % increase in long-term mortality risk for each level increase in stage of disease and a 113 % increase in long-term mortality risk for TAG-72 positivity) and the 15-year interval (with a 82 % increase in long-term mortality risk for each level increase in stage of disease and a 104 % increase in long-term mortality risk for TAG-72 positivity). The authors concluded that the absence of detectable TAG-72 antigen within the surgical field at the completion of radioimmunoguided surgical procedure for primary colorectal cancer was of significant prognostic value and conferred a long-term and sustainable survival advantage to those patients in whom complete surgical removal of all tissues with detectable radiolabeled anti-TAG-72 murine MAb (i.e., detectable TAG-72 antigen) was accomplished.

Several other groups of investigators have utilized ^{125}I-CC49 murine MAb in radioimmunoguided surgery for colorectal cancer [1, 125–130].

In 1997, Manayan et al. [125] from Swedish Hospital Medical Center (Seattle, Washington, USA) evaluated radioimmunoguided surgery in colorectal cancer patients using ^{125}I-CC49 murine MAb. Patients were intravenously injected with 2 mCi (74 MBq) of ^{125}I-CC49 murine MAb, and for which the subsequent time to surgery was not reported. There were 26 evaluable colorectal cancer patients, including 19 with primary colorectal cancer and 7 with recurrent colorectal cancer. All patients underwent surgical exploration using traditional inspection and palpation, followed by a systematic re-exploration of the surgical field using a commercially available gamma detection probe system. Tumor localization of ^{125}I-CC49 murine MAb was demonstrated in 14 of 19 (73 %) patients with primary colorectal cancer and in all 7 (100 %) patients with recurrent colorectal cancer. Overall, occult sites of ^{125}I-CC49 murine MAb uptake, which were not detected by traditional inspection and palpation, were identified by radioimmunoguided surgery in a total of 33 sites from among 15 of 26 (58 %) patients, including 12 of 19 (63 %) primary colorectal cancer patients and 3 of 7 (43 %) recurrent colorectal cancer patients. The finding of occult disease by radioimmunoguided surgery resulted in a change in therapeutic decision-making in 6 of 26 (23 %) cases. The author concluded that radioimmunoguided surgery provided additional intraoperative information for better determination of the stage of disease and was impactful on therapeutic decision-making.

From 1997 to 2001, additional investigations into radioimmunoguided surgery in colorectal cancer patients using ^{125}I-CC49 murine MAb were reported by Schneebaum et al. [1, 126–130] at Tel-Aviv University (Tel-Aviv, Israel). Overall, they evaluated a total of 58 patients with recurrent colorectal cancer who were intravenously injected with 2 mCi (74 MBq) of ^{125}I-CC49 murine MAb at approximately 24 days prior to surgery. All patients underwent surgical exploration using traditional inspection and palpation, followed by a systematic re-exploration of the surgical field using a commercially available gamma detection probe system. Tumor localization of ^{125}I-CC49 murine MAb was seen in 54 of 58 patients (96 %). While traditional surgical exploration identified 117 suspected tumor sites, radioimmunoguided surgery identified 177 suspected tumor sites. Histologic H&E confirmation of tumor was confirmed in 131 suspected tumor sites. In 17 of 58 patients (29.3 %), there was at least one occult tumor site identified by radioimmunoguided surgery and subsequent histologic H&E confirmation which was not initially identified by traditional surgical exploration. The finding of occult disease by radioimmunoguided surgery resulted in a major change in the intraoperative surgical decision-making in 16 of 58 (27.6 %) cases. Additionally, they reported that there was a difference in histologic H&E confirmation of radioimmunoguided surgery-positive excised tissues (i.e., "radioimmunoguided surgery performance") for non-lymphoid tissues versus lymphoid tissues, with a positive predictive value and a negative predictive value for radioimmunoguided surgery of 96 % and 90 % in non-lymphoid tissues as compared to 40 % and 100 % in lymphoid tissues, respectively. The author concluded that radioimmunoguided surgery increased the chance of intraoperatively finding occult disease and resultantly provided additional information that affected intraoperative surgical decision-making and postoperative therapy planning.

24.6.1.4 Radioimmunoguided Surgery Using Humanized CC49 Monoclonal Antibody

The third-generation radiolabeled anti-TAG-72 MAb utilized in radioimmunoguided surgery was ^{125}I-labeled humanized C_H2 domain-deleted CC49 MAb (^{125}I-HuCC49ΔC_H2 MAb) [1, 59, 134]. In 2004, the results of a phase I pilot clinical trial conducted at The Ohio State University (Columbus, Ohio, USA) using ^{125}I-HuCC49ΔC_H2 MAb was reported for assessing the clearance, safety, and effectiveness of localization of this humanized domain-deleted anti-TAG-72 MAb during radioimmunoguided surgery [134]. Study eligibility included patients with recurrent colorectal cancer undergoing a surgical exploration and excluded those patients with any prior exposure to murine antibodies. A total of 20 patients with recurrent colorectal cancer were evaluated. All patients were intravenously injected with 2 mCi (74 MBq) of ^{125}I-HuCC49ΔC_H2 MAb. HAMA determinations were obtained at baseline, as well as at 4–6 weeks and 12 weeks post-injection of the ^{125}I-HuCC49ΔC_H2 MAb. At the time of their subsequent surgery, patients underwent surgical exploration using traditional inspection and palpation techniques, followed by a systematic re-exploration of the surgical field using a commercially available gamma detection probe system. All suspicious tissues were biopsied or excised to determine the presence of absence of carcinoma, and the findings were analyzed to determine the sensitivity and positive predictive value of traditional surgical exploration versus radioimmunoguided surgery exploration with the gamma detection probe. Of the 20 recurrent colorectal cancer patients evaluated, the first 15 patients had their surgical procedures performed at various time intervals (3, 5, 7, 9, 11, and 13 days) after the injection of ^{125}I-HuCC49ΔC_H2 MAb and independent of the precordial counts. For the remaining 5 patients, surgery was performed after the precordial counts fell below 30 counts per two seconds, thus signifying an optimal level of clearance of the ^{125}I-HuCC49 ΔC_H2 MAb from the blood-pool background, which took place at 10–24 days after the injection of the ^{125}I-HuCC49ΔC_H2 MAb. This level of clearance of the blood-pool background of the ^{125}I-HuCC49ΔC_H2 MAb in these 5 patients allowed for intraoperative differentiation of radioimmunoguided surgery-positive tissue compared to normal adjacent tissue. Among those 5 patients with optimized clearance, there were 17 suspicious tissue sites identified using traditional surgical exploration and 21 suspicious tissue sites identified by radioimmunoguided surgery exploration with the gamma detection probe. Approximately 90 % of the sampled suspicious tissue sites identified by both traditional surgical exploration and by radioimmunoguided surgery exploration with the gamma detection probe were histologically confirmed to contain tumor. Of the 6 suspicious tissue sites which were identified only by radioimmunoguided surgery exploration with the gamma detection probe and not by traditional surgical exploration, 5 suspicious tissue sites were sampled, and all 5 were histologically confirmed to contain tumor. The sensitivity and the positive predictive value of ^{125}I-HuCC49ΔC_H2 MAb for identifying recurrent colorectal cancer was 64 % versus 92 % and 90 % versus 100 %, respectively, for traditional surgical exploration versus radioimmunoguided surgery exploration with the gamma detection probe. There was no significant degree of HAMA response detected in any of the pilot study patients. The rate of tumor localization and detection of occult disease was similar that was previously reported by Arnold et al. [118] for the ^{125}I-CC49 murine MAb but was without any evidence of a detectable HAMA response in the current phase I pilot clinical trial [134]. The authors concluded that this pilot study demonstrated the safety and utility of ^{125}I-HuCC49ΔC_H2 MAb in radioimmunoguided surgery for colorectal cancer patients. Despite these promising results, no further clinical trials specifically utilizing HuCC49ΔC_H2 MAb were subsequently conducted secondary to corporate funding deficiencies in ongoing research and development directed toward ^{125}I-HuCC49ΔC_H2 MAb.

24.6.1.5 Radioimmunoguided Surgery Using Anti-CEA Murine Monoclonal Antibodies

There have been multiple groups of investigators who have limitedly evaluated the utility of radioimmunoguided surgery using various radiolabeled anti-CEA murine MAbs for colorectal cancer [1, 69, 70, 106–113, 116, 135–141].

In 1990, Curtet et al. [135] from the French Institute of Health and Medical Research (INSERM, Nantes, France) evaluated 10 patients with colorectal cancer, including 6 primary colorectal cancer patients and 4 recurrent colorectal cancer who were intravenously injected with 2.0–4.8 mCi (74–178 MBq) of ^{111}In-anti-CEA murine MAb fragment (^{111}In-G15) at a time of approximately 2–6 days prior to surgery. Colon tumor and normal colon counts were comparatively recorded in 7 of the 10 evaluated patients, with all 7 demonstrating a colon tumor-to-normal colon count ratio greater than or equal to 1.2 and with 3 of those 7 patients demonstrating a colon tumor-to-normal colon count ratio greater than or equal to 2.6. In contrast, the colon tumor-to-normal liver count ratio was generally less than 1.0, again emphasizing the limitation of all ^{111}In-labeled MAb in radioguided surgery secondary to the nonspecific accumulation of any given ^{111}In-labeled MAb conjugate within the liver, thus making it difficult to identify suspicious liver lesions and limiting its application to only the identification of extrahepatic sites of disease [117, 135]. The authors concluded that other radionuclides would be more suitable than ^{111}In for optimizing radioimmunoguided surgery.

In 1991, Dawson et al. [1, 69] from Charing Cross Hospital (London, United Kingdom) evaluated 43 patients undergoing surgery with primary colorectal cancer and 9 patients undergoing second-look laparotomy for recurrent colorectal cancer who were intravenously injected with 2 mCi (74 MBq) of ^{125}I-anti-CEA murine MAb (^{125}I-A_5B_7) at a time of approximately 3–10 days prior to surgery. Tumor localization of ^{125}I-A_5B_7 was seen in 42 of 43 patients (97.7 %) with primary tumors and 8 of 9 patients (88.9 %) with recurrent disease undergoing a second-look procedure. Additional information concerning extent of disease was revealed by radioimmunoguided surgery in 11 of 43 (25.6 %) primary colorectal cancer patients and in 5 of 9 (55.6 %) recurrent colorectal cancer patients. Likewise, they found that the use of radioimmunoguided surgery altered the final surgical procedure undertaken in 2 of 43 cases (4.7 %) of primary colorectal cancer and in 3 of 9 cases (33.3 %) of recurrent colorectal cancer. The authors concluded that radioimmunoguided surgery had the greatest potential for altering the behavior of the surgeon during second-look procedures for recurrent colorectal cancer.

In 1995, Lechner et al. [1, 136–138] from Community Hospital of Klosterneuburg (Klosterneuburg, Austria) evaluated 20 patients with primary colorectal cancer in a prospective feasibility clinical trial who were intravenously injected with 25 mCi (925 MBq) of ^{99}Tc-anti-CEA murine MAb fragment (^{99}Tc-IMMU-4) at a time of approximately 24 h prior to surgery. Patients underwent preoperative external planar radioimmunoscintigraphy approximately 1 h after injection and single-photon emission computed tomography (SPECT) imaging approximately 4–8 h after injection. Tumor localization of ^{99}Tc-IMMU-4 was seen on preoperative external planar radioimmunoscintigraphy and SPECT imaging in a total of 19 of 20 patients (95 %). Tumor localization of ^{99}Tc-IMMU-4 was demonstrated during radioimmunoguided surgery in all 20 patients (100 %), with radioimmunoguided surgery demonstrating the additional localization of a second synchronous tumor (previously unrecognized by colonoscopy or by preoperative external planar radioimmunoscintigraphy and SPECT imaging) within the ascending colon of a patient with a known primary rectal cancer. Additionally, radioimmunoguided surgery demonstrated N1 lymph node metastases in 2 patients, N2/3 lymph node metastases in 3 patients, liver metastases in 1 patient, and peritoneal carcinomatosis in 1 patient, all of which were not seen on preoperative external planar radioimmunoscintigraphy and SPECT imaging. Thus, the authors demonstrated that radioimmunoguided surgery assessment using ^{99}Tc-IMMU-4 resulted in the upstaging of disease in 7 of 20 patients (35 %). The authors concluded that radioimmunoguided surgery was helpful for more accurate staging of disease and was resultantly important for decision-making regarding postoperative adjuvant therapy planning.

In 1995, Di Carlo et al. [106–108] from University of Milan (Milan, Italy) evaluated radioimmunoguided surgery using ^{125}I-labeled biotinylated anti-CEA murine MAb fragment (^{125}I-biotinylated F023C5) in a cumulative series of 15 colorectal cancer patients, including 12 primary colorectal cancer patients and 3 recurrent colorectal cancer patients. Patients were intravenously injected with 2 mCi (74 MBq) of ^{125}I-biotinylated F023C5 murine MAb fragment, followed by 2 sequential intravenous injections of avidin for promoting more rapid clearance of the MAb from the blood-pool circulation, and followed by subsequent surgery performed approximately 6 days after the initial ^{125}I-biotinylated F023C5 murine MAb fragment injection. Intraoperative tumor localization with a gamma detection probe was successful in 8 of 12 (67 %) primary colorectal cancer patients and in 2 of 3 (67 %) recurrent colorectal cancer patients. The intraoperative gamma detection probe findings were instrumental in modifying the surgical approach in 3 of 15 (20 %) of patients, including 2 of 12 (17 %) primary colorectal cancer patients and 1 of 3 (33 %) recurrent colorectal cancer patients and thus leading to removal of occult sites of disease that would have otherwise gone unrecognized by traditional intraoperative inspection and palpation techniques alone.

In 1998, Percivale et al. [1, 109–111] from University of Genoa (Genoa, Italy) evaluated radioimmunoguided surgery with ^{125}I-F023C5 murine MAb fragment in a group of 34 patients with recurrent or metastatic colorectal cancer using a commercially available gamma detection probe system. Patients were intravenously injected with 2 mCi (74 MBq) of ^{125}I-F023C5 murine MAb fragment at a mean of 10.9 ± 0.8 days prior to surgery. A total of 54 histologically confirmed tumor sites were identified at by traditional surgical exploration and radioimmunoguided surgery. Intraoperative gamma detection probe assessment at the time of radioimmunoguided surgery identified 52 sites of ^{125}I-F023C5 murine MAb fragment uptake. Therefore, radioimmunoguided surgery correctly identified tumor in 50 of 54 (93 %) histologically confirmed tumor sites, with only 2 of 52 (4 %) false-negative results. Based upon the findings of intraoperative gamma detection probe assessment alone, radioimmunoguided surgery identified additional occult sites of disease in 3 of 34 patients (9 %) which was not detected by traditional surgical exploration alone. The authors concluded that radioimmunoguided surgery with ^{125}I-F023C5 murine MAb fragment provided essential information in selected cases for patients with recurrent or metastatic colorectal cancer.

In 1998, Renda et al. [1, 112] from University of Naples Federico II (Naples, Italy) reported on the detection of ^{99m}Tc-anti-CEA murine MAb radioimmunoguided surgery in 10 patients with colorectal cancer. Patients were intravenously injected with a nonspecified dose of ^{99m}Tc-anti-CEA murine MAb at approximately 24 h prior to surgery. Radioimmunoguided surgery successfully identified tumor in 6 of 10 (60 %) ^{99m}Tc-anti-CEA murine MAb patients. The authors were unable to draw any significant conclusions from their radioimmunoguided surgery experience and recommended the evaluation of newer MAbs.

In 1999, Veroux et al. [113] from University of Catania (Catania, Italy) evaluated 15 colorectal cancer patients (including 10 primary colorectal cancer patients and 5 recurrent colorectal cancer patients) who were intravenously injected with 2–3 mCi (74–111 MBq) of ^{125}I-anti-CEA murine MAb fragment (^{125}I-F023C5) at approximately 24–48 h prior to surgery. Radioimmunoguided surgery successfully identified tumor in 12 of 15 patients (80 %), including 9 of 10 (90 %) primary colorectal cancer patients and 3 of 5 (60 %) recurrent colorectal cancer patients [Personal communication: Massimiliano Veroux, University Hospital of Catania, Catania, Italy, veroux@unict.it, January 8, 2015].

In 2000, Mayer et al. [139] from University College London (London, United Kingdom) evaluated 33 colorectal cancer patients, including 17 primary tumors, 16 with liver metastases, and 1 with an anastomotic recurrence, who were intravenously injected with 1.5–7.7 mCi (57–285 MBq) of ^{125}I-anti-CEA murine single-chain monoclonal antibody fragment (^{125}I-MFE-23-his) at a time of 1–6 days prior to surgery. A total of 51 sites were intraoperatively assessed with a commercially available gamma detection probe system. They demonstrated that 82 % of probed sites were true positives, with a sensitivity of 84 %, positive predictive value of 100 %, and overall accuracy of 84 %.

In 2001, Hladik et al. [1, 116] from Charles University/Faculty of Medicine in Hradec Králové (Hradec Králové, Czech Republic) evaluated the detection of ^{99}Tc-IMMU-4 murine MAb fragment by preoperative radioimmunoscintigraphy, radioimmunoguided surgery, and histology (H&E and immunohistochemistry) in 65 patients with either primary or recurrent colorectal cancer. Patients were intravenously injected with 18.9–24.3 mCi (700–900 MBq) of ^{99}Tc-IMMU-4 murine MAb fragment at a time of approximately 24 h prior to surgery. Preoperative radioimmunoscintigraphy identified primary or recurrent tumor in 60 of 65 (92 %) patients. They determined that preoperative radioimmunoscintigraphy using ^{99}Tc-IMMU-4 murine MAb fragment led to a sensitivity and accuracy for the detection of primary tumor or local recurrence of 92 % and 92 %, for the detection of hepatic metastases of 75 % and 92 %, and for the detection of extrahepatic metastases of 57 % and 78 %, respectively. Intraoperative gamma detection probe assessment identified radioimmunoguided surgery-positive lymph nodes in 23 of 65 (35 %) patients. Of the 23 radioimmunoguided surgery-positive lymph node of the patients, 19 (82 %) were confirmed positive for lymph node involvement by histology, including histologic confirmation recognized by immunohistochemistry alone in 3 of 19 (16 %) histologically confirmed lymph node-positive patients. The authors concluded that radioimmunoguided surgery was potentially useful in the surgical management of primary colorectal patients by improving the intraoperative assessment of the extent of disease and staging of disease as a result of more accurately identifying occult lymph node disease.

In 2002 and 2007, Gioffrè Florio et al. [140, 141] from University of Messina (Messina, Italy) sequentially reported upon a cumulative series of 25 patients with colorectal cancer, including 8 primary colorectal cancer patients and 17 recurrent colorectal cancer patients who were intravenously injected with approximately 20–30 mCi (750–1110 MBq) of ^{99m}Tc-IMMU-4 murine MAb fragment at a time of approximately 24 h prior to surgery. Patients also underwent preoperative radioimmunoscintigraphy at 2–4 h after injection and again repeated at 8 and 24 h after injection in selected cases. Preoperative radioimmunoscintigraphy demonstrated tumor localization in 24 of 25 patients. Intraoperative gamma detection probe assessment demonstrated tumor localization in all 25 patients. The authors concluded that radioimmunoguided surgery was useful for directing removal of tumor, verifying complete resection and assessing negative margin status, and demonstrated the ability to identify metastatic tumor foci of less than 1 cm^3 in size.

Finally, in 2003, Gu et al. [1, 70] from Beijing Cancer Hospital of Peking University (Beijing, China) evaluated 29 patients with primary colorectal cancer who were injected with 1 mCi (37 MBq) of ^{125}I-anti-CEA murine MAb (^{125}I-CL58) into the colonic submucosa at the tumor surrounding areas (at 2, 4, 6, 8, 10, and 12 o'clock locations) via colonoscopy at a time of approximately 3–14 days prior to surgery. Tumor localization of ^{125}I-CL58 with a commercially available gamma detection probe system was seen in 27 of 29 (93.1 %) patients, and radioimmunoguided surgery correctly identified negative surgical resection margins in 42 of 44 (95.5 %) H&E-negative surgical resection margin specimens. In this study, the authors reported that the sensitivity (92.0 % vs. 60.0 %; $p=0.0087$) and specificity (87.8 % vs. 79.2 %; $p=0.0117$) of radioimmunoguided surgery versus traditional surgical exploration for correctly identifying lymph node metastases was statistically significantly greater for radioimmunoguided surgery.

24.6.1.6 Radioimmunoguided Surgery Using Anti-A33 Transmembrane Glycoprotein Antigen Humanized Monoclonal Antibody

In 2008, Strong et al. [142] at Memorial Sloan-Kettering Cancer Center (New York, New York, USA) reported on 2 patients with colorectal cancer undergoing radioimmunoguided surgery using ^{124}I-huA33 MAb, a humanized MAb directed against the A33 transmembrane glycoprotein antigen. Both patients were intravenously injected with 4 mCi (148 MBq) of ^{124}I-huA33 MAb at approximately 7 days prior to surgery. Whole-body positron emission tomography (PET) imaging was performed within 4 h after ^{124}I-huA33 MAb injection and again at approximately 7 days after ^{124}I-huA33MAb injection (but within 3 h of the start of surgery). Radioimmunoguided surgery was undertaken using a commercially available high-energy gamma detection probe and a commercially available beta detection probe, with *in situ* tumor counts, *in situ* background, and *ex situ* tumor counts taken. Postoperative specimen PET imaging was performed on surgically resected tissue. They reported a significantly greater tumor-to-background count ratio for the beta detection probe (approximately 6.2-to-1 to 6.3-to-1) as compared to the high-energy gamma detection probe (approximately 2.5-to-1 to 3.7-to-1).

24.6.1.7 Radioimmunoguided Surgery Using a Multiple Monoclonal Antibody "Cocktail"

Clinical investigations into the use of a multiple MAb "cocktail" in radioimmunoguided surgery are limited to the reported experience of a group of investigators from University of Milan (Milan, Italy) [108, 143].

In 1995, Di Carlo et al. [108] from University of Milan (Milan, Italy) evaluated radioimmunoguided surgery using a doublet MAb "cocktail" of ^{125}I-biotinylated B72.3 murine MAb and ^{125}I-biotinylated F023C5 murine MAb in 16 colorectal cancer patients, including 6 with primary colorectal cancer and 10 with recurrent colorectal cancer. The patients were intravenously injected with a total dose of approximately 2 mCi (74 MBq) of this MAb "cocktail", consisting of ^{125}I-biotinylated B72.3 murine MAb and ^{125}I-biotinylated F023C5 murine MAb, sequentially followed by a subsequent intravenous injection of 1 mg of avidin 48 h after the initial MAb "cocktail" intravenous injection and an additional intravenous injection of 3 mg of avidin 24–48 h prior to surgery for promoting more rapid clearance of the MAb "cocktail" from the blood-pool circulation and subsequent surgery performed approximately 6 days after the initial MAb "cocktail" intravenous injection. Tumor localization of the doublet MAb "cocktail" with a gamma detection probe was successful in 12 of 16 (75 %) patients, including in 5 of 6 (83 %) primary colorectal cancer patients and in 7 of 10 (70 %) recurrent colorectal cancer patients. The intraoperative gamma detection probe findings were instrumental in modifying the surgical therapeutic approach in 4 of 10 (40 %) recurrent colorectal cancer patients, thus leading to removal of occult sites of disease that would have otherwise gone unrecognized by traditional intraoperative inspection and palpation techniques alone.

In 1997, de Nardi et al. [143] from University of Milan (Milan, Italy) evaluated radioimmunoguided surgery using a triplet MAb "cocktail" of ^{125}I-biotinylated B72.3 murine MAb, ^{125}I-biotinylated F023C5 murine MAb, and ^{125}I-biotinylated F023C3 murine MAb in 14 colorectal cancer patients, including 8 with primary colorectal cancer and 6 with recurrent colorectal cancer. The patients were intravenously injected with a total dose of approximately 2 mCi (74 MBq) of this MAb "cocktail", consisting of ^{125}I-biotinylated B72.3 murine MAb, ^{125}I-biotinylated F023C5 murine MAb, and ^{125}I-biotinylated F023C3 murine MAb, followed by a subsequent intravenous injection of 1 mg of avidin 24–48 h after the initial MAb "cocktail" intravenous injection for promoting more rapid clearance of the MAb "cocktail" from the blood-pool circulation (with a second and third intravenous injection of avidin, if needed) and subsequent surgery performed approximately 4 days after the initial MAb "cocktail" intravenous injection. Tumor localization of the triplet MAb "cocktail" with a gamma detection probe was successful in 10 of 14 (71 %) patients, including in 6 of 8 (75 %) primary colorectal cancer patients and in 4 of 6 (67 %) recurrent colorectal cancer patients. The intraoperative gamma detection probe findings were instrumental in modifying the surgical therapeutic approach in 2 of 6 (33 %) recurrent colorectal cancer patients, thus leading to removal of occult sites of disease that would have otherwise gone unrecognized by traditional intraoperative inspection and palpation techniques alone. The author postulated that radioimmunoguided surgery using a MAb "cocktail" could improve the sensitivity of tumor detection by allowing binding to more antigenic sites.

24.6.2 Gastric Cancer

The feasibility of radioimmunoguided surgery for gastric cancer has been evaluated in a somewhat limited fashion by several groups of investigators [1, 98, 144–148].

In 1988, Martin et al. [1, 98] at The Ohio State University (Columbus, Ohio, USA) evaluated ^{125}I-B72.3 murine MAb in 5 patients with gastric cancer (including 3 primary gastric cancer patients and 2 recurrent gastric cancer patients) undergoing radioimmunoguided surgery. The patients were intravenously injected with approximately 4–5 mCi (148–185 MBq) of ^{125}I-B72.3 murine MAb at a time of 5–23 days (mean 15 days) prior to surgery. Intraoperative finding at the time of gamma detection probe assessment revealed tumor localization in 4 of 5 gastric cancer patients (80 %), including correctly identifying lymph node metastases in 4 of 5 patients (80 %).

In 1994, Xu et al. [1, 144] and Liu et al. [1, 145] from Beijing Cancer Hospital of Peking University (Beijing, China) evaluated ^{131}I-3H11, a murine MAb raised against human gastric cancer cells, in 23 patients with primary gastric cancer undergoing radioimmunoguided surgery. There were 19 patients who received an endoscopic submucosal injection of 0.25–0.8 mCi (9.25–29.6 MBq) of ^{131}I-3H11 at 4 points around the tumor, as well as 4 patients who received an intravenous injection of a nonspecified dose of ^{131}I-3H11. Of the 19 patients receiving an endoscopic submucosal injection of ^{131}I-3H11, 18 patients underwent intraoperative gamma detection probe assessment. They reported an ability to detect "cancer infiltration of the gastric wall" with a sensitivity of 94.6 %, specificity of 96.7 %, and accuracy of 95.9 %. They reported detection of metastatic lymph nodes with a sensitivity of 99.2 %, specificity of 97.7 %, and accuracy of 98.8 %. The authors concluded that radioimmunoguided surgery "may improve the radical resectability rate and possibly the overall survival rate in patients with gastric cancer."

In 1998, Lucisano et al. [1, 146] from University of Genoa (Genoa, Italy) evaluated ^{125}I-B72.3 murine MAb in 7 patients with gastric cancer undergoing radioimmunoguided surgery. The patients were intravenously injected with approximately 2 mCi (74 MBq) of ^{125}I-B72.3 murine MAb at a time of 14–30 days (mean 19 days) prior to surgery. The correct radioimmunoguided surgery *in situ* identification of the primary tumor was seen in 4 of 7 patients (57 %) and of metastatic lymph nodes in 2 of 4 patients (50 %).

Also, in 1998, Mussa et al. [147] from University of Turin (Turin, Italy) evaluated ^{111}In-B72.3 murine MAb in 3 patients with gastric cancer undergoing radioimmunoguided surgery. The patients were intravenously injected with approximately 5 mCi (185 MBq) of ^{111}In-B72.3 murine MAb at a time of 7 days prior to surgery. Intraoperative gamma detection probe assessment confirmed *in situ* tumor-to-background counts of greater than 2 in all 3 cases and, based upon all primary tumor site and lymph node basins examined, demonstrated a sensitivity of 100 %, specificity of 72 %, and no false-negative findings.

Finally, in 2000, Wang et al. [148] from Beijing Medical University (Peking, China) evaluated ^{125}I-3H11 murine MAb in 35 patients with primary gastric cancer undergoing radioimmunoguided surgery. All patients received an endoscopic submucosal injection of a nonspecified dose of ^{125}I-3H11 around the tumor at a time of 4–11 days prior to surgery. Of the 35 patients injected, 33 underwent subsequent successful radioimmunoguided surgery. They demonstrated a sensitivity of 83.6 %, specificity of 95.0 %, and accuracy of 91.3 % for the detection of lymph node metastases. The presence of micrometastatic lymph node disease was verified immunohistochemically in 10 of 19 (52.6 %) lymph nodes that were radioimmunoguided surgery positive but were H&E negative.

Despite these early promising results, no further clinical investigations into the clinical utility of radioimmunoguided surgery for gastric cancer have been subsequently pursued.

24.6.3 Pancreatic Cancer

The feasibility of radioimmunoguided surgery for pancreatic cancer has been previously evaluated in an extremely limited fashion [1, 139, 149].

In 1997, LaValle et al. [1, 149] from The Ohio State University (Columbus, Ohio, USA) evaluated radioimmunoguided surgery for assessing of the extent of disease in 10 cases of pancreatic adenocarcinoma that were deemed resectable by preoperative CT scan, including 9 patients with primary lesions and 1 patient with a presumed solitary hepatic metastasis at a time of 1 year following prior pancreaticoduodenectomy. The patients were intravenously injected with 2 mCi (74 MBq) of ^{125}I-CC49 murine MAb and then underwent surgery after adequate clearance of the blood-pool background was determined by precordial gamma detection probe counts at a mean time of 26.1 days (range 7–35 days) after injection. At the time of surgery, patients underwent surgical exploration at the time of laparotomy using traditional inspection and palpation, followed by a systematic re-exploration of the surgical field using a commercially available gamma detection probe system. There were 3 patients who ultimately underwent pancreatic resection for locoregional disease, whereas the other 7 patients had visceral metastases, carcinomatosis, or both that were detected at the time of laparotomy. All sites suspicious for tumor by traditional inspection and palpation assessment of the abdomen were verified to be radioimmunoguided surgery positive. However, additional occult pancreatic adenocarcinoma was identified by radioimmunoguided surgery assessment alone, demonstrating dissemination of disease to both the abdominal viscera and lymph nodes. Radioimmunoguided surgery assessment detected significantly more total sites (viscera and lymph node sites) of metastatic disease than traditional inspection and palpation assessment (73 sites vs. 31 sites for radioimmunoguided surgery assessment vs. traditional inspection and palpation assessment, respectively, $p<0.05$), with the greatest difference being observed for lymph node metastases (44 sites vs. 6 sites for radioimmunoguided surgery assessment vs. traditional inspection and palpation assessment, respectively, $p<0.001$).

In 2000, Mayer et al. [139] from University College London (London, United Kingdom) evaluated ^{125}I-MFE-23-his, an anti-CEA murine single-chain monoclonal antibody fragment, in a single patient with hepatic metastases from pancreatic cancer undergoing radioimmunoguided surgery, as well as in addition to 34 other patients with colorectal cancer. However, the details regarding the radioimmunoguided surgery procedure findings for the single patient with hepatic metastases from pancreatic cancer were not described in this report.

Despite these early promising results, no further clinical investigations into the clinical utility of radioimmunoguided surgery for pancreatic cancer have been subsequently pursued.

24.6.4 Breast Cancer

The feasibility of radioimmunoguided surgery for breast cancer has been evaluated in a somewhat limited fashion by several groups of investigators [1, 98, 110, 150–153].

In 1989, Nieroda et al. [1, 98, 150] from The Ohio State University (Columbus, Ohio, USA) evaluated radioimmunoguided surgery for the intraoperative assessment of 14 patients with breast cancer undergoing either modified radical mastectomy or breast-conserving surgery and axillary lymph node dissection. All patients were intravenously injected with 5 mCi (185 MBq) of ^{125}I-B72.3 murine MAb at a time of 6–24 days prior to surgery. A commercially available gamma detection probe system was used intraoperatively for determining *in situ* and *ex situ* probe counting within the breast tissue and the axillary tissue. Gamma probe counting correctly identified histologically confirmed tumor in 7 of 8 patients (88 %) with an intact breast tumor and correctly confirmed the absence of tumor in 4 of 6 patients (67 %) with no residual intact breast tumor (secondary to a prior diagnostic surgical excisional breast biopsy). Gamma probe counting within the breast tissue was suspicious in 2 of 14 patients in which histopathology could not confirm residual tumor within the breast tissue. Unexpected occult breast tumor was identified in 3 of 14 patients (21 %). In the axillary tissues, probe counting identified 1 of 2 cases (50 %) of histologically confirmed lymph node involvement and confirmed the absence of lymph node involvement in 8 of 12 patients (67 %). Gamma probe counting within the axillary tissues was suspicious for lymph node involvement in 4 of 14 patients (29 %) in which histopathology could not confirm lymph node involvement. The authors concluded that radioimmunoguided surgery appeared to be useful for identification of residual, subclinical, and multicentric carcinoma of the breast and accurately delineates the pattern of antigenic drainage of tumor into the regional lymph nodes.

In 1996 and again identically re-reported in 1998, Percivale et al. [1, 151], Badellino et al. [1, 152], and Bertoglio et al. [110] from University of Genoa (Genoa, Italy) evaluated radioimmunoguided surgery for the intraoperative assessment of 21 patients with locally advanced breast cancer who underwent 3 cycles of neoadjuvant fluorouracil, epidoxorubicin, and cyclophosphamide prior to surgery with modified radical mastectomy. Patients were intravenously injected with either 1.5 mCi (56 MBq) of ^{125}I-B72.3 murine MAb ($n=11$) or 1.5 mCi (56 MBq) of ^{125}I- F023C5 (an anti-CEA murine MAb fragment) ($n=10$) at a mean time of 21.7 or 10.3 days, respectively, prior to the surgical procedure. A commercially available gamma detection probe system was used intraoperatively for determining *in situ* and *ex situ* gamma probe counting within the breast tissue, axillary region, and internal mammary region. In the ^{125}I-B72.3 murine MAb group, radioimmunoguided surgery correctly identified the primary breast tumor in 7 of 11 patients (64 %) and identified occult multicentric disease in 2 of 4 patients (50 %). Likewise, in the ^{125}I-B72.3 murine MAb group, there were 8 of 11 patients (73 %) who had histologically confirmed lymph node involvement, with 3 of 8 such patients (38 %) correctly identified by radioimmunoguided surgery. In the ^{125}I- F023C5 group, radioimmunoguided surgery correctly identified the primary breast tumor in 4 of 10 patients (40 %) and identified occult multicentric disease in 1 of 2 patients (50 %). Likewise, in the ^{125}I-F023C5 group, there were 9 of 10 patients (90 %) who had histologically confirmed lymph node involvement, with 3 of 9 such patients (33 %) correctly identified by radioimmunoguided surgery. There were no false-positive results observed in either group. The authors concluded that radioimmunoguided surgery appeared to be safe and reliable technique for intraoperative assessment of breast cancer; however, since radioimmunoguided surgery did not identify all neoplastic tissue, further investigations using other more breast-specific MAbs would be warranted.

In 2001, Burak et al. [1, 153] from The Ohio State University (Columbus, Ohio, USA) evaluated radioimmunoguided surgery for the intraoperative assessment of 10 patients with breast cancer undergoing primary tumor excision. Patients were intravenously injected with 2 mCi (74 MBq) of ^{125}I-labeled NR-LU-10, an anti-17-1A murine MAb fragment, at 2, 4, or 7 days prior to surgery. Preoperative pharmacokinetics were evaluated. A commercially available gamma detection probe system was used for determining *in situ* and *ex situ* gamma probe counting of the primary breast tumor, as well as *in situ* gamma probe counting of the resection cavity and *ex situ* gamma probe counting of excised cavity resection margin specimens. Gamma probe counting of the breast tumor *in situ* was able to distinguish tumor from surrounding nonmalignant background tissues in only 7 of 10 patients (70 %), secondary to elevated levels of the gamma probe counts noted within the surrounding nonmalignant background tissues in those 3 cases. Normal surrounding nonmalignant breast tissues had the highest relative amount of radioactivity within the central/periareolar breast region. However, *ex situ* gamma probe counting of the breast tumor after tumor excision in those 3 cases subsequently showed elevated tumor-to-surrounding nonmalignant background tissue gamma probe count ratios. There were 12 of 38 H&E-negative excised cavity resection margin specimens which showed elevated levels of the gamma probe counts, representing only a 32 % specificity. The authors concluded that ^{125}I-labeled NR-LU-10 had favorable pharmacokinetics and tumor-binding ability as a targeting agent for breast cancer; yet its binding to in situ surrounding nonmalignant breast tissue and elevated gamma probe counts in H&E-negative excised cavity resection margin specimens limited its potential role for intraoperative *in situ* tumor identification and evaluation of tumor surgical resection margins.

At the current time, despite the development of MAbs targeted against human epidermal growth factor receptor 2 (Her2/neu) and for which Her2/neu is overexpressed in approximately 15–30 % of breast cancers, there have been no subsequent clinical investigations into the potential feasibility and role of radioimmunoguided surgery using MAbs targeted against Her2/neu in Her2/neu-positive breast cancer patients.

24.6.5 Ovarian Cancer

The feasibility of radioimmunoguided surgery for ovarian cancer has been previously evaluated in a limited fashion by various groups of investigators [1, 98, 114, 154–160]. The first description of radioimmunoguided surgery for ovarian cancer was reported in 1988 by Martin et al. [1, 98] at The Ohio State University (Columbus, Ohio, USA). Patients planned for a second-look laparotomy after postoperative systemic chemotherapy were intravenously injected with approximately 4–5 mCi (148–185 MBq) of ^{125}I-B72.3 murine MAb at a time of 7–20 days (mean 13 days) prior to surgery. Intraoperative findings at the time of gamma detection probe assessment using a commercially available gamma detection probe system were mixed, revealing definite tumor localization in only 4 of 8 ovarian cancer patients (50 %), with 1 patient having borderline tumor localization and with 3 patients having no tumor localization by radioimmunoguided surgery. Of the 3 patients having no tumor localization by radioimmunoguided surgery, 1 patient had micrometastatic disease detected at second-look laparotomy, and 2 patients had obvious tumor at the time of traditional inspection and palpation assessment during second-look laparotomy.

In 1989, Gitsch et al. [154–156] from University of Vienna (Vienna, Austria) evaluated radioimmunoguided surgery in 12 patients with ovarian cancer, including 4 patients with primary ovarian cancer and 8 patients strongly suspected to have recurrent ovarian cancer who were undergoing second-look laparotomy. Patients were intravenously injected with 3 mCi (111 MBq) of ^{131}I-OC-125 (an anti-CA-125 murine MAb which is specifically targeted against the MUC16 antigen) at a time of up to 8 days prior to surgery. A prototype gamma detection probe system was utilized for intraoperative tumor localization. The presence of tumor localization with ^{131}I-OC-125 was correctly confirmed in 6 of 8 patients (75 %) with histologically confirmed disease, and the absence of tumor localization with ^{131}I-OC-125 was correctly confirmed in all 4 patients (100 %) without any histologically confirmed disease.

In 1990, Bell et al. [157] from The Ohio State University (Columbus, Ohio, USA) and Riverside Methodist Hospital (Columbus, Ohio, USA) evaluated radioimmunoguided surgery in 9 patients suspected of recurrent ovarian cancer who were undergoing second-look laparotomy and who were intravenously injected with approximately 4–5 mCi (148–185 MBq) of ^{125}I-B72.3 murine MAb at a time of 12–28 days (mean 14 days) prior to surgery. Intraoperative findings using a commercially available gamma detection probe system were again mixed. Gamma detection probe assessment correctly detected true positive counts in 3 of 6 evaluable patients (50 %) with histologically confirmed disease. There was 1 patient with histologically confirmed disease who was unevaluable secondary to high background counts. Conversely, gamma detection probe assessment correctly detected true negative counts in 1 of 2 evaluable patients (50 %) without histologically confirmed disease.

In 1990, Jäger et al. [158] from University of Erlangen-Nürnberg (Erlangen, Germany) evaluated radioimmunoguided surgery in 22 patients with suspected recurrent ovarian cancer undergoing a planned second-look laparotomy after prior administration of postoperative systemic chemotherapy using a ^{131}I-OC-125 murine monoclonal antibody fragment (^{131}I-IMACIS II). Patients were intravenously injected with approximately 1.9–3.0 mCi (70–110 MBq) of ^{131}I-IMACIS II MAb at a time of 4–13 days (mean 8 days) prior to surgery. Histologic confirmation of recurrent disease at second-look laparotomy was found in 10 of 22 patients (45 %). At the time of second-look laparotomy, traditional inspection and palpation assessment identified the histologically confirmed disease in only 4 of those 10 patients (40 %), while radioimmunoguided surgery identified the histologically confirmed disease in 9 of those 10 patients (90 %), with histologically confirmed disease being identified solely by radioimmunoguided surgery in 6 of those 10 patients (60 %). Although there were 7 of 12 patients (58 %) without histologically confirmed disease who had elevated gamma probe counts at the time of radioimmunoguided surgery, it is very noteworthy to emphasize that 6 of those 7 patients (85 %) without histologically confirmed disease but who had elevated gamma probe counts at radioimmunoguided surgery developed clinically detectable signs of disease progression within a 4-month time frame after their second-look laparotomy procedure. The authors concluded that radioimmunoguided surgery was potentially helpful for detecting cancerous tissues at the time of second-look laparotomy and for defining patients at increased risk for early recurrence of disease.

In 1992, Krag et al. [114] from University of California at Davis (Sacramento, California, USA) and University of Vermont (Burlington, Vermont, USA) evaluated radioimmunoguided surgery in 5 patients with suspected recurrent ovarian cancer undergoing a planned second-look laparotomy after prior postoperative systemic chemotherapy using ^{111}In-CYT-103. Patients were intravenously injected with approximately 5 mCi (185 MBq) of ^{111}In-CYT-103 at a time of 4–15 days prior to surgery. At the time of surgery, patients underwent surgical exploration at the time of laparotomy using traditional inspection and palpation, followed by a systematic re-exploration of the surgical field using a commercially available gamma detection probe system. However, the authors did not perform a subgroup analysis of their data for the 5 patients with suspected recurrent ovarian cancer as compared to the other 8 included patients with colorectal cancer, thus making it impossible to gleam any information regarding their radioimmunoguided surgery experience specifically with ovarian cancer.

In 1994, Ind et al. [159] from Saint Bartholomew's Hospital (London, United Kingdom) evaluated radioimmunoscintigraphy and radioimmunoguided surgery in 16 patients with proven or suspected ovarian cancer, specifically using ^{99m}Tc-SM3 murine MAb (which binds with an epitope on polymorphic epithelial mucin, MUC1) in 15 patients and ^{99m}Tc-H17E2 murine MAb (which binds with an epitope on placental-derived and germ cell-derived alkaline phosphatase) in 1 patient. Patients were intravenously injected with 16.2 mCi (600 MBq) of ^{99m}Tc-SM3 or ^{99m}Tc-H17E2 at a time of approximately 24–30 h prior to radioimmunoguided surgery. Radioimmunoscintigraphy was performed 10 min, 4–6 h, and 20–24 h after injection of the ^{99m}Tc-labeled murine MAb. Radioimmunoscintigraphy demonstrated tumor localization of ^{99m}Tc-SM3 in 8 of 8 patients with ovarian cancer, in 3 of 6 patients with benign ovarian tumors, and in 1 patient with an ovarian metastasis from colonic adenocarcinoma. Radioimmunoscintigraphy demonstrated tumor localization of ^{99m}Tc-H17E2 in the 1 patient with an ovarian cancer. The authors' presentation of their gamma detection probe data was somewhat restricted, thus limiting an in-depth analysis of their result. However, the authors did report that the use of the gamma detection probe during radioimmunoguided surgery had an 82 % sensitivity and a 72 % specificity for detecting malignancy when the tumor-to-background uptake ratio exceeded 1.5-to-1.0 and had a 68 % sensitivity and an 81 % specificity for detecting malignancy when the tumor-to-background uptake ratio exceeded 2.3-to-1.0. The authors concluded that radioimmunoscintigraphy and radioimmunoguided surgery had potential clinical benefit for perioperative localization of ovarian cancer at laparotomy.

In 1997, McIntosh et al. [160] from the University of Nebraska (Omaha, Nebraska, USA) evaluated 10 patients with ovarian cancer undergoing a planned second-look laparotomy after completing prior primary treatment using ^{125}I-CC49 murine MAb. Patients were intravenously injected with approximately 2 mCi (74 MBq) of ^{125}I-CC49 murine MAb at a time of 23–27 days (mean 24.5 days) prior to surgery. At the time of surgery, patients underwent surgical exploration at the time of laparotomy using traditional inspection and palpation, followed by a systematic re-exploration of the surgical field using a commercially available gamma detection probe system. At the time of second-look laparotomy, 6 of 10 patients were ultimately found to have histologically confirmed disease, and 4 of 10 patients were ultimately not found to have histologically confirmed disease. At the time of second-look laparotomy, traditional inspection and palpation assessment deemed 4 of 10 patients as cancer positive, with all 4 of those patients having histologically confirmed disease but with only 2 of those 4 patients being assessed as gamma detection probe positive. At the time of second-look laparotomy, traditional inspection and palpation assessment deemed 6 of 10 patients as cancer negative, with 4 of 6 of those patients having no histologically confirmed disease. Whereas, radioimmunoguided surgery with the gamma detection probe judged 5 of those 6 traditional inspection- and palpation-assessed cancer-negative patients as gamma detection probe positive, with 2 of those 5 gamma detection probe-positive but traditional inspection- and palpation-assessed cancer-negative patients having histologically confirmed disease. Of those 4 patients who were ultimately not found to have histologically confirmed disease at the time of second-look laparotomy (and who incidentally all initially judged as cancer negative by traditional inspection and palpation assessment), 3 patients were initially judged as gamma detection probe positive. Interestingly, 2 of those 3 gamma detection probe-positive patients without histologically confirmed disease at the time of second-look laparotomy went on to develop clinical/radiographic detectable recurrent disease at 24 and 42 months after radioimmunoguided surgery. The authors concluded that radioimmunoguided surgery permitted occult disease detection that could potentially lead to beneficial changes in patient management.

Despite these multiple early reports showing promising results, no further clinical investigations into the clinical utility of radioimmunoguided surgery for ovarian cancer have been subsequently pursued.

24.6.6 Prostate Cancer

The feasibility of radioimmunoguided surgery for prostate cancer has been previously evaluated in an extremely limited fashion, consisting of a small clinical report using ^{125}I-B72.3 murine MAb [1, 161] and a single patient case report using ^{111}In-capromab pendetide [1, 162].

In 1993, Badalament et al. [1, 161] from The Ohio State University (Columbus, Ohio, USA) reported on the feasibility of radioimmunoguided surgery in a clinical series of 10 patients with prostate cancer who were planned for radical retropubic prostatectomy and bilateral pelvic lymphadenectomy. Patients were intravenously injected with approximately 2 mCi (74 MBq) of ^{125}I-CC49 murine MAb at a time of 17–38 days (mean 26.3 days) prior to surgery. Intraoperative gamma detection probe assessment during radioimmunoguided surgery successfully localized tumor within the prostate of all 10 patients. Likewise, intraoperative gamma detection probe assessment was able to identify otherwise clinically occult bilateral intraprostatic tumor in 3 patients. Furthermore, intraoperative gamma detection probe assessment was able to correctly identified regional lymph node metastases in 2 patients. The authors concluded that radioimmunoguided surgery was technically feasible during radical prostatectomy and pelvic lymphadenectomy and could be a future useful adjunctive tool during laparoscopic pelvic lymphadenectomy.

In 2000, Anderson et al. [1, 162] from Anderson Regional Medical Center (Meridian, Mississippi, USA) reported on a single patient with suspected metastatic prostate cancer. The patient was intravenously injected with 5 mCi (185 MBq) of ^{111}In-capromab pendetide, a murine MAb that recognizes prostate-specific membrane antigen. Planar gamma camera imaging and SPECT was undertaken on day 0 and day 4, showing uptake within the prostate, mesenteric lymph nodes, right pulmonary hilum, and the left supraclavicular region. In order to confirm a diagnosis of metastatic prostate cancer, the patient subsequently received a repeat intravenous injection of 5 mCi (185 MBq) of ^{111}In-capromab pendetide and then underwent radioimmunoguided surgery at a time of 4 days after the repeat ^{111}In-capromab pendetide injection. At the time of radioimmunoguided surgery, successful gamma detection probe-directed surgical excision of a gamma detection probe-positive (but clinically occult) left supraclavicular lymph node was accomplished. The gamma detection probe-positive left supraclavicular lymph node contained metastatic prostate cancer, thus providing histologic confirmation of the diagnosis of metastatic prostate cancer.

Despite these two early promising reports, no further clinical investigations into the clinical utility of radioimmunoguided surgery for prostate cancer have been subsequently pursued.

24.6.7 Clear Cell Renal Cell Cancer

The feasibility of radioimmunoguided surgery for clear cell renal cell cancer has been previously evaluated in a limited fashion, consisting of two small case series reports [1, 84, 142].

In 2008, Strong et al. [1, 142] at Memorial Sloan-Kettering Cancer Center (New York, New York, USA) reported on 2 patients with clear cell renal cell cancer undergoing radioimmunoguided surgery using ^{124}I-cG250 MAb. Both patients were intravenously injected with 5 mCi (185 MBq) of ^{124}I-cG250 approximately 7 days prior to surgery. Whole-body PET imaging was performed within 4 h after ^{124}I-cG250 MAb injection and again at approximately 7 days after ^{124}I-cG250 MAb injection (but within 3 h of the start of surgery). Radioimmunoguided surgery was undertaken using a commercially available high-energy gamma detection probe and a commercially available beta detection probe, with *in situ* tumor counts, *in situ* background, and *ex situ* tumor counts taken. Postoperative specimen PET imaging was performed on surgically resected tissue. There was no significant difference in the tumor-to-background count ratio detected by the high-energy gamma detection probe (approximately 2.8-to-1 to 3.5-to-1) as compared to the beta detection probe (approximately 2.2-to-1 to 2.4-to-1).

In 2013, Povoski et al. [84] from The Ohio State University (Columbus, Ohio, USA) reported on a multimodal imaging and detection approach in 2 patients with clear cell renal cell cancer using ^{124}I-cG250 MAb. Patient 1 was intravenously injected with 5.4 mCi (200 MBq) of ^{124}I-cG250 at 4 days prior to surgery. Patient 1 underwent preoperative PET imaging, followed by a laparoscopic right radical nephrectomy with retroperitoneal lymph node dissection, with intraoperatively utilization of a commercially available laparoscopic gamma detection probe for *in situ* and *ex situ* counting. The laparoscopic gamma detection probe correctly identified increased ^{124}I-cG250 MAb activity within the primary tumor of the right kidney, as well as within adjacent retroperitoneal lymph node tissues. Postoperative specimen PET imaging was performed on intact excised right radical nephrectomy specimen and the intact excised retroperitoneal lymph node dissection specimen, clearly identifying the sites of disease within both excised specimens. Patient 2 was intravenously injected with 5.2 mCi (192 MBq) of ^{124}I-cG250 at 5 days prior to surgery. Patient 2 underwent preoperative PET imaging, followed by an open right partial nephrectomy of the inferior pole of the right kidney. At the discretion of the operating surgeon, an intraoperative gamma detection probe was not utilized during the surgical procedure. However, postoperative specimen PET imaging was performed on both the intact excised right partial nephrectomy specimen and on the excised right partial nephrectomy specimen after post-excisional specimen bisection, clearly identifying the tumor size and tumor location within the intact and bisected specimens and the relationship of the tumor to the adjacent normal parenchymal surgical resection margin surface within the bisected specimen. In their report, Povoski et al. [84] discussed that this innovative ^{124}I-cG250 MAb multimodal imaging and detection approach appeared to be useful for accurate preoperative and intraoperative localization and confirmation of complete removal of all sites of disease during both laparoscopic and open surgical resection of clear cell renal cell cancer and for cases with or without known/suspected regional lymph node involvement. Furthermore, they went on to concluded that (1) as specifically pertaining to laparoscopic surgical resection of clear cell renal cell cancer, this approach could allow for identification and complete surgical resection of the known primary tumor and of any sites of occult disease (i.e., regional lymph node metastases) by a minimally invasive laparoscopic surgical approach, which otherwise would not be technically feasible without the aid of the ^{124}I-cG250 MAb targeting agent; (2) as specifically pertaining to attempted partial nephrectomy by either laparoscopic or open surgical resection for patients with early-stage clear cell renal cell cancer, this approach could improve the success rate of complete surgical resection by providing supplemental confirmatory information to the urologic surgeon and the pathologist about the kidney parenchyma surgical resection margin status; and (3) as specifically pertaining to radical nephrectomy by either laparoscopic or open surgical resection of more advanced-stage but still potentially surgically resectable disease (i.e., such as larger primary tumors and/or bulky regional lymph node involvement), this approach could be advantageous for providing intraoperative guidance to the urologic surgeon for assessing the exact extent of disease and for confirming completeness of surgical resection.

Despite these two promising reports, no further clinical investigations into the clinical utility of radioimmunoguided surgery for clear cell renal cell cancer have been subsequently described.

24.6.8 Lung Cancer

The feasibility of radioimmunoguided surgery for lung cancer has been previously investigated in an extremely limited fashion by two groups of investigators [1, 163, 164].

In 1998, Grazia et al. [1, 163] from University of Bologna (Bologna, Italy) reported on the feasibility of radioimmunoguided surgery in a small clinical series of 8 patients with primary adenocarcinoma of the lung using ^{125}I-B72.3 murine MAb. Patients were intravenously injected with

0.9–1.5 mCi (33–56 MBq) of ^{125}I-B72.3 murine MAb at a time of 11–44 days (mean 20.4 days) prior to surgery. Tumor localization of ^{125}I-B72.3 murine MAb was demonstrated during radioimmunoguided surgery in all 8 patients (100 %) with histologically confirmed primary adenocarcinoma of the lung. However, they did encounter persistently elevated precordial counts over the region of the heart in 2 of 8 patients with primary adenocarcinoma of the lung. The authors concluded that this high radioactive background count activity found over the region of the heart within these two particular cases could represent a potential limiting factor for successful gamma detection probe assessment within the thorax.

In 1998, Mansi et al. [1, 164] from Second University of Naples (Naples, Italy) reported on radioimmunoguided surgery performed on a single patient with primary non-small cell lung cancer using ^{125}I-B72.3 murine MAb and on a single patient with squamous cell lung cancer using ^{99m}Tc-F023C5 murine MAb fragment. The patient with primary non-small cell lung cancer was intravenously injected with 2 mCi (74 MBq) of ^{125}I-B72.3 murine MAb and underwent radioimmunoguided surgery 29 days following injection, and for which there was no *in situ* selective localization of ^{125}I-B72.3 murine MAb detected within the area of the primary lung tumor with the gamma detection probe at the time of surgery. The patient with squamous cell lung cancer was intravenously injected with 15 mCi (555 MBq) of ^{99m}Tc-F023C5 murine MAb fragment and underwent radioimmunoguided surgery 36 h following injection. In this particular patient, there was no *in situ* selective localization of ^{99m}Tc-F023C5 murine MAb fragment to the primary lung tumor, but for which there was *in situ* selective localization of ^{99m}Tc-F023C5 murine MAb fragment to a small lymph node metastasis detected by the gamma detection probe at the time of surgery (and for which this small lymph node metastasis was not previously identifiable on preoperative diagnostic computed tomography or radioimmunoscintigraphy). Furthermore, the authors reported that the resected primary lung tumor and the resected small lymph node metastasis from this patient both demonstrated a 2:1 tumor-to-background count ratio on *ex situ* counting with the gamma detection probe.

24.6.9 Squamous Cell Cancer of the Skin of the Face and Scalp

The feasibility of radioimmunoguided surgery for squamous cell carcinoma of the skin has been limited to a single published report in the literature by Argenzio et al. [1, 165] from Second University of Naples (Caserta, Italy) in 1999. In this report, they described 2 patients with squamous cell carcinoma of the skin of the face and scalp region who were intravenously injected with 15 mCi (555 MBq) of ^{99m}Tc-F023C5, a ^{99m}Tc-anti-CEA murine MAb fragment. Diagnostic gamma camera imaging was performed at 4 and 12 h after injection of ^{99m}Tc-F023C5. Subsequently, 36 h after injection of ^{99m}Tc-F023C5, intraoperative gamma detection probe assessment was performed using a commercially available gamma detection probe system to define the boundaries of the primary tumor, guide the extent of the surgical resection, and assess the adequacy of the surgical resection margins. The authors reported that a tumor-to-background tissue ratio of greater than 2 was a clearly discriminate value for defining diseased tissue and concluded that radioimmunoguided surgery had a potential role in the surgical management of squamous cell carcinoma of the skin. However, no other such reports have been published since that time.

24.6.10 Recurrent Medullary Thyroid Cancer

The feasibility of radioimmunoguided surgery for recurrent medullary thyroid cancer has been evaluated in a limited fashion by several groups of investigators [1, 166–168].

From 1993 to 1998, Peltier, Barbet, and colleagues [1, 166, 167] from multiple medical institutions across France reported on radioimmunoguided surgery using a combination of four different handheld gamma detection probe systems and a 2-step radioimmunotargeting agent system in a cumulative series of 14 patients with a history of medullary thyroid cancer who had elevated calcitonin level after undergoing prior total thyroidectomy and accompanying partial or complete cervical lymph node dissection resection. This 2-step radioimmunotargeting agent system consisted of (1) an unradiolabeled bispecific antibody complex (which was itself comprised of a fragment of anti-CEA IgG1 murine MAb that was coupled chemically with a fragment of anti-diethylenetriaminepentaacetic acid (anti-DTPA) IgG1 murine MAb) and (2) an ^{111}In-labeled bivalent hapten (^{111}In-di-DTPA-tyrosyl-lysine). Patients were first intravenously injected with 0.1 mg/kg of body weight of the unradiolabeled bispecific antibody complex. Then, approximately 4–5 day thereafter, patients were subsequently intravenously injected with 2.7–5.4 mCi (100–200 MBq) of the ^{111}In-labeled bivalent hapten. Radioimmunoguided surgery was then performed approximately 3–7 days after the injection of the ^{111}In-labeled bivalent hapten. Intraoperative tumor localization with a gamma detection probe was demonstrated in 12 of 14 patients (86 %), with those 2 patients without radioimmunoguided surgery tumor localization having no histologically confirmed tumor identified at the time of surgery. Likewise, radioimmunoguided surgery localized occult disease in 4 of 12 patients (33 %) with histologically confirmed tumor which was not recognized by traditional surgical inspection and palpation alone. The authors concluded that radioimmunoguided surgery could improve the therapeutic management of recurrent medullary thyroid cancer.

In 2000, de Labriolle-Vaylet et al. [1, 168] from multiple medical institutions across France reported on radioimmunoguided surgery using this same 2-step radioimmunotargeting agent system in which *in situ* gamma detection probe counting was recorded from a total of 208 sites within 11 patients with suspected recurrent or metastatic medullary thyroid cancer. Patients were first intravenously injected with 0.1 mg/kg of body weight of the unradiolabeled bispecific antibody complex. Then, approximately 3–5 days thereafter, patients were subsequently intravenously injected with 3.2–10.0 mCi (118–370 MBq) of the ^{111}In-labeled bivalent hapten. Radioimmunoguided surgery was then performed approximately 2–4 days after the injection of the ^{111}In-labeled bivalent hapten. For the 208 total sites of suspected recurrent or metastatic disease, histologic confirmation verified that *in situ* gamma detection probe assessment resulted in 46 (22.1 %) true positives, 134 (64.4 %) true negatives, 15 (7.2 %) false negatives, and 13 (6.4 %) false positives, thus giving an accuracy of 86 %, sensitivity of 75 %, and specificity of 90 %. The authors concluded that radioimmunoguided surgery provided added value to the overall surgical management of suspected recurrent or metastatic medullary thyroid cancer by allowing for identification of occult disease which was not otherwise identifiable at the time of conventional surgery.

24.7 Bridging the Gap between the Histologic Identification of Malignant Cells and the Detection of Tumor-Specific Antigens within Radioimmunoguided Surgery-Positive Resected Tissues: A Changing Dictum toward the Concept of Antigen-Directed Cancer Surgery

There has been a major ongoing debate which has existed since the inception of the concept of radioimmunoguided surgery. That debate has been as to whether tissues recognized as positive by a handheld gamma detection probe at the time of radioimmunoguided surgery (i.e., radioimmunoguided surgery-positive tissues), but for which malignant cells cannot be histologically confirmed within those same tissues at the time of pathologic evaluation, represent false positive results or true positive results with respect to radioimmunoguided surgery [1, 19, 118–120, 124, 131, 169–177]. Therefore, the question that is raised in this ongoing debate is as to what is most important, the histologic identification of malignant cells within radioimmunoguided surgery-positive resected tissues or simply the detection of tumor-specific antigens within radioimmunoguided surgery-positive resected tissues? The answer to this question, while not always well recognized by those that continue to debate this issue, has already been answered within this chapter.

The best illustration of this debate regarding the histologic identification of malignant cells versus the detection of tumor-specific antigens within radioimmunoguided surgery-positive resected tissues can be garnered from the collaborative work of Cote et al. [169, 170, 173, 176]. In 1996, Cote et al. [176] reported on the cumulative evaluation of a total of 57 paraffin-embedded lymph nodes (including 39 radioimmunoguided surgery-positive lymph nodes) which were removed at the time of radioimmunoguided surgery and which underwent histologic evaluation with (1) routine H&E, (2) serial section immunohistochemistry using a cocktail of MAb (AE1/Cam 5.2) to cytokeratin, and (3) immunohistochemistry using CC49 murine MAb from a group of 16 colorectal cancer patients preoperatively intravenously injected with ^{125}I-CC49 murine MAb. From this group of 57 lymph nodes evaluated, there were 15 radioimmunoguided surgery-negative/routine H&E-negative lymph nodes, 3 radioimmunoguided surgery-negative/routine H&E-positive lymph nodes, 25 radioimmunoguided surgery-positive/routine H&E-negative lymph nodes, and 14 radioimmunoguided surgery-positive/routine H&E-positive lymph nodes. Thus, from the entire group of 57 lymph nodes evaluated, a total of 17 lymph nodes were identified as positive for malignant cells by routine H&E evaluation alone. Of the 40 lymph nodes identified as negative for malignant cells by routine H&E evaluation alone, serial section cytokeratin immunohistochemistry evaluation revealed occult malignant cells in 10 of these routine H&E-negative lymph nodes, thus identifying a total of 27 metastatic lymph nodes from among the 57 lymph nodes evaluated. Furthermore, while only 17 (63 %) of the 27 metastatic lymph nodes were assessed as positive for malignant cells by routine H&E evaluation alone, 24 (89 %) of the 27 metastatic lymph nodes were identified as radioimmunoguided surgery-positive lymph nodes ($p < 0.05$). Along similar lines, serial section cytokeratin immunohistochemistry evaluation revealed occult malignant cells in 10 (40 %) of 25 lymph nodes that were characterized as radioimmunoguided surgery-positive/routine H&E-negative lymph nodes. In 15 of the 25 radioimmunoguided surgery-positive/routine H&E-negative lymph nodes, no malignant cells could be identified after combined routine H&E and serial section cytokeratin immunohistochemistry. In 5 of those 15 radioimmunoguided surgery-positive/routine H&E-negative lymph nodes in which no malignant cells could be identified after combined routine H&E and serial section cytokeratin immunohistochemistry, CC49 murine MAb immunohistochemistry revealed CC49 murine MAb immunoreactivity within histiocytes, interfollicular zones, or subcapsular sinuses. In striking contrast, none of the 15 radioimmunoguided surgery-negative/routine H&E-negative lymph nodes were found to contain any evidence of CC49 murine MAb immunoreactivity. The striking contrast between the findings in these radioimmunoguided surgery-positive/histologic-negative tissues and radioimmunoguided surgery-negative/histologic-negative tissues highlight the potential important role of detecting tumor-specific antigens within radioimmunoguided surgery-positive tissues in the absence of finding malignant cells on histologic evaluation.

Although not representing radioimmunoguided surgery, there have been 2 published reports describing the utilization of *ex vivo* radioimmunodetection with a handheld gamma detection probe in the pathology department for identification of *ex vivo* radioimmunodetection-positive lymph nodes from within the mesocolons of the resected colorectal specimens [178, 179] that complement the work reported by Cote et al. [169, 170, 173, 176]. These 2 reports examining *ex vivo* radioimmunodetection are noteworthy of discussion, as they further illustrate the importance of detection of tumor-specific antigens versus the histologic detection of malignant cells. In

1993, Abdel-Nabi et al. [178] from University of Buffalo (Buffalo, New York, USA) reported on the evaluation of a total of 628 lymph nodes within resected colorectal specimens using *ex vivo* radioimmunodetection with a handheld gamma detection probe in the pathology department 2-to-1 from 13 colorectal cancer patients preoperatively intravenously injected with one of two ^{111}In-anti-CEA murine MAbs (^{111}In-IVP ZCE 025 or ^{111}In-CYT-372). Only 93 lymph nodes (15 %) were palpable (i.e., ≥5 mm) within the mesocolons of the resected colorectal specimens, while 535 lymph nodes (85 %) were nonpalpable (i.e., <5 mm) and were only identified within the mesocolons of the resected colorectal specimens following performance of fat dissolution/clearance of the resected colorectal specimens. A total of 44 lymph nodes within the mesocolons were histologically positive for malignant cells within 8 of the 13 resected colorectal specimens. This included 19 of 93 palpable (i.e., ≥5 mm) lymph nodes which were histologically positive for malignant cells and 25 of the 535 nonpalpable (i.e., <5 mm) lymph nodes which were histologically positive for malignant cells. A total of 47 lymph nodes within the mesocolons were identified as *ex vivo* radioimmunodetection-positive lymph nodes using the handheld gamma detection probe in the pathology department, including 22 palpable (i.e., ≥5 mm) *ex vivo* radioimmunodetection-positive lymph nodes and 25 nonpalpable (i.e., <5 mm) *ex vivo* radioimmunodetection-positive lymph nodes. There were 19 of 22 palpable (i.e., ≥ 5 mm) *ex vivo* radioimmunodetection-positive lymph nodes (86 %) which were histologically positive for malignant cells and 25 of 25 nonpalpable (i.e., <5 mm) *ex vivo* radioimmunodetection-positive lymph nodes (100 %) which were histologically positive for malignant cells. In 2007, Sézeur et al. [179] from multiple medical institutions across France reported on the evaluation of a total of 705 lymph nodes within resected colorectal specimens using the fat dissolution/clearance method and using an *ex vivo* radioimmunodetection method (with a handheld gamma detection probe on a square centimeter coordinate grid using a tumor-to-nontumor count ratio of 2.5-to-1) in the pathology department from 16 colorectal cancer patients preoperatively intravenously injected with a bispecific anti-CEA/anti-diethylenetriaminepentaacetic acid (DTPA) murine MAb followed 4 days later by a ^{111}In-labeled bivalent hapten di-DTPA-TL. There were 308 lymph nodes (44 %) measuring <2 mm, 256 lymph nodes (36 %) measuring 2 to <4 mm, and 141 lymph nodes (20 %) measuring ≥4 mm which were identified within the mesocolons of the resected colorectal specimens of 7 of the 16 resected colorectal specimens using the fat dissolution/clearance method for detection. There were 29 total sites of metastatic disease identified within the mesocolons of the resected colorectal specimens using the fat dissolution/clearance method for detection, including 17 lymph node metastases and 12 metastatic deposits without structural features of a lymph node (i.e., extranodal mesocolon metastatic deposits) identified. Evaluation by H&E alone detected only 10 of 29 total sites of metastatic disease, including 8 of 17 lymph node metastases and only 2 of 12 extranodal mesocolon metastatic deposits. Based upon the *ex vivo* radioimmunodetection with a handheld gamma detection probe and using the square centimeter grid coordinate method of detection, the blocks of mesocolon with significant radioactivity contained 226 lymph nodes and 24 sites of metastatic disease, including 16 of 17 lymph node metastases and 8 of 12 extranodal mesocolon metastatic deposits. Evaluation by the *ex vivo* radioimmunodetection method provided significantly better detection ($p<0.001$) than evaluation by H&E alone. Both of these reports [178, 179] demonstrate the utility of *ex vivo* radioimmunodetection of lymph nodes from within the mesocolons of the resected colorectal specimens and its improved correlation to true histologically positive lymph node metastases.

Taking this one step further and as eluded to within the previously described work reported by Cote et al. [169, 170, 173, 176], the more important question is whether it is the detection and surgical resection of tumor cells within radioimmunoguided surgery-positive tissues which is ultimately most important or whether it is simply the detection and surgical resection of a tumor-specific antigen within radioimmunoguided surgery-positive tissues which is ultimately most important? The answer to important question has long been best illustrated by radioimmunoguided surgery directed against the TAG-72 antigen, particularly related to findings within lymph nodes and other tissues surgically resected or not surgically resected at the time of anti-TAG-72 radioimmunoguided surgery, and the resultant impact of those findings on long-term patient outcomes. The clinical trials addressing this specific question were previously described in great detail within a prior section of this chapter (i.e., Sect. 25.6.1.3). However, to reiterate, the answer to this important question culminates with the findings already outlined in the most recent long-term survival analysis [133] performed at The Ohio State University (Columbus, Ohio, USA) regarding primary colorectal cancer patients with a minimum 15-year duration of patient follow-up after radioimmunoguided surgery with ^{125}I-labeled anti-TAG-72 murine MAb (^{125}I-CC49 murine MAb and ^{125}I-CC83 murine MAb). This long-term survival analysis specifically compared TAG-72-negative patients with no evidence of detectable TAG-72 antigen-bearing tissues upon completion of the operation to TAG-72-positive patients with evidence of persistent detectable TAG-72 antigen-bearing tissues upon completion of the operation and clearly demonstrated that the absence of detectable TAG-72 antigen within the surgical field at the completion of radioimmunoguided surgical procedure was of significant prognostic value, showing significantly improved median and time-dependent survival, most notably for advanced-stage disease, and with time-dependent multivariate Cox proportional hazards regression analysis demonstrating the significance of both pathologic stage of disease and TAG-72 positivity status upon long-term mortality risk. The authors concluded that the absence of detectable TAG-72 antigen within the surgical field at the completion of radioimmunoguided surgical procedure for primary colorectal cancer conferred a long-term and sustainable survival advantage to those patients in whom complete surgical removal of all tissues with detectable radiolabeled anti-TAG-72 murine MAb (i.e., detectable TAG-72 antigen) was accomplished. Clearly then, it is not what is surgically removed at the time of cancer surgery which is ultimately of most importance, but it is rather what is left behind at the time of cancer surgery which is ultimately of most importance. Therefore, one can postulate that surgical clearance of all radioimmunoguided surgery-positive tissues (i.e., surgical clearance of all detectable tumor antigen within the tissues) is what is ultimately important, independent of whether or not malignant cells can be histologically identified within those surgically resected tissues. Thus, if it is to again become clinically relevant, radioimmunoguided surgery, as it was once known, will need to move toward new lines of thinking, both on a molecular level and in an attempt to change the dictum for the surgical treatment of cancer toward a concept of antigen-directed cancer surgery. With the ongoing advancements and developments in diagnostic imaging technology and therapeutics, antigen-directed cancer surgery can represent an important advancement in oncologic theranostics and realistically contribute in a positive fashion to patient outcomes [180].

24.8 Concluding Remarks

From a historical perspective, it is clear that radioimmunoguided surgery represents one of the most important developments in the realm of all radioguided surgery applications, as the genesis and predominant clinical utilization of radioimmunoguided surgery during the 1980s and 1990s was fundamentally important in the later technological development and refinement of all currently commercially available radiation detection devices used so commonplace in the multitude of present-day radioguided surgery applications. It is a fair statement to say that if it was not for the development of radioimmunoguided surgery during the 1980s and the subsequent technological advancements in radiation detection device design, it would be quite possible that the rapid emergence of radioguided sentinel lymph node biopsy technology for both breast cancer and melanoma that ensued in the 1990s would have not been fully realized until a much later time. In order for radioimmunoguided surgery to again become clinically relevant in the future, we must direct our attention toward the molecular basis of cancer, incorporate cancer diagnostics and cancer therapeutics in an oncologic theranostics fashion, and fully realize and embrace radioimmunoguided surgery as a powerful form of antigen-directed cancer surgery.

References

1. Povoski SP, Neff RL, Mojzisik CM, O'Malley DM, Hinkle GH, Hall NC, Murrey Jr DA, Knopp MV, Martin Jr EW. A comprehensive overview of radioguided surgery using gamma detection probe technology. World J Surg Oncol. 2009;7:11.
2. Ghose T, Tai J, Aquino J, Norvell S, MacDonald A. Tumor localization of 131I-labeled antibodies by radionuclide imaging. Radiology. 1975;116:445–8.
3. Ghose T, Guclu A, Tai J, MacDonald AS, Norvell ST, Aquino J. Antibody as carrier of 131I in cancer diagnosis and treatment. Cancer. 1975;36:1646–57.
4. Belitsky P, Ghose T, Aquino J, Tai J, MacDonald AS. Radionuclide imaging of metastases from renal-cell carcinoma by 131I-labeled antitumor antibody. Radiology. 1978;126:515–7.
5. Belitsky P, Ghose T, Aquino J, Norvell ST, Blair AH. Radionuclide imaging of primary renal-cell carcinoma by I-131-labeled antitumor antibody. J Nucl Med. 1978;19:427–30.
6. Goldenberg DM, DeLand F, Kim E, Bennett S, Primus FJ, van Nagell JR, Jr EN, DeSimone P, Rayburn P. Use of radiolabeled antibodies to carcinoembryonic antigen for the detection and localization of diverse cancers by external photoscanning. N Engl J Med. 1978;298:1384–6.
7. Carey LC. Foreward. In: Martin Jr EW, editor. Radioimmunoguided surgery (RIGS) in the detection and treatment of colorectal cancer. 1st ed. Austin: R.G. Landes Company; 1994. p. xiii–xiv.
8. Aitken DR, Thurston MO, Hinkle Jr GH, Martin DT, Haagensen Jr DE, Houchens D, Tuttle SE, Martin Jr EW. Portable gamma probe for radioimmune localization of experimental colon tumor xenografts. J Surg Res. 1984;36:480–9.
9. Aitken DR, Hinkle GH, Thurston MO, Tuttle SE, Martin DT, Olsen J, Haagensen Jr DE, Houchens D, Martin Jr EW. A gamma-detecting probe for radioimmune detection of CEA-producing tumors. Successful experimental use and clinical case report. Dis Colon Rectum. 1984;27:279–82.
10. Martin DT, Hinkle GH, Tuttle S, Olsen J, Nabi H, Houchens D, Thurston M, Martin Jr EW. Intraoperative radioimmunodetection of colorectal tumors with a hand-held radiation detector. Am J Surg. 1985;150:672–5.
11. Martin Jr EW, Hinkle G, Mojzisik C, Thurston MO. Radioimmunoguided surgery: a new intraoperative approach to the detection of tumor. Cancer Treat Res. 1990;51:387–411.
12. Martin Jr EW, Tuttle SE, Rousseau M, Mojzisik CM, O'Dwyer PJ, Hinkle GH, Miller EA, Goodwin RA, Oredipe OA, Barth RF, Olsen JO, Houchens D, Jewell SD, Bucci DM, Adams D, Steplewski Z, Thurston MO. Radioimmunoguided surgery: intraoperative use of monoclonal antibody 17-1A in colorectal cancer. Hybridoma. 1986;5 Suppl 1:S97–S108.
13. Hinkle GH, Laven DL. Radionucleotides. In: Martin Jr EW, editor. Radioimmunoguided surgery (RIGS) in the detection and treatment of colorectal cancer. 1st ed. Austin: R.G. Landes Company; 1994. p. 29–39.
14. Hinkle G, Houchens D, Miller E, Nines R, Nabi H, Thurston M, Tuttle S, Mojzisik C, Martin EW Jr. Preferential localization of antibody combinations in tumor xenografts in nude mice. In: Rygaard J, Brünner N, Graem N, Spang-Thomsen M, editors. Immune-deficient animals in biomedical research. Copenhagen: 5th Int. Workshop on Immune-Deficient Animals; 1987. p. 248–50.
15. Thurston MO. Development of the gamma-detecting probe for radioimmunoguided surgery. In: Martin EW, editor. Radioimmunoguided surgery (RIGS) in the detection and treatment of colorectal cancer. 1st ed. Austin: R.G. Landes Company; 1994. p. 41–65.
16. Berens A, Mosic J. The RIGS patient in the clinical setting. In: Martin EW, editor. Radioimmunoguided surgery (RIGS) in the detection and treatment of colorectal cancer. 1st ed. Austin: R.G. Landes Company; 1994. p. 107–23.
17. Nieroda CA, Milenic DE, Colcher D, Schlom J. Monoclonal antibodies for use in radioimmunoguided surgery (RIGS). In: Martin Jr EW, editor. Radioimmunoguided surgery (RIGS) in the detection and treatment of colorectal cancer. 1st ed. Austin: R.G. Landes Company; 1994. p. 7–27.
18. Hinkle GH, Houchens DP, Sampsel J, Schneebaum S. The RIGS system using animal models. In: Martin Jr EW, editor. Radioimmunoguided surgery (RIGS) in the detection and treatment of colorectal cancer. 1st ed. Austin: R.G. Landes Company; 1994. p. 67–80.
19. Sun D, Bloomston M, Hinkle G, Al-Saif OH, Hall NC, Povoski SP, Arnold MW, Martin EW. Radioimmunoguided surgery (RIGS), PET/CT image-guided surgery, and fluorescence image-guided surgery: past, present, and future. J Surg Oncol. 2007;96:297–308.
20. Leenaars M, Hendriksen CF. Critical steps in the production of polyclonal and monoclonal antibodies: evaluation and recommendations. ILAR J. 2005;46:269–79.

21. Schwaber J, Cohen EP. Human x mouse somatic cell hybrid clone secreting immunoglobulins of both parental types. Nature. 1973;244(5416):444–7.
22. Schwaber J, Cohen EP. Pattern of immunoglobulin synthesis and assembly in a human-mouse somatic cell hybrid clone. Proc Natl Acad Sci U S A. 1974;71:2203–7.
23. Köhler G, Milstein C. Continuous cultures of fused cells secreting antibody of predefined specificity. Nature. 1975;256:495–7.
24. Schroff RW, Foon KA, Beatty SM, Oldham RK, Morgan Jr AC. Human anti-murine immunoglobulin responses in patients receiving monoclonal antibody therapy. Cancer Res. 1985;45:879–85.
25. Morrison SL, Johnson MJ, Herzenberg LA, Oi VT. Chimeric human antibody molecules: mouse antigen-binding domains with human constant region domains. Proc Natl Acad Sci U S A. 1984;81:387–411.
26. Riechmann L, Clark M, Waldmann H, Winter G. Reshaping human antibodies for therapy. Nature. 1988;332(6162):323–7.
27. Tamura M, Milenic DE, Iwahashi M, Padlan E, Schlom J, Kashmiri SVS. Structural correlates of an anticarcinoma antibody: identification of a specificity-determining residues (SDRs) and development of a minimally immunogenic antibody variant by retention of SDRs only. J Immunol. 2000;164:1432–41.
28. Bruggeman M, Neuberger MS. Strategies for expressing human antibody repertoires in transgenic mice. Immunol Today. 1996;17:391–7.
29. Mendez MJ, Green LL, Corvalan JR, Jia XC, Maynard-Currie CE, Yang XD, Gallo ML, Louie DM, Lee DV, Erickson KL, Luna J, Roy CM, Abderrahim H, Kirschenbaum F, Noguchi M, Smith DH, Fukushima A, Hales JF, Klapholz S, Finer MH, Davis CG, Zsebo KM, Jakobovits A. Functional transplant of megabase human immunoglobulin loci recapitulates human antibody response in mice. Nat Genet. 1997;15:146–56.
30. McCafferty J, Griffiths AD, Winter G, Chiswell DJ. Phage antibodies: filamentous phage displaying antibody variable domains. Nature. 1990;348(6301):552–4.
31. Winter G, Griffiths AD, Hawkins RE, Hoogenboom HR. Making antibodies by phage display technology. Annu Rev Immunol. 1994;12:433–55.
32. Burton DR, Barbas III CF. Human antibodies from combinatorial libraries. Adv Immunol. 1994;57:191–280.
33. Martin Jr EW, Barnes JA, Thurston MO. Introduction: the RIGS concept. In: Martin Jr EW, editor. Radioimmunoguided surgery (RIGS) in the detection and treatment of colorectal cancer. 1st ed. Austin: R.G. Landes Company; 1994. p. 1–6.
34. Martin Jr EW, Thurston MO. The use of monoclonal antibodies (MAbs) and the development of an intraoperative hand-held probe for cancer detection. Cancer Invest. 1996;14:560–71.
35. Martin Jr EW, Thurston MO. Intraoperative radioimmunodetection. Semin Surg Oncol. 1998;15:205–8.
36. Paganelli G, Magnani P, Fazio F. Pretargeting of carcinomas with the avidin-biotin system. Int J Biol Markers. 1993;8:155–9.
37. Boerman OC, van Schaijk FG, Oyen WJ, Corstens FH. Pretargeted radioimmunotherapy of cancer: progress step by step. J Nucl Med. 2003;44:400–11.
38. Gruaz-Guyon A, Janevik-Ivanovska E, Raguin O, De Labriolle-Vaylet C, Barbet J. Radiolabeled bivalent haptens for tumor immunodetection and radioimmunotherapy. Q J Nucl Med. 2001;45:201–6.
39. Goldenberg DM, Rossi EA, Sharkey RM, McBride WJ, Chang CH. Multifunctional antibodies by the dock-and-lock method for improved cancer imaging and therapy by pretargeting. J Nucl Med. 2008;49:158–63.
40. Johnson VG, Schlom J, Paterson AJ, Bennett J, Magnani JL, Colcher D. Analysis of a human tumor-associated glycoprotein (TAG-72) identified by monoclonal antibody B72.3. Cancer Res. 1986;46:850–7.
41. Sheer DG, Schlom J, Cooper HL. Purification and composition of the human tumor-associated glycoprotein (TAG-72) defined by monoclonal antibodies CC49 and B72.3. Cancer Res. 1988;48:6811–8.
42. Loy TS, Nashelsky MB. Reactivity of B72.3 with adenocarcinomas. An immunohistochemical study of 476 cases. Cancer. 1993;72:2495–8.
43. Colcher D, Milenic D, Roselli M, Raubitschek A, Yarranton G, King D, Adair J, Whittle N, Bodmer M, Schlom J. Characterization and biodistribution of recombinant and recombinant/chimeric constructs of monoclonal antibody B72.3. Cancer Res. 1989;49:1738–45.
44. Stramignoni D, Bowen R, Atkinson BF, Schlom J. Differential reactivity of monoclonal antibodies with human colon adenocarcinomas and adenomas. Int J Cancer. 1983;31:543–52.
45. Ohuchi N, Simpson JF, Colcher D, Schlom J. Complementation of anti-CEA and anti-TAG-72 monoclonal antibodies in reactivity to human gastric adenocarcinomas. Int J Cancer. 1987;40:726–33.
46. Thor A, Gorstein F, Ohuchi N, Szpak CA, Johnston WW, Schlom J. Tumor-associated glycoprotein (TAG-72) in ovarian carcinomas defined by monoclonal antibody B72.3. J Natl Cancer Inst. 1986;76:995–1006.
47. Nuti M, Teramoto YA, Mariani-Costantini R, Hand PH, Colcher D, Schlom J. A monoclonal antibody (B72.3) defines patterns of distribution of a novel tumor-associated antigen in human mammary carcinoma cell populations. Int J Cancer. 1982;29:539–45.
48. Thor A, Ohuchi N, Szpak CA, Johnston WW, Schlom J. Distribution of oncofetal antigen tumor-associated glycoprotein-72 defined by monoclonal antibody B72.3. Cancer Res. 1986;46:3118–24.
49. Colcher D, Hand PH, Nuti M, Schlom J. A spectrum of monoclonal antibodies reactive with human

antibody (B72.3) used for the in situ radioimmunodetection of human colon carcinoma xenografts. Cancer Res. 1984;44:5744–9.
97. Sickle-Santanello BJ, O'Dwyer PJ, Mojzisik C, Tuttle SE, Hinkle GH, Rousseau M, Schlom J, Colcher D, Thurston MO, Nieroda C, Sardi A, Farrar WB, Minton JP, Martin Jr EW. Radioimmunoguided surgery using the monoclonal antibody B72.3 in colorectal tumors. Dis Colon Rectum. 1987;30:761–4.
98. Martin Jr EW, Mojzisik CM, Hinkle GH, Sampsel J, Siddiqi M, Tuttle SE, Sickle-Santanello B, Colcher D, Thurston MO, Bell J, Farrar WB, Schlom J. Radioimmunoguided surgery using monoclonal antibody. Am J Surg. 1988;156:386–92.
99. Tuttle SE, Jewell SD, Mojzisik CM, Hinkle GH, Colcher D, Schlom J, Martin EW. Intraoperative radioimmunolocalization of colorectal carcinoma with a hand-held gamma probe and MAb B72.3: comparison of in vivo gamma probe counts with in vitro MAb radiolocalization. Int J Cancer. 1988;42:352–8.
100. Nieroda CA, Mojzisik C, Sardi A, Ferrara P, Hinkle G, Thurston MO, Martin Jr EW. Radioimmunoguided surgery in primary colon cancer. Cancer Detect Prev. 1990;14:651–6.
101. Martin Jr EW, Carey LC. Second-look surgery for colorectal cancer. Ann Surg. 1991;214:321–5; discussion 326–7.
102. Cohen AM, Martin Jr EW, Lavery I, Daly J, Sardi A, Aitken D, Bland K, Mojzisik C, Hinkle G. Radioimmunoguided surgery using iodine 125 B72.3 in patients with colorectal cancer. Arch Surg. 1991;126:349–52.
103. Di Carlo V, Stella M, De Nardi P, Baratti D, Sassi I, Mangili F, Zito M, Badellino F, Dionigi R, Fazio F. The role of B72.3 125-I monoclonal antibody in the radioimmunoguided surgery of colorectal neoplasms. Ann Ital Chir. 1991;62:245–9.
104. Stella M, De Nardi P, Paganelli G, Sassi I, Zito M, Magnani P, Baratti D, Mangili F, Spagnolo W, Siccardi AG, Fazio F, Di Carlo V. Surgery for colorectal cancer guided by radiodetecting probe. Clinical evaluation using monoclonal antibody B72.3. Eur J Surg. 1991;157:485–8.
105. Di Carlo V, Badellino F, Stella M, De Nardi P, Fazio F, Percivale P, Bertoglio S, Schenone F, Benevento A, Carcano G, Dominioni L, Dionigi R. Role of B72.3 iodine 125-labeled monoclonal antibody in colorectal cancer detection by radioimmunoguided surgery. Surgery. 1994;115:190–8.
106. Stella M, De Nardi P, Paganelli G, Magnani P, Mangili F, Sassi I, Baratti D, Gini P, Zito F, Cristallo M, Fazio F, Di Carlo V. Avidin-biotin system in radioimmunoguided surgery for colorectal cancer. Advantages and limits. Dis Colon Rectum. 1994;37:335–43.
107. Paganelli G, Stella M, Zito F, Magnani P, De Nardi P, Mangili F, Baratti D, Veglia F, Di Carlo V, Siccardi AG, Fazio F. Radioimmunoguided surgery using iodine-125-labeled biotinylated monoclonal antibodies and cold avidin. J Nucl Med. 1994;35:1970–5.
108. Di Carlo V, Stella M, De Nardi P, Fazio F. Radioimmunoguided surgery: clinical experience with different monoclonal antibodies and methods. Tumori. 1995;81(3 Suppl):98–102.
109. Bertoglio S, Benevento A, Percivale P, Cafiero F, Moresco L, Peressini A, Dionigi R, Badellino F. Radioimmunoguided surgery benefits in carcinoembryonic antigen-directed second-look surgery in the asymptomatic patient after curative resection of colorectal cancer. Semin Surg Oncol. 1998;15:263–7.
110. Bertoglio S, Percivale P, Schenone F, Peressini A, Murolo C, Badellino F. Role of tumor-associated antigen expression in radioimmunoguided surgery for colorectal and breast cancer. Semin Surg Oncol. 1998;15:249–53.
111. Percivale P, Bertoglio S, Meszaros P, Schenone F, Gipponi M, Moresco L, Cosso M, Badellino F. Radioimmunoguided surgery with different iodine-125 radiolabeled monoclonal antibodies in recurrent colorectal cancer. Semin Surg Oncol. 1998;15:231–4.
112. Renda A, Iovino F, Capasso L, Ricciardelli L, Tammaro V, Acampa W. Radioimmunoguided surgery in colorectal cancer: a 6-year experience with four different technical solutions. Semin Surg Oncol. 1998;15:226–30.
113. Veroux G, Nicosia A, Veroux P, Cardillo P, Veroux M, Amodeo C. Radioimmunoguided surgery. Hepatogastroenterology. 1999;30:3099–108.
114. Krag DN, Haseman MK, Ford P, Smith L, Taylor MH, Schneider P, Goodnight JE. Gamma probe location of 111indium-labeled B72.3: an extension of immunoscintigraphy. J Surg Oncol. 1992;51:226–30.
115. Muxi A, Pons F, Vidal-Sicart S, Setoain FJ, Herranz R, Novell F, Fernandez RM, Trias M, Setoain J. Radioimmunoguided surgery of colorectal carcinoma with an 111In-labelled anti-TAG72 monoclonal antibody. Nucl Med Commun. 1999;20:123–30.
116. Hladik P, Vizda J, Bedrna J, Simkovic D, Strnad L, Smejkal K, Voboril Z. Immunoscintigraphy and intra-operative radioimmunodetection in the treatment of colorectal carcinoma. Colorectal Dis. 2001;3:380–6.
117. Collier BD, Abdel-Nabi H, Doerr RJ, Harwood SJ, Olsen J, Kaplan EH, Winzelberg GG, Grossman SJ, Krag DN, Mitchell EP. Immunoscintigraphy performed with In-111-labeled CYT-103 in the management of colorectal cancer: comparison with CT. Radiology. 1992;185:179–86.
118. Arnold MW, Schneebaum S, Berens A, Petty L, Mojzisik C, Hinkle G, Martin Jr EW. Intraoperative detection of colorectal cancer with radioimmunoguided surgery and CC49, a second-generation monoclonal antibody. Ann Surg. 1992;216:627–32.
119. Arnold MW, Schneebaum S, Berens A, Mojzisik C, Hinkle G, Martin Jr EW. Radioimmunoguided

surgery challenges traditional decision making in patients with primary colorectal cancer. Surgery. 1992;112:624–9; discussion 629–30.
120. Arnold MW, Young DC, Hitchcock CL, Schneebaum S, Martin Jr EW. Radioimmunoguided surgery in primary colorectal carcinoma: an intraoperative prognostic tool and adjuvant to traditional staging. Am J Surg. 1995;170:315–8.
121. Bertsch DJ, Burak WE, Young DC, Arnold MW, Martin Jr EW. Radioimmunoguided surgery system improves survival for patients recurrent colorectal cancer. Surgery. 1995;118:634–8.
122. Arnold MW, Hitchcock CL, Young DC, Burak Jr WE, Bertsch DJ, Martin Jr EW. Intra-abdominal patterns of disease dissemination in colorectal cancer identified using radioimmunoguided surgery. Dis Colon Rectum. 1996;39:509–13.
123. Bertsch DJ, Burak Jr WE, Young DC, Arnold MW, Martin Jr EW. Radioimmunoguided surgery for colorectal cancer. Ann Surg Oncol. 1996;3:310–6.
124. Arnold MW, Young DC, Hitchcock CL, Barberá-Guillem E, Nieroda C, Martin Jr EW. Staging of colorectal cancer: biology vs. morphology. Dis Colon Rectum. 1998;41:1–6.
125. Manayan RC, Hart MJ, Friend WG. Radioimmunoguided surgery for colorectal cancer. Am J Surg. 1997;173:386–9.
126. Schneebaum S, Papo J, Graif M, Baratz M, Baron J, Skornik Y. Radioimmunoguided surgery benefits for recurrent colorectal cancer. Ann Surg Oncol. 1997;4:371–6.
127. Avital S, Haddad R, Troitsa A, Kashtan H, Brazovsky E, Gitstein G, Skornick Y, Schneebaum S. Radioimmunoguided surgery for recurrent colorectal cancer manifested by isolated CEA elevation. Cancer. 2000;89:1692–8.
128. Schneebaum S, Troitsa A, Avital S, Haddad R, Kashtan H, Gitstein G, Baratz M, Brazovsky E, Papo J, Skornick Y. Identification of lymph node metastases in recurrent colorectal cancer. Recent Results Cancer Res. 2000;157:281–92.
129. Haddad R, Avital S, Troitsa A, Chen J, Baratz M, Brazovsky E, Gitstein G, Kashtan H, Skornick Y, Schneebaum S. Benefits of radioimmunoguided surgery for pelvic recurrence. Eur J Surg Oncol. 2001;27:298–301.
130. Schneebaum S, Troitsa A, Haddad R, Avital S, Kashtan H, Baratz M, Brazovsky E, Papo J, Skornick Y. Immunoguided lymph node dissection in colorectal cancer: a new challenge? World J Surg. 2001;25:1495–8; discussion 1499.
131. Quinlan D, Davidson A, Gamponia E, Lindley J, Doshi H. Detection of tumor-associated glycoprotein-72 (TAG-72) in short-term and long-term surviving colon cancer patients using a first- and second-generation monoclonal antibody. Proc Am Assoc Cancer Res. 1991;32:271.
132. Burak Jr WE, Schneebaum S, Kim JA, Arnold MW, Hinkle G, Berens A, Mojzisik C, Martin Jr EW. Pilot study evaluating the intraoperative localization of radiolabeled monoclonal antibody CC83 in patients with metastatic colorectal carcinoma. Surgery. 1995;118:103–8.
133. Povoski SP, Hatzaras IS, Mojzisik CM, Arnold MW, Hinkle GH, Hitchcock CL, Young DC, Martin Jr EW. Antigen-directed cancer surgery for primary colorectal cancer: 15-year survival analysis. Ann Surg Oncol. 2012;19:131–8.
134. Agnese DM, Abdessalam SF, Burak WE, Arnold MW, Soble D, Hinkle GH, Young D, Kazaeli MB, Martin Jr EW. Pilot study using a humanized CC49 monoclonal antibody (HuCC49ΔC_H2) to localize recurrent colorectal carcinoma. J Surg Oncol. 2004;11:197–202.
135. Curtet C, Vuillez JP, Daniel G, Aillet G, Chetanneau A, Visset J, Kremer M, Thédrez P, Chatal JF. Feasibility study of radioimmunoguided surgery of colorectal carcinomas using indium-111 CEA-specific monoclonal antibody. Eur J Nucl Med. 1990;17:299–304.
136. Lechner P, Lind P, Binter G. Tc-99m-labeled anti-CEA antibodies in intraoperative diagnosis of colorectal cancer. Nuklearmedizin. 1995;34:8–14. [German].
137. Lechner P. Probe-guided surgery of colorectal carcinoma. Acta Med Austriaca. 1997;24:68–72. [German].
138. Lechner P, Lind P, Snyder M, Haushofer H. Probe-guided surgery for colorectal cancer. Recent Results Cancer Res. 2000;157:273–80.
139. Mayer A, Tsiompanou E, O'Malley D, Boxer GM, Bhatia J, Flynn AA, Chester KA, Davidson BR, Lewis AA, Winslet MC, Dhillon AP, Hilson AJ, Begent RH. Radioimmunoguided surgery in colorectal cancer using a genetically engineered anti-CEA single-chain Fv antibody. Clin Cancer Res. 2000;6:1711–9.
140. Gioffrè Florio MA, Baldari S, Famà F, Giacobbe G, Pollicino A. Radioimmunoguided surgery (R.I.G.S.) in colorectal cancer. Preliminary results. Chir Ital. 2002;54:323–9. [Italian].
141. Gioffrè Florio MA, Famà F, Gullo G, Mazzei S, Pollicino A, Scarfò P, Vindigni A. Personal experience using radioimmunoguided surgery (RIGS). Ann Ital Chir. 2007;78:433–7. [Italian].
142. Strong VE, Humm J, Russo P, Jungbluth A, Wong WD, Daghighian F, Old L, Fong Y, Larson SM. A novel method to localize antibody-targeted cancer deposits intraoperatively using handheld PET beta and gamma probes. Surg Endosc. 2008;22:386–91.
143. de Nardi P, Stella M, Magnani P, Paganelli G, Mangili F, Fazio F, di Carlo V. Combination of monoclonal antibodies for radioimmunoguided surgery. Int J Colorectal Dis. 1997;12:24–8.
144. Xu G, Zhang M, Liu B, Li Z, Lin B, Xu X, Jin M, Li J, Wu J, Dong Z. Radioimmunoguided surgery in gastric cancer using 131-I labeled monoclonal antibody 3H11. Semin Surg Oncol. 1994;10:88–94.
145. Liu BG, Xu GW, Zhang MY. A clinical trial of radioimmunoguided surgery for gastric cancer. Zhonghua Zhong Liu Za Zhi. 1994;16:284–7. [Chinese].

146. Lucisano E, Bertoglio S. Role of radioimmunoguided surgery using iodine-125-labeled B72.3 monoclonal antibody in gastric cancer surgery. Semin Surg Oncol. 1998;15:212–4.
147. Mussa A, Sandrucci S, Mobiglia A, Baccega M, Mussa B, De Filippi PG. Role of radioimmunolocalization in the staging of gastric carcinoma. Semin Surg Oncol. 1998;15:209–11.
148. Wang C, Wang Y, Su X, Lin B, Xu X, Zhang M, Li J, Xu G. Iodine-125 labeled monoclonal antibody 3H11: in radioimmunoguided surgery for primary gastric cancer. Zhonghua Wai Ke Za Zhi. 2000;38:507–9. [Chinese].
149. LaValle GJ, Martinez DA, Sobel D, DeYoung B, Martin Jr EW. Assessment of disseminated pancreatic cancer: a comparison of traditional exploratory laparotomy and radioimmunoguided surgery. Surgery. 1997;122:867–71; discussion 871–3.
150. Nieroda CA, Mojzisik C, Sardi A, Farrar WB, Hinkle G, Siddiqi MA, Ferrara PJ, James A, Schlom J, Thurston MO, Martin Jr EW. Staging of carcinoma of the breast using a hand-held gamma detecting probe and monoclonal antibody B72.3. Surg Gynecol Obstet. 1989;169:35–40.
151. Percivale P, Bertoglio S, Meszaros P, Canavese G, Cafiero F, Gipponi M, Campora E, Gasco M, Badellino F. Radioimmunoguided surgery after primary treatment of locally advanced breast cancer. J Clin Oncol. 1996;14:1599–603.
152. Badellino F, Bertoglio S, Mariani G, Meszaros P, Canavese G, Percivale P. Use of radioimmunoguided surgery after induction chemotherapy in locally advanced breast cancer. Semin Surg Oncol. 1998;15:245–8.
153. Burak Jr WE, DePalatis L, Mosic JL, Soble D, Hinkle G, Hitchcock CL. Radioimmunoguided breast surgery using radiolabeled antibody NR-LU-10 FAB: a pilot study. Tumori. 2001;87:142–6.
154. Gitsch E, Pateisky N, Schatten C. Diagnostic and intraoperative immunoscintigraphy in ovarian cancer. Eur J Obstet Gynecol Reprod Biol. 1989;32:33–7.
155. Gitsch E, Pateisky N. Radio-immunoscintigraphy and intraoperative tumour detection by means of anti-tumour antibodies in patients with ovarian cancer. Baillieres Clin Obstet Gynaecol. 1989;3:31–6.
156. Pateisky N, Gitsch E. Immunoscintigraphy and intraoperative tumor search in ovarian cancer. Arch Gynecol Obstet. 1989;245:606–9. [German].
157. Bell J, Mojzisik C, Hinkle Jr G, Derman H, Schlom J, Martin E. Intraoperative radioimmunodetection of ovarian cancer using monoclonal antibody B72.3 and a portable gamma-detecting probe. Obstet Gynecol. 1990;76:607–11.
158. Jäger W, Feistel H, Paterok EM, Ronay G, Tulusan AH, Wolf F, Lang N. Resection guided by antibodies (REGAJ): a diagnostic procedure during second-look operation in ovarian cancer patients. Br J Cancer Suppl. 1990;10:18–20.
159. Ind TE, Granowska M, Britton KE, Morris G, Lowe DG, Hudson CN, Shepherd JH. Peroperative radioimmunodetection of ovarian carcinoma using a hand-held gamma detection probe. Br J Cancer. 1994;70:1263–6.
160. McIntosh DG, Colcher D, Seemayer T, Smith ML. The intraoperative detection of ovarian adenocarcinoma using radiolabeled CC49 monoclonal antibody and a hand-held gamma-detecting probe. Cancer Biother Radiopharm. 1997;12:287–94.
161. Badalament RA, Burgers JK, Petty LR, Mojzisik CM, Berens A, Marsh W, Hinkle GH, Martin Jr EW. Radioimmunoguided radical prostatectomy and lymphadenectomy. Cancer. 1993;71:2268–75.
162. Anderson RS, Eifert B, Tartt S, King P. Radioimmunoguided surgery using indium-111 capromab pendetide (PROSTASCINT) to diagnose supraclavicular metastasis from prostate cancer. Urology. 2000;56:669xii–v.
163. Grazia M, Bini A, Stella F, Pagani D, Bazzocchi R. Radioimmunoguided surgery and intraoperative lung cancer staging. Semin Surg Oncol. 1998;15:215–9.
164. Mansi L, Di Lieto E, Rambaldi PF, Bergaminelli C, Fallanca F, Vicidomini G, Cuccurullo V, Mancusi R. Preliminary experience with radioimmunoguided surgery of primary neoplasms of the lung. Minerva Chir. 1998;53:369–72. [Italian].
165. Argenzio V, Rambaldi PF, Iorio G, Cuccurullo V, Cascini G, Argenzio G, Mansi L. Radioimmunoguided surgery in squamous cell carcinoma. J Am Soc Plast Surg. 1999;103:749–51.
166. Peltier P, Curtet C, Chatal JF, Le Doussal JM, Daniel G, Aillet G, Gruaz-Guyon A, Barbet J, Delaage M. Radioimmunodetection of medullary thyroid cancer using a bispecific anti-CEA/anti-indium-DTPA antibody and an indium-111-labeled DTPA dimer. J Nucl Med. 1993;34:1267–73.
167. Barbet J, Peltier P, Bardet S, Vuillez JP, Bachelot I, Denet S, Olivier P, Leccia F, Corcuff B, Huglo D, Proye C, Rouvier E, Meyer P, Chatal JF. Radioimmunodetection of medullary thyroid carcinoma using indium-111 bivalent hapten and anti-CEA x anti-DTPA-indium bispecific antibody. J Nucl Med. 1998;39:1172–8.
168. de Labriolle-Vaylet C, Cattan P, Sarfati E, Wioland M, Billotey C, Brochériou C, Rouvier E, de Roquancourt A, Rostène W, Askienazy S, Barbet J, Milhaud G, Gruaz-Guyon A. Successful surgical removal of occult metastases of medullary thyroid carcinoma recurrences with the help of immunoscintigraphy and radioimmunoguided surgery. Clin Cancer Res. 2000;6:363–71.
169. Houchens D, Cote R, Saad A, Nines R, Berens A, Sampsel J, Crockford D, Schneebaum S, Arnold M, Martin Jr E. Presence of occult tumor detected by 125I-labeled monoclonal antibody CC49. Proc AACR. 1992;33:317.
170. Houchens D, Cote R, Saad A, Nines R, Berens A, Crockford D, Rojas-Corona R. Schneebaum S,

Arnold M, Martin E, Jr. Radioimmunoguided surgery in colorectal cancer: histologic and immunohistochemical analysis of lymph nodes from patients injected with 125I-labeled monoclonal antibody CC49. Presented at the Seventh International Conference on Monoclonal Antibody Immunoconjugates for Cancer, San Diego; 5–7 Mar 1992.
171. Stephens AD, Punja U, Sugarbaker PH. False-positive lymph nodes by radioimmunoguided surgery: report of a patient and analysis of the problem. J Nucl Med. 1993;34:804–8.
172. Greenson JK, Isenhart CE, Rice R, Mojzisik C, Houchens D, Martin Jr EW. Identification of occult micrometastases in pericolic lymph nodes of Duke's B colorectal cancer patients using monoclonal antibodies against cytokeratin and CC49. Correlation with long-term survival. Cancer. 1994;73:563–9.
173. Hitchcock CL, Greenson JK, Sampsel JW, Houchens DP, Saad AD, Isenhart CE Schneebaum S, Seethi S, Cote RJ. RIGS pathology and the biologic staging of colorectal cancer. In: Martin EW, editor. Radioimmunoguided surgery (RIGS) in the detection and treatment of colorectal cancer. 1st ed. Austin: R.G. Landes Company; 1994. p. 147–60.
174. Schneebaum S, Arnold MW, Houchens DP, Greenson JK, Cote RJ, Hitchcock CL, Young DC, Mojzisik CM, Martin Jr EW. The significance of intraoperative periportal lymph node metastasis identification in patients with colorectal carcinoma. Cancer. 1995;75:2809–17.
175. Hitchcock CL, Arnold MW, Young DC, Schneebaum S, Martin Jr EW. TAG-72 expression in lymph nodes and RIGS. Dis Colon Rectum. 1996;39:473–5.
176. Cote RJ, Houchens DP, Hitchcock CL, Saad AD, Nines RG, Greenson JK, Schneebaum S, Arnold MW, Martin Jr EW. Intraoperative detection of occult colon cancer micrometastases using 125 I-radiolabled monoclonal antibody CC49. Cancer. 1996;77:613–20.
177. Barbera-Guillem E, Arnold MW, Nelson MB, Martin Jr EW. First results for resetting the antitumor immune response by immune corrective surgery in colon cancer. Am J Surg. 1998;176:339–43.
178. Abdel Nabi H, Doerr RJ, Balu D, Rogan L, Farrell EL, Evans NH. Gamma probe assisted ex vivo detection of small lymph node metastases following the administration of indium-111-labeled monoclonal antibodies to colorectal cancers. J Nucl Med. 1993;34:1818–22.
179. Sézeur A, Châtelet FP, Cywiner C, de Labriolle-Vaylet C, Chastang C, Billotey C, Malafosse M, Gallot D, Betton P, Montravers F, Carvajal-Gonzalez S, Askienazy S, Talbot JN, Rain JD, Milhaud G, Saumon G, Barbet J, Gruaz-Guyon A. Pathology underrates colon cancer extranodal and nodal metastases; ex vivo radioimmunodetection helps staging. Clin Cancer Res. 2007;13(18 Pt 2):5592s–7.
180. Povoski SP, Hatzaras IS, Mojzisik CM, Martin Jr EW. Oncologic theranostics: recognition of this concept in antigen-directed cancer therapy for colorectal cancer with anti-TAG-72 monoclonal antibodies. Expert Rev Mol Diagn. 2011;11:667–70.

^{18}F-FDG-Directed Surgery and ^{18}F-FDG-Directed Interventional Procedures

25

Stephen P. Povoski, Douglas A. Murrey Jr., and Nathan C. Hall

Contents

S.P. Povoski, MD (✉)
Division of Surgical Oncology, Department of Surgery, Arthur G. James Cancer Hospital and Richard J. Solove Research Institute and Comprehensive Cancer Center, The Ohio State University, Columbus, OH 43210, USA
e-mail: stephen.povoski@osumc.edu

D.A. Murrey Jr., MD
Department of Radiology, The Ohio State University, Columbus, OH 43210, USA
e-mail: douglas.murrey@osumc.edu

N.C. Hall, MD, PhD
Department of Radiology, University of Pennsylvania, Philadelphia, PA 19104, USA
e-mail: nathan.hall@uphs.upenn.edu

Portions of the contents of this chapter are adapted from 5 prior Open Access articles:

1. Povoski et al.: A comprehensive overview of radioguided surgery using gamma detection probe technology. *World Journal of Surgical Oncology*, 2009, **7**:11.; doi:10.1186/1477-7819-7-11; http://www.wjso.com/

K. Herrmann et al. (eds.), *Radioguided Surgery: Current Applications and Innovative Directions in Clinical Practice*, DOI 10.1007/978-3-319-26051-8_25

content/pdf/1477-7819-7-11.pdf; © 2009 Povoski et al; licensee BioMed Central Ltd. This is an Open Access article distributed under the terms of the Creative Commons Attribution License (http://creativecommons.org/licenses/by/2.0), which permits unrestricted use, distribution, and reproduction in any medium, provided the original work is properly cited.
2. Povoski et al.: Multimodal imaging and detection approach to ^{18}F-FDG-directed surgery for patients with known or suspected malignancies: a comprehensive description of the specific methodology utilized in a single-institution cumulative retrospective experience. *World Journal of Surgical Oncology*, 2011, **9:**152.; doi:10.1186/1477-7819-9-152; http://www.wjso.com/content/pdf/1477-7819-9-152.pdf; © 2011 Povoski et al; licensee BioMed Central Ltd. This is an Open Access article distributed under the terms of the Creative Commons Attribution License (http://creativecommons.org/licenses/by/2.0), which permits unrestricted use, distribution, and reproduction in any medium, provided the original work is properly cited.
3. Povoski et al.: ^{18}F-FDG PET/CT oncologic imaging at extended injection-to-scan acquisition time intervals derived from a single institution ^{18}F-FDG-directed surgery experience: feasibility and quantification of ^{18}F-FDG accumulation within ^{18}F-FDG-avid lesions and background tissues. *BMC Cancer* 2014 **14:**453.; doi:10.1186/1471-2407-14-453; http://www.biomedcentral.com/content/pdf/1471-2407-14-453.pdf; © 2014 Povoski et al; licensee BioMed Central Ltd. This is an Open Access article distributed under the terms of the Creative Commons Attribution License (http://creativecommons.org/licenses/by/4.0), which permits unrestricted use, distribution, and reproduction in any medium, provided the original work is properly cited.
4. Chapman et al.: Comparison of two threshold detection criteria methodologies for determination of probe positivity for intraoperative in situ identification of presumed abnormal ^{18}F-FDG avid tissue sites during radioguided oncologic surgery. *BMC Cancer.* 2014 **14:**667.; doi:10.1186/1471-2407-14-667; http://www.biomedcentral.com/content/pdf/1471-2407-14-667.pdf; © 2014 Chapman et al; licensee BioMed Central Ltd. This is an Open Access article distributed under the terms of the Creative Commons Attribution License (http://creativecommons.org/licenses/by/4.0), which permits unrestricted use, distribution, and reproduction in any medium, provided the original work is properly cited.
5. Povoski et al.: Feasibility of a multimodal ^{18}F-FDG-directed lymph node surgical excisional biopsy approach for appropriate diagnostic tissue sampling in patients with suspected lymphoma. *BMC Cancer* 2015 **15:**378.; doi:10.1186/s12885-015-1381-z; http://www.biomedcentral.com/content/pdf/s12885-015-1381-z.pdf; © 2015 Povoski et al; licensee BioMed Central Ltd. This is an Open Access article distributed under the terms of the Creative Commons Attribution License (http://creativecommons.org/licenses/by/4.0), which permits unrestricted use, distribution, and reproduction in any medium, provided the original work is properly cited.

Abstract

The use of positron-emitting and high-energy gamma photon-emitting radiopharmaceuticals, like fluorine-18 fluorodeoxyglucose (^{18}F-FDG), for real-time cancer detection and surgical guidance within the operating room and for real-time guidance of diagnostic and therapeutic interventional procedures within the interventional radiology suite, has great clinical potential. This technology may allow for (1) real-time intraoperative staging of the extent of disease; (2) real-time intraoperative surgical planning and execution of the necessary and most appropriate operation, determination of the extent of surgical resection, and determination of the completeness of surgical resection; (3) real-time pathologic evaluation of intact surgical resected specimens for the confirmation of completeness of surgical resection and for surgical margin assessment; (4) real-time pathologic evaluation of diagnostically biopsied tissues for confirmation of correctness of tissue diagnosis; and (5) real-time guidance of diagnostic and therapeutic interventional procedures within the interventional radiology suite. This chapter discusses (1) the history and development of positron imaging and detection, (2) the fundamental basis for the use of ^{18}F-FDG in positron imaging and detection strategies, (3) the inherent limitations of ^{18}F-FDG in positron imaging and detection strategies, (4) radiation detection devices utilized during ^{18}F-FDG-directed surgery, (5) the clinical applications of real-time ^{18}F-FDG-directed surgery and real-time ^{18}F-FDG-directed interventional procedures, (6) timing issues related to ^{18}F-FDG-directed surgery, (7) the inherent challenge of in situ detection of ^{18}F-FDG with a gamma photon detection device, and (8) occupational radiation exposure during ^{18}F-FDG radioguided surgical procedures.

25.1 The History of the Development of Positron Imaging and Detection

The theoretical physics framework behind the implementation of positron imaging and detection is the basic concept of electron-positron annihilation [1–6], which was first realized in the 1930s. Within any given biological system, electron-positron annihilation results when a positron (i.e., a positively charged antimatter counterpart of an electron), emitted from the nucleus of a radionuclide and travels only a few millimeters, collides with an electron (i.e., a negative charged particle) within a biological tissue and generates two resultant high-energy 511 keV gamma photons traveling in opposite directions.

The development of clinical applications of positron imaging and detection has its origins in the early 1950s [7, 8] and occurred far before the subsequent availability of fluorine-18 fluorodeoxyglucose (^{18}F-FDG) in the late 1970s [9, 10]. The first reported clinical application of positron imaging technology in humans was published by Gordon L. Brownell and William H. Sweet at the Massachusetts General Hospital (Boston, Massachusetts, USA) in 1953 and consisted of the collection of three-dimensional data using a prototype positron imaging device on patients with brain tumors who were intravenously injected with arsenic-74 [7, 8]. Subsequent technologic advancements over the ensuing two decades culminated in the development of the first commercially available positron emission tomography (PET) device by the early 1970s for generating whole-body positron transaxial tomographs [7, 11–14], thus representing the antecedent of current-day PET imaging devices.

Currently, positron imaging and detection, in the specific form of ^{18}F-FDG PET imaging, is a well-established cancer imaging modality that is routinely used in the clinical management of a wide variety of solid malignancies [6, 15–25]. ^{18}F-FDG PET is generally combined with "anatomical" imaging, by way of computed tomography (CT), for attempting to maximize the geographic localization and spatial recognition of sites of ^{18}F-FDG avidity to corresponding anatomic structures. A wide range of diagnostic utilities of ^{18}F-FDG PET/CT have been clinically investigated and implemented [6, 15–25]. Those diagnostic clinical applications include (1) initial cancer diagnosis, (2) initial cancer staging, (3) subsequent cancer restaging, (4) therapy planning, (5) monitoring therapy response, (6) surveillance for cancer survivors, and (7) cancer screening for at-risk populations. As a step beyond these diagnostic clinical cancer imaging utilities, there has been emergent interest in the feasibility of utilizing ^{18}F-FDG for real-time cancer detection and surgical guidance within the operating room [6, 26–76] and for real-time guidance of diagnostic and therapeutic interventional procedures within the interventional radiology suite [6, 77–95].

25.2 The Fundamental Basis for the Use of ^{18}F-FDG in Positron Imaging and Detection Strategies

The radionuclide ^{18}F has a relatively short physical half-life of approximately 110 min [6, 96, 97]. The radioactive decay pattern of ^{18}F is predominantly (97 %) by way of positron emission (i.e., beta plus decay emission). The maximum positron radiation emission energy of ^{18}F is approximately 635 keV, giving ^{18}F a relatively low maximum positron radiation emission energy level as compared to other positron-emitting radionuclides. As a result, the positron emitted from the nucleus of ^{18}F travels only a very short distance (i.e., approximately 1–2 mm) within a biological tissue before interacting/colliding with an electron (i.e., a negative charged particle). This interaction/collision of the emitted positron with the electron and the resultant electron-positron annihilation within a biological tissue generates two resultant high-energy 511 keV gamma photons traveling in opposite directions [1–6, 96, 97]. These resultant high-energy 511 keV gamma photons can travel many, many centimeters within a biological tissue. As based upon the initial positron emission and subsequent electron-positron annihilation process which occurs by ^{18}F, the detection of ^{18}F within biological tissues can potentially be accomplished by one of two mechanisms: (1) a direct mechanism of detection of positron emissions (i.e., beta plus decay emissions) using a beta plus detection device or (2) an indirect mechanism of detection of the resultant high-energy 511 keV gamma photons arising from electron-positron annihilation process using a gamma photon detection device [6].

Dating back to the work of Otto Heinrich Warburg in the early 1930s from the Kaiser-Wilhelm-Gesellschaft zur Förderung der Wissenschaften (Berlin-Dahlem, Germany), it has long been recognized that malignant tumors have an accelerated rate of glucose metabolism and have an increased rate of glucose transport and glucose utilization [6, 98–101]. The biochemical transport and processing mechanisms related to ^{18}F-FDG, a non-physiologic ^{18}F-labeled analog of glucose, within malignant cells are also well described within the scientific literature [6, 102–104]. ^{18}F-FDG within the circulatory system is transported into cells (both malignant cells and normal cells) by a facilitated diffusion mechanism involving specific glucose transporters (i.e., GLUT transporters). Once it is within the cell, ^{18}F-FDG is phosphorylated to ^{18}F-FDG-6-phosphate by the enzyme hexokinase. However, unlike ^{18}F-FDG, ^{18}F-FDG-6-phosphate cannot be readily transported across the cellular membrane of either malignant cells or normal cells, thus essentially entrapping the ^{18}F-FDG-6-phosphate within those cells. The enzyme glucose-6-phosphatase is responsible for dephosphorylating ^{18}F-FDG-6-phosphate back to ^{18}F-FDG within the intracellular environment and is present in relatively lower levels within malignant cells as opposed to normal cells. Additionally, unlike glucose-6-phosphate, ^{18}F-FDG-6-phosphate cannot be utilized as a substrate in the metabolic steps of glycolysis, hence attributing to the further accumulation of ^{18}F-FDG-6-phosphate within those cells. This overall process which results in the intracellular accumulation ^{18}F-FDG-6-phosphate is thought to occur more readily in malignant cells than in normal cells secondary to the combination of the overexpression of the glucose transporters GLUT 1 and GLUT 3 by malignant cells, the higher level of hexokinase within malignant cells, and the lower level of glucose-6-phosphatase within malignant cells, thus leading to proportionally greater accumulation of ^{18}F-FDG-6-phosphate within malignant cells as compared to normal cells. This elegantly elucidated biochemical transport and processing mechanism represents the fundamental basis behind the clinical application of ^{18}F-FDG for the detection of malignant tumor using positron imaging and detection strategies (i.e., diagnostic PET imaging technology and various radiation detection probe technologies) [6, 98–104].

25.3 Inherent Limitations for the Use of ^{18}F-FDG in Positron Imaging and Detection Strategies

Despite the fact that these biochemical transport and processing mechanisms lead to the greater accumulation of the phosphorylated form of ^{18}F-FDG within malignant cells as compared to normal cells, there are several inherent limitations regarding the utilization of ^{18}F-FDG for the detection of malignant tumor using positron imaging and detection strategies [6, 75, 102, 105–107]. First, ^{18}F-FDG can readily accumulate within various normal tissues (i.e., brain, heart, mucosa and smooth muscle of the stomach, small intestines and colon, thyroid, liver, spleen, and brown fat) which typically have physiologic propensity for ^{18}F-FDG accumulation. Second, ^{18}F-FDG can also readily accumulate within tissues representing benign disease processes (i.e., infection, inflammation, and trauma). The basis for these first two limitations is the fact that ^{18}F-FDG is not a cancer-specific imaging and detection agent. Third, ^{18}F-FDG is excreted by way of the urinary tract (kidneys, ureters, and bladder), thus leading to accumulation within those structures. Fourth, alterations in tissue uptake of ^{18}F-FDG can occur in patients with elevated blood glucose levels/impaired glucose metabolism, in patients receiving insulin, and in obese patients. An accumulation of ^{18}F-FDG within normal tissues leads to intrinsically higher background levels of ^{18}F-FDG activity within normal tissues located in proximity to adjacent sites of elevated ^{18}F-FDG activity representing malignant tumor. This may be particularly challenging when the malignant tumor site itself has a relatively low level of ^{18}F-FDG activity, leading to a relatively low target-to-background ratio (i.e., low tumor-to-background ratio) of the radiation emissions of ^{18}F-FDG.

25.4 Radiation Detection Devices Utilized during ^{18}F-FDG-Directed Surgery: Mechanisms for the Detection of ^{18}F-FDG and Device Specifications

25.4.1 General Considerations

As previously mentioned, there are two mechanisms for how ^{18}F-FDG within biological tissues can be detected by a radiation detection device: (1) the direct detection of positron emissions (i.e., beta plus decay emissions) using a beta plus detection device and (2) the detection of the resultant high-energy 511 keV gamma photons arising from electron-positron annihilation process using a gamma photon detection device [6]. The ability to successfully detect ^{18}F-FDG within a site of suspected malignancy is highly dependent upon the specific type of radiation detection device utilized and its performance parameters [6, 108]. The most important performance parameters for any given radiation detection device are (1) overall sensitivity (i.e., efficiency, detected count rate per unit of activity), (2) spatial selectivity (i.e., radial sensitivity distribution), (3) spatial resolution (i.e., lateral sensitivity distribution), (4) energy resolution (i.e., spectral discrimination), and (5) contrast.

Radiation detection devices are categorized as either scintillation detectors or semiconductor ionization detectors [6, 108]. The basis for how a scintillation-type detection system works is that the radiation emitted from the radionuclide excites atoms within the scintillation crystal, producing visible light in proportion to the energy absorbed, and for which a photomultiplier enhances the resultant visible light and converts it into an electrical pulse which is quantified by a detection unit. Examples of inorganic scintillation materials used in scintillation detectors include thallium-activated sodium iodide (NaI[Tl]), thallium-activated cesium iodide (CsI[Tl]), sodium-activated cesium iodide (CsI[Na]), samarium-activated lutetium orthooxysilicate (LSO), bismuth germanate (BGO), cerium-activated gadolinium orthosilicate (GSO[Ce]), cerium-activated lutetium yttrium orthosilicate (LYSO[Ce]), and cerium-activated lutetium gadolinium oxyorthosilicate (LGSO[Ce]). Examples of organic ("plastic") scintillation materials used in scintillation detectors include anthracene ($C_{14}H_{10}$), stilbene ($C_{14}H_{12}$), and naphthalene ($C_{10}H_8$). The basis for how a semiconductor ionization-type detection system works is that the radiation emitted from the radionuclide produces free electrons as it passes through and ionizes the semiconductor crystal, creating an electrical pulse which is quantified by a detection unit. Examples of crystalline materials used in semiconductor ionization detectors include cadmium telluride (CdTe), cadmium zinc telluride (CdZnTe), mercuric iodide (HgI_2), and silicon.

There are advantageous and disadvantageous features to both the scintillation-type detection system design and the semiconductor ionization-type detection system design [6, 108]. On one hand, scintillation-type detection systems have higher sensitivity (especially for medium-energy to high-energy gamma photons) but have poorer energy resolution and scatter rejection. Likewise, scintillation-type detection probes tend to have a much bulkier and heavier probe head profile. On the other hand, semiconductor ionization-type detection systems have higher-energy resolution and scatter rejection but have lower sensitivity (especially for medium-energy to high-energy gamma photons). Likewise, semiconductor ionization-type detection probes tend to have a much more compact and light-weight probe head profile.

25.4.2 Gamma Photon Detection

The detector component of a gamma detection probe generally consists of an inorganic scintillator detector or a semiconductor ionization detector [6, 108]. Most commercially available handheld gamma detection probes are generally designed for detecting radioisotopes of gamma-ray energies in the low-energy emission (0–150 keV) range and medium-energy emission (150–400 keV) range, thus allowing successful detection of radioisotopes such as technetium-99 m (^{99m}Tc; 140 keV and 142 keV), indium-111 (^{111}In; 171 keV and 247 keV), iodine-123 (^{123}I; 159 keV), and iodine-125 (^{125}I; 35 keV) [6, 76, 108]. However, most commercially available handheld gamma detection probes are not specifically designed for detecting resultant high-energy 511 keV gamma emissions emanating from the electron-positron annihilation process that is characteristic of high-energy gamma photon-emitting radionuclides, like ^{18}F. As a result, there has been a recent appearance of commercially available handheld gamma detection probes that are specifically intended for attempting to detect high-energy 511 keV gamma emissions, and for which these high-energy gamma detection probes have been designated as "PET" probes. The overall weight and physical dimensions of any such "PET" probe is generally a function of the thickness of side and back shielding (with materials like lead, tungsten, gold, or platinum) and the length of collimation (i.e., extension of shielding in a forward direction beyond the distal face of the detector in the direction of the radiation source being counted) that is thought to be necessary to block adjacent background radiation, to limit the field-of-view, and to collimate the head of the probe, with the intention of limiting the area of tissue contributing to the probe count rate and of providing better spatial resolution between areas of tissue of differing radioactivity levels [6, 73, 108, 109]. All conventional attempts to improve upon the current "PET" probe design by further increasing the degree of side/back shielding or the collimation length to further block adjacent background radiation, or by increasing crystal diameter/thickness to capture a greater percentage of 511 keV gamma emissions, are generally counterproductive, as such conventional approaches will simply result in a "PET" probe configuration that is prohibitively too large in physical size, too heavy in weight, and potentially of significant greater cost. Alternatively, in order to attempt to bypass these physical barriers related to the degree of side and back shielding, collimation, and crystal diameter/thickness in designing handheld gamma detection probes specifically intended for the detection of 511 KeV gamma emissions, efforts have been redirected toward engineering more novel "PET" probe designs for which their efficacy is not dependent upon side and back shielding, collimation, or crystal diameter/thickness. Several examples of alternative design concepts for "PET" probe include secondary K-alpha x-ray fluorescence [73, 76, 109], active electronic collimation [39, 61, 64, 66, 70, 76, 110–112], and other crystal geometry designs using multiple small crystals with specific novel geometric configurations [76, 113, 114] for optimizing and maximizing background rejection capabilities. These innovative alternative design concepts for improving the efficacy of detection of high-energy gamma photon-emitting/positron-emitting radionuclides, some of which have already been successfully applied to handheld gamma detection probe systems, are also the focus of current preclinical research that is actively looking at developing small platform, portable perioperative and intraoperative patient and ex vivo surgical specimen imaging devices which possess similar capabilities for detecting high-energy gamma photon-emitting/positron-emitting radionuclides [76]. However, such small platform, portable perioperative and intraoperative patient and ex vivo surgical specimen imaging devices have not yet been fully realized or made commercially available for use in the setting of clinical medicine.

25.4.3 Beta plus Decay (i.e., Positron) Detection

The detector component of a beta plus detection probe generally consists of a semiconductor ionization detector or an organic ("plastic") scintillator detector but for which an inorganic scintillator detector can also be utilized [6, 45, 52, 108, 115–127]. As previously mentioned, whereas high-energy 511 keV gamma photons can travel many, many centimeters within biological tissues, positrons travels only very short distances (i.e., approximately 1–2 mm) within biological tissues before they are annihilated. This difference in the distances traveled by positrons as opposed to resultant high-energy 511 keV gamma photons within biologic tissues contributes to both the advantages and disadvantages of direct detection of positrons by a handheld beta plus detection probe. Thus, handheld beta plus detection probes can be small in physical size and light in weight secondary to the fact that whereas gamma photon detection of high-energy 511 keV gamma photons relies heavily on the thickness of side and back shielding and the length of collimation, beta plus decay detection of positrons does not require any significant degree of side and back shielding or collimation. However, whereas gamma photon detection of high-energy 511 keV gamma photons is less effected by the distance from the source of 511 keV gamma emissions to the proximity of the head of the handheld gamma detection probe, beta plus decay detection requires close apposition of the head of the handheld beta plus detection probe to the source of the positrons emitted from the biologic tissue. As a result, if the head of the handheld beta plus detection probe is not in direct contact with the biologic tissue emitting positrons, or if the source of the positrons emitted from the biologic tissue is located several millimeters below of the surface of that biologic tissue, the handheld beta plus detection probe will be unable to detect such ^{18}F-FDG-avid tissues. Along similar lines, the simple placement of a sterile disposable barrier sheath over the handheld beta plus detection probe significantly reduces the overall sensitivity for the detection of ^{18}F-FDG-avid tissues by such a device.

25.5 Clinical Applications of Real-Time ^{18}F-FDG-Directed Surgery and Real-Time ^{18}F-FDG-Directed Interventional Procedures (Tables 25.1 and 25.2)

The principal motivation behind the use of ^{18}F-FDG for providing for real-time cancer detection and guidance within the operating room has been multifactorial, including exploring its applicability for real-time intraoperative staging, surgical planning and execution, and determination of completeness of surgical resection [6]. The clinical application of ^{18}F-FDG-directed surgery was first described in 1999 by Desai et al. from the Ohio State University (Columbus, Ohio, USA) for colorectal cancer [6, 26, 27]. In this first clinical description of ^{18}F-FDG-directed surgery, a total of 15 colorectal cancer patients received an intravenous injection of 4.0–5.7 mCi (148–211 MBq) of ^{18}F-FDG at a time of 58–110 min prior to intraoperative evaluation with a commercially available gamma detection probe. Fourteen of these 15 patients had undergone a prior preoperative diagnostic ^{18}F-FDG PET scan. A single or multiple tumor foci were identified with the gamma detection probe as ^{18}F-FDG-avid tissue in 14 of the 15 patients receiving an intravenous injection of ^{18}F-FDG on the day of surgery. Likewise, a single or multiple tumor foci were correctly identified with the gamma detection probe as ^{18}F-FDG-avid tissue in 13 of 14 patients undergoing a prior preoperative diagnostic ^{18}F-FDG PET scan, correctly correlating to the sites of hypermetabolic activity seen on the prior preoperative diagnostic ^{18}F-FDG PET imaging.

Table 25.1 All reported published series for real-time ^{18}F-FDG-directed surgery

Primary author	Reference(s)	Year(s)	Location(s)	Number of patients	Known malignancies in patients evaluated	^{18}F-FDG dose	Injection-to-operation start time / Injection-to-probing time / Injection-to-postoperative specimen imaging time	Probe type(s)	Detection threshold criteria method (DTCM) and findings for ^{18}F-FDG-avid lesions with probe(s)
Desai	[26, 27]	1999, 2000	Columbus, OH, USA	15	Colorectal	Range, 4.0–5.7 mCi (Range, 148–211 MBq)	IOST: 40–100 min IPT: 58–110 min IPOSIT: ND	GDP	DTCM for GDP: three-sigma criteria Reported three-sigma criteria identified ^{18}F-FDG-avid lesions in 14 of 15 patients
Zervos	[28]	2001	Columbus, OH, USA	10	Colorectal	Range, 5–10 mCi (Range, 185–370 MBq)	IOST: NS IPT: NS IPOSIT: ND	GDP BDP	DTCM for GDP: three-sigma criteria and T/B ratio Reported three-sigma criteria identified ^{18}F-FDG-avid lesions in 5 of 5 patients for GDP Reported mean (range) T/B ratios 1.53:1 (1.25:1–1.78:1) for ^{18}F-FDG-avid lesions for GDP DTCM for BDP: T/B ratio Reported mean (range) T/B ratios 1.64:1 (1.11:1–2.17:1) for ^{18}F-FDG-avid lesions for BDP
Essner	[29, 30]	2001	Santa Monica, CA, USA	8	Colorectal, melanoma	Range, 7–10 mCi (Range, 259–370 MBq)	IOST: "up to 3 h" IPT: "up to 4 h later" IPOSIT: ND	GDP	DTCM for GDP: T/B ratio $\geq$ 1.5:1 Reported T/B ratio $\geq$ 1.5:1 identified 11 of 17 ^{18}F-FDG-avid lesions Reported range T/B ratios in vivo: 1.16:1–7.92:1 for ^{18}F-FDG-avid lesions

Yen	[32]	2004	Taoyuan, Taiwan	2	Cervical	2 and 5 mCi (74 and 185 MBq)	IOST: NS IPT: NS IPOSIT: ND	GDP BDP	DTCM for GDP: T/B ratio DTCM for BDP: T/B ratio Reported T/B ratios: 1.78:1 and 1.53:1 for ^{18}F-FDG-avid lesions, but not specified for which probe type
Franc	[36]	2005	San Francisco, CA, USA	5	Melanoma	Mean, 14.6 (±3.2) mCi (Mean, 540 (±118) MBq)	IOST: 178–240 min IPT: NS IPOSIT: ND	HEGDP BDP	DTCM for GDP: T/B ratio DTCM for BDP: T/B ratio Reported identified 3 of 5 ^{18}F-FDG-avid lesions, but not specified for which probe type Reported range T/B ratios: 1.2:1–10:1 for ^{18}F-FDG-avid lesions, but not specified for which probe type
Kraeber-Bodéré	[37, 41]	2005, 2007	Nantes, France	10	Thyroid	Mean, 7.2 (4.5–14.2) mCi (Mean, 265 (165–526) MBq)	IOST: ≈30 min IPT: NS	GDP	DTCM for GDP: T/B ratio Reported mean(range) T/B ratios in vivo: 1.40:1 (0.76:1–2.59:1) for ^{18}F-FDG-avid lesions Reported mean(range) T/B ratios ex vivo: 2.44:1 (1.18:1–7.89:1) for ^{18}F-FDG-avid lesions
Gulec	[38, 43]	2006	Santa Monica, CA, USA	40	Breast, colorectal, lymphoma, melanoma, seminoma, thyroid	Range, 7–10 mCi (Range, 259–370 MBq)	IOST: 1–4 h IPT: NS IPOSIT: ND	HEGDP	DTCM for HEGDP: T/B ratio ≥ 1.5:1 Reported T/B ratio ≥ 1.5:1 identified 40 of 40 ^{18}F-FDG-avid lesions (cumulatively from in situ and ex vivo T/B ratios Reported mean (range) T/B ratios in situ: 1.9:1 (1.4:1–2.5:1) for ^{18}F-FDG-avid lesions Reported mean (range) T/B ratios ex vivo: 2.1:1 (1.5:1–3.3:1) for ^{18}F-FDG-avid lesions

(continued)

Table 25.1 (continued)

Primary author	Reference(s)	Year(s)	Location(s)	Number of patients	Known malignancies in patients evaluated	^{18}F-FDG dose	Injection-to-operation start time Injection-to-probing time Injection-to-postoperative specimen imaging time	Probe type(s)	Detection threshold criteria method (DTCM) and findings for ^{18}F-FDG-avid lesions with probe(s)
Nwogu	[40]	2006	Buffalo, NY, USA	10	Lung	10 mCi (370 MBq)	IOST: "within 4 h" IPT: NS IPOSIT: ND	GDP	DTCM for GDP: T/B ratio Reported T/B ratio ≥ 3.0:1 ex vivo for primary tumor site in 10 of 10 cases and T/B ratio ≥ 2.0:1 ex vivo for lymph nodes in 8 of 10 cases
Gulec	[42, 43]	2007	Goshen, IN, USA	25	Adrenocortical, breast, carcinoma of unknown primary, colorectal, gastric, GIST, head and neck, lung, lymphoma, melanoma, ovarian, thyroid	Range, 5–15 mCi (Range, 185–555 MBq)	IOST: 2–6 h IPT: NS IPOSIT: ND	HEGDP	DTCM for HE GDP: T/B ratio ≥ 1.5:1 Reported T/B ratio ≥ 1.5:1 identified 24 of 25 ^{18}F-FDG-avid lesions Reported range T/B ratios: 1.5 to 3.8 for ^{18}F-FDG-avid lesions
Povoski	[6, 44, 46–51, 53, 54, 56, 67, 71, 73–76]	2007–2015	Columbus, OH, USA	157	Breast, cervical, colorectal, eccrine, endometrial, head and neck, lung lymphoma, melanoma, ovarian, plasmacytoma, sarcoma, thyroid, urothelial	Mean, 15.1 (4.6–26.1) mCi (Mean, 559 (170–966) MBq)	IOST: NS IPT: mean (range): 286 (176–532) minutes IPOSIT: mean (range): 389 (86–741) minutes on diagnostic scanner and mean (range): 458 (272–656) minutes on micro scanner	GDP HEGDP	DTCM for GDP: Three-sigma criteria and T/B ratio DTCM for HEGDP: three-sigma criteria and T/B ratio Reported ^{18}F-FDG-avid lesions identified in 156 of 157 patients, but the details for identification of the ^{18}F-FDG-avid lesions was not specifically delineated according to probe type or DTCM

Piert	[45, 52]	2007	Munich, Germany	17	Breast, colorectal, esophageal, gastric, gastroesophageal, melanoma, thyroid	Range, 1–3 mCi (Range, 36.6–110.6 MBq)	IOST: NS IPT: mean (range): 184 (19–365) minutes IPOSIT: ND	HEGDP BDP	DTCM for HEGDP: NS DTCM for BDP: T/B ratio ≥ 1.5:1 Reported T/B ratio ≥ 1.5:1 identified 16 of 17 ^{18}F-FDG-avid lesions for BDP Reported mean (range) T/B ratios ex vivo: 6.6:1 (1.3:1–17.2:1) for ^{18}F-FDG-avid lesions for BDP
Van Baardwijk	[55]	2008	Maastricht, The Netherlands	5	Lung	Median, 0.97 (0.92–1.24) mCi (Median, 36 (34–46) MBq)	IOST: ND IPT: ND IPOSIT: median (range): 180 (150–300) minutes	ND	ND (no intraoperative probing performed, and only postoperative specimen imaging performed) The ^{18}F-FDG-avid lesion(s) was identified in 5 of 5 cases on postoperative specimen imaging
Gollub	[57]	2009	New York, NY, USA	5	Colorectal, colonic polyps	Range, 15–20 mCi (Range, 555–740 MBq)	IOST: ND IPT: ND IPOSIT: mean (range): 195 (169–223) minutes	ND	ND (no intraoperative probing performed, and only postoperative specimen imaging performed) The ^{18}F-FDG-avid lesion(s) was identified in 5 of 5 cases on postoperative specimen imaging
Molina[a]	[58]	2009	Miami, Florida, USA	10	Breast, gastric, lymphoma, melanoma	Range, 10–12 mCi (Range, 370–444 MBq)	IOST: 3–4 h IPT: NS IPOSIT: ND	HEGDP	DTCM for HEGDP: NS Reported that HEGDP correctly identified 14 ^{18}F-FDG-avid lesions

(continued)

Table 25.1 (continued)

Primary author	Reference(s)	Year(s)	Location(s)	Number of patients	Known malignancies in patients evaluated	^{18}F-FDG dose	Injection-to-operation start time Injection-to-probing time Injection-to-postoperative specimen imaging time	Probe type(s)	Detection threshold criteria method (DTCM) and findings for ^{18}F-FDG-avid lesions with probe(s)
De Jong	[61]	2010	Groningen, Germany	3	Testicular	0.14 mCi/kg body weight (5 MBq/kg body weight)	IOST: 3 h IPT: NS IPOSIT: ND	HEGDP	DTCM for HEGDP: T/B ratio ≥ 1.5:1 Reported T/B ratio ≥ 1.5:1 identified in 4 ^{18}F-FDG-avid lesions, with T/B ratio ≥ 5.0:1 in all cases
Lee	[62]	2010	San Francisco, CA, USA	2	Melanoma	11.4 and 16.6 mCi (422 and 614 MBq)	IOST: NS IPT: NS IPOSIT: ND	HEGDP	DTCM for HEGDP: T/B ratio Reported T/B ratios: 4.4:1 and 2.2:1 for ^{18}F-FDG-avid lesions
García	[64]	2011	Barcelona, Spain	7	Colorectal, ovarian, thyroid	Mean, 10.0 (9.5–10.5) mCi (Mean, 370 (352–389) MBq)	IOST: 3–5 h IPT: NS IPOSIT: ND	HEGDP	DTCM for HEGDP: T/B ratio Reported T/B ratio ≥ 1.5:1 identified 14 of 16 ^{18}F-FDG-avid lesions Reported range T/B ratios: 1.5–2.5 for ^{18}F-FDG-avid lesions

Kim	[65]	2011	Dauegu, Seoul, and Jeju, Korea	12	Thyroid	Mean, 9.8 (6.1–15.4) mCi (Mean, 363 (227–570) MBq)	IOST: mean (range): 228 (134–395) minutes IPT: NS IPOSIT: ND	HEGDP	DTCM for HEGDP: T/B ratio >1.3:1 Reported mean (range) T/B ratios ex vivo for confirmed tumor sites: 1.51:1 (1.17:1–4.03:1) for ^{18}F-FDG-avid lesions Reported mean (range) T/B ratios ex vivo for confirmed benign sites: 1.14 (1.01 :1–1.48:1) for ^{18}F-FDG-avid lesions
Francis	[68]	2012	Little Rock, AK, USA Hershey, PA, USA	4	Thyroid	NS	IOST: "at least 2 h" IPT: NS IPOSIT: ND	GDP HEGDP	DTCM for GDP: NS DTCM for HEGDP: NS No specific probe localization data was reported
Vos	[70]	2012	Amsterdam, The Netherlands	9	Breast, colorectal, esophageal, skin, lymphoma, melanoma, thyroid	0.095 mCi/kg body weight (3.5 MBq/kg body weight)	IOST: ≈4 h IPT: NS IPOSIT: ND	HEGDP	DTCM for HEGDP: NS Reported that HEGDP identified ^{18}F-FDG-avid lesions in 9 of 9 patients

All reported series in Table 25.1 represent those reported series with greater than one reported patient in their series, and for which any additional references representing single case reports and/or review papers from the same institution were also added to any reported series with greater than one reported patient in their series

For all reported series in Table 25.1 in which there were multiple reports from the same institution and in which it appeared that the study patients were derived from the same overall patient population, these reported series were combined under the name of the predominant primary author from that institution, and the total "number of patients" from that institution was estimated as based upon the available data within all the reports from that same institution which appeared to be derived from the same overall patient population

Abbreviations: *BDP* beta plus detection probe, *DTCM* detection threshold criteria method, *^{18}F-FDG* fluorine-18 fluorodeoxyglucose, *GDP* gamma detection probe, *GIST* gastrointestinal stromal tumor, *HEGDP* high-energy gamma detection probe ("PET probe"), *IOST* injection-to-operation start time, *IPOSI* injection-to-postoperative specimen imaging time, *IPT* injection-to-probing time, *MBq* megabecquerels, *mCi* millicuries, *NS* not clearly specified in the reported series, *ND* not done in the reported series, *SUVmax* maximum standardized uptake value, *T/B ratio* target-to-background ratio for detection of ^{18}F-FDG-avid lesion

[a]Personal communication from Manuel A. Molina (Lakeland Regional Cancer Center, Lakeland, Florida, USA, manmolina@hotmail.com, February 25, 2015) confirms a total of 14 ^{18}F-FDG-avid lesions identified from among a total of 10 patients undergoing ^{18}F-FDG-directed surgery (and with 2 patients having no ^{18}F-FDG-avid lesion identifiable with the HEGDP at the time of ^{18}F-FDG-directed surgery)

Table 25.2 All reported published series for real-time ^{18}F-FDG-directed diagnostic and interventional procedures

Primary author	Reference(s)	Year(s)	Location(s)	Interventional procedure	Number of patients	Known malignancies in patients evaluated	^{18}F-FDG dose	Injection-to-scan time Injection-to-procedure time	^{18}F-FDG-avid lesion SUVmax
Klaeser	[79, 80]	2009, 2010	Bern, Switzerland	Biopsies	28	Breast, cervical, lung, lymphoma, melanoma, ovarian, sarcoma	Range, 0.08–0.19 mCi/kg body weight (Range, 3–7 MBq/kg body weight)	IST: 60–180 min IPT: NS	NS
Tatli	[81]	2011	Boston, MA, USA	Biopsies	12	Breast, colorectal, lung, melanoma, ovarian, lymphoma	Mean, 20.6 (16.6–23.9) mCi (Mean, 762 (614–884) MBq)	IST: 61–78 min IPT: ≈120 min	3.9–19.1
Shyn	[82, 83, 89, 90]	2011–2014	Boston, MA, USA	Biopsies and ablations	12	Breast, colorectal, esophageal, lung, ovarian, sarcoma	Mean, 14.7 (10.4–16.8) mCi (Mean, 544 (385–622) MBq)	IST: 78–130 min IPT: ≈120 min	1.5–23.1
Ryan	[85, 86]	2013	New York, NY, USA	Ablations	23	Colorectal, endometrial, head and neck, hepatocellular, lung, melanoma, pancreas, sarcoma	Pre-ablation dose: median, 4.2 (3. 6–4.4) mCi (median, 155 (133–163) MBq) Post-ablation assessment dose: median 8.4 (7.6–8.8) mCi (median 310 (281–326) MBq)	IST: 40–143 min (for pre-ablation scan) IPT: NS IST: NS (for post-ablation assessment scan)	NS
Cerci[a]	[87, 91]	2013, 2014	Curitiba, Parcanà, Brazil	Biopsies	126	Breast, carcinoma of unknown primary, cervical, colorectal, gastric, head and neck, lung, lymphoma, melanoma, other, prostate,	Range, 8–12 mCi (Range, 296–444 MBq)	IST: ≈60 –90 min IPT: NS	3.5–27.6

Aparici	[88, 92, 93]	2013, 2014	San Francisco, CA, USA	Biopsies	4	Esophageal, lymphoma, prostate	5 mCi (185 MBq)	IST: 60 min IPT: NS	NS
Cornelis	[95]	2014	New York, NY, USA	Biopsies	105	Breast, colorectal, endometrial, esophageal, gastric, germ cell, head and neck, lung, lymphoma, melanoma, pancreas, plasmacytoma, prostate, renal cell, sarcoma, skin, small bowel, thyroid, vulva	Mean, 6.9 (3.9–13.2) mCi (Mean, 255 (144–288) MBq)	IST: 35–183 min IPT: NS	1.9–44.4

All reported series in Table 25.2 represent those reported series with greater than one reported patient in their series, and for which any additional references representing single case reports and/or review papers from the same institution were also added to any reported series with greater than one reported patient in their series

For all reported series in Table 25.2 in which there were multiple reports from the same institution and in which it appeared that the study patients were derived from the same overall patient population, these reported series were combined under the name of the predominant primary author from that institution, and the total "number of patients" from that institution was estimated as based upon the available data within all the reports from that same institution which appeared to be derived from the same overall patient population

Abbreviations: *^{18}F-FDG* fluorine-18 fluorodeoxyglucose, *IPT* injection-to-procedure time, *IST* injection-to-scan time, *MBq* megabecquerels, *mCi* millicuries, *NS* not clearly specified in the reported series, *SUVmax* maximum standardized uptake value

[a]Cerci et al. [91] mention "update of our group's result" as "217 PET/CT-guided biopsies performed," but without formal presentation of accompanying data

Subsequent to the first report of ^{18}F-FDG-directed surgery in 1999 [6, 26, 27], multiple groups of investigators from across the globe have collectively investigated the utility of real-time ^{18}F-FDG-directed surgery and real-time ^{18}F-FDG-directed diagnostic and therapeutic interventional procedures in regard to a wide range of solid malignancies, including colorectal cancer, gastric cancer, gastroesophageal cancer, pancreatic cancer, melanoma, lymphoma, breast cancer, ovarian cancer, endometrial cancer, cervical cancer, vulvar cancer, testicular cancer, prostate cancer, head and neck malignancies (squamous cell cancer of the oral cavity, oropharynx, hypopharynx, and laryngeal regions, iodine-negative recurrent papillary thyroid cancer, and recurrent medullary thyroid cancer), lung cancer, squamous cell cancer of the skin, GIST (gastrointestinal stromal tumor tumors), sarcoma, adrenocortical carcinoma, and carcinoma of unknown primary [6, 28–95]. Table 25.1 summarizes all reported real-time ^{18}F-FDG-directed surgery series in the literature [6, 26–76]. Table 25.2 summarizes all reported real-time ^{18}F-FDG-directed diagnostic and therapeutic interventional procedure series in the literature [6, 77–95]. It is worth noting a substantial portion of the clinical investigations into the use of ^{18}F-FDG for real-time detection and guidance during cancer surgery for a variety of solid malignancies have been conducted at the Ohio State University (Columbus, Ohio, USA) [6, 26–28, 44, 46–51, 53, 54, 56, 59, 67, 71–76].

Our own experience with utilizing ^{18}F-FDG for real-time cancer detection and guidance within the operating room at the Ohio State University (Columbus, Ohio, USA) [6, 26–28, 44, 46–51, 53, 54, 56, 59, 67, 71–76] has strengthened our long-standing contention regarding the importance of implementing a multimodal imaging and detection approach to ^{18}F-FDG-directed surgery [50, 67, 74, 76]. Since 2005, the general structure of this multimodal approach has incorporated various components, including (1) same-day preoperative patient diagnostic whole-body PET/CT imaging, (2) intraoperative gamma detection probe assessment, (3) specimen imaging of surgically resected specimens with both a clinical PET/CT unit and a micro PET/CT unit, (4) radioactivity counting of selected portion of surgically resected specimens by an automatic gamma well counter, and (5) same-day postoperative patient diagnostic limited field-of-view PET/CT imaging [67].

On the day of the anticipated ^{18}F-FDG-directed surgery procedure, patients fasted for a minimum of 6 h before undergoing the same-day preoperative diagnostic whole-body ^{18}F-FDG PET/CT scan [67, 74]. Each patient received a same-day, single-dose, preoperative, intravenous injection of ^{18}F-FDG, consisting of an averaged recommended dose in the range of approximately 15 mCi (555 MBq). The ^{18}F-FDG dosing at the Ohio State University (Columbus, Ohio, USA) was based upon the standard-of-care practice guidelines set in the USA by the Society of Nuclear Medicine, the American College of Radiology, and the Society for Pediatric Radiology for diagnostic ^{18}F-FDG PET/CT image acquisition (i.e., 10–20 mCi (370–740 MBq) of ^{18}F-FDG in adults) [128, 129]. The same-day, single-dose, preoperative, intravenous dose of ^{18}F-FDG was generally administered approximately 75 min prior to the planned time of the same-day preoperative diagnostic whole-body ^{18}F-FDG PET/CT scan, which was performed within the time frame recognized by the standard-of-care practice guidelines set in the USA by the Society of Nuclear Medicine, the American College of Radiology, and the Society for Pediatric Radiology for diagnostic ^{18}F-FDG PET/CT image acquisition [128, 129]. The same-day preoperative diagnostic whole-body ^{18}F-FDG PET/CT scan usually consisted of 6–8 field-of-view PET bed positions and with 2 min of PET imaging for each field-of-view PET bed position. Patients then proceeded to the operating room for their anticipated surgical procedure and completed standard postoperative recovery in the postanesthesia care unit. The same-day postoperative diagnostic limited field-of-view ^{18}F-FDG PET/CT scan was generally restricted to those field-of-view PET bed positions encompassing the immediate area of the surgical field (usually consisting of 1–3 field-of-view PET bed positions, in order to limit overall patient radiation exposure for the CT portion of the PET/CT, and with 10 min of PET imaging for each field-of-view PET bed position).

Our multimodal imaging and detection approach to ^{18}F-FDG-directed surgery at the Ohio State University (Columbus, Ohio, USA) [50, 67, 74, 76] demonstrated technical and logistical feasibility for coordination of services by the surgeon, nuclear medicine physician, and pathologist in a same-day fashion. It allowed for (1) real-time intraoperative staging of the extent of disease; (2) real-time intraoperative surgical planning and execution of the necessary and most appropriate operation, determination of the extent of surgical resection, and determination of the completeness of surgical resection; (3) real-time pathologic evaluation of intact surgical resected specimens for the confirmation of completeness of surgical resection and for surgical margin assessment; and (4) real-time pathologic evaluation of diagnostically biopsied tissues for confirmation of correctness of tissue diagnosis.

25.6 Timing Issues Related to ^{18}F-FDG-Directed Surgery: Impact of Length of Time from Injection of ^{18}F-FDG to the Performance of Intraoperative Gamma Detection Probing

Numerous investigators have evaluated the concept of delayed phase and dual-time-point diagnostic ^{18}F-FDG PET imaging [74] in which a portion of the diagnostic ^{18}F-FDG PET imaging sequence is extended temporally out further than is generally recommended by the standard-of-care practice guidelines for diagnostic ^{18}F-FDG PET/CT image acquisition [128, 129]. Remarkably, several of these groups of investigators have performed delayed phase diagnostic ^{18}F-FDG PET imaging out to ultra-extended injection-to-scan acquisition time intervals ranging to 6–9 h after the initial ^{18}F-FDG injection dose is administered [31, 74, 130–134].

In contrast to the innumerous work done on extended injection-to-scan acquisition time intervals for diagnostic ^{18}F-FDG PET imaging, there has been very little data or discussion in the literature regarding the equivalent scenario of extended injection-to-probing time intervals as it pertains to gamma detection probing of patients intravenously injected with ^{18}F-FDG [31, 38, 42, 43, 74]. Therefore, it is reasonable to say that the optimal length of time from the injection of ^{18}F-FDG to the performance of intraoperative gamma detection probing has yet to be determined.

In 2004, Higashi et al. [31, 74] examined the question of "appropriate timing" for "postinjection" gamma detection probing using phantom studies and a limited series of 3 patients with "superficially located malignant lesions." For the phantom studies, they used 5 liter plastic barrels filled with saline containing varying-dose "background" ^{18}F-FDG as the "body trunk" phantom, 0.2 liter plastic bottles filled with saline containing varying-dose ^{18}F-FDG as the "kidney" phantom, and 2 fixed-dose ^{18}F-FDG sources to simulate "superficially located tumor nodules." For the 3 patients with "superficially located malignant lesions," they performed "preoperative" gamma detection probing at the skin surface at 1, 3, 5, 6, and/or 7 h after receiving an intravenous injection of 2–10 mCi (74–370 MBq) of ^{18}F-FDG (and for which no intraoperative gamma detection probing was undertaken). In their limited patient data set, they showed that the tumor-to-background ratios of ^{18}F-FDG by gamma detection probing at the skin surface remained relatively stable at the measured time intervals and remained relatively stable up to the 7-h postinjection time interval. However, they were concerned that the overall lower ^{18}F-FDG count rates encountered at time intervals of 6–7 h postinjection of ^{18}F-FDG, secondary to the normal physical decay pattern of ^{18}F-FDG, "would be problematic" when applied to a clinical application of intraoperative gamma detection probing. Therefore, they concluded that the clinical application of intraoperative gamma detection probing was "more suitable" at 1–3 h postinjection of ^{18}F-FDG as compared to 6–7 h postinjection of ^{18}F-FDG.

In 2006 and 2007, Gulec et al. [38, 42, 43, 74] reported on two consecutive series of patients, including 40 patients undergoing intraoperative gamma detection probing after receiving an intravenous injection of 7–10 mCi (259–370 MBq) of ^{18}F-FDG [38] and 25 patients undergoing intraoperative gamma detection probing after receiving an intravenous injection of 5–15 mCi (185–555 MBq) of ^{18}F-FDG [42]. In both series, Gulec et al. [38, 42, 43] reported observing a nonsignificant trend toward an increased tumor-to-background ratio of ^{18}F-FDG as the duration of time from the ^{18}F-FDG injection to performing intraoperative gamma detection probing increased, with satisfactory count rates and lesion detection capabilities up to 6 h of time after injection of ^{18}F-FDG. Therefore, regarding intraoperative gamma detection probing during ^{18}F-FDG-directed surgery, they concluded that longer injection-to-probing time intervals "accentuated" the tumor-to-background ratio of ^{18}F-FDG and resulted in "better lesion detection" [38, 42]. However, they also stated that "more delayed intervals between FDG injection and imaging might compromise image quality as a result of lower count rates" [42].

Most recently, in 2014, our group at the Ohio State University (Columbus, Ohio, USA) [74] examined the question of extended injection-to-scan acquisition time intervals in a retrospective data analysis of a subset of patients undergoing ^{18}F-FDG-directed surgery. This data analysis specifically looked at preoperative ^{18}F-FDG PET/CT imaging and postoperative ^{18}F-FDG PET/CT imaging of 32 individual ^{18}F-FDG-avid lesions (from among a total of 7 patients) which were not surgically manipulated or altered during ^{18}F-FDG-directed surgery, and, for which, all of these 32 individual ^{18}F-FDG-avid lesions were visualized on both same-day preoperative ^{18}F-FDG PET/CT imaging and same-day postoperative ^{18}F-FDG PET/CT imaging. In this retrospective data analysis, both ^{18}F-FDG-avid lesions and their corresponding background tissues were assessed on same-day preoperative and postoperative ^{18}F-FDG PET/CT scans. This data analysis demonstrated several important time-dependent observations. First, ^{18}F-FDG PET/CT imaging performed at extended injection-to-scan acquisition times of up to a mean time of 530 min (i.e., approximately five half-lives for ^{18}F-FDG) was able to maintain a designation of good/adequate diagnostic image quality deemed necessary for clinical interpretation. Second, the mean ^{18}F-FDG-avid lesion SUV_{max} value increased significantly from preoperative to postoperative ^{18}F-FDG PET/CT imaging (mean ^{18}F-FDG-avid lesion SUV_{max} value; 7.7 preoperative to 11.3 postoperative; P <0.001). Third, mean background SUV_{max} value decreased significantly from preoperative to postoperative ^{18}F-FDG PET/CT imaging (mean background SUV_{max} value; 2.3 preoperative to 2.1 postoperative; $P=0.017$). Fourth, the mean lesion-to-background SUV_{max} ratio increased significantly from preoperative to postoperative ^{18}F-FDG PET/CT imaging (mean lesion-to-background SUV_{max} ratio; 3.7 preoperative to 5.8 postoperative; P <0.001).

The far-reaching implications of these collective time-dependent observations [74] appear highly influential for guiding future direction in ^{18}F-FDG-directed procedural and surgical applications, as well as ^{18}F-FDG PET/CT oncologic imaging. First and foremost, these time-dependent observations justify the more widespread and integrated, real-time use of diagnostic ^{18}F-FDG PET/CT imaging in conjunction with ^{18}F-FDG-directed interventional radiology diagnostic biopsy procedures and therapeutic ablation procedures, as well as with ^{18}F-FDG-directed surgical procedures. These sorts of integrated, real-time utilities for diagnostic ^{18}F-FDG PET/CT imaging would facilitate periprocedural verification of appropriate tissue targeting during ^{18}F-FDG-directed interventional radiology diagnostic biopsy procedures and therapeutic ablation procedures and for perioperative verification of appropriate tissue targeting and completeness of resection during ^{18}F-FDG-directed surgical procedures. Secondly but still importantly, these time-dependent observations could have far-reaching impact on potentially reshaping future thinking regarding what represents the "most optimal" injection-to-scan acquisition time interval for all routine diagnostic ^{18}F-FDG PET/CT oncologic imaging.

25.7 Inherent Challenge of In Situ Detection of ^{18}F-FDG with a Gamma Photon Detection Device When Encountering a Low Target-to-Background Ratio of ^{18}F-FDG and the Impact of Threshold Detection Criteria Methodology on the Determination of Gamma Detection Probe Positivity for Intraoperative In Situ Identification of ^{18}F-FDG-Avid Tissue Sites during ^{18}F-FDG-Directed Surgery

A significant challenge faced during attempted intraoperative in situ identification of ^{18}F-FDG-avid tissue sites with a gamma photon detection device during ^{18}F-FDG-directed surgery is a scenario in which a low target-to-background ratio (i.e., low tumor-to-background ratio) of high-energy 511 keV gamma photon emissions is encountered within the surgical field [6, 31, 38, 42, 43, 45, 52, 73, 75, 115–126]. As previously discussed, a low target-to-background ratio of high-energy 511 keV gamma photon emissions can results from a multitude of factors, including the marginal ^{18}F-FDG uptake by certain tumor-bearing tissues, the distribution and degree of intrinsic physiologic background ^{18}F-FDG activity within adjacent surrounding tissues which do not represent tumor-bearing tissues, and innumerable factors related to the technical specifications of the specific gamma photon detection device used for generating the counts per second measurements [75]. In this regard, some investigators have suggested that a minimum in situ target-to-background ratio of 1.5-to-1 for ^{18}F-FDG is necessary for allowing the surgeon to comfortably differentiate tumor-bearing tissues from normal tissue during ^{18}F-FDG-directed surgery [38, 42, 43, 73, 75]. However, a target-to-background ratio of 1.5-to-1 simply represents an arbitrary and fixed ratio determination.

Our personal experience with ^{18}F-FDG-directed surgery at the Ohio State University (Columbus, Ohio, USA) [6, 26–28, 44, 46–51, 53, 54, 56, 59, 67, 71–76] clearly indicates that the observed in situ target-to-background ratio of ^{18}F-FDG-avid tissue sites is frequently less than 1.5-to-1 and is highly dependent upon the specific gamma photon detection device utilized. Resultantly, when intraoperative detection of in situ ^{18}F-FDG-avid tissue sites relies solely on a fixed target-to-background ratio (i.e., a ratiometric threshold method) as the threshold for probe positivity, the success of intraoperative detection can be limited and provide unsatisfactory results to the surgeon [73, 75]. Therefore, our own group has long contended that improved intraoperative in situ identification of ^{18}F-FDG-avid tissue sites during ^{18}F-FDG-directed surgery can be better accomplished by the use of the three-sigma statistical threshold criteria method for determination of gamma detection probe positivity. The three-sigma statistical threshold criteria defines any given tissue as being probe positive when the count rate in that tissue exceeds three standard deviations above the mean count rate detected within normal adjacent tissue.

In order to comparatively assess the efficacy of the 1.5-to-1 ratiometric threshold criteria method and the three-sigma statistical threshold criteria method for determination of gamma detection probe positivity for intraoperative in situ detection of ^{18}F-FDG-avid tissue sites during ^{18}F-FDG-directed surgery, we evaluated a total of 401 intraoperative gamma detection probe measurement sets of in situ counts per second measurements collected from our prospective, pilot study database and performed our analysis in a manner that was completely independent of the specific type of gamma detection probe system that was used for determination of the counts per second measurements [75]. Our data analysis demonstrated that the three-sigma statistical threshold criteria method was significantly better than the 1.5-to-1 ratiometric threshold criteria method (P <0.001) for determining gamma detection probe positivity for intraoperative in situ detection of ^{18}F-FDG-avid tissue sites during

^{18}F-FDG-directed surgery. Likewise, the three-sigma statistical threshold criteria method was able to detect true positive results at target-to-background counts ratios that were much lower than could be detected by a ratiometric threshold criteria method that set the target-to-background count ratio cutoff at 1.5-to-1. Thus, if a surgeon utilized a gamma detection probe system with high count rate sensitivity, it was theoretically feasible that target-to-background count ratios as low as 1.1-to-1 could be identified as in situ probe positive when applying the three-sigma statistical threshold criteria method. Therefore, use of the three-sigma statistical threshold criteria for determination of gamma detection probe positivity for intraoperative in situ detection of ^{18}F-FDG-avid tissue sites during ^{18}F-FDG-directed surgery proved instrumental for overcoming the commonly encountered scenario of a low target-to-background ratio (i.e., low tumor-to-background ratio).

25.8 Occupational Radiation Exposure to Intraoperative and Perioperative Personnel from ^{18}F-FDG Radioguided Surgical Procedures

Occupational radiation exposure incurred by intraoperative and perioperative personnel participating in surgical cases has been previously evaluated by several groups of investigators [37, 41, 44–46, 52, 54, 55, 57, 60, 61, 64, 67, 135–137]. These investigators have reported data based upon several different study-design scenarios, including utilizing simulated surgical cases [46, 135, 136], surgical cases in which the patient was injected with ^{18}F-FDG but in which actual ^{18}F-FDG-directed surgery with intraoperative utilization of radiation detection probes was not undertaken for assisting in the surgical procedure [55, 57, 137], and actual ^{18}F-FDG-directed surgery cases [37, 41, 44, 45, 52, 54, 60, 61, 64, 67].

The most comprehensive evaluation of occupational radiation exposure to intraoperative and perioperative personnel participating in ^{18}F-FDG-directed surgery cases was published in 2008 by our group at the Ohio State University (Columbus, Ohio, USA) [54, 67]. In this comprehensive study, 10 actual ^{18}F-FDG-directed surgery cases were evaluated. A mean dose of 18.9 mCi (699 MBq) of ^{18}F-FDG was intravenously injected at a mean time of 142 min prior to surgery. The resultant mean deep dose equivalent per case for the surgeon, anesthetist, scrub technologist, postoperative nurse, circulating nurse, and preoperative nurse was 164, 119, 92, 63, 54, and 48 μSv, respectively.

The results of this comprehensive evaluation were used to determine the estimated number of ^{18}F-FDG-directed surgery cases per year and the estimated number of hours of exposure per year that could be theoretically incurred by the surgeon, anesthetist, scrub technologist, postoperative nurse, circulating nurse, and preoperative nurse in both the USA and internationally [54, 67]. Based upon the established annual occupational exposure limit for adults within the USA of a total effective dose equivalent of 50,000 μSv (as defined by the US Nuclear Regulatory Commission) [54, 138], the estimated number of ^{18}F-FDG-directed surgery cases per year and the estimated number of hours of exposure per year that could be theoretically incurred by the surgeon, anesthetist, scrub technologist, postoperative nurse, circulating nurse, and preoperative nurse were 305 cases and 820 h, 420 cases and 1020 h, 543 cases and 2083 h, 794 cases and 1471 h, 926 cases and 2941 h, and 1042 cases and 602 h, respectively [54]. In contrast to the annual occupational exposure limit for adults within the USA, the annual occupational exposure limit for the adult international community outside the USA (as defined by the International Commission on Radiological Protection (ICRP)) is more stringent and complex, with the annual occupational exposure limit for adults to be a total effective dose equivalent of 20,000 μSv per year, averaged over a 5-year period (100,000 μSv in 5 years), with further provision that the total effective dose equivalent should not exceed 50,000 μSv in any single year [54, 139, 140]. Based upon the established annual occupational exposure limit for the adult international community outside the USA defined by the International Commission on Radiological Protection (ICRP), the estimated number of ^{18}F-FDG-directed surgery cases per year and the estimated number of hours of exposure per year that could be theoretically incurred by the surgeon, anesthetist, scrub technologist, postoperative nurse, circulating nurse, and preoperative nurse were 122 cases and 328 h, 168 cases and 408 h, 217 cases and 833 h, 317 cases and 588 h, 370 cases and 1176 h, and 417 cases and 241 h, respectively [54]. The data outlined in this comprehensive evaluation [54, 67] clearly illustrated that the absorbed radiation dose received by both intraoperative and perioperative personnel involved in ^{18}F-FDG-directed surgery cases was relatively low per case and allows for all such personnel to participate in multiple cases and still remain well below regulatory standards set for occupational radiation exposure limits.

25.9 Concluding Remarks

The use of positron-emitting and high-energy gamma photon-emitting radiopharmaceuticals, like ^{18}F-FDG, for real-time cancer detection and surgical guidance within the operating room and for real-time guidance of diagnostic and therapeutic interventional procedures within the interventional radiology suite, has great clinical potential. When a multimodal imaging and detection approach to ^{18}F-FDG-directed surgery is utilized, thus coordinating of services provided by the surgeon, nuclear medicine physician, and pathologist, this integrated approach has the potential for allowing (1) real-time intraoperative staging of the extent of disease; (2) real-time intraoperative surgical planning and execution of the necessary and most appropriate operation, determination of the extent of surgical resection, and determination of the completeness of surgical resection; (3) real-time pathologic evaluation of intact surgical resected specimens for the confirmation of completeness of surgical resection and for surgical margin assessment; (4) real-time pathologic evaluation of diagnostically biopsied tissues for confirmation of correctness of tissue diagnosis; and (5) real-time guidance of diagnostic and therapeutic interventional procedures within the interventional radiology suite. However, major hurdles still exist for maximizing the clinical potential of these technologies. The greatest challenges that remain involve the need for the development of more technically optimized handheld radiation detection probes for positron-emitting and high-energy gamma photon-emitting radiopharmaceuticals, like ^{18}F-FDG, as well as the need for the development of portable positron and high-energy gamma photon imaging devices that can be fully integrated into the operative/perioperative arena for real-time intraoperative/perioperative patient and specimen imaging. If these hurdles can be overcome, the use of positron-emitting and high-energy gamma photon-emitting radiopharmaceuticals for real-time cancer detection and surgical guidance within the operating room and for real-time guidance of diagnostic and therapeutic interventional procedures within the interventional radiology suite can become more fully realized and potentially impactful upon the long-term outcome for cancer patients.

References

1. Joliot F. Preuve expérimentale de l'annihilation des electrons positifs. CR Acad Sci. 1933;197:1622–5.
2. Thibaud J. L'annihilation des positrons au contact de la matière et la radiation qu'en resulte. CR Acad Sci. 1933;197:1629–32.
3. Klemperer O. On the annihilation radiation of the positron. Math Proc Camb Phil Soc. 1934;30:347–54.
4. Berriger R, Montgomery CG. The angular distribution of positron annihilation radiation. Phys Rev. 1942;61: 222–4.
5. Wrenn Jr FR, Good ML, Handler P. The use of positron-emitting radioisotopes for the localization of brain tumors. Science. 1951;113(2940):525–7.
6. Povoski SP, Neff RL, Mojzisik CM, O'Malley DM, Hinkle GH, Hall NC, Murrey Jr DA, Knopp MV, Martin Jr EW. A comprehensive overview of radioguided surgery using gamma detection probe technology. World J Surg Oncol. 2009;7:11.
7. Brownell GL. A history of positron imaging. October 15, 1999. http://neurosurgery.mgh.harvard.edu/docs/PEThistory.pdf.
8. Brownell GL, Sweet WH. Localization of brain tumors with positron emitters. Nucleonics. 1953;11: 40–5.

9. Gallagher BM, Ansari A, Atkins H, Casella V, Christman DR, Fowler JS, Ido T, MacGregor RR, Som P, Wan CN, Wolf AP, Kuhl DE, Radiopharmaceuticals RM, XXVII. 18F-labeled 2-deoxy-2-fluoro-d-glucose as a radiopharmaceutical for measuring regional myocardial glucose metabolism in vivo: tissue distribution and imaging studies in animals. J Nucl Med. 1977;18:990–6.
10. Ido T, Wan CN, Casella V, Fowler JS, Wolf AP, Reivich M, Kuhl DE. Labeled 2-deoxy-D-glucose analogs: 18F-labeled 2-deoxy-2-fluoro-D-glucose, 2-deoxy-2-fluoro-D-mannose and 14C-2-deoxy-2-fluoro-D-glucose. J Label Compd Radiopharm. 1978;24:174–83.
11. Chesler DA. Three-dimensional activity distribution from multiple positron scintigraphs. J Nucl Med. 1971;12:347–8 [Abstract].
12. Chesler DA. Positron tomography and three-dimensional reconstruction technique. In: Freedman GS, editor. Tomographic imaging in nuclear medicine. 1st ed. New York, NY: Society of Nuclear Medicine; 1973. p. 176–83.
13. Ter-Pogossian MM, Phelps ME, Hoffman EJ, Mullani NA. A positron-emission transaxial tomograph for nuclear imaging (PETT). Radiology. 1975;114: 89–98.
14. Hoffmann EJ, Phelps ME, Mullani NA, Higgins CS, Ter-Pogossian MM. Design and performance characteristics of a whole-body positron transaxial tomograph. J Nucl Med. 1976;17:493–502.
15. Hillner BE, Siegel BA, Liu D, Shields AF, Gareen IF, Hanna L, Stine SH, Coleman RE. Impact of positron emission tomography/computed tomography and positron emission tomography (PET) alone on expected management of patients with cancer: initial results from the National Oncologic PET Registry. J Clin Oncol. 2008;26:2155–61.
16. Hillner BE, Siegel BA, Shields AF, Liu D, Gareen IF, Hanna L, Stine SH, Coleman RE. The impact of positron emission tomography (PET) on expected management during cancer treatment: findings of the National Oncologic PET Registry. Cancer. 2009; 115:410–8.
17. Poeppel TD, Krause BJ, Heusner TA, Boy C, Bockisch A, Antoch G. PET/CT for the staging and follow-up of patients with malignancies. Eur J Radiol. 2009;70:382–92.
18. Stroobants S. To PET or not to PET: what are the indications? Eur J Cancer. 2011;47 Suppl 3:S304–5.
19. Czernin J, Allen-Auerbach M, Nathanson D, Herrmann K. PET/CT in oncology: current status and perspectives. Curr Radiol Rep. 2013;1:177–90.
20. Schöder H, Gönen M. Screening for cancer with PET and PET/CT: potential and limitations. J Nucl Med. 2007;48 Suppl 1:4S–18.
21. Kojima S, Zhou B, Teramukai S, Hara A, Kosaka N, Matsuo Y, Suzuki H, Torigoe S, Suzuki T, Uno K, Fukushima M. Cancer screening of healthy volunteers using whole-body 18F-FDG-PET scans: The Nishidai clinic study. Eur J Cancer. 2007;43:1842–8.
22. Minamimoto R, Senda M, Uno K, Jinnouchi S, Iinuma T, Ito K, Okuyama C, Oguchi K, Kawamoto M, Suzuki Y, Tsukamoto E, Terauchi T, Nakashima R, Nishio M, Nishizawa S, Fukuda H, Yoshida T, Inoue T. Performance profile of FDG-PET and PET/CT for cancer screening on the basis of a Japanese Nationwide Survey. Ann Nucl Med. 2007;21:481–98.
23. Terauchi T, Murano T, Daisaki H, Kanou D, Shoda H, Kakinuma R, Hamashima C, Moriyama N, Kakizoe T. Evaluation of whole-body cancer screening using 18F-2-deoxy-2-fluoro-D-glucose positron emission tomography: a preliminary report. Ann Nucl Med. 2008;22:379–85.
24. Lee JW, Kang KW, Paeng JC, Lee SM, Jang SJ, Chung JK, Lee MC, Lee DS. Cancer screening using 18F-FDG PET/CT in Korean asymptomatic volunteers: a preliminary report. Ann Nucl Med. 2009;23:685–91.
25. Nishizawa S, Kojima S, Teramukai S, Inubushi M, Kodama H, Maeda Y, Okada H, Zhou B, Nagai Y, Fukushima M. Prospective evaluation of whole-body cancer screening with multiple modalities including [18F]fluorodeoxyglucose positron emission tomography in a healthy population: a preliminary report. J Clin Oncol. 2009;27:1767–73.
26. Desai D, Arnold M, Saha S, Hinkle G, Soble D, Frye J, DePalatis L, Mantil J, Satter M, Martin E. Intraoperative gamma detection of FDG distribution in colorectal cancer. Clin Positron Imaging. 1999;2:325.
27. Desai DC, Arnold M, Saha S, Hinkle G, Soble D, Fry J, DePalatis LR, Mantil J, Satter M, Martin EW. Correlative whole-body FDG-PET and intraoperative gamma detection of FDG distribution in colorectal cancer. Clin Positron Imaging. 2000;3: 189–96.
28. Zervos EE, Desai DC, DePalatis LR, Soble D, Martin EW. 18F-labeled fluorodeoxyglucose positron emission tomography-guided surgery for recurrent colorectal cancer: a feasibility study. J Surg Res. 2001;97:9–13.
29. Essner R, Hsueh EC, Haigh PI, Glass EC, Huynh Y, Daghighian F. Application of an [(18)F] fluorodeoxyglucose-sensitive probe for the intraoperative detection of malignancy. J Surg Res. 2001;96: 120–6.
30. Essner R, Daghighian F, Giuliano AE. Advances in FDG PET probes in surgical oncology. Cancer J. 2002;8:100–8.
31. Higashi T, Saga T, Ishimori T, Mamede M, Ishizu K, Fujita T, Mukai T, Sato S, Kato H, Yamaoka Y, Matsumoto K, Senda M, Konishi J. What is the most appropriate scan timing for intraoperative detection of malignancy using 18F-FDG-sensitive gamma probe? Preliminary phantom and preoperative patient study. Ann Nucl Med. 2004;18:105–14.
32. Yen TC, See LC, Lai CH, Yah-Huei CW, Ng KK, Ma SY, Lin WJ, Chen JT, Chen WJ, Lai CR, Hsueh S. 18F-FDG uptake in squamous cell carcinoma of the cervix is correlated with glucose transporter 1 expression. J Nucl Med. 2004;45:22–9.

33. Yap JT, Carney JP, Hall NC, Townsend DW. Image-guided cancer therapy using PET/CT. Cancer J. 2004;10:221–33.
34. Barranger E, Kerrou K, Petegnief Y, David-Montefiore E, Cortez A, Daraï E. Laparoscopic resection of occult metastasis using the combination of FDG-positron emission tomography/computed tomography image fusion with intraoperative probe guidance in a woman with recurrent ovarian cancer. Gynecol Oncol. 2005;96:241–4.
35. Carrera D, Fernandez A, Estrada J, Martin-Comin J, Gamez C. [Detection of occult malignant melanoma by 18F-FDG PET-CT and gamma probe]. Rev Esp Med Nucl. 2005;24:410–3. [Spanish].
36. Franc BL, Mari C, Johnson D, Leong SP. The role of a positron- and high-energy gamma photon probe in intraoperative localization of recurrent melanoma. Clin Nucl Med. 2005;30:787–91.
37. Kraeber-Bodéré F, Cariou B, Curtet C, Bridji B, Rousseau C, Dravet F, Charbonnel B, Carnaille B, Le Néel JC, Mirallié E. Feasibility and benefit of fluorine 18-fluoro-2-deoxyglucose-guided surgery in the management of radioiodine-negative differentiated thyroid carcinoma metastases. Surgery. 2005;138:1176–82.
38. Gulec SA, Daghighian F, Essner R. PET-Probe. Evaluation of technical performance and clinical utility of a handheld high-energy gamma probe in oncologic surgery. Ann Surg Oncol. 2006 [Epub ahead of print].
39. Meller B, Sommer K, Gerl J, von Hof K, Surowiec A, Richter E, Wollenberg B, Baehre M. High energy probe for detecting lymph node metastases with 18F-FDG in patients with head and neck cancer. Nuklearmedizin. 2006;45:153–9.
40. Nwogu C, Fischer G, Tan D, Glinianski M, Lamonica D, Demmy T. Radioguided detection of lymph node metastasis in non-small cell lung cancer. Ann Thorac Surg. 2006;82:1815–20; discussion 1820.
41. Curtet C, Carlier T, Mirallié E, Bodet-Milin C, Rousseau C, Barbet J, Kraeber-Bodéré F. Prospective comparison of two gamma probes for intraoperative detection of 18F-FDG: in vitro assessment and clinical evaluation in differentiated thyroid cancer patients with iodine-negative recurrence. Eur J Nucl Med Mol Imaging. 2007;34:1556–62.
42. Gulec SA, Hoenie E, Hostetter R, Schwartzentruber D. PET probe-guided surgery: applications and clinical protocol. World J Surg Oncol. 2007;5:65.
43. Gulec SA. PET probe-guided surgery. J Surg Oncol. 2007;96:353–7.
44. Hall NC, Povoski SP, Murrey DA, Knopp MV, Martin EW. Combined approach of perioperative 18F-FDG PET/CT imaging and intraoperative 18F-FDG handheld gamma probe detection for tumor localization and verification of complete tumor resection in breast cancer. World J Surg Oncol. 2007;5:143.
45. Piert M, Burian M, Meisetschlager G, Stein HJ, Ziegler S, Nahrig J, Picchio M, Buck A, Siewert JR, Schwaiger M. Positron detection for the intraoperative localisation of cancer deposits. Eur J Nucl Med Mol Imaging. 2007;34:1534–44.
46. Sarikaya I, Povoski SP, Al-Saif OH, Kocak E, Bloomston M, Marsh S, Cao Z, Murrey DA, Zhang J, Hall NC, Knopp MV, Martin EW. Combined use of preoperative 18F FDG-PET imaging and intraoperative gamma probe detection for accurate assessment of tumor recurrence in patients with colorectal cancer. World J Surg Oncol. 2007; 5:80.
47. Sun D, Bloomston M, Hinkle G, Al-Saif OH, Hall NC, Povoski SP, Arnold MW, Martin EW. Radioimmunoguided surgery (RIGS), PET/CT image-guided surgery, and fluorescence image-guided surgery: past, present, and future. J Surg Oncol. 2007;96:297–308.
48. Agrawal A, Hall NC, Ringel MD, Povoski SP, Martin Jr EW. Combined use of perioperative TSH-stimulated 18F-FDG PET/CT imaging and gamma probe radioguided surgery to localize and verify resection of iodine scan-negative recurrent thyroid carcinoma. Laryngoscope. 2008;118:2190–4.
49. Cohn DE, Hall NC, Povoski SP, Seamon LG, Farrar WB, Martin Jr EW. Novel perioperative imaging with 18F-FDG PET/CT and intraoperative 18F-FDG detection using a handheld gamma probe in recurrent ovarian cancer. Gynecol Oncol. 2008;110: 152–7.
50. Hall NC, Povoski SP, Murrey DA, Knopp MV, Martin EW. Bringing advanced medical imaging into the operative arena could revolutionize the surgical care of cancer patients. Expert Rev Med Devices. 2008;5:663–7.
51. Moffatt-Bruce SD, Povoski SP, Sharif S, Hall NC, Ross Jr P, Johnson MA, Martin Jr EW. A novel approach to positron emission tomography in lung cancer. Ann Thorac Surg. 2008;86:1355–7.
52. Piert M, Carey J, Clinthorne N. Probe-guided localization of cancer deposits using [(18)F]fluorodeoxyglucose. Q J Nucl Med Mol Imaging. 2008;52: 37–49.
53. Povoski SP, Hall NC, Martin EW, Walker MJ. Multimodality approach of perioperative ^{18}F-FDG PET/CT imaging, intraoperative ^{18}F-FDG handheld gamma probe detection, and intraoperative ultrasound for tumor localization and verification of resection of all sites of hypermetabolic activity in a case of occult recurrent metastatic melanoma. World J Surg Oncol. 2008;6:1.
54. Povoski SP, Sarikaya I, White WC, Marsh SG, Hall NC, Hinkle GH, Martin Jr EW, Knopp MV. Comprehensive evaluation of occupational radiation exposure to intraoperative and perioperative personnel from 18F-FDG radioguided surgical procedures. Eur J Nucl Med Mol Imaging. 2008;35:2026–34.
55. van Baardwijk A, Bosmans G, van Suylen RJ, van Kroonenburgh M, Hochstenbag M, Geskes G, Lambin P, De Ruysscher D. Correlation of intra-tumour heterogeneity on 18F-FDG PET with pathologic features in non-small cell lung cancer: a feasibility study. Radiother Oncol. 2008;87:55–8.

56. Murrey Jr DA, Bahnson EE, Hall NC, Povoski SP, Mojzisik CM, Young DC, Sharif S, Johnson MA, Abdel-Misih S, Martin Jr EW, Knopp MV. Perioperative (18)F-fluorodeoxyglucose-guided imaging using the becquerel as a quantitative measure for optimizing surgical resection in patients with advanced malignancy. Am J Surg. 2009;198:834–40.
57. Gollub MJ, Akhurst TJ, Williamson MJ, Shia J, Humm JL, Wong WD, Paty PB, Guillem JG, Weiser MR, Temple LK, Dauer LT, Jhanwar SC, Kronman RE, Montalvo CV, Miller AR, Larson SM, Margulis AR. Feasibility of ex vivo FDG PET of the colon. Radiology. 2009;252:232–9.
58. Molina MA, Goodwin WJ, Moffat FL, Serafini AN, Sfakianakis GN, Avisar E. Intra-operative use of PET probe for localization of FDG avid lesions. Cancer Imaging. 2009;9:59–62.
59. Hall NC, Povoski SP, Murrey DA, Martin Jr EW, Knopp MV. Ex vivo specimen FDG PET/CT imaging for oncology. Radiology. 2010;255:663–4.
60. Nalley C, Wiebeck K, Bartel TB, Bodenner D, Stack Jr BC. Intraoperative radiation exposure with the use of (18)F-FDG-guided thyroid cancer surgery. Otolaryngol Head Neck Surg. 2010;142:281–3.
61. de Jong JS, van Ginkel RJ, Slart RH, Lemstra CL, Paans AM, Mulder NH, Hoekstra HJ. FDG-PET probe-guided surgery for recurrent retroperitoneal testicular tumor recurrences. Eur J Surg Oncol. 2010;36:1092–5.
62. Lee GO, Costouro NG, Groome T, Kashani-Sabet M, Leong SPL. The use of intraoperative PET probe to resect metastatic melanoma. BMJ Case Reports. 2010. doi:10.1136/bcr.12.2009.2593.
63. Hartemink KJ, Muller S, Smulders YM, Petrousjkavandentol M, Comans EF. [Fluorodeoxyglucose F18(FDG)-probe guided biopsy]. Ned Tijdschr Geneeskd. 2010;154:A1884. [Dutch].
64. García JR, Fraile M, Soler M, Bechini J, Ayuso JR, Lomeña F. [PET/CT-guided salvage surgery protocol. Results with ROLL Technique and PET probe]. Rev Esp Med Nucl. 2011;30:217–22. [Spanish].
65. Kim WW, Kim JS, Hur SM, Kim SH, Lee SK, Choi JH, Kim S, Choi JY, Lee JE, Kim JH, Nam SJ, Yang JH, Choe JH. Radioguided surgery using an intraoperative PET probe for tumor localization and verification of complete resection in differentiated thyroid cancer: A pilot study. Surgery. 2011;149: 416–24.
66. Manca G, Biggi E, Lorenzoni A, Boni G, Roncella M, Ghilli M, Volterrani D, Mariani G. Simultaneous detection of breast tumor resection margins and radioguided sentinel node biopsy using an intraoperative electronically collimated probe with variable energy window: a case report. Clin Nucl Med. 2011;36:e196–8.
67. Povoski SP, Hall NC, Murrey Jr DA, Chow AZ, Gaglani JR, Bahnson EE, Mojzisik CM, Kuhrt MP, Hitchcock CL, Knopp MV, Martin Jr EW. Multimodal imaging and detection approach to 18F-FDG-directed surgery for patients with known or suspected malignancies: a comprehensive description of the specific methodology utilized in a single-institution cumulative retrospective experience. World J Surg Oncol. 2011;9:152.
68. Francis CL, Nalley C, Fan C, Bodenner D, Stack Jr BC. 18F-fluorodeoxyglucose and 131I Radioguided Surgical Management of Thyroid Cancer. Otolaryngol Head Neck Surg. 2012;146:26–32.
69. Bains S, Reimert M, Win AZ, Khan S, Aparici CM. A patient with psoriatic arthritis imaged with FDG-PET/CT demonstrated an unusual imaging pattern with muscle and fascia involvement: a case report. Nucl Med Mol Imaging. 2012;46:138–43.
70. Vos CG, Hartemink KJ, Muller S, Oosterhuis JW, Meijer S, van den Tol MP, Comans EF. Clinical applications of FDG-probe guided surgery. Acta Chir Belg. 2012;112:414–8.
71. Hall N, Murrey D, Povoski S, Barker D, Zhang J, Bahnson E, Chow A, Martin EW, Knopp MV. Evaluation of 18FDG PET/CT image quality with prolonged injection-to-scan times. Mol Imaging Biol. 2012;14(2, supplement):P610.
72. Hall NC, Povoski SP, Zhang J, Knopp MV, Martin Jr EW. Use of intraoperative nuclear medicine imaging technology: strategy for improved patient management. Expert Rev Med Devices. 2013;10:149–52.
73. Povoski SP, Chapman GJ, Murrey Jr DA, Lee R, Martin Jr EW, Hall NC. Intraoperative detection of ^{18}F-FDG-avid tissue sites using the increased probe counting efficiency of the K-alpha probe design and variance-based statistical analysis with the three-sigma criteria. BMC Cancer. 2013;13:98.
74. Povoski SP, Murrey Jr DA, Smith SM, Martin Jr EW, Hall NC. 18F-FDG PET/CT oncologic imaging at extended injection-to-scan acquisition time intervals derived from a single-institution 18F-FDG-directed surgery experience: feasibility and quantification of 18F-FDG accumulation within 18F-FDG-avid lesions and background tissues. BMC Cancer. 2014;14:453.
75. Chapman GJ, Povoski SP, Hall NC, Murrey Jr DA, Lee R, Martin Jr EW. Comparison of two threshold detection criteria methodologies for determination of probe positivity for intraoperative in situ identification of presumed abnormal 18F-FDG-avid tissue sites during radioguided oncologic surgery. BMC Cancer. 2014;14:667.
76. Povoski SP, Hall NC, Murrey Jr DA, Wright CL, Martin Jr EW. Feasibility of a multimodal 18F-FDG-directed lymph node surgical excisional biopsy approach for appropriate diagnostic tissue sampling in patients with suspected lymphoma. BMC Cancer. 2015;15:378.
77. Prior JO, Kosinski M, Delaloye AB, Denys A. Initial report of PET/CT-guided radiofrequency ablation of liver metastases. J Vasc Interv Radiol. 2007; 18:801–3.
78. Mallarajapatna GJ, Kallur KG, Ramanna NK, Susheela SP, Ramachandra PG. PET/CT-guided percutaneous biopsy of isolated intramuscular metastases from postcricoid cancer. J Nucl Med Technol. 2009;37:220–2.

79. Klaeser B, Mueller MD, Schmid RA, Guevara C, Krause T, Wiskirchen J. PET-CT-guided interventions in the management of FDG-positive lesions in patients suffering from solid malignancies: initial experiences. Eur Radiol. 2009;19:1780–5.
80. Klaeser B, Wiskirchen J, Wartenberg J, Weitzel T, Schmid RA, Mueller MD, Krause T. PET/CT-guided biopsies of metabolically active bone lesions: applications and clinical impact. Eur J Nucl Med Mol Imaging. 2010;37:2027–36.
81. Tatli S, Gerbaudo VH, Feeley CM, Shyn PB, Tuncali K, Silverman SG. PET/CT-guided percutaneous biopsy of abdominal masses: initial experience. J Vasc Interv Radiol. 2011;22:507–14.
82. Shyn PB, Tatli S, Sainani NI, Morrison PR, Habbab F, Catalano P, Silverman SG. Minimizing image misregistration during PET/CT-guided percutaneous interventions with monitored breath-hold PET and CT acquisitions. J Vasc Interv Radiol. 2011;22:1287–92.
83. Sainani NI, Shyn PB, Tatli S, Morrison PR, Tuncali K, Silverman SG. PET/CT-guided radiofrequency and cryoablation: is tumor fluorine-18 fluorodeoxyglucose activity dissipated by thermal ablation? J Vasc Interv Radiol. 2011;22:354–60.
84. Werner MK, Aschoff P, Reimold M, Pfannenberg C. FDG-PET/CT-guided biopsy of bone metastases sets a new course in patient management after extensive imaging and multiple futile biopsies. Br J Radiol. 2011;84:e65–7.
85. Schoellnast H, Larson SM, Nehmeh SA, Carrasquillo JA, Thornton RH, Solomon SB. Radiofrequency ablation of non-small-cell carcinoma of the lung under real-time FDG PET CT guidance. Cardiovasc Intervent Radiol. 2011;34 Suppl 2:S182–5.
86. Ryan ER, Sofocleous CT, Schöder H, Carrasquillo JA, Nehmeh S, Larson SM, Thornton R, Siegelbaum RH, Erinjeri JP, Solomon SB. Split-dose technique for FDG PET/CT-guided percutaneous ablation: a method to facilitate lesion targeting and to provide immediate assessment of treatment effectiveness. Radiology. 2013;268:288–95.
87. Cerci JJ, Pereira Neto CC, Krauzer C, Sakamoto DG, Vitola JV. The impact of coaxial core biopsy guided by FDG PET/CT in oncological patients. Eur J Nucl Med Mol Imaging. 2013;40:98–103.
88. Win AZ, Aparici CM. Real-time FDG PET/CT-guided bone biopsy in a patient with two primary malignancies. Eur J Nucl Med Mol Imaging. 2013; 40:1787–8.
89. Shyn PB. Interventional positron emission tomography/computed tomography: state-of-the-art. Tech Vasc Interv Radiol. 2013;16:182–90.
90. Shyn PB, Tatli S, Sahni VA, Sadow CA, Forgione K, Mauri G, Morrison PR, Catalano PJ, Silverman SG. PET/CT-guided percutaneous liver mass biopsies and ablations: targeting accuracy of a single 20 s breath-hold PET acquisition. Clin Radiol. 2014;69: 410–5.
91. Cerci JJ, Huber FZT, Bogoni M. PET/CT-guided biopsy of liver lesions. Clin Transl Imaging. 2014;2:157–63.
92. Aparici CM, Win AZ. Use of positron emission tomography/CT to perform biopsy of a mesenteric mass. J Vasc Interv Radiol. 2014;25:1609.
93. Aparici CM, Aslam R, Win AZ. Initial experience of utilizing real-time intra-procedural PET/CT biopsy. J Clin Imaging Sci. 2014:4:54.
94. Chakraborty PS, Dhull VS, Karunanithi S, Verma S, Kumar R. Malignant melanoma with cavitary pulmonary metastasis: Diagnostic dilemma resolved by FDG PET/CT guided biopsy. Indian J Nucl Med. 2014;29:196–7.
95. Cornelis F, Silk M, Schoder H, Takaki H, Durack JC, Erinjeri JP, Sofocleous CT, Siegelbaum RH, Maybody M, Solomon SB. Performance of intraprocedural 18-fluorodeoxyglucose PET/CT-guided biopsies for lesions suspected of malignancy but poorly visualized with other modalities. Eur J Nucl Med Mol Imaging. 2014;41:2265–72.
96. Syder SE, Kilbourne MR. Chemistry of fluorine-18 radiopharmaceuticals. In: Welch MJ, Redvanly CS, editors. Handbook of radiopharmaceuticals: radiochemistry and applications. 1st ed. Hoboken: John Wiley and Sons, Ltd; 2003. p. 195–228.
97. Fowler JS, Fowler JS, Ido T. Design and synthesis of 2-deoxy-2-[18F] fluoro-D-glucose (18FDG). In: Welch MJ, Redvanly CS, editors. Handbook of radiopharmaceuticals: radiochemistry and applications. 1st ed. Hoboken: John Wiley and Sons, Ltd; 2003. p. 307–22.
98. Warburg O, Posener K, Negelein E. The metabolism of the carcinoma cell. In: Warburg O, editor. The mechanism of tumors. 1st ed. New York: Richard R. Smith, Inc; 1931. p. 129–69.
99. Warburg O. On the origin of cancer cells. Science. 1956;123(3191):309–14.
100. Weber G. Enzymology of cancer cells. N Engl J Med. 1977;296:486–93.
101. Merrall NW, Plevin R, Gould GW. Growth factors, mitogens, oncogenes and the regulation of glucose transport. Cell Signal. 1993;5:667–75.
102. Pauwels EK, Ribeiro MJ, Stoot JH, McCready VR, Bourguignon M, Mazière B. FDG accumulation and tumor biology. Nucl Med Biol. 1998;25: 317–22.
103. Gambhir SS. Molecular imaging of cancer with positron emission tomography. Nat Rev Cancer. 2002;2:683–93.
104. Buck AK, Reske SN. Cellular origin and molecular mechanisms of 18F-FDG uptake: is there a contribution of the endothelium? J Nucl Med. 2004;45: 461–3.
105. Otsuka H, Graham M, Kubo A, Nishitani H. Clinical utility of FDG PET. J Med Invest. 2004;51:14–9.
106. Otsuka H, Morita N, Yamashita K, Nishitani H. FDG-PET/CT for cancer management. J Med Invest. 2007;54:195–9.
107. Büsing KA, Schönberg SO, Brade J, Wasser K. Impact of blood glucose, diabetes, insulin, and obesity on standardized uptake values in tumors and healthy organs on 18F-FDG PET/CT. Nucl Med Biol. 2013;40:206–13.

108. Heller S, Zanzonico P. Nuclear probes and intraoperative gamma cameras. Semin Nucl Med. 2011;41:166–81.
109. Martin EW, Chapman GJ, Subramaniam VV, Povoski SP. Intraoperative detection of gamma emissions using K-alpha X-ray fluorescence. Expert Rev Med Devices. 2010;7:431–4.
110. GFE Gesellschaft für Forschungs und Entwicklungsservice mbH; Gamma Locator DXI. http://www.gfe-service.de/en/ylocator.php.
111. Gerl J, Ameil F, Kojouharov Z, Surowiec D. High energy gamma probe with position sensing capability. European Patent EP 1 596 223 B1; Filed May 10, 2005; Published January 21, 2009.
112. Gerl J. Kojouharov Z, Ameil E, Surowiec D. High energy gamma probe with position sensing capability. United States Patent US 7,312,460 B2; Filed May 10, 2005; Published December 25, 2007.
113. Lecomte R, Schmitt D, Lamoureux G. Geometry study of a high resolution PET detection system using small detectors. IEEE Trans Nucl Sci. 1984;31:556–61.
114. Levin CS. New imaging technologies to enhance the molecular sensitivity of positron emission tomography. Proc IEEE. 2008;96:439–67.
115. Raylman RR, Wahl RL. A fiber-optically coupled positron-sensitive surgical probe. J Nucl Med. 1994;35:909–13.
116. Daghighian F, Mazziotta JC, Hoffman EJ, Shenderov P, Eshaghian B, Siegel S, Phelps ME. Intraoperative beta probe: a device for detecting tissue labeled with positron or electron emitting isotopes during surgery. Med Phys. 1994;21:153–7.
117. Raylman RR, Fisher SJ, Brown RS, Ethier SP, Wahl RL. Fluorine-18-fluorodeoxyglucose-guided breast cancer surgery with a positron-sensitive probe: validation in preclinical studies. J Nucl Med. 1995;36:1869–74.
118. Raylman RR, Wahl RL. Evaluation of ion-implanted-silicon detectors for use in intraoperative positron-sensitive probes. Med Phys. 1996;23:1889–95.
119. Raylman RR. A solid-state intraoperative beta probe system. (Nuclear Science) IEEE Trans Nucl Sci. 2000;47:1696–703.
120. Yasuda S, Makuuchi H, Fujii H, Nakasaki H, Mukai M, Sadahiro S, Tajima T, Ide M, Shohtsu A, Suzuki Y. Evaluation of a surgical gamma probe for detection of 18F-FDG. Tokai J Exp Clin Med. 2000;25:93–9.
121. Raylman RR. Performance of a dual, solid-state intraoperative probe system with 18F, 99mTc, and (111)In. J Nucl Med. 2001;42:352–60.
122. Raylman RR, Srinivasan A. Endoprobe: a system for radionuclide-guided endoscopy. Med Phys. 2004;31:3306–13.
123. Yamamoto S, Matsumoto K, Senda M. Optimum threshold setting for a positron-sensitive probe with background rejection capability. Ann Nucl Med. 2004;18:251–6.
124. Yamamoto S, Matsumoto K, Sakamoto S, Tarutani K, Minato K, Senda M. An intra-operative positron probe with background rejection capability for FDG-guided surgery. Ann Nucl Med. 2005;19: 23–8.
125. Yamamoto S, Higashi T, Matsumoto K, Senda M. Development of a positron-imaging detector with background rejection capability. Ann Nucl Med. 2006;20:655–62.
126. Strong VE, Galanis CJ, Riedl CC, Longo VA, Daghighian F, Humm JL, Larson SM, Fong Y. Portable PET probes are a novel tool for intraoperative localization of tumor deposits. Ann Surg Innov Res. 2009;3:2.
127. Singh B, Stack Jr BC, Thacker S, Gaysinskiy V, Bartel T, Lowe V, Cool S, Entine G, Nagarkar V. A hand-held beta imaging probe for FDG. Ann Nucl Med. 2013;27:203–8.
128. Delbeke D, Coleman RE, Guiberteau MJ, Brown ML, Royal HD, Siegel BA, Townsend DW, Berland LL, Parker JA, Hubner K, Stabin MG, Zubal G, Kachelriess M, Cronin V, Holbrook S. Procedure guideline for tumor imaging with 18F-FDG PET/CT 1.0. J Nucl Med. 2006;47:885–95.
129. American College of Radiology (ACR) and the Society for Pediatric Radiology (SPR) Practice Parameter for Performing FDG-PET/CT in Oncology, Res. 24 – 2012, Amended 2014 (Res. 39). http://www.acr.org/~/media/ACR/Documents/PGTS/guidelines/FDG_PET_CT.pdf.
130. Lodge MA, Lucas JD, Marsden PK, Cronin BF, O'Doherty MJ, Smith MA. A PET study of 18FDG uptake in soft tissue masses. Eur J Nucl Med. 1999;26:22–30.
131. Spence AM, Muzi M, Mankoff DA, O'Sullivan SF, Link JM, Lewellen TK, Lewellen B, Pham P, Minoshima S, Swanson K, Krohn KA. 18F-FDG PET of gliomas at delayed intervals: improved distinction between tumor and normal gray matter. J Nucl Med. 2004;45:1653–9.
132. Basu S, Kung J, Houseni M, Zhuang H, Tidmarsh GF, Alavi A. Temporal profile of fluorodeoxyglucose uptake in malignant lesions and normal organs over extended time periods in patients with lung carcinoma: implications for its utilization in assessing malignant lesions. Q J Nucl Med Mol Imaging. 2009;53:9–19.
133. Horky LL, Hsiao EM, Weiss SE, Drappatz J, Gerbaudo VH. Dual phase FDG-PET imaging of brain metastases provides superior assessment of recurrence versus post-treatment necrosis. J Neurooncol. 2011;103:137–46.
134. Prieto E, Martí-Climent JM, Domínguez-Prado I, Garrastachu P, Díez-Valle R, Tejada S, Aristu JJ, Peñuelas I, Arbizu J. Voxel-based analysis of dual-time-point 18F-FDG PET images for brain tumor identification and delineation. J Nucl Med. 2011;52:865–72.

135. Heckathorne E, Dimock C, Dahlbom M. Radiation dose to surgical staff from positron-emitter-based localization and radiosurgery of tumors. Health Phys. 2008;95:220–6.
136. Heckathorne E, Dimock C, Dahlbom M, Daghighian F. Radiation dose to surgical staff from PET-based localization and radiosurgery of tumors. Health Phys. 2007;93:S45.
137. Andersen PA, Chakera AH, Klausen TL, Binderup T, Grossjohann HS, Friis E, Palnaes Hansen C, Schmidt G, Kjaer A, Hesse B. Radiation exposure to surgical staff during F-18-FDG-guided cancer surgery. Eur J Nucl Med Mol Imaging. 2008;35:624–9.
138. United States Nuclear Regulatory Commission (1991). Section 20.1201 – occupational dose limits for adults, subpart C – occupational dose limits, part 20 – Standards for Protection Against Radiation, Chapter I – Nuclear Regulatory Commission, NRC Regulations Title 10 of the Code of Federal Regulations. http://www.nrc.gov/reading-rm/doc-collections/cfr/part020/full-text.html.
139. ICRP. Publication 60. The 1990 recommendations of the international commission on radiological protection. Ann ICRP. 1991;21(1–3):1–201.
140. ICRP. Publication 103. The 2007 recommendations of the international commission on radiological protection (chapters 5 and 6). Ann ICRP. 2007;37(2-4):81–123.

Part XI

Outlook: New Techniques, Image Fusion, Optical Imaging

Fluorescent Tracers, Hybrid Tracers

26

Dawid Murawa and Karol Połom

Contents

Abstract

Fluorophores used in near-infrared emission spectra have recently gained a significant interest. The increased attention given to fluorophores over the last decade results from their possible substantial impact on patient care. The new era of surgical molecular navigation may help with real-time visualization of tumors, lymph nodes, nerves, vital structures, or blood vessels. All of this in overlying colors may help in faster and even safer tumor resection, allowing preservation of important structures in human body. We can observe a paradigm shift in cancer surgery improving safety of the operation, patient outcome, and from the financial point of view, the cost of medical treatment.

26.1 Introduction

Fluorophores used in near-infrared emission spectra have recently gained a significant interest. The increased attention given to fluorophores over the last decade results from their possible substantial impact on patient care. The new era of surgical molecular navigation may help with real-time visualization of tumors, lymph nodes, nerves, vital structures, or blood vessels. All of this in overlying colors may help in faster and even safer tumor resection, allowing preservation of important structures in human body. We can observe a paradigm shift in cancer surgery

Project supported by the Wroclaw Centre of Biotechnology, program The Leading National Research Centre (KNOW) for years 2014–2018.

D. Murawa (✉)
Ist Department of Surgical Oncology and General Surgery, Greater Poland Cancer Center, ul. Garbary 15, Poznan 61-866, Poland

Regional Specialist Hospital in Wroclaw, Research and Development Centre, ul. Kamieńskiego 73a, Wrocław 51-124, Poland
e-mail: dmurawa@gmail.com

K. Połom
Ist Department of Surgical Oncology and General Surgery, Greater Poland Cancer Center, ul. Garbary 15, Poznan 61-866, Poland

K. Herrmann et al. (eds.), *Radioguided Surgery: Current Applications and Innovative Directions in Clinical Practice*, DOI 10.1007/978-3-319-26051-8_26

improving safety of the operation, patient outcome, and from the financial point of view, the cost of medical treatment.

During the last century, five imaging techniques have been applied in patient care: X-ray (along with it, the entire spectrum including plain film, fluoroscopy, and computed tomography (CT)), magnetic resonance imaging (MRI), ultrasonography (US), single-photon emission computed tomography (SPECT) including handheld gamma cameras, and positron emission tomography (PET) [1]. All these techniques helped in preoperative diagnosis of patients. For image-guided surgery, ultrasonography, fluoroscopy, and handheld gamma cameras are widely used. Also, intraoperative use of MRI or CT and even PET have slowly started playing an important role, in particular in neurosurgery and laryngology [2]. The new technology which can really revolutionize surgical guidance in real-time is the use of fluorophores that are not visible in daylight, but are only visible in the near-infrared (NIR) light range (spectra of 700–900 nm). Fluorophores have minimal interfering absorption and fluorescence from biological samples. Likewise, they allow for imaging with the use of inexpensive laser diode excitation, reduced scattering, and enhanced tissue penetration depth. As visible light can travel through the tissue in a microscale, the near-infrared light has the potential to penetrate the tissue in millimeters or even centimeters. A significant piece of information is that tissues exhibit almost no autofluorescence in NIR light. Resultantly, the signal-to-background ratio can be maximized using fluorescent agents, creating "white stars in the black sky" [3] (Table 26.1).

After injection of a fluorophore into the tissue, charge-coupled device (CCD) cameras and light-emitting diodes (LEDs) can be used to detect fluorophore (in some cameras, the operation theater light has to be turned off). The structure of CCD consists of three main components: an NIR-sensitive image intensifier, 16-bit dynamic-range frame transfer CCD camera, and LEDs [4]. In order to detect fluorescence from fluorophore, LEDs produce one wavelength of an invisible NIR beam onto the substance. In response, fluorophore emits back another wavelength of an invisible NIR beam (Stokes shift) which is detected by the intensifier and displayed on the camera [5, 6]. It takes milliseconds, enabling real-time guidance during surgery.

The history of fluorescence-guided surgery started in 1948 when the first nontargeted fluorescence-guided surgery was performed by Moore and Peyton [7]. They used fluorescein and an ultraviolet light Wood's lamp for localizing brain tumors during brain surgery. Another important breakthrough was the use of targeted fluorescence surgical imaging by Folli et al. in 1992 [8]. They used carcinoembryonic antigen-targeted antibodies labeled with fluorescein for in vivo visualization of colorectal cancer. The next significant step forward was the use of ICG in the sentinel lymph node biopsy procedure by Kitai et al. in 2005, with a charge-couple device and light-emitting diodes [9]. In 2011, van Dam et al. presented their experience in the use of folate receptor-α-targeted antibodies labeled with fluorescein for in vivo visualization of ovarian cancer [10].

During last several years, a large number of new molecules have been developed, and we now have targeted molecules for cancer cells [11], sentinel lymph node biopsy [12], molecules cleared by liver into bile for bile duct imaging [13], molecules cleared by kidneys for ureter imaging [14], agents used in cardiovascular diseases [15], neurological diseases [16], skeletal disorders [17], and agents for nerve visualization [18].

This near-infrared fluorescence (NIRF)-guided surgery may play such a significant role, especially when we realize that resection of a solid tumor during surgery with clear margins is responsible for curative treatment. This is extremely important as we analyze situations in which it is difficult to differentiate cancer tissue from normal tissue, like in breast cancer where a positive margin after breast-conserving therapy might be reported in from 5 % up to 49 % of cases [19, 20]. Another example where a cancer margin plays an important role in planning the surgery is neurosurgery. As the tumor is situated close to important structures, the differentiation between cancer tissue and healthy tissue could be critical. Most likely, the use of NIRF-guided surgery will lead to improvement of patient outcomes due to implementation of this technology

Table 26.1 Fluorescent contrast agents

Contrast agent	Emission wavelength	Usage
ICG	820–830	Ophthalmic angiography and for determining cardiac output, hepatic function, and liver blood flow and off-label/research use to monitor fluid (e.g., blood, lymph, cerebrospinal fluid, or urine)-filled structures or as a vascular, renal, or excretory pathway contrast agent, tumor detection
IRDye 800CW	789	Imaging agents in clinical studies for detection of disease and its progression and for monitoring of treatment and drug efficacy
CF770	797	Imaging agents in clinical studies for detection of disease and its progression and for monitoring of treatment and drug efficacy
CF790	806	Imaging agents in clinical studies for detection of disease and its progression and for monitoring of treatment and drug efficacy
Alexa Fluor 790	814	Dye conjugated to a variety of antibodies, peptides, proteins, tracers, and amplification substrates optimized for cellular labeling and detection
Cy7	775	Produce cyanine7-labeled biomolecules for subsequent use in various in vivo research, and drug design-related experiments
IR-783	798	Dye conjugated to a variety of antibodies, peptides, proteins, tracers, and amplification substrates optimized for cellular labeling and detection
Fluorescein Sodium	520	Diagnostic fluorescein for angiography or angioscopy of the retina and iris vasculature. Off-label/research use to monitor fluid (e.g., blood, lymph, cerebrospinal fluid, or urine)-filled structures or as a vascular, renal, or excretory pathway contrast agent
Methylene Blue	680–700	For drug-induced methemoglobinemia. Research use as an intraluminal gastrointestinal tract contrast agent and SNB
Acriflavine	510	DNA intercalator and nuclear stain
5-ALA and its esters	635	Approved as a topical solution. Aminolevulinic acid hydrochloride as a topical solution plus blue light illumination using the BLU-U (Blue Light Photodynamic Therapy Illuminator) is indicated for the treatment of minimally to moderately thick actinic keratoses (grade 1 or 2) of the face or scalp. Its metabolite is fluorescent – for tumor visualization (neurosurgery)
5-ALA		Unclear mechanism of accumulation in tumors
cRGD	Varies	Connection to integrins presented on certain tumor cells
Folate	Varies	In an oral formulation for contraception (combination with ethinyl estradiol and drospirenone). Available as a dietary supplement. Binds to FRα- overexpressed by some cancer cells
Chlorotoxin	Varies	Mechanism of targeting, which may involve MMP2
Cyclic RPMC	Varies	RPMC-F peptide may bind to an integrin, specifically $\alpha5\beta1$
NP41	Varies	Connection to the extracellular matrix of the epi-/peri- and endoneurium of nerves

(continued)

Table 26.1 (continued)

Contrast agent	Emission wavelength	Usage
BMB	540	Connection to myelin, passes to the central nervous system, cannot detect nonmyelinated nerves
GE3082	600	Connection to myelin, passes to the central nervous system, cannot detect nonmyelinated nerves
Technetium-99 m tilmanocept	Varies	Lymphatic mapping for SNB in breast cancer or melanoma. Binds to mannose receptors of lymphatic-resident reticuloendothelial cells
ACPP	Varies	Employs to protease activity present in the microenvironment of tumors and atherosclerotic plaques to accumulate fluorescence. Possible combination with chemotherapeutic or photodynamic agents
ProSense MMPSense	700 780	Employs to protease activity present in the microenvironment of tumors and atherosclerotic plaques to accumulate fluorescence
GB119	Cy5 (680 nm)	Employs to cathepsin protease activity present in the tumor microenvironment to dequench fluorescence
BMV083	Cy5 (680 nm)	Employs to cathepsin-S protease activity in the tumor microenvironment to dequench fluorescence
γGlu-HMRG	515–550	Topically active fluorogenic substrate for γ-glutamyltranspeptidase
Anti-CA19-9	Varies	Binds to CA19-9 (expressed on some cancer cells)
Anti-CEA	Varies	Binds to CEA (expressed on some cancer cells)
Anti-EPCAM	Varies	Binds to EPCAM (expressed on some cancer cells)
Anti-PSMA	Varies	Binds to PSMA (expressed on some cancer cells)
Anti-EGFR	Varies	Binds to EGFR (expressed on some cancer cells)

during difficult surgical cases for which the outcome of the surgical procedure is based on surgical skills and experience of the surgeon. Currently, for surgeries with a high number of cancer-positive margins, like malignant gliomas, prostate cancer, and breast cancer, implementation of NIRF-guided surgery might be a significant step forward for improving long-term patient outcomes.

The next important field of NIRF-guided surgery is preservation of important structures. In cancer surgery, not only radical cancer resection but also postoperative morbidity with limiting iatrogenic injuries is responsible for the final outcome of the patient [6, 21–23]. In this case, visualization of nerves is very important since their injury will lead to postoperative morbidity, in particular injury to motor nerves [24]. Fluorescent molecules which bind with nerves and help identify these structures will lead to improvement in surgical techniques. Currently, untargeted indocyanine green (ICG) helps visualize ureters, bile ducts, blood vessels, lymphatic vessels, and lymph nodes.

Of course, enthusiasm for use of this technique should be tempered due to physics behind NIRF. The laws of physics are responsible for small depth of detection that is about 5–8 mm; however, this could be improved by better equipment and more advanced molecules. The depth of penetration limitation for NIRF imaging has been a major obstacle to implementation of NIRF imaging during surgery. However, continued clinical research effort are slowly impacting upon the adoption of NIRF imaging for surgical applications.

In a review paper by Nguyen and Tsien, adoption of the following terms was proposed for clinical use – live molecular navigation (LMN) in cases where we image in vivo targeted tracers and a term of fluorescence-guided surgery (FGS) in cases where we image ex vivo resected specimen [23]. For fluorescence-guided surgery, we require just a fluorescent molecule to visualize structures in near-infrared light, but in the case of LMN fluorescent molecules, we will have to specifically localize targeted tissue in living patient [23]. This will be a step toward fluorescent-based molecularly targeted visualization in real-time between healthy tissue and cancer tissue.

26.2 Clinical Application of NIRF Molecules

The mystery of visualization of normally unseen agents in visible light lies in fluorophores and a camera where LEDs produce one wavelength of an invisible NIR beam onto the fluorophore [6, 21, 22]. The molecule responses and emits back another wavelength of an invisible NIR beam (Stokes shift) [5, 86]. This is detected by the intensifier of the system and displayed on the camera.

Today, the most widely used fluorophore tracer is ICG. It is the only 800 nm NIRF agent approved by the US Food and Drug Administration (FDA) and the European Medicines Agency (EMA). ICG is a water-soluble, anionic, amphiphilic tricarbocyanine tracer with a hydrodynamic diameter of 1.2 nm, molecular mass of 776 Da, and excitation and emission wavelengths in serum at 778 and 830, respectively [25, 26]. In the clinical practice, ICG has been used for many decades in hepatic function, cardiac output, and ophthalmic perfusion [27–29]. Recently, it has proven its practical usage in surgical oncology, secondary to its NIRF properties. In the literature, it demonstrates a high safety profile with just a few reported adverse reactions. Serious anaphylactic complications were reported in about 0.05 % of cases [30]. The toxicity was observed only in cases of higher dose intake than that approved by the US FDA. As compared to radiolabeled colloids that are used in sentinel lymph node (SLN) biopsy procedures, ICG does not represent a radiation material exposure risk.

Another tracer which demonstrates NIR properties is methylene blue (MB). It has been used for many years as a visible contrast agent (dark blue) especially in SLN biopsy. MB can reach about 700 nm emission with a molecular weight of only 320 Da.

Another tracer used in NIRF is 5-aminolevulinic acid (5-ALA). It is used for protoporphyrin synthesis as well as for tumor detection and tumor treatment – in this case, its photodynamic properties are taken advantage of. After topical or oral administration, 5-ALA starts synthesis and concentration of protoporphyrin IX (PpIX) in epithelia and neoplastic tissues. The PpIX has fluorescent properties. The use of 5-ALA has primarily been limited to the localization of malignant gliomas and meningiomas during neurosurgery cases. From the physical point of view, PpIX has two fluorescence emission peaks; for NIRF-guided surgery, 700 nm is used.

Lastly, sodium fluorescein has been used for many decades in various medical applications. Its usage is approved for diagnostic angiography and for angioscopy, in order to visualize the retina and iris vasculature [32].

26.3 Nanoparticles (NPs) Used in Biomedicine

In recent years, a large number of different substances have been proposed for biomedical imaging. They can be divided into metal-based, carbon-based, polymer-based, biological-based, and lipid-based nanoparticles. According to Choi and Frangioni, we can arrange them into subgroups [33]:

1. Metal oxide nanoparticles – an iron (Fe) core and a polymeric coating builds spherical ferromagnetics which are used in biomedical imaging, cell tracking, and monitoring of drug delivery [34]. Iron oxide NPs are classified by size and coating monocrystalline iron oxide nanocolloid (MION, 5–30 nm), cross-linked iron oxide (CLIO,10–50 nm), and superparamagnetic iron oxide (SPIO, >50 nm). These NPs are used in MRI as contrast-enhancing tracers [35].
2. Gold-containing nanostructures – they create different 3D structures like nanorods (a nanoobject with two similar external dimensions in the nanoscale and the third dimension significantly larger than the other two external dimensions), nanofibers (flexible nanorods), nanoshells (hollow NPs), and nanocages (porous wall-covered nanoshell structures). The use of gold NPs in medicine is various; it has been applied to and has been used for a long time as drug delivery, imaging, tumor therapy, and radiation sensitization. They have not only been used in NIRF imaging, but also in noninvasive photothermal ablation of tumors. These NPs are excited by ultrasound and microwaves. The usage is limited by their toxicity, especially regarding gold salts accumulation in the body [36].
3. Quantum dots (QDs) – they are known also as semiconductor nanocrystals. They consist of inorganic core, with or without a shell and a biocompatible coating. Their size is small and ranges from 5 to 50 nm. These NPs are widely used for tracking biochemical pathways and cancer metastases in animals [37]. QDs, in comparison with organic fluorophores, exhibit higher photostability, extinction coefficient, and quantum yield, and can also provide broadband absorption, narrow and tunable emission spectra, and multivalent ligand conjugation. Secondary to their small size and proper physical parameters, they are widely used in NIRF research. Due to the toxic element in the core of the QDs and in vivo stability, their clinical translation is not currently possible.
4. Silica NPs – it is a popular component of core-shell biodegradable NPs. They are widely used mainly due to their chemical and biological inert nature. The structure of silica NPs can be modified using siloxane-based cross-linkers. We can use metals to compose silica-based nanoshells and to improve its fluorescence ability. When the fluorophore is encapsulated in a silica NP shell, it shows high fluorescence emission intensity, excellent photostability, and water solubility. The limitations to using silica NPs may be their yet undetermined toxicity profile.
5. Molecular dots – these small molecules are built of calcium phosphatate with biocompatible, multilayer nanocomposites. The advantage is the low toxicity of the calcium phosphatate core. Another advantage is its bioresorbable and biodegradable structure. Limitations of these NPs include final large size (20–100 nm) and difficult surface modifications.

6. Carbon-based NPs – hollow containers built of C60 buckyballs and cylindrical single-walled (SWNT) or multi-walled carbon nanotubes (MWNT) are used as diagnostic and therapeutic agents. Their size is between 3 and 100 nm. Due to their solely carbon structure, they are strongly hydrophobic, leading to aggregation and nonspecific binding to plasma proteins. After surface modification, they exhibit extraordinary strength, electrical properties, and thermal conductivities. Again, limitations in clinical usage include their toxicity (with presented induced inflammation or even cell death), as well as difficulties in surface modifications [38].
7. Nanowires – these metal-based semiconductors are built of silicon, carbon, and other materials. The size is 2–5 nm; however, adding water soluble coating will increase the size from 10 up to 300 nm. One of the limitations into clinical translation of these NPs is a needlelike shape of nanowires (the same as carbon nanotubes), which are similar to asbestos fibers causing mesothelioma.
8. Biological NPs – they are built of nanoscale components, like peptides, proteins, enzymes, antibodies, lipoproteins, viruses, and natural polymer. The most commonly used tissue-derived components are collagen and hyaluronate. They cause minimal response and after small surface modifications are used as imaging tracers. After conjugation of peptides and antibodies with biological fluorophores, they can be used as targeted tracer. Another group of biological NPs are long half-life biological NP agents like albumin, lipoproteins, chitosan, dextran (a-1,6 polyglucose), and dextrin (a-1,4 polyglucose), which can be used as templates for carrying drugs and constrast agents. One additional example of biological agents is alginate and agarose, which are used in drug delivery and tissue engineering. For now, the biggest challenge is poor physical strength, difficulty in controlling the size and shape of NPs, and additional difficulty in controlling degradation, sometimes even immunogenicity [39].
9. Polymer nanospheres – synthetic polymers like poly(lactic acid) (PLA),poly(lactide-co-glycolide) (PLGA), poly(vinyl alcohol), poly(acrylic acid), poly(vinylpyrrolidone), poly(ethyleneimine), poly(amino acids), poly(L-lysine), poly(glutamic acid), poly (malic acid), poly(aspartamides), poly(methyl methacrylate), poly(methylcyanoacrylate), poly (ethylcyanoacrylate), poly(isobutylcyanoacrylate), and poly(isohexylcyanoacrylate) are widely used in creating NPs delivering drugs into site. These polymers can be coated with other functional polymers. To release its cargo, a trigger stimulus is needed, such as a change in pH, temperature, or chemical environment [40]. By coating other NPs, like Au, QDs, and silica with polymers, we can obtain better stability and longer blood half-life.
10. Dendrimers – are spherical macromolecules with treelike branched internal structure. With globular shape and internal cavities, dendrimers can encapsulate therapeutic agents either in their interior or on their surface.
11. Liposomes – with approachable synthesis and significant cargo capacity, they are widely used as delivery remedium for drugs, diagnostic agents, peptides, antibodies, hormones, and macromolecules after encapsulation by their lipid membranes [41]. Limitations of liposomes include poor vehicle stability and outbreak leakage. By adding biodegradable coating, we can improve stabilization of the membrane.

26.4 Translation into Clinical Usage

ICG is the most commonly used dye in NIRF researches. With implementation of newer cameras and after primary research, we can observe more dyes with additional conjugation to improve detection as well as coming into targeted molecules.

Nowadays, NIRF-guided surgery has been implemented in different areas.

26.4.1 Sentinel Lymph Node Biopsy

As first described by Kitai et al. in 2005 and Murawa et al. in 2009, SLN biopsy using ICG has been investigated [9, 42]. Additionally, the use of hybrid tracer with human serum albumin (i.e., ICG:HAS) has been proposed. According to Ohnishi et al., ICG combined with HSA improves its quantum yield (QY) described as "the brightness" of ICG approximately threefold, also increasing the molecular weight; this in turn improves ICG retention in the SLNs [26]. Polom et al. [51] and Schaafsma et al. [53] described the clinical use of ICG:HAS for SLN biopsy in melanoma and vulvar cancer respectively. Another step in improving stability and visualization of the NIRF tracer in SLN biopsy was the use of multimodal ICG-(99 m) Tc-nanocolloid in prostate cancer patients proposed by van der Poel et al. [43]. In recent years, many papers have been published regarding SLN biopsy using NIRF tracers for many different malignancies, including breast cancer [44–47, 49] as well as in colorectal cancer [45, 48, 49], skin cancer [50, 51], cervical cancer [52], vulvar cancer [53], head and neck cancer [54], lung cancer [55, 56], penile cancer [57], endometrial cancer [58], gastric cancer [59], and esophageal cancer [60].

In comparison with blue dye, NIRF-guided SLN biopsy seems to be a better option due to increased tissue penetration depth and lack of staining of the patient. A novel strategy for attempting to increase lymph node retention has been developed by Vera et al. by creating a lymphatic tracer which is specific for a receptor (mannose-binding protein) found on reticuloendothelial cells of lymph nodes [61].

26.4.2 Tumor Imaging

NIRF-guided surgery has also proved to be useful in tumor detection. This was first described by Ishizawa et al. [62] for primary and metastatic liver tumors, and later described by other groups for multiple other tumors [63–71]. The most significant issue with NIRF imaging is the depth of penetration of NIRF imaging, such that deeper placed tumors cannot be visualized. According to the published data, the approximate maximum depth of penetration of NIRF imaging is about 8 mm from the surface. In case of tumors located on the surface of liver or closely to the surface, they are easily detected in NIRF visualization. This is particularly useful in case of colorectal cancer metastases of the liver, as they are mostly located on the surface of the liver parenchyma [62, 63].

In case of insulinoma, one of the methods developed for localizing insulinomas is the intra-arterial injection of a high dose of MB [64]. Another study presented by Hutteman et al. showed useful demarcation of the tumor in other pancreatic tumors, including adenocarcinoma ($n=6$), neuroendocrine tumor ($n=1$), and adenomatous polyp ($n=1$) [65]. NIRF-guided surgery has also proved to be useful in case of parathyroid gland resection using MB as a fluorescent dye [66]. NIRF tracers can be also used in marking in endoscopy intestinal tumors, in particular by tattooing the tumor position [67]. Also in endoscopy of gastric cancer, ICG can be used to differentiate mucosal gastric cancer from submucosal cancer and even deeper cancers, which represents a risk factor for lymph node metastasis and can lead to additional surgical treatment [68]. One additional area of interest is the use of ICG in a prototype fluorescence mammographic imaging system. Hagen et al. and Poellinger et al. used ICG to discriminate between malignant and benign lesions in breast tissue [69, 70]. Recently, Tummers et al. proposed intraoperative detection of breast cancer during breast-conserving therapy and also for detection of free margins using MB and an NIRF-guided surgical approach [71].

26.4.3 Angiography

ICG is a very good tracer to visualize blood vessel structures. ICG usage in angiography imaging, as it pertains to coronary artery bypass grafts, peripheral vascular disease, and solid organ transplantation [72–74]. ICG-assisted angiography imaging could be also used to show good vasculature of the gastrointestinal tract anastomosis. Murawa et al. demonstrated intraoperatively that assessing NIR-guided ICG angiography in case of esophageal cancer may play a role in determining the vascular integrity of an anastomosis [75]. NIRF angiography has also been used to evaluate colon cancer anastomosis [76]. NIRF angiography can also be applied in reconstructive surgery in order to show intraoperative evaluation of tissue flap viability. The evaluation of tissue flaps during reconstructive surgery is critical, and the loss of tissue flap viability can be devastating. During the surgery, we can visualize arterial inflow, venous return, and tissue perfusion, prior to harvest and after flap transfer [77, 78]. This NIRF angiography technique is not only useful to plan the reconstruction, but also after transplantation. NIRF angiography can detect impaired flap blood flow and can be helpful for differentiating among poor arterial inflow, poor venous outflow, or poor perfusion [77, 78]. Upon recognition of the problem, intraoperative solution can be implemented. It is also useful in recognition of microvascular thrombosis [78].

26.4.4 Preservation of Normal Tissues

A good target for NIRF imaging might be nerves. During surgery, it is sometimes very difficult to differentiate nerves from other tissues and their resultant iatrogenic injury can result in increased morbidity. The initial study by Gibbs-Strauss et al. showed a good visualization of nerves in the case of using fluorophores targeted against myelin from sheath on axons [102]. Another study by KleinJan et al. described the in vivo nerve-staining capabilities of locally administered fluorescent lectin analogs [24]. Further investigations are needed to evaluate the utility of NIRF imaging in identifying autonomic nerves which must be preserved during rectal cancer and prostate cancer surgery which are responsible for preserving urinary continence and erectile function.

26.5 Hybrid Tracers

Hybrid tracers, composed of both a radioactive tracer component and a fluoresent dye component, have been developed in order to allow for desired preoperative nuclear medicine imaging capabilities as well have high sensitivity intraoperative NIRF imaging capabilities.

Currently, the best known hybrid tracer used in clinical studies is ICG-^{99m}Tc-nanocolloid. This was first used in prostate cancer [43], and is now being widely clinically applied to other malignancies. One aspect worth noticing is that this hybrid tracer has proven similar drainage pattern as pure ^{99m}Tc-nanocolloid [79, 80]. Another important issue is that in one injection of this tracer, we can use a combination of preoperative nuclear medicine imaging of radioactive compound and intraoperative radio- and fluorescence guidance surgery for SLN biopsy. From the chemical point of view, the combination of both dyes into one hybrid is based on non-covalent self-assembly [81]. This works only when we combine ICG with an organic nanocolloid. When we try to combine ICG with an inorganic ^{99m}Tc-sulfur colloid, such a combination is not possible and leads to a decreased intensity of the fluorescent dye [4].

A combination of a radioactive and fluorescent dye is also possible with MB. MB iodization leads to creation of ^{125}I-methylene blue. Its clinical usage was proven in breast cancer studies but only using its radioactive and optical properties [82, 83].

A hybrid tracer like ICG-^{99m}Tc-nanocolloid can be used in areas with a complex anatomy or in areas where the SLN is near the injection site [43, 79, 80]. It is worth pointing out that the fluorescent dye component of the hybrid tracer has a higher identification rate in comparison with blue dye alone. In vulvar cancer, the SLN identification rate was 96 % using fluorescent image-guided surgery in comparison with 65 % of successful identification using just optical properties of a blue dye [84].

Fluorophores can be combined with antibodies, and can be used for targeted imaging. Sampath et al. proposed conjugation of multimodal mAb – trastuzumab – for Her receptor using IRDye 800CW with diethylenetriaminepentaacetic acid (DTPA) for 111In radiolabeling [85]. They showed that NIRF proved to have similar target-to-background ratio as SPECT image. Another conjugation of trastuzumab with different fluorophores was also proposed by Ogawa et al. and Aldrich et al. [5, 86, 87]. In a paper by Xu et al., the authors proposed a conjugation of cetuximab together with trastuzumab to the fluorophore Cy7 and 111In-DTPA through a novel modular synthetic strategy, resulting in mAb-based imaging probe libraries [88]. All these combinations were also seen in SPECT imaging secondary to radioactive properties of some elements. In addition to other visualization technologies, we can also use PET imaging in order to improve sensitivity of these hybrid tracers. The first demonstration of that targeted hybrid tracer was using anti-CD20 murine mAb NuB2 for targeting CD20 positive cells [89]. Likewise, after successfully visualizing their targeted hybrid tracer on SPECT and NIRF imaging, Sampath et al. [90] developed an analog trastuzumab targeted hybrid tracer that was capable of being visualized on PET and NIRF imaging. The hybrid tracer was 64Cu-DOTA and IRDye 800CW to detect the metastatic breast cancer cells. Another study aiming to prove an expression of EpCAM on prostate cancer and for circulating tumor cells is currently under investigation in some clinical trials. In a paper by Hall et al., mAbs against EpCAM were dual labeled with IRDye 800CW and with 64Cu-DOTA for metastatic lymph node detection in prostate cancer [91].

Another area of research is peptide-based targeting. The majority of targets are based on characterized radiopeptides that bind αvβ3 integrins, somatostatin receptors (SSTRs), and matrix metalloproteinases (MMPs). New vessel formation was studied by targeting αvβ3integrin with its peptide sequence Arg-Gly-Asp (RGD). For targeting RGD, Huston et al. proposed DTPA, IRDye 800CW, and 111In conjugation for both radioactive and NIRF imaging [92]. In a paper by Ye et al., a new particle for RGD imaging was proposed as in model of delivery of desferrioxamine to tumor cells with additional chelation of radiometals [93]. In the case of using SSTRs for neuroendocrine tumor imaging, Edwards et al. proposed a dual-labeled SSTR agent by attaching the NIRF dye cypate to the C-terminus of DOTA-octreotate and radiolabeling with 64Cu [94]. Another marker – MMP-9 for heterotopic ossification, was combined together with DOTA and IRDye 800CW, followed by labeling with 64Cu for early detection of new bone formation by PET imaging [95]. Another multimodal peptide agent was proposed for detecting interleukin-11 receptor-α, which was dual labeled using an 111In-DTPA chelate and IR-783 [96]. In another study, non-peptide conjugation of bisphosphonate with IRDye 800CW was used in the detection of breast cancer microcalcifications [97]. An additional targeting tracer which might help decrease the number of positive margins in breast cancer cases was proposed on a mouse model by Nguyen et al. [98]. They used peptides which are responsive to tumor-associated matrix metalloproteinases (MMPs). In research done by Rosbach et al. on fresh resected human specimen, multiple biomarkers of epithelial neoplasia were evaluated by using combined antibodies [99]. Overexpression of γ-glutamyltranspeptidase (GGT) in ovarian cancer was a target for γ-glutamyltranspeptidase-activated fluorescent tracer sprayed topically in a mouse model [100]. The first in-human use of an NIRF tracer in ovarian cancer was reported by von Dam et al. [10], in which they utilized folate receptor-α-targeted antibodies labeled with fluorescein for in vivo visualization of ovarian cancer. Most targeted NIRF tracers have been evaluated on animal models. The only NIRF-directed surgery which proved to increased tumor-free survival was the administration of 5-ALA, which is an agent that starts synthesis and results in concentration of protoporphyrin IX (PpIX) in epithelia and neoplastic tissues in malignant glioblastoma [101]. It is worth mentioning at this point that when using all these targeted NIRF tracers, we have to remember about the heterogeneity of various malignancies. In the case of ovarian cancer, expression of FRα is present in 72 % of primary and 81 % of recurrent epithelial ovarian cancer. Likewise, regarding gliomas, the use of 5-ALA (which had such a positive result on tumor-free survival) is possible only in 57 % of grade III or grade IV gliomas and only in 6 % of grade II gliomas, due to the fact that these tumors were positive for 5-ALA target-protoporphyrin IX.

References

1. Frangioni JV. New technologies for human cancer imaging. J Clin Oncol. 2008;26:4012–21.
2. Kubben PL, et al. Intraoperative MRI-guided resection of glioblastoma multiforme: a systematic review. Lancet Oncol. 2011;12:1062–70. PubMed: 21868286.

3. Frangioni JV. In vivo near-infrared fluorescence imaging. Curr Opin Chem Biol. 2003;7:626–34.
4. Sevick-Muraca EM, Sharma R, Rasmussen JC, Marshall MV, Wendt JA, Pham HQ, et al. Imaging of lymph flow in breast cancer patients after microdose administration of a near-infrared fluorophore: feasibility study. Radiology. 2008;246:734–41.
5. Ogawa M, Regino CA, Choyke PL, Kobayashi H. In vivo target-specific activatable near-infrared optical labeling of humanized monoclonal antibodies. Mol Cancer Ther. 2009;8:232–9.
6. Polom K, Murawa D, Rho Y, Nowaczyk P, Hünerbein M, Murawa P. Current trends and emerging future of indocyanine green usage in surgery and oncology: a literature review. Cancer. 2011;117(21):4812–22.
7. Moore GE, Peyton WT. The clinical use of fluorescein in neurosurgery; the localization of brain tumors. J Neurosurg. 1948;5:392–8.
8. Folli S, et al. Immunophotodiagnosis of colon carcinomas in patients injected with fluoresceinated chimeric antibodies against carcinoembryonic antigen. Proc Natl Acad Sci U S A. 1992;89:7973–7.
9. Kitai T, Inomoto T, Miwa M, Shikayama T. Fluorescence navigation with indocyanine green for detecting sentinel lymph nodes in breast cancer. Breast Cancer. 2005;12:211–5.
10. von Dam GM, et al. Intraoperative tumor-specific fluorescence imaging in ovarian cancer by folate receptor-α targeting: first in-human results. Nat Med. 2011;17:1315–9.
11. Choi HS, et al. Targeted zwitterionic near-infrared fluorophores for improved optical imaging. Nat Biotechnol. 2013;31:148–53.
12. Emerson DK, et al. A receptor-targeted fluorescent radiopharmaceutical for multireporter sentinel lymph node imaging. Radiology. 2012;265:186–93.
13. Figueiredo JL, Siegel C, Nahrendorf M, Weissleder R. Intraoperative near-infrared fluorescent cholangiography (NIRFC) in mouse models of bile duct injury. World J Surg. 2010;34:336–43.
14. Choi HS, et al. Synthesis and in vivo fate of zwitterionic near-infrared fluorophores. Angew Chem Int Ed Engl. 2011;50:6258–63.
15. Sosnovik DE, et al. Fluorescence tomography and magnetic resonance imaging of myocardial macrophage infiltration in infarcted myocardium in vivo. Circulation. 2007;115:1384–91.
16. Hyde D, et al. Hybrid FMT-CT imaging of amyloid-beta plaques in a murine Alzheimer's disease model. Neuroimage. 2009;44:1304–11.
17. Wunder A, Tung CH, Müller-Ladner U, Weissleder R, Mahmood U. In vivo imaging of protease activity in arthritis: a novel approach for monitoring treatment response. Arthritis Rheum. 2004;50: 2459–65.
18. Whitney MA, et al. Fluorescent peptides highlight peripheral nerves during surgery in mice. Nat Biotechnol. 2011;29:352–6.
19. Rizzo M, et al. The effects of additional tumor cavity sampling at the time of breast-conserving surgery on final margin status, volume of resection, and pathologist workload. Ann Surg Oncol. 2010;17:228–34.
20. McLaughlin SA. Surgical management of the breast: breast conservation therapy and mastectomy. Surg Clin North Am. 2013;93:411–28.
21. Vahrmeijer AL1, Hutteman M, van der Vorst JR, van de Velde CJ, Frangioni JV. Image-guided cancer surgery using near-infrared fluorescence. Nat Rev Clin Oncol. 2013;10(9):507–18. doi:10.1038/nrclinonc.2013.123. Epub 2013 Jul 23.
22. Schaafsma BE, Mieog JS, Hutteman M, van der Vorst JR, Kuppen PJ, Löwik CW, Frangioni JV, van de Velde CJ, Vahrmeijer AL. The clinical use of indocyanine green as a near-infrared fluorescent contrast agent for image-guided oncologic surgery. J Surg Oncol. 2011;104(3):323–32. doi:10.1002/jso.21943.
23. Nguyen QT, Tsien RY. Fluorescence –guided surgery with live molecular navigation- a new cutting edge. Nat Rev Cancer. 2013;13(9):653–62.
24. KleinJan GH, Buckle T, van Willigen DM, van Oosterom MN, Spa SJ, Kloosterboer HE, van Leeuwen FW. Fluorescent lectins for local in vivo visualization of peripheral nerves. Molecules. 2014;19(7):9876–92. doi:10.3390/molecules19079876.
25. Kirchherr AK, Briel A, Mader K. Stabilization of indocyanine green by encapsulation within micellar systems. Mol Pharm. 2009;6:480–91.
26. Ohnishi S, Lomnes SJ, Laurence RG, Gogbashian A, Mariani G, Frangioni JV. Organic alternatives to quantum dots for intraoperative near-infrared fluorescent sentinel lymph node mapping. Mol Imaging. 2005;4:172–81.
27. Kang SW, Chung SE, Shin WJ, Lee JH. Polypoidal choroidal vasculopathy and late geographic hyperfluorescence on indocyanine green angiography. Br J Ophthalmol. 2009;93:759–64.
28. Tanaka E, Chen FY, Flaumenhaft R, Graham GJ, Laurence RG, Frangioni JV. Real-time assessment of cardiac perfusion, coronary angiography, and acute intravascular thrombi using dual-channel near-infrared fluorescence imaging. J Thorac Cardiovasc Surg. 2009;138:133–40.
29. Deja M, Ahlers O, Macguill M, et al. Changes in hepatic blood flow during whole body hyperthermia. Int J Hyperthermia. 2010;26:95–100.
30. Olsen TW, Lim JI, Capone Jr A, Myles RA, Gilman JP. Anaphylactic shock following indocyanine green angiography. Arch Ophthalmol. 1996;114:97.
31. Stummer W, Novotny A, Stepp H, Goetz C, Bise K, Reulen HJ. Fluorescence-guided resection of glioblastoma multiforme by using 5-aminolevulinic acid-induced porphyrins: a prospective study in 52 consecutive patients. J Neurosurg. 2000;93:1003–13.
32. Kuroda K, et al. Intra-arterial injection fluorescein videoangiography in aneurysm surgery. Neurosurgery. 2012;72:141–50.
33. Choi HS, Frangioni JV. Nanoparticles for biomedical imaging: fundamentals of clinical translation. Mol Imaging. 2010;9(6):291–310.

34. McCarthy JR, Kelly KA, Sun EY, Weissleder R. Targeted delivery of multifunctional magnetic nanoparticles. Nanomedicine. 2007;2(2):153–67.
35. Liau J, Shiehmorteza M, Girard OM, Sirlin CB, Bydder M. Evaluation of MRI fat fraction in the liver and spine pre and post SPIO infusion. Magn Reson Imaging. 2013;31(6):1012–6. doi:10.1016/j.mri.2013.01.016.
36. Fadeel B, Garcia-Bennett AE. Better safe than sorry: understanding the toxicological properties of inorganic nanoparticles manufactured for biomedical applications. Adv Drug Deliv Rev. 2010;62(3):362–74.
37. Cai W, Shin DW, Chen K, et al. Peptide-labeled near-infrared quantum dots for imaging tumor vasculature in living subjects. Nano Lett. 2006;6(4):669–76.
38. Kostarelos K. The long and short of carbon nanotube toxicity. Nat Biotechnol. 2008;26(7):774–6.
39. Langer R. Drug delivery and targeting. Nature. 1998;392(6679 Suppl):5–10.
40. Chan JM, Zhang L, Yuet KP, et al. PLGA-lecithin-PEG core-shell nanoparticles for controlled drug delivery. Biomaterials. 2009;30(8):1627–34.
41. Mulder WJ, Strijkers GJ, van Tilborg GA, et al. Nanoparticulate assemblies of amphiphiles and diagnostically active materials for multimodality imaging. Acc Chem Res. 2009;42(7):904–14.
42. Murawa D, Hirche C, Dresel S, Hunerbein M. Sentinel lymph node biopsy in breast cancer guided by indocyanine green fluorescence. Br J Surg. 2009;96(11):1289–94.
43. van der Poel HG, Buckle T, Brouwer OR, Valdés Olmos RA, van Leeuwen FW. Intraoperative laparoscopic fluorescence guidance to the sentinel lymph node in prostate cancer patients: clinical proof of concept of an integrated functional imaging approach using a multimodal tracer. Eur Urol. 2011;60(4):826–33.
44. Hirche C, Murawa D, Mohr Z, Kneif S, Hunerbein M. ICG fluorescence – guided sentinel node biopsy for axillary nodal staging in breast cancer. Breast Cancer Res Treat. 2010;121(2):373–8.
45. Hirche C, Mohr Z, Kneif S, Murawa D, Hunerbein M. High rate of solitary sentinel node metastases identification by fluorescence-guided lymphatic imaging in breast cancer. J Surg Oncol. 2012;105(2):162–6.
46. Jung SY, Kim SK, Kim SW, Kwon Y, Lee ES, Kang HS, Ko KL, Shin KH, Lee KS, Park IH, Ro J, Jeong HJ, Joo J, Kang SH, Lee S. Comparison of sentinel lymph node biopsy guided by the multimodal method of indocyanine green fluorescence, radioisotope, and blue dye versus the radioisotope method in breast cancer: a randomized controlled trial. Ann Surg Oncol. 2014;21(4):1254–9.
47. Verbeek FP, Troyan SL, Mieog JS, Liefers GJ, Moffitt LA, Rosenberg M, Hirshfield-Bartek J, Gioux S, van de Velde CJ, Vahrmeijer AL, Frangioni JV. Near-infrared fluorescence sentinel lymph node mapping in breast cancer: a multicenter experience. Breast Cancer Res Treat. 2014;143(2):333–42.
48. Ankersmit M, van der Pas MH, van Dam DA, Meijerink WJ. Near infrared fluorescence lymphatic laparoscopy of the colon and mesocolon. Colorectal Dis. 2011;13 Suppl 7:70–3.
49. Hirche C, Mohr Z, Kneif S, Doniga S, Murawa D, Strik M, Hunerbein M. Ultrastaging of colon cancer by sentinel node biopsy using fluorescence navigation with indocyanine green. Int J Colorectal Dis. 2012;27(3):319–24.
50. Cloyd JM, Wapnir IL, Read BM, Swetter S, Greco RS. Indocyanine green and fluorescence lymphangiography for sentinel lymph node identification in cutaneous melanoma. J Surg Oncol. 2014;110(7):888–92.
51. Polom K, Murawa D, Rho YS, Spychala A, Murawa P. Skin melanoma sentinel lymph node biopsy using real-time fluorescence navigation with indocyanine green and indocyanine green with human serum albumin. Br J Dermatol. 2012;166(3):682–3.
52. Jewell EL, Huang JJ, Abu-Rustum NR, Gardner GJ, Brown CL, Sonoda Y, Barakat RR, Levine DA, Leitao Jr MM. Detection of sentinel lymph nodes in minimally invasive surgery using indocyanine green and near-infrared fluorescence imaging for uterine and cervical malignancies. Gynecol Oncol. 2014;133(2):274–7.
53. Schaafsma BE, Verbeek FP, Peters AA, van der Vorst JR, de Kroon CD, van Poelgeest MI, Trimbos JB, van de Velde CJ, Frangioni JV, Vahrmeijer AL, Gaarenstroom KN. Near-infrared fluorescence sentinel lymph node biopsy in vulvar cancer: a randomised comparison of lymphatic tracers. BJOG. 2013;120(6):758–64.
54. Nakamura Y, Fujisawa Y, Nakamura Y, Maruyama H, Furuta J, Kawachi Y, Otsuka F. Improvement of the sentinel lymph node detection rate of cervical sentinel lymph node biopsy using real-time fluorescence navigation with indocyanine green in head and neck skin cancer. J Dermatol. 2013;40(6):453–7.
55. Oh Y, Lee YS, Quan YH, Choi Y, Jeong JM, Kim BM, Kim HK. Thoracoscopic color and fluorescence imaging system for sentinel lymph node mapping in porcine lung using indocyanine green-neomannosyl human serum albumin: intraoperative image-guided sentinel nodes navigation. Ann Surg Oncol. 2014;21(4):1182–8.
56. Gilmore DM, Khullar OV, Jaklitsch MT, Chirieac LR, Frangioni JV, Colson YL. Identification of metastatic nodal disease in a phase 1 dose-escalation trial of intraoperative sentinel lymph node mapping in non-small cell lung cancer using near-infrared imaging. J Thorac Cardiovasc Surg. 2013;146(3):562–70.
57. Brouwer OR, van den Berg NS, Mathéron HM, van der Poel HG, van Rhijn BW, Bex A, van Tinteren H, Valdés Olmos RA, van Leeuwen FW, Horenblas S. A hybrid radioactive and fluorescent tracer for sentinel node biopsy in penile carcinoma as a potential replacement for blue dye. Eur Urol. 2014;65(3):600–9.

58. Sinno AK, Fader AN, Roche KL, Giuntoli 2nd RL, Tanner EJ. A comparison of colorimetric versus fluorometric sentinel lymph node mapping during robotic surgery for endometrial cancer. Gynecol Oncol. 2014;134(2):281–6.
59. Yoshida M, Kubota K, Kuroda J, Ohta K, Nakamura T, Saito J, Kobayashi M, Sato T, Beck Y, Kitagawa Y, Kitajima M. Indocyanine green injection for detecting sentinel nodes using color fluorescence camera in the laparoscopy-assisted gastrectomy. J Gastroenterol Hepatol. 2012;27 Suppl 3:29–33.
60. Kubota K, Yoshida M, Kuroda J, Okada A, Ohta K, Kitajima M. Application of the HyperEye Medical System for esophageal cancer surgery: a preliminary report. Surg Today. 2013;43(2):215–20.
61. Vera DR, Wallace AM, Hoh CK, Mattrey RF. A synthetic macromolecule for sentinel node detection: (99 m)Tc-DTPA-mannosyl-dextran. J Nucl Med. 2001;42:951–9.
62. Ishizawa T, Fukushima N, Shibahara J, et al. Real-time identification of liver cancers by using indocyanine green fluorescent imaging. Cancer. 2009;115:2491–504.
63. Gotoh K, Yamada T, Ishikawa O, et al. A novel image-guided surgery of hepatocellular carcinoma by indocyanine green fluorescence imaging navigation. J Surg Oncol. 2009;100:75–9.
64. Winer JH, Choi HS, Gibbs-Strauss SL, Ashitate Y, Colson YL, Frangioni JV. Intraoperative localization of insulinoma and normal pancreas using invisible near-infrared fluorescent light. Ann Surg Oncol. 2010;17(4):1094–100.
65. Hutteman M, van der Vorst JR, Mieog JS, Bonsing BA, Hartgrink HH, Kuppen PJ, Löwik CW, Frangioni JV, van de Velde CJ, Vahrmeijer AL. Near-infrared fluorescence imaging in patients undergoing pancreaticoduodenectomy. Eur Surg Res. 2011;47(2):90–7.
66. McWade MA, Paras C, White LM, Phay JE, Solórzano CC, Broome JT, Mahadevan-Jansen A. Label-free Intraoperative Parathyroid Localization with Near-Infrared Autofluorescence Imaging. J Clin Endocrinol Metab. 2014;99(12):4574–80. jc20142503. [Epub ahead of print].
67. Lee JG, Low AH, Leung JW. Randomized comparative study of indocyanine green and India ink for colonic tattooing: an animal survival study. J Clin Gastroenterol. 2000;31:233–6.
68. Kimura T, Muguruma N, Ito S, et al. Infrared fluorescence endoscopy for the diagnosis of superficial gastric tumors. Gastrointest Endosc. 2007;66:37–43.
69. Hagen A, Grosenick D, Macdonald R, et al. Late-fluorescence mammography assesses tumor capillary permeability and differentiates malignant from benign lesions. Opt Express. 2009;17:17016–33.
70. Poellinger A, Burock S, Grosenick D, et al. Breast cancer: early- and late-fluorescence near-infrared imaging with indocyanine green – a preliminary study. Radiology. 2011;258(2):409–16.
71. Tummers QR, Verbeek FP, Schaafsma BE, Boonstra MC, van der Vorst JR, Liefers GJ, van de Velde CJ, Frangioni JV, Vahrmeijer AL. Real-time intraoperative detection of breast cancer using near-infrared fluorescence imaging and methylene blue. Eur J Surg Oncol. 2014;40(7):850–8.
72. Reuthebuch O, Haussler A, Genoni M, et al. Novadaq SPY: intraoperative quality assessment in off-pump coronary artery bypass grafting. Chest. 2004;125:418–24.
73. Sekijima M, Tojimbara T, Sato S, et al. An intraoperative fluorescent imaging system in organ transplantation. Transplant Proc. 2004;36:2188–90.
74. Kang Y, Lee J, Kwon K, et al. Dynamic fluorescence imaging of indocyanine green for reliable and sensitive diagnosis of peripheral vascular insufficiency. Microvasc Res. 2010;80:552–5.
75. Murawa D, Huenerbein M, Spychala A, et al. Indocyanine green angiography for evaluation of gastric conduit perfusion during esophagectomy. Acta Chir Belg. 2012;112(4):275–80.
76. Kudszus S, Roesel C, Schachtrupp A, Höer JJ. Intraoperative laser fluorescence angiography in colorectal surgery: a noninvasive analysis to reduce the rate of anastomotic leakage. Langenbecks Arch Surg. 2010;395(8):1025–30.
77. Komorowska-Timek E, Gurtner GC. Intraoperative perfusion mapping with laser-assisted indocyanine green imaging can predict and prevent complications in immediate breast reconstruction. Plast Reconstr Surg. 2010;125:1065–73.
78. Holm C, Dornseifer U, Sturtz G, Ninkovic M. Sensitivity and specificity of ICG angiography in free flap reexploration. J Reconstr Microsurg. 2010;26:311–6.
79. Brouwer OR, Buckle T, Vermeeren L, Klop WM, Balm AJ, van der Poel HG, et al. Comparing the hybrid fluorescent-radioactive tracer indocyanine green-99mTc-nanocolloid with 99mTc-nanocolloid for sentinel node identification: a validation study using lymphoscintigraphy and SPECT/CT. J Nucl Med. 2012;53:1034–40.
80. Brouwer OR, Klop WM, Buckle T, Vermeeren L, van den Brekel MW, Balm AJ, et al. Feasibility of sentinel node biopsy in head and neck melanoma using a hybrid radioactive and fluorescent tracer. Ann Surg Oncol. 2012;19:1988–94.
81. van Leeuwen AC, Buckle T, Bendle G, Vermeeren L, Valdes Olmos R, van de Poel HG, et al. Tracer-cocktail injections for combined pre- and intraoperative multimodal imaging of lymph node (s) in a spontaneous mouse prostate tumor model. J Biomed Opt. 2011;16:016004.
82. Cundiff JD, Wang YZ, Espenan G, Maloney T, Camp A, Lazarus L, et al. A phase I/II trial of 125I methylene blue for one-stage sentinel lymph node biopsy. Ann Surg. 2007;245:290–6.
83. Harkrider WW, Diebold AE, Maloney T, Espenan G, Wang YZ, Stafford SJ, et al. An extended phase II trial of iodine-125 methylene blue for sentinel lymph node identification in women with breast cancer. J Am Coll Surg. 2013;216:599–605.

84. Mathéron HM, van den Berg NS, Brouwer OR, Kleinjan GH, van Driel WJ, Trum JW, Vegt E, Kenter G, van Leeuwen FW, Valdés Olmos RA. Multimodal surgical guidance towards the sentinel node in vulvar cancer. Gynecol Oncol. 2013; 131(3):720–5.
85. Sampath L, Kwon S, Ke S, Wang W, Schiff R, Mawad ME. Sevick- Muraca EM. Dual-labeled trastuzumab-based imaging agent for the detection of human epidermal growth factor receptor 2 overexpression in breast cancer. J Nucl Med. 2007; 48(9):1501–10.
86. Ogawa M, Regino CA, Seidel J, Green MV, Xi W, Williams M, Kosaka N, Choyke PL, Kobayashi H. Dual-modality molecular imaging using antibodies labeled with activatable fluorescence and a radionuclide for specific and quantitative targeted cancer detection. Bioconjug Chem. 2009;20(11): 2177–84.
87. Aldrich MB, Wang X, Hart A, Kwon S, Sampath L, Marshall MV. Sevick-Muraca EM () Assessment of free dye in solutions of dual labeled antibody conjugates for in vivo molecular imaging. Mol Imaging Biol. 2011;13(1):32–42.
88. Xu H, Eck PK, Baidoo KE, Choyke PL, Brechbiel MW. Toward preparation of antibody-based imaging probe libraries for dual-modality positron emission tomography and fluorescence imaging. Bioorg Med Chem. 2009;17(14):5176–81.
89. Paudyal P, Paudyal B, Iida Y, Oriuchi N, Hanaoka H, Tominaga H, Ishikita T, Yoshioka H, Higuchi T, Endo K. Dual functional molecular imaging probe targeting CD20 with PET and optical imaging. Oncol Rep. 2009;22(1):115–9.
90. Sampath L, Kwon S, Hall MA, Price RE, Sevick-Muraca EM. Detection of cancer metastases with a dual-labeled near-infrared/positron emission tomography imaging agent. Transl Oncol. 2010;3(5):307–217.
91. Hall MA, Kwon S, Robinson H, Lachance PA, Azhdarinia A, Ranganathan R, Price RE, Chan W, Sevick-Muraca EM. Imaging prostate cancer lymph node metastases with a multimodality contrast agent. Prostate. 2012;72(2):129–46.
92. Houston JP, Ke S, Wang W, Li C, Sevick-Muraca EM. Quality analysis of in vivo near-infrared fluorescence and conventional gamma images acquired using a dual-labeled tumor-targeting probe. J Biomed Opt. 2005;10(5):054010.
93. Ye Y, Bloch S, Xu B, Achilefu S. Novel near-infrared fluorescent integrin-targeted DFO analogue. Bioconjug Chem. 2008;19(1):225–34.
94. Edwards WB, Xu B, Akers W, Cheney PP, Liang K, Rogers BE, Anderson CJ, Achilefu S. Agonist–antagonist dilemma in molecular imaging: evaluation of a monomolecular multimodal imaging agent for the somatostatin receptor. Bioconjug Chem. 2008;19(1):192–200.
95. Rodenberg E, Azhdarinia A, Lazard Z, Hall M, Kwon S, Wilganowski N, Merched-Sauvage M, Salisbury EA, Davis AR, Sevick-Muraca EM, Olmsted-Davis E. MMP-9 as a biomarker of heterotopic ossification. Tissue Eng Part A. 2011; 17(19–20):2487–96.
96. Wang W, Ke S, Kwon S, Yallampalli S, Cameron AG, Adams KE, Mawad ME, Sevick-Muraca EM. A new optical and nuclear dual-labeled imaging agent targeting interleukin 11 receptor alpha chain. Bioconjug Chem. 2007;18(2):397–402.
97. Bhushan KR, Misra P, Liu F, Mathur S, Lenkinski RE, Frangioni JV. Detection of breast cancer microcalcifications using a dual modality SPECT/NIR fluorescent probe. J Am Chem Soc. 2008;130(52): 17648–9.
98. Nguyen QT, Olson ES, Aguilera TA, Jiang T, Scadeng M, Ellies LG, Tsien RY. Surgery with molecular fluorescence imaging using activatable cell-penetrating peptides decreases residual cancer and improves survival. Proc Natl Acad Sci U S A. 2010;107:4317–22.
99. Rosbach KJ, Williams MD, Gillenwater AM, Richards-Kortum RR. Optical molecular imaging of multiple biomarkers of epithelial neoplasia: epidermal growth factor receptor expression and metabolic activity in oral mucosa. Transl Oncol. 2012;5: 160–71.
100. Urano Y, Sakabe M, Kosaka N, Ogawa M, Mitsunaga M, Asanuma D, Kamiya M, Young MR, Nagano T, Choyke PL, Kobayashi H. Rapid cancer detection by topically spraying a γ-glutamyltranspeptidase-activated fluorescent probe. Sci Transl Med. 2011; 3:110ra119.
101. Stummer W, Pichlmeier U, Meinel T, Wiestler OD, Zanella F, Reulen HJ, ALA-Glioma Study Group. Fluorescence-guided surgery with 5-aminolevulinic acid for resection of malignant glioma: a randomised controlled multicentre phase III trial. Lancet Oncol. 2006;7:392–401.
102. Gibbs-Strauss SL, Nasr KA, Fish KM, Khullar O, Ashitate Y, Siclovan TM, Johnson BF, Barnhardt NE, Tan Hehir CA, Frangioni JV. Nerve-highlighting fluorescent contrast agents for image-guided surgery. Mol Imaging. 2011;10:91–101.

Magnetic Advances in Cancer Surgery

27

B. Anninga, M. Ahmed, and Michael Douek

Contents

Abstract

Sentinel lymph node biopsy (SLNB) provides prognostic information in the management of solid tumours. Currently, the 'combined technique' using radioisotope and blue dye is considered the 'gold standard'. This technique has drawbacks due to radioisotope dependence and adverse reactions to blue dye. Novel alternatives have been developed, but the established 'gold standard' method for SLNB has not changed. This chapter covers the clinical experience with the magnetic technique, which was developed as an alternative to radioisotope dependence for SLNB in breast cancer. It also discusses its application to other cancers and assesses the published literature for current and potential future work. The magnetic technique has been proven to be non-inferior to the combined technique for SLNB in breast cancer and has consequently been extended to concurrent breast lesion localisation and SLNB in melanoma. Superparamagnetic iron oxide (SPIO)-enhanced MRI has proven applications in axillary staging of breast cancer and could prove a viable, non-invasive alternative to SLNB. The magnetic technique has demonstrated promising results when applied to cancer surgery. Further assessment within well-constructed randomised controlled trials is now necessary to bring this innovative application into routine clinical practice.

B. Anninga • M. Ahmed
Research Oncology, Division of Cancer Studies, King's College London, London SE1 9RT, UK

M. Douek, MD, FRCS (Eng), FRCS (Gen) (✉)
Research Oncology KCL, Division of Cancer Studies, Guy's Hospital, King's College London, 3rd Floor Bermondsey Wing, Great Maze Pond, London SE1 9RT, UK
e-mail: michael.douek@kcl.ac.uk

K. Herrmann et al. (eds.), *Radioguided Surgery: Current Applications and Innovative Directions in Clinical Practice*, DOI 10.1007/978-3-319-26051-8_27

27.1 Introduction

Radioactive tracers have long been established for guiding cancer surgery, through assessment of the extent of tumour spread. Correctly detecting and histologically assessing the first draining lymph node in solid tumours, such as breast cancer and melanoma, are crucial in determining the stage of disease and planning of further treatment. The concept of a sentinel lymph node (SLN) was first described in a large group of penile cancer patients by Cabanas in 1977 [1]. Morton et al. published the blue dye approach in 1992 for melanoma [2] and standardised this technique. The idea of using a radioactive tracer (99-m technetium), published first by Alex et al. in 1993 for melanoma [3], made sentinel lymph node biopsy (SLNB) more accurate and widely available to surgeons. Krag et al. [4] in 1993 and Giuliano et al. [5] in 1994 confirmed these findings in breast cancer patients by using radioactive tracer in 22 patients and blue dye in 174 patients, respectively.

27.2 Current Evidence on Radioactive Approach

Kim et al. performed a systematic review and meta-analysis in 2006 looking at SLNB in patients with early-stage breast cancer. This analysis evaluated successful mapping of SLNs and the false-negative rate (FNR) of the radioactive and blue dye procedure. A total of 8059 patients were included, of which 7765 had a successfully mapped SLN resulting in a mean identification rate of 96 % [6]. The FNR ranged from 0 to 29 %, with an overall mean of 7.3 %. A total of 68 studies were included of which 18 used blue dye alone, 16 used radioactive tracer alone and 34 studies used the combined technique. The FNR was favourable for studies that used the combined technique (7.0 %) compared to blue dye alone (10.9 %) or radioactive tracer alone (8.8 %), a difference which was statistically significant ($P=0.047$) [6]. Similar success rates of mapping of the SLN can be found in melanoma, as assessed by Valsecchi et al. in 2011 [7]. Including a total of 71 studies and 25,240 patients, the mean success rate was 98.1 % (95 % CI: 97.3–98.6 %) and increased with the more recent year of publication. The FNR of SLNB in melanoma ranged from 0.0 to 34.0 %, with an overall mean of 12.5 % (95 % CI: 11–14.2 %) [7]. All studies in this analysis used the radioactive tracer (in combination with lymphoscintigraphy), and blue dye was added in 89 % of the studies. Consequently, the combined technique of radioactive tracer and blue dye is now considered the gold standard for performing SLNB in breast cancer and melanoma.

The use of a radioactive tracer was expanded into other applications, such as radioguided occult lesion localisation (ROLL) for the management of non-palpable breast cancers, first being described in 1998 [8]. In ROLL, a small quantity of radioactive tracer is injected into the lesion during ultrasonic examination. A gamma probe is used intraoperatively to guide the surgical removal of the lesion. This was subsequently extended to perform occult lesion localisation in conjunction with SLNB. This technique, also referred to as sentinel node and occult lesion localisation (SNOLL), has been evaluated in several studies to date, including two randomised controlled trials (RCTs). Successful complete resection rate is between 82.0 and 90.5 % with a SLNB success rate of between 88.2 and 100 % [9]. An alternative localisation technique subsequently developed using small titanium seeds (4 × 0.8 mm), labelled with I-125. The seed is introduced into the lesion percutaneously by either stereotactic or ultrasound guidance via a standard 18-gauge needle. Surgery can then proceed with the gamma probe used to direct the surgeon to the localised site. I-125 emits 27 Kev gamma rays compared to ^{99}Tc, which emits 140 KeV [10]. This means that by altering the sensitivity on the gamma probe, it is possible to differentiate between radioactive emissions from the localised lesion and the SLNs irrespective of the site of the primary lesion. A meta-analysis of this technique has demonstrated reduced reoperation rates for involved surgical margins and reduced operating times compared to conventional wire-guided surgery [10].

27.3 A Novel Magnetic Technique for SLNB

Radioactive techniques suffer from significant drawbacks. The use of radioisotopes expose patients and healthcare workers to radiation. Therefore, the use of radioisotopes is heavily controlled by legislation (both on the specific training for surgeons and on the subsequent disposal of surgical waste). Also, preoperative planar imaging (lymphoscintigraphy) with radioisotopes, which provides only 2D imaging, can be of limited usefulness and can provide limited image quality and resolution. As a result of the latter, some centres have completely stopped undertaking routine preoperative planar lymphoscintigraphy in breast cancer patients. The blue dye injection can obscure the surgical field and frequently leaves a blue skin staining, which can take months to fade or can be permanent. There is also up to a 0.9 % risk [11] of an adverse reaction to patent blue V dye, as a result of which some centres have stopped using it routinely. There is thus a clinical need to develop a new technique for detecting and identifying SLNs without these drawbacks.

Non-radioactive alternatives to using radioisotope have been developed, including a magnetic technique for identifying SLNs using a superparamagnetic iron oxide (SPIO) contrast agent injected subcutaneously into the breast and then detected using a handheld magnetometer (see Fig. 27.1a). Proof of principle for identifying SLNs was demonstrated using a prototype magnetometer and a SPIO contrast agent (Endorem, Guerbet, France) [12, 13]. The magnetic technique provides a colour change (brown or black, see Fig. 27.1b) in the lymph nodes and allows localisation using a handheld magnetometer probe. This research work led to the development of two medical devices: a handheld magnetometer (SentiMag, Endomagnetics Ltd., UK) and an injectable magnetic tracer (Sienna+, Endomagnetics Ltd., UK). Sienna+, a blackish-brown sterile aqueous suspension of superparamagnetic carboxydextran-coated iron oxide particles, is 60 nm (Z-averaged diameter; <0.25 polydispersity), ideally suited for SLNB. This diameter enables the SLNs to selectively filter out the particles and is similar to the particle size of standard radioisotope tracers (60 nm).

27.4 Trials Evaluating the Magnetic Technique

The international phase II non-randomized SentiMAG Multicentre Trial was the first to evaluate the magnetic technique for SLNB against the standard (radioisotope with or without patent blue V dye) [14]. It was an academically run trial, adopted by the National Institute for Health Research (NIHR). The trial compared the sentinel node identification rate with the new magnetic technique against that of the standard technique in 170 patients. The magnetic technique was found to have a SLN identification rate that was non-inferior to the standard technique [14]. The SLN identification rate was 95.0 % with the standard technique and 94.4 % with the magnetic technique (0.62 % difference; 95 % upper confidence limit 4.4 %; 6.88 % discordance). A total of 404

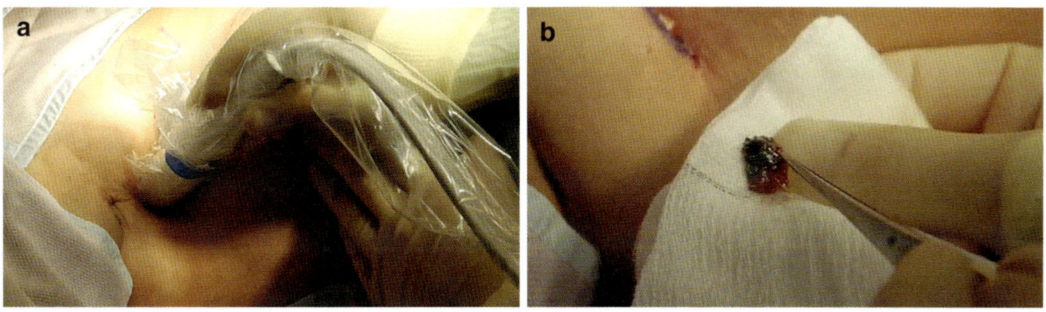

Fig. 27.1 Transcutaneous SLN localisation in the axilla, using the magnetic technique (**a**). The SLN identified in this case was blue, hot on the gamma probe and brown discoloured (**b**) due to the magnetic tracer

SLNs were removed, and the lymph node retrieval rate was also no different (1.9 lymph nodes per patient with the standard and 2.0 with the magnetic techniques). Although the results of this phase II non-randomized clinical trial [14] were very encouraging, they were not sufficient to justify changing from the standard of practice utilization of radioisotope (+/- blue dye) to that of the magnetic tracer technique. The Central-European SentiMag Study [15] subsequently confirmed this in 150 patients, who underwent SLNB, with the magnetic and radioisotope technique only (no blue dye). This study reported a SLN identification rate of 97.3 % for radioisotope alone versus 98.0 % for the magnetic technique and mean SLN retrieval of 1.8 versus 1.9, respectively. A third study, performed by Rubio et al. [16], prospectively evaluated the magnetic technique for SLNB in 120 patients with clinically node-negative early breast cancer also without the use of blue dye. They found no drainage in two patients by either technique, leaving 118 patients for analysis. They also concluded that detection of SLNs using SPIO is a not inferior to the radiotracer technique. The radiotracer technique resulted in a 95.7 % identification rate compared to a 98.3% identification rate using SPIO with the magnetic technique. One further small study published by Shiozawa et al. [17] was conducted in 30 patients who underwent the magnetic technique with blue dye, but no radioisotope, and reported a SLN identification rate of 77 %, 80 %, and 90 % for the magnetic technique, blue dye only, and magnetic technique with blue dye, respectively.

27.5 Trials Evaluating Further Applications of the Magnetic Technique

The magnetic technique has other potential clinical applications beyond SLNB. Annually, 50,000 patients are diagnosed with breast cancer within the United Kingdom, and over one-third of these are diagnosed with non-palpable or clinically occult lesions on breast imaging [18]. The introduction of greater numbers of screening programmes worldwide and increasingly advanced breast imaging modalities, such as MRI, mean that these figures are likely to continue rising further. The standard treatment for these non-palpable lesions is surgical excision using wire-guided localisation (WGL) and axillary staging using SLNB. However, despite being the current standard, WGL is limited by poor patient satisfaction, technical difficulties (such as wire migration, poor cosmetic outcome, high reoperation rates, diathermy burns), and negative impacts upon operative theatre scheduling due to the necessity of radiology input on the day of surgery [19]. This has resulted in alternative localisation techniques being developed, which have demonstrated benefits over WGL in systematic review and meta-analyses [10, 19], but their uptake has been limited due to their dependence upon radioisotopes and its associated legislative implications for handling and disposal [20]. The MagSNOLL Multicentre Trial aims to use a single ultrasound-guided intratumoural injection of 0.5 mL of magnetic tracer to localise the non-palpable lesion and perform concurrent SLNB. Once the magnetic tracer is injected, the patient may proceed to the operative theatre and using the handheld magnetometer to identify the peak 'hot spot' within the breast (which corresponds to the site of injection), the lesion can be identified intraoperatively and subsequently excised. Concurrent SLNB is performed as per the standard magnetic technique used in the SentiMAG Multicentre Trial. This technique could potentially eliminate the requirement for wire insertion, the need of radioisotopes for SLNB, as well as allowing localisation and axillary staging to be performed after a single injection. Further assessment of the retention of the magnetic tracer at the site of injection is required to determine further potential applications for the magnetic tracer as a biopsy marker, which on confirmation of malignancy could avoid the need for an additional localisation procedure. The initial results of the MagSNOLL trial were presented at the 37th San Antonio Breast Cancer Symposium, Texas, USA, between 9 and 13 December 2014 [21]. They demonstrated the successful localisation of all breast cancers in a small cohort of 20 non-palpable breast cancers, with re-excision for involved margins in two patients. The SLN identification rate with the magnetic tracer alone was inferior to the combined technique of radioisotope and blue dye (85 % versus 97 %, respectively). This demonstrated the successful radioisotope-independent localisation of breast cancers as well as the limitations of an intratumoural injection for SLNB, which requires further optimisation [22].

SLNB is used as a prognostic test in melanoma patients with stage pT2a-pT3b melanoma of any anatomic site. The gold standard for SLNB in melanoma is currently the combined technique; a preoperative injection of radioisotope followed by preoperative lymphoscintigraphy and intraoperative injection of patent blue V dye and gamma probe guided localisation of the SLN. The SLNB procedure is carried out at the same time as definitive wider excision of the primary melanoma. Patients with melanoma of Breslow thickness 1.2–3.5 mm and a positive SLNB have a 72.3±4.6 % 5-year survival compared to 90.2±1.3 % if the SLNB is negative [23]. SLNB in these patients provides important prognostic information and identifies patients with SLN metastasis who may benefit from further surgery to the affected nodal basin.

After establishing feasibility in breast cancer with the SentiMAG Multicentre Trial, Douek et al. [25] aimed to extend the indication for use of the magnetic technique to melanoma. Localisation of the correct lymphatic basin to operate on, particularly in primary trunk lesions where a multi-basin lymphatic drainage pattern can occur in 29 % of patients [24], is crucial in melanoma SLNB. The MELAMAG Trial evaluates the magnetic technique for SLNB against the standard technique (radioisotope and patent blue dye) [25]. Intraoperative localisation of the SLN was performed using the handheld magnetometer after intradermal administration of the magnetic tracer. Patients with primary cutaneous melanoma who were scheduled for SLNB and clinically AJCC stage IB-IIC [26] were eligible to be recruited into this international multicentre trial. The MELAMAG Trial evaluated the proportion of SLNs detected (detection rate) with either the standard or the magnetic technique. In addition, an MRI subprotocol evaluated the accuracy of MRI for the localisation of SLNs. The first results of this study were presented at the European Society of Surgical Oncology meeting in Liverpool. A total of 133 patients were recruited and 129 patients were available for analysis (four excluded). The SLN identification rate was 97.7 % (126/129) with the standard combined technique and 95.3 % (123/129) with the magnetic technique (2.3 difference; 95 % upper CI of 6.4 %, 5.4 % discordance) [27]. With radioisotope alone, the SLN identification rate was 95.3 % (123/129) and compared favourable with the magnetic technique (0.0 % difference; 95 % upper CI of 4.5 %; 7.8 discordance).

27.6 The Role of Axillary MRI Using Contrast-Enhanced SPIO

Axillary MRI provides an alternative to SLNB in determining axillary burden. Data from studies using intravenously administered SPIO indicates that these contrast agents have sensitivity and specificity for the detection of axillary involvement of 98 and 96 %, respectively [28]. Meng et al. [29] assessed the cost-effectiveness of MRI and PET for the evaluation of axillary lymph nodes in early breast cancer. They found that if MRI could accurately diagnose axillary involvement, the most cost-effective strategy was to replace SLNB with axillary MRI. With this strategy, true-positive patients would undergo a single surgical procedure, axillary lymph node dissection (ALND), replacing two sequential surgical procedures (SLNB followed by ALND). True-negative patients would not require any surgery. The challenge of applying this into routine clinical practice is the false-positive rate of 6.3 % for MRI versus 0.2 % for SLNB [29]. Harnan et al. [28] in their systematic review considered the use of MRI assessment of axillary lymph node status in early breast cancer and recorded a mean sensitivity and specificity of 90 and 95 %, respectively. The highest mean sensitivity and specificity was seen with SPIO-enhanced MRI, with values of 98 and 96 %, respectively.

Johnson et al. studied the distribution of SPIO within lymph nodes in a cohort of breast cancer patients undergoing SLNB using the magnetic technique [30] and showed that the 13 lymph nodes containing metastases had variable quantities of iron within them, but the iron was not present in the areas of the lymph node containing the metastasis. This study therefore demonstrated that areas of non-enhancement within SLNs and non-SLNs on contrast-enhanced MRI indicated a metastatic focus. This technique could potentially identify patients with significant axillary involvement preoperatively, who therefore require ALND and also lead to the concept of 'selective axillary surgery' of involved lymph nodes only combining preoperative imaging with novel techniques to guide surgeons intraoperatively [31].

27.7 Changing Practice in Cancer Surgery

The magnetic technique for SLNB, using SPIO, has been developed primarily to provide an alternative to radioisotope dependency and subsequently increase uptake of this 'gold standard' procedure. The magnetic technique has been demonstrated to be non-inferior to the standard radioisotope (+/- blue dye) technique within multicentre trials and is the most promising technique that does not depend on radioisotopes [32]. This magnetic technique is also been evaluated in melanoma [25] and for lesion localisation and concurrent SLNB in breast cancer [33].

All metal retractors have to be removed from the surgical field in order to successfully perform magnetic guided surgery. Plastic retractors, such as the Doxpal® self-retaining retractor (Swemac Innovation AB, Linköping, Sweden), as demonstrated in Fig. 27.2, were introduced to replace the existing conventional metallic retractors.

The magnetic technique has not been evaluated on its own before (i.e. without blue dye or radioisotope), as this can only be achieved within a randomised controlled trial. There is now a clinical need for an academically run (independent) and non-commercial randomised controlled trial to establish if the magnetic technique should be used routinely. This Phase III trial will need to be designed with a tight margin for non-inferiority in order to address this reliably. This trial will be the largest trail of the magnetic technique and the most important trial of a non-radioisotope technique for SLNB. This trial could also change practice across several other tumour types, since SLNB is now also performed in colorectal [34], penile [35], and anal [36] cancers.

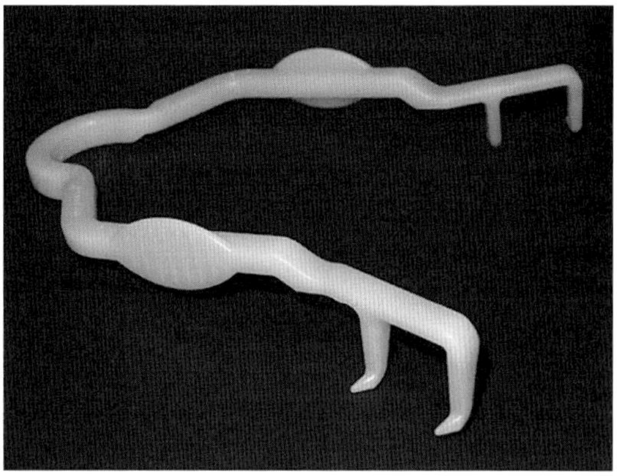

Fig. 27.2 The Doxpal® self-retaining plastic retractor used during magnetic guided surgery to replace the conventional metallic retractors

Conclusion

The magnetic technique, using SPIO, provides a credible alternative to radioisotope dependence in the performance of lymphatic mapping across a range of cancer types. It also provides the opportunity for extended applications including the use of MRI for axillary staging, 'selective axillary surgery', and localisation surgery for clinically occult lesions. Further assessment within clinical trials is necessary to bring these innovative applications to clinical practice.

Acknowledgements The authors are trialists within the academically run and sponsored SentiMAG, MELAMAG and MagSNOLL trials.

Conflict of Interest Statement The authors have no disclosures to make concerning financial and personal relationships with other people or organisations that could inappropriately influence their work. No ethical approval was requested for this work.

References

1. Cabanas RM. An approach for the treatment of penile carcinoma. Cancer. 1977;39:456–66.
2. Morton DL, Wen DR, Wong JH, et al. Technical details of intraoperative lymphatic mapping for early stage melanoma. Arch Surg. 1992;127:392–9.

3. Alex JC, Weaver DL, Fairbank JT, Rankin BS, Krag DN. Gamma-probe-guided lymph node localization in malignant melanoma. Surg Oncol. 1993;2:303–8.
4. Krag DN, Weaver DL, Alex JC, Fairbank JT. Surgical resection and radiolocalization of the sentinel lymph node in breast cancer using a gamma probe. Surg Oncol. 1993;2:335–9; discussion 340.
5. Giuliano AE, Kirgan DM, Guenther JM, Morton DL. Lymphatic mapping and sentinel lymphadenectomy for breast cancer. Ann Surg. 1994;220:391–8; discussion 398–401.
6. Kim T, Giuliano AE, Lyman GH. Lymphatic mapping and sentinel lymph node biopsy in early-stage breast carcinoma: a metaanalysis. Cancer. 2006;106:4–16.
7. Valsecchi ME, Silbermins D, de Rosa N, Wong SL, Lyman GH. Lymphatic mapping and sentinel lymph node biopsy in patients with melanoma: a meta-analysis. J Clin Oncol. 2011;29:1479–87.
8. Zurrida S, Galimberti V, Monti MC, Luini A. Radioguided localization of occult breast lesions. Breast. 1998;7:11–3.
9. Ahmed M, Douek M. Sentinel node and occult lesion localization (SNOLL): a systematic review. Breast. 2013;22:1034–40.
10. Ahmed M, Douek M. Radioactive seed localisation (RSL) in the treatment of non-palpable breast cancers: Systematic review and meta-analysis. Breast. 2013; 22:383–8.
11. Barthelmes L, Goyal A, Newcombe RG, et al. Adverse reactions to patent blue V dye – the new start and almanac experience. Eur J Surg Oncol. 2010; 36:399–403.
12. Joshi T, Pankhurst QA, Hattersley S, Douek M. Magnetic nanoparticles for detecting cancer spread. Breast Cancer Res Treat. 2007;1006 Suppl 1:S129.
13. Johnson L, Douek M. Magnetic sentinel lymph node detection for breast cancer. Cancer Res. 2010;70:140s.
14. Douek M, Klaase J, Monypenny I, et al. Sentinel node biopsy using a magnetic tracer versus standard technique: the SentiMAG multicentre trial. Ann Surg Oncol. 2014;21:1237–45.
15. Thill M, Kurylcio A, Welter R, et al. The Central-European SentiMag study: sentinel lymph node biopsy with superparamagnetic iron oxide (SPIO) vs. radioisotope. Breast. 2014. doi:10.1016/j.breast.2014.01.004.
16. Rubio IT, Diaz-Botero S, Esgueva A, et al. The superparamagnetic iron oxide is equivalent to the Tc99 radiotracer method for identifying the sentinel lymph node in breast cancer. Eur J Surg Oncol. 2015; 41:46–51.
17. Shiozawa M, Lefor AT, Hozumi Y, et al. Sentinel lymph node biopsy in patients with breast cancer using superparamagnetic iron oxide and a magnetometer. Breast Cancer. 2013;20:223–9.
18. Lovrics PJ, Cornacchi SD, Farrokhyar F, et al. The relationship between surgical factors and margin status after breast-conservation surgery for early stage breast cancer. Am J Surg. 2009;197:740–6.
19. Ahmed M, van Hemelrijck M, Douek M. Systematic review of radioguided versus wire-guided localization in the treatment of non-palpable breast cancers. Breast Cancer Res Treat. 2013;140:241–52.
20. Mayes E, Douek M, Pankhurst Q. Magnetic nanoparticles: from fabrication to clinical applications. New York: CRC Press; 2012.
21. Ahmed M, Esposito E. Report from the 37th San Antonio Breast Cancer Symposium, 9–13th December 2014, Texas, USA. Ecancermedicalscience. 2015; 9:508.
22. Ahmed M, Anninga B, Goyal S, et al. Magnetic Sentinel Node and Occult Lesion Localization in breast cancer (MagSNOLL trial). Br J Surg. 2015;102(6):646–52.
23. Morton DL, Thompson JF, Cochran AJ, et al. Sentinel-node biopsy or nodal observation in melanoma. N Engl J Med. 2006;355:1307–17.
24. Federico AC, Chagpar AB, Ross MI, et al. Effect of multiple-nodal basin drainage on cutaneous melanoma. Arch Surg. 2008;143:632–7; discussion 637–8.
25. Douek, M. MELAMAG Trial: a prospective multicentre feasibility non-randomised clinical trial to compare sentinel node biopsy using magnetic nanoparticles vs. standard technique in melanoma 2014. See http://public.ukcrn.org.uk/search/StudyDetail.aspx?StudyID=14011 for further details. Accessed 25 Feb 2014.
26. Balch CM, Gershenwald JE, Soong SJ, et al. Final version of 2009 AJCC melanoma staging and classification. J Clin Oncol. 2009;2009(27):6199–206.
27. Douek M, Anninga B, White S, et al. Sentinel lymph node biopsy for melanoma using a magnetic technique: Primary outcome of the MELAMAG Multicentre Trial. Eur J Surg Oncol. 2014;40:S50.
28. Harnan SE, Cooper KL, Meng Y, et al. Magnetic resonance for assessment of axillary lymph node status in early breast cancer: a systematic review and meta-analysis. Eur J Surg Oncol. 2011;37:928–36.
29. Meng Y, Ward S, Cooper K, Harnan S, Wyld L. Cost-effectiveness of MRI and PET imaging for the evaluation of axillary lymph node metastases in early stage breast cancer. Eur J Surg Oncol. 2011;37:40–6.
30. Johnson L, Pinder SE, Douek M. Deposition of superparamagnetic iron-oxide nanoparticles in axillary sentinel lymph nodes following subcutaneous injection. Histopathology. 2013;62:481–6.
31. Ahmed M, Usiskin SI, Hall-Craggs MA, Douek M. Is imaging the future of axillary staging in breast cancer? Eur Radiol. 2013. doi:10.1007/s00330-013-3009-5.
32. Ahmed M, Purushotham AD, Douek M. Novel techniques for sentinel lymph node biopsy in breast cancer: a systematic review. Lancet Oncol. 2014; 15(8):e351–62.
33. Douek, M. Magnetic Sentinel Node and Occult Lesion Localisation (MagSNOLL): a feasibility study using magnetic nanoparticles for sentinel node biopsy and localisation of occult breast cancers. 2014. See http://public.ukcrn.org.uk/Search/StudyDetail.aspx?StudyID=14979 for further details. Accessed 25 Feb 2014.
34. van der Zaag ES, Bouma WH, Tanis PJ, Ubbink DT, Bemelman WA, Buskens CJ. Systematic review of

sentinel lymph node mapping procedure in colorectal cancer. Ann Surg Oncol. 2012;19:3449–59.
35. Papes D, Altarac S, Arslani N, Rajkovic Z, Antabak A, Cacic M. Melanoma of the glans penis and urethra. Urology. 2014;83:6–11.
36. Tehranian S, Treglia G, Krag DN, et al. Sentinel node mapping in anal canal cancer: systematic review and meta-analysis. J Gastrointestin Liver Dis JGLD. 2013;22:321–8.

Ultrasound Fusion (SPECT/US) 28

Martin Freesmeyer and Thomas Winkens

Contents

Abstract

This chapter is about initial experiences regarding the feasibility and applicability of quasi-integrated freehand (fh) single-photon emission computed tomography (SPECT)/ultrasonography (US) fusion imaging in patients undergoing sentinel lymph node (SLN) imaging or in patients with thyroid disease. The principles of radioguided surgery can be applied to this technology. The successful and emerging concept of hybrid imaging is applied to US imaging, resulting in a tool that combines the delivery of functional information (SLN, thyroid tissue) with excellent visualization of morphology. The medium-term goal of fhSPECT/US fusion imaging is to enhance diagnostic accuracy; however, further improvements are necessary to overcome technical limitations regarding the quality of co-registration and fhSPECT resolution.

28.1 Introduction

Radioguided surgery is a surgical methodology which involves the administration of a radionuclide and the subsequent intraoperative identification and surgical removal of resultant radiolabeled structures. Radioguided surgery involves the use of hand held gamma detection probes, as well as may incorporate the use of

M. Freesmeyer (✉) • T. Winkens
Clinic of Nuclear Medicine, Jena University Hospital, Bachstraße 18, Jena 07743, Germany
e-mail: martin.freesmeyer@med.uni-jena.de; thomas.winkens@med.uni-jena.de

K. Herrmann et al. (eds.), *Radioguided Surgery: Current Applications and Innovative Directions in Clinical Practice*, DOI 10.1007/978-3-319-26051-8_28

portable gamma cameras for optimizing intraoperative detection. Recently, it has become possible not only to identify a radiolabeled structure in the body during radioguided surgery, but also to perform intraoperative cross-sectional imaging combined with visualization and display of the radioactivity distribution on a monitor screen – based on the freehand SPECT (fhSPECT) system, as previously described in the literature [1–4]. Therefore, the incorporation of intraoperative cross-sectional imaging (which can be performed in a multimodal approach) into the standard radioguided surgery methodology can potentially provide additional valuable intraoperative information for optimizing the surgical outcome for patients. This is the subject of the current chapter.

Multimodal cross-sectional diagnostics fusion imaging has gained importance over the past 10 years [5–8]. The use of PET/CT and SPECT/CT has spread rapidly as these hybrid techniques offer advantages over separately undertaken diagnostic procedures (e.g., PET and CT). The benefits of PET/MR are currently being assessed in clinical studies. In addition, technical prerequisites have been addressed with a view to integrating ultrasound (US) into hybrid imaging strategies and enabling its combination with existing cross-sectional image datasets (PET, SPECT, CT, MR) [9–12]. This will permit the advantages of US, in particular its superior soft tissue contrast and high spatial resolution, to be utilized in a hybrid imaging setting.

The technique of combining fhSPECT with US has the potential to become an accurate and useful method to improve preoperative surgical planning. For example, in breast cancer, a sentinel lymph node (SLN) can be accurately identified prior to axillary lymph node dissection after injecting a specific radiopharmaceutical. The fhSPECT/US fusion technique can then be used both to target the appropriate radiolabeled lymph node and subsequently allow examination using US.

Furthermore, in addition to its preoperative use, fhSPECT/US can exclusively be employed in a diagnostic capacity to combine information from any nuclear medicine imaging examination with US data. This instantaneous combination of data would be desirable especially for thyroid diagnostics, as standard and separate diagnostic examination with $^{99m}TcO_4$ and thyroid US can occasionally yield ambiguous results [13].

The medium-term goals of the fusion concept presented in this chapter are, on the one hand, to improve diagnostic accuracy and, on the other, to optimize patient selection for therapeutic procedures and better plan interventions.

28.2 Technical Foundations

28.2.1 fhSPECT

Freehand SPECT is a three-dimensional cross-sectional imaging technique that is based on measurement of the radioactivity distribution of a radionuclide with a gamma detection probe [1]. After administration of a radiopharmaceutical, the gamma detection probe, with its attached localization markers, is moved in different planes around the examination region in a meandering fashion (around the axilla in the case of a breast SLN examination and around the neck in the case of a thyroid examination) and measures the radiation emitted (Fig. 28.1a–c). Using a video camera and an optical positioning system that are mounted above the patient, the position of the gamma detection probe is registered, and the activity distribution is spatially allocated. In addition, the patient is marked with localization markers (shared sensor) to minimize the influence of patient movements on registration accuracy (Fig. 28.1a). After data acquisition, a three-dimensional SPECT cross-sectional image dataset is reconstructed in DICOM format and subsequently displayed on a monitor screen (Fig. 28.1c).

28.2.2 Navigated US

Navigated US is based on the positioning of the two-dimensional US images within a virtual three-dimensional space. For this purpose, two positioning markers are attached to the US probe, which are detected using a magnetic field generated by an electromagnetic transmitter next to the

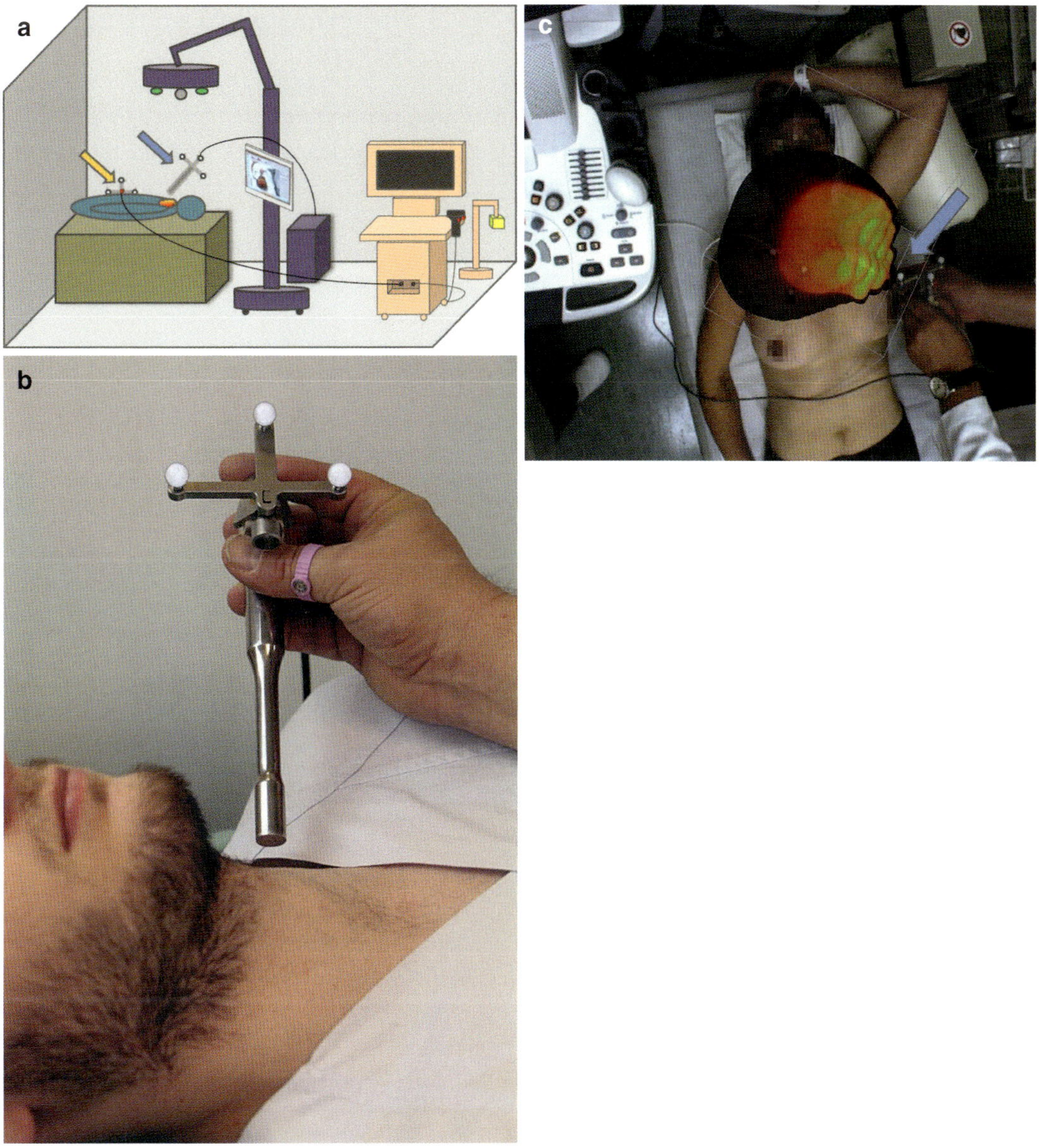

Fig. 28.1 (**a**) fhSPECT examination setup. The radiation that is emitted from the body (here the thyroid gland) is measured using a gamma detection probe (*blue arrow*). The position of the gamma detection probe is recorded with optical markers (*white spheres*) and an optical tracking system (*green*), which is mounted above the patient. In addition, the patient is monitored with an optical tracker (*orange arrow*), to register and correct minor patient movements and enable US data fusion in the second examination step. The activity distribution is projected onto a video image of the patient that is captured by a camera (*gray circle*) mounted above the patient and is initially displayed on a screen. (**b**) Depiction of the gamma detection probe. The gamma detection probe has three optical markers attached at defined distances, which allow precise spatial localization. (**c**) Video recording of an fhSPECT examination of an SLN. The scanned region is represented in color within a virtual space (*cube*). The handheld gamma detection probe (*blue arrow*) traces around the respective region (here the left axilla)

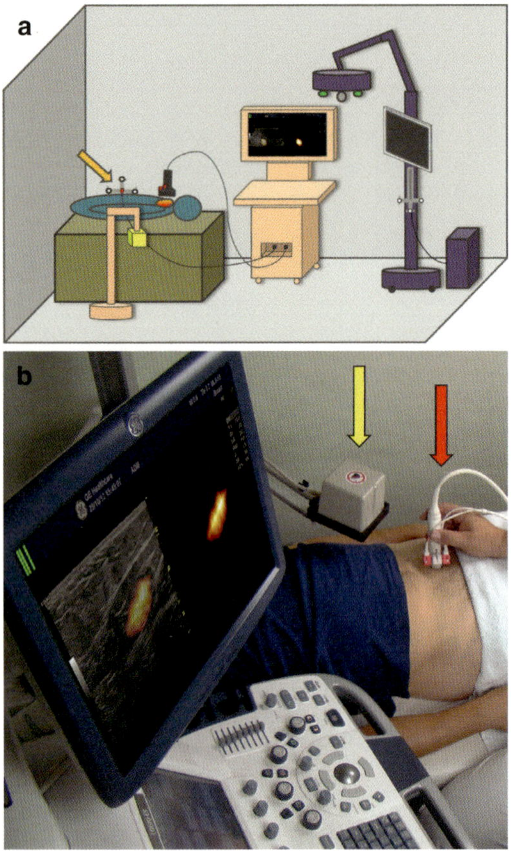

Fig. 28.2 (**a**) Setup of fhSPECT/US fusion imaging during US examination. The position of the US probe within the magnetic field that is generated by the transmitter (*yellow*) is detected using the attached markers (*red*). This enables identification of the plane of the US image and superimposition of it onto the previously recorded fhSPECT dataset. The fhSPECT/US fusion images are displayed in nearly real time on the screen of the US device, both in the semitransparent overlay mode (screen left) and as the SPECT image on its own (screen right). The optical tracker of the patient (*orange arrow*) is equipped with an additional electromagnetic sensor that allows detection within the magnetic field. This tracker is connected to the US device. When moving the US probe, the movement can be traced in the US image as well as in the fhSPECT dataset. (**b**) Freehand SPECT/US examination. The image shows the US probe (*red arrow*) with two red localization markers and the electromagnetic transmitter (*yellow arrow*). Nearly real-time visualization of fusion imaging is depicted on the screen of the US device (**b**: From Freesmeyer et al. [14]. *Image Courtesy: Schattauer Verlag*)

patient's bed (Fig. 28.2a, b) [15]. The allocation of these markers allows the US image to be mapped to a given plane within the virtual three-dimensional space.

28.2.3 Fusion Imaging: Examination Protocol

The fusion of fhSPECT and US is carried out via a complex but manageable (within the clinical routine) sequence of steps, as explained below.

1. *Acquisition of fhSPECT data*
   First, the activity distribution is measured, as described above. It is important that the patient does not move at this stage, if possible. To reduce the influence of minor patient movements, the gamma detection probe and the patient are marked with optical position markers, which allow unequivocal mapping of the activity distribution in space, and the automatic correction of data obtained during minor involuntary changes in patient position. To ensure precise matching between the US (performed later) and fhSPECT examination data, the patient's optical position marker for fhSPECT is equipped with an additional electromagnetic sensor that allows detection within the magnetic field during the entire fhSPECT/US procedure (Fig. 28.1a, Fig. 28.2b).
2. *Reconstruction of fhSPECT data*
   Data reconstruction is carried out with a modified iterative algorithm (maximum likelihood expectation maximization) for nonuniform limited-angle projections and can be either projected as a maximum intensity projection onto a video image of the patient or visualized as a three-dimensional cross-sectional dataset in DICOM format (Fig. 28.1c, Fig. 28.2a) [1].
3. *Transfer of fhSPECT data to the US instrument*
   The fhSPECT dataset is transferred to the US instrument using a USB stick. The subsequent processing and fusion is carried out "online" (live) on the US device.
4. *Image fusion on the US device*
   The fhSPECT dataset is opened on the US system and can be viewed on its computer screen. As soon as the navigation software of the instrument is turned on, the US image within the electromagnetic field is displayed simultaneously with the corresponding sectional plane of the fhSPECT data in split-screen mode.

The registration of both datasets is achieved using the shared patient sensor, which serves as a reference point for both examination modes, as described above (Fig. 28.2a). Apart from the side-by-side display of both datasets (split-screen mode), it is also possible to overlay both imaging modalities in a semitransparent fashion, which allows exact localization of radiolabeled structures with the corresponding anatomical correlates (Fig. 28.2a). When the US probe is moved within the electromagnetic field, a congruent shift of the fhSPECT image occurs, which results in a "live" overlay of fhSPECT and US data. Throughout the US, examination of the corresponding sectional plane of the fhSPECT is simultaneously shown, making it possible to precisely overlay activity distribution onto the anatomical structure.

5. *Data storage*
   As with conventional US images, the split-screen and overlay images can be saved as screenshots and as such permanently archived. In addition, it is possible to record moving images as image stacks (loops) that allow subsequent inspection of the entire region captured by fhSPECT/US.

28.3 fhSPECT/US Fusion for Breast Cancer and Melanoma SLN Examination

Just as preoperative lymphoscintigraphy and portable intraoperative gamma cameras play an important role in the identification and removal of SLNs, preoperative US plays an important role in the diagnostics of breast cancer and melanoma [16, 17]. Preoperative diagnostic ultrasound is useful in the identification of anatomically abnormal lymph nodes within lymph node basins draining the region of a tumour, thus signifying possible metastatic lymph node involvement. However, the information provided by preoperative lymphoscintigraphy and diagnostic US tends to be separate and disconnected. On the one hand, conventional diagnostic US examination can only assess the morphology of all visible lymph nodes; yet it cannot identify the exact SLN into which the primary lymph drainage from the tumor will occur. On the other hand, preoperative lymphoscintigraphy can be used to identify the SLNs with confidence, but morphological assessment of those lymph nodes is not possible. Thus, the combined information from both examination methods would allow for targeted SLN-specific sonographic characterization and would help optimize the surgical management of the lymph nodes.

We undertook a pilot study in our clinic to evaluate the feasibility and applicability of fhSPECT/US fusion imaging in patients with breast cancer and melanoma [14]. Initially, one or more SLNs were identified through planar lymphoscintigraphy of the lymphatic-draining region. Immediately afterward, an fhSPECT examination of the same region was carried out. Patients with breast cancer who presented axillary SLNs were examined in the lateral body position with the arm elevated. Patients with melanoma were examined in a position depending on the localization of the lymph-draining region, such that the respective lymph nodes were easily accessible for US examination. The subsequent fhSPECT examination was carried out in accordance with the previously described protocol (Fig. 28.3).

In this pilot study [14], the following points were also considered: (1) the resolution and the quality of the three-dimensional fhSPECT reconstruction, (2) the accuracy of the signal registration (did the focal accumulation in the fhSPECT image correspond to a lymph node in the US image?), (3) a thorough examination of criteria for malignancy in the respective lymph node, and (4) retrospective comparison of the US result with the histological diagnosis.

All examinations in this pilot study [14] were technically successful. Artifacts that led to limited visualization of the SLN were observed in approximately 33 % of cases. These were caused by a superimposed injection site, insufficient resolution of two foci in close proximity, or central void areas in the activity distribution within focal maxima. In approximately 70 % of cases, we observed a good correlation between the two

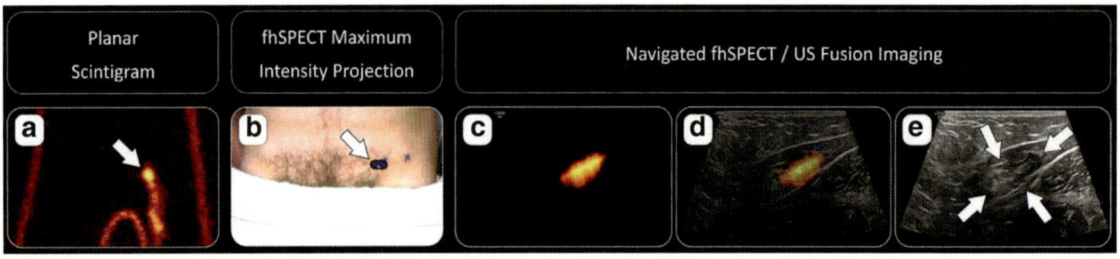

Fig. 28.3 Example of an fhSPECT/US examination of an SLN in a patient with malignant melanoma on the left lower leg. (**a**) Planar scintigram after injection of 100 MBq Nanocoll, showing the SLN and the respective draining lymph vessel (*white arrow*). (**b**) The fhSPECT reconstruction and overlay with the video image of the patient shows focal activity accumulation in the left inguinal region in the projection. (**c–e**) fhSPECT/US fusion imaging with fhSPECT (**c**), semitransparent overlay of fhSPECT and US (fhSPECT/US) (**d**), and US (**e**). A lymph node with no signs of malignancy can be seen in the ultrasound image at the location of highest activity (*white arrows*; **e**). Both datasets are almost exactly aligned and show no spatial incongruence (From Freesmeyer et al. [14]. *Image courtesy: Schattauer Verlag*)

datasets, with a spatial deviation of <1 cm. According to US criteria, one lymph node in a total of 18 patients was classified as potentially malignant. In total, lymph node metastases were detected in 5/18 patients by histopathology. However, these were not suspicious in the preoperative fhSPECT/US examination.

Thus, it can be concluded that for preoperative SLN visualization, fhSPECT/US can be successfully performed at a technical level and, with reasonable organizational effort, can be integrated into the clinical routine. In individual cases, the concept might also aid in preoperative planning. In this pilot study [14], we performed the method in a small patient group, but could not demonstrate its clinical benefit.

There is further potential to optimize the registration accuracy of both imaging modalities. Furthermore, additional steps are necessary to improve the three-dimensional reconstruction quality of fhSPECT data, as well as the spatial resolution.

28.4 fhSPECT/US Fusion Imaging in Thyroid Disease Diagnostics

In addition to measuring thyroid hormones in blood, US and thyroid scintigraphy play key roles in thyroid diagnostics [18]. The radiopharmaceutical of choice is $^{99m}TcO_4$, which enters thyroid cells via the sodium-iodide integral membrane protein symporter. Following administration of the radiopharmaceutical, subsequent planar thyroid scintigraphy shows functional thyroid tissue. Due to image capture using the summation technique, abnormal regions that are completely surrounded by normal tissue or those located at the organ periphery may escape reliable detection. Likewise, when several thyroid nodules in close proximity are detected by US, it becomes difficult to match them with the correct functional state. In particular, in the case of thyroid carcinomas that present exclusively as hypofunctional tissue, accurate matching between the functional state and morphology is essential for diagnosis (Fig. 28.4) [19].

The second component of thyroid diagnostics in any patient with suspected thyroid disease is US [18]. Special attention is paid to thyroid volume and the existence of thyroid nodules. However, analogous to the preoperative US examination of the axillary lymph nodes in breast cancer, the information from radiopharmaceutical imaging is missing. US alone cannot reveal whether a thyroid nodule represents hypofunctional, normal, or hyperfunctional tissue. This distinction is essential to determine the subsequent therapeutic approach. Hypoactive thyroid nodules need to be monitored, punctured, or removed. Thyroid nodules with normal tissue activity usually do not require therapeutic intervention, whereas hyperfunctional thyroid nodules need either radioiodine therapy or removal. In particular, when planning a fine-needle aspiration biopsy of several thyroid nodules in close proximity, the accurate allocation of functional state to morphol-

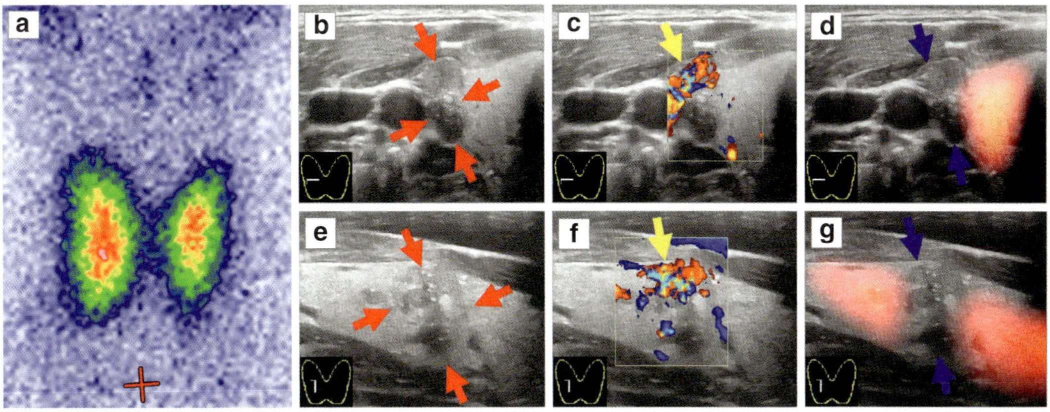

Fig. 28.4 Example of US fusion imaging in a patient with thyroid cancer. Small papillary thyroid cancer allocated laterally in the right thyroid lobe. Thyroid scintigraphy (**a**) does not show a clear focal abnormality, B-mode ultrasonography (**b**, **e**) revealed an irregular hypoechoic area (*red arrows*), and color Doppler sonography (**c**, **f**) showed partial hyperperfusion (*yellow arrows*) within a regular-size right lobe (5 mL). The lesion consisted of two differently configured areas: ventrally, a hypoechoic part with a distinct margin, and dorsally, a more hypoechoic, probably necrotic part with an irregular margin. Magnetic sensor-navigated ^{124}I-PET/US fusion (**d**, **g**) confirmed that the sonographic finding was clearly ^{124}I-negative (hypofunctional, *blue arrows*) (From Freesmeyer et al. [19]). ^{124}I depicts thyroid metabolism in a very similar way as ^{99m}TcO4 does. As a PET-tracer, ^{124}I is superior to ^{99m}TcO4 SPECT imaging regarding spatial resolution. 124I was chosen in this example to demonstrate the usefulness of fusion imaging with ultrasound

ogy is essential for selection of the correct puncture sites.

The almost simultaneous performance of fhSPECT and US examination assists in overcoming the uncertainties in correlating scintigraphic data with US information since it allows: (1) three-dimensional visualization of the activity distribution, (2) free of superimposition artifacts, and (3) unambiguous colocalization with a specific anatomical structure as detected by US.

In the diagnostic thyroid imaging setting, a thyroid fhSPECT/US examination can be performed as based upon the same does of ^{99m}TcO4 that is given for the performance of the standard of care recommendation for thyroid scintigraphy. Thus, such a combined examination approach of standard thyroid scintigraphy and thyroid fhSPECT/US examination adds no additional radiation exposure to the patient as compared to standard thyroid scintigraphy alone. Therefore, the fhSPECT examination can be carried out immediately after standard thyroid scintigraphy in planar imaging mode. The gamma detection probe is moved around the patient's neck in a meandering fashion in order to capture the activity distribution in three dimensions. The positioning of the gamma detection probe/camera is analogous to the technique described for SLN visualization. A further important aspect of thyroid examination is the positioning of the patient. We have found it advantageous to position the neck as freely as possible, in order to be able to measure the radioactivity emitted from the thyroid gland from as many angles and directions as possible. Analogous to the SLN fhSPECT/US examination, the following steps are required: acquisition of the raw data, reconstruction, data transfer to the US device, and image fusion on the screen of the US system (Fig. 28.5).

The fhSPECT/US examination of the thyroid gland was evaluated in a proof-of-concept study [20]. Its technical feasibility was demonstrated in all the examinations carried out. The registration accuracy was always <1 cm. However, artifacts appeared in the thyroid fhSPECT that prevented the correct assignment of the functional state to the matching morphological correlate. In one case, apparent radiotracer uptake outside the thyroid tissue was observed; in another case, two focal maxima were reconstructed even though planar thyroid scintigraphy only showed one maximum. Furthermore, the marginal areas of the thyroid gland were sometimes insufficiently depicted.

In summary, we conclude that fhSPECT/US examination of the thyroid gland is applicable

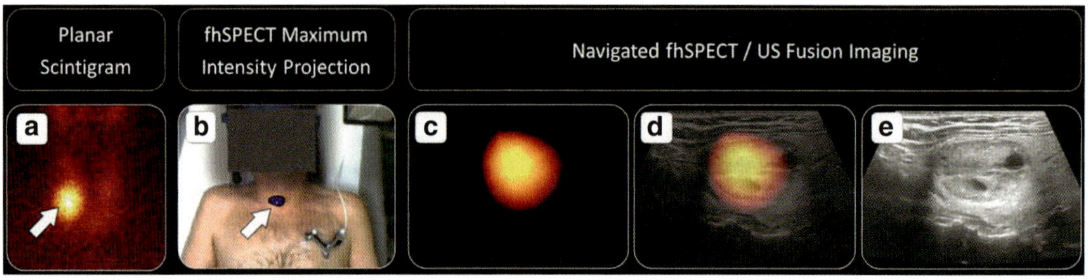

Fig. 28.5 Example of an fhSPECT/US examination of the thyroid gland. (**a**) Planar thyroid scintigram depicting an autonomous adenoma in the right thyroid lobe (*white arrow*). The surrounding thyroid tissue is almost completely suppressed. (b) The fhSPECT reconstruction and overlay with the video image of the patient shows focal activity accumulation in the right neck region in the projection. (**c**–**e**) fhSPECT/US fusion imaging with fhSPECT, (**c**) semitransparent overlay of fhSPECT and US (fhSPECT/US) (**d**), and US (**e**). At the location of the focal activity, there is a hypoechoic, partially cystic nodule with a halo, without signs of malignancy, which sonographically matches an adenoma. As can be seen in **d**, the two datasets are almost exactly superimposed (From Freesmeyer et al. [20]. *Image courtesy: Radiology; Radiological Society of North America*)

and feasible. Moreover, it can be integrated with moderate effort into the clinical routine. It is also important to emphasize that patients are not exposed to additional radiation.

28.5 Summary

Freehand SPECT/US is technically feasible and easily executable. Our pilot studies have demonstrated the applicability of the method in small groups of patients [14, 20]. Proof of clinical benefit of the method is a topic for further needed studies that should, in particular, focus on its possible role in clinical care and its potential contribution in improving therapeutic decision-making.

The fact that the fhSPECT component of fhSPECT/US is carried out immediately before the US examination, within one examination session and with the patient in the same position, significantly reduces the negative influence that different patient positioning in two separate examinations has on registration accuracy. Therefore, fhSPECT/US is a one-time, albeit sequential, examination procedure comparable to hybrid imaging such as SPECT/CT, PET/CT, and PET/MRI.

The fhSPECT/US method presented here fits in with similar hybrid imaging approaches that include US. Initially, CT and MRI datasets were fused with US data for prostate and liver examinations [15, 21–24]. Later, PET data were added for fusion imaging, a topic that has been described extensively by Ewertsen et al. and has been further evaluated by several subsequent studies related to nuclear medicine [10, 25–28]. Galdames et al. fused previously recorded and segmented DMSA SPECT datasets of the kidney "offline" with separately collected US datasets on a dedicated workstation [11]. In a further development of this approach, Bucki et al. fused SPECT with US datasets using optical markers that were attached to the patient's bed during both examinations [9]. This concept already included "live" visualization of both datasets on the screen of the US instrument.

However, the fhSPECT/US concept does have several limitations that need to be taken into account:

1. *Slight to moderate inaccuracy of data registration*: Although fhSPECT and US are carried out in immediate succession, some inaccuracies can still occur due to minor patient movements. This limitation is why fhSPECT/US imaging can only be classified as nearly real-time and not simply as real-time. This effect can be amplified by the fact that the fhSPECT examination is carried out without direct skin contact, while US examination requires gentle pressure on the skin. This can lead to slight tissue displacement in the axillary region (SLN) and in the soft tissue in the neck region (thyroid gland), which also contributes to the inaccuracies.

2. *Insufficient fhSPECT resolution when relative activity differences are small*: In the thyroid gland, areas of different activities can occur at close proximity. Furthermore, the signal to noise ratio in the thyroid gland is significantly lower than in an SLN. This leads, at times, to an unsatisfactory reconstruction of thyroid activity.
3. *Artifacts in dorsal thyroid gland reconstruction*: Although the activity distribution is recorded from different directions and under different angles, the spatial resolution of the fhSPECT system in the depth of the tissue is insufficient. This is a problem particularly for structures located in the dorsal part of the thyroid gland.

Therefore, further optimization of fhSPECT instrumentation is necessary to improve image acquisition, including spatial resolution of the distribution of radioactivity within the field being examined. A miniaturized handheld gamma camera can potentially achieve additional improvement in image acquisition. Furthermore, it would be useful to develop a detector that simultaneously records and displays the US image as well as the radioactivity distribution in a true real-time fashion. Such a concept has recently been introduced as rthESA (real-time handheld emission spot allocator) [29].

References

1. Wendler T, Hartl A, Lasser T, Traub J, Daghighian F, Ziegler SI, et al. Towards intra-operative 3D nuclear imaging: reconstruction of 3D radioactive distributions using tracked gamma probes. Med Image Comput Comput Assist Interv. 2007;10:909–17.
2. Wendler T, Herrmann K, Schnelzer A, Lasser T, Traub J, Kutter O, et al. First demonstration of 3-D lymphatic mapping in breast cancer using freehand SPECT. Eur J Nucl Med Mol Imaging. 2009;37(8):1452–61.
3. Wendler T, Traub J, Freesmeyer M, Wiesner S. Inventors; hybrides bildgebungssystem für intraoperative. Interventionelle und diagnostische anwendungen. patent application 2012. Deutsches Patent- und Markenamt.
4. Wiesner S, Dressel P, Friebe M, Freesmeyer M, Navab N, Wendler T, et al. Registration Free SPECT and Ultrasound Imaging. The 23rd Conference of the Society for Medical Innovation and Technology (SMIT); Tel Aviv. Israel 2011.
5. Beyer T, Townsend DW, Brun T, Kinahan PE, Charron M, Roddy R, et al. A combined PET/CT scanner for clinical oncology. J Nucl Med. 2000;41(8):1369–79. Epub 2000/08/17.
6. Hasegawa BH, Wong KH, Iwata K, Barber WC, Hwang AB, Sakdinawat AE, et al. Dual-modality imaging of cancer with SPECT/CT. Technol Cancer Res Treat. 2002;1(6):449–58. Epub 2003/03/11.
7. Seo Y, Mari C, Hasegawa BH. Technological development and advances in single-photon emission computed tomography/computed tomography. Semin Nucl Med. 2008;38(3):177–98. Epub 2008/04/09.
8. Townsend DW. Dual-modality imaging: combining anatomy and function. J Nucl Med. 2008;49(6):938–55. Epub 2008/05/17.
9. Bucki M, Chassat F, Galdames F, Asahi T, Pizarro D, Lobo G. Real-time SPECT and 2D ultrasound image registration. In: Ayache N, Ourselin S, Maeder A, editors. Medical image computing and computer-assisted intervention – MICCAI 2007. Berlin/Heidelberg: Springer; 2007. p. 219–26.
10. Ewertsen C. Image fusion between ultrasonography and CT, MRI or PET/CT for image guidance and intervention - a theoretical and clinical study. Dan Med Bull. 2010;57(9):B4172. Epub 2010/09/08.
11. Galdames FJ, Perez CA, Estevez PA, Held CM, Jaillet F, Lobo G, et al. Registration of renal SPECT and 2.5D US images. Comput Med Imaging Graph. 2011;35(4):302–14.
12. Péria O, Chevalier L, Francois-Joubert A, Caravel J, Dalsoglio S, Lavallée S, et al. Using a 3D Position Sensor for Registration of SPECT and US Images of the Kidney. Comput Vis Virtual Real Robot Med. 1995;905:23–9.
13. Darr AM, Opfermann T, Niksch T, Driesch D, Marlowe RJ, Freesmeyer M. Low-activity 124I-PET/Low-dose CT versus 99mTc-pertechnetate planar scintigraphy or 99mTc-pertechnetate single-photon emission computed tomography of the thyroid: a pilot comparison. Clin Nucl Med. 2013.
14. Freesmeyer M, Winkens T, Opfermann T, Elsner P, Runnebaum I, Darr A. Real-time ultrasound and freehand-SPECT. Experiences with sentinel lymph node mapping. Nuklearmedizin. 2014;53(6):259–64.
15. Jung EM, Friedrich C, Hoffstetter P, Dendl LM, Klebl F, Agha A, et al. Volume navigation with contrast enhanced ultrasound and image fusion for percutaneous interventions: first results. PLoS One. 2012;7(3).
16. Cools-Lartigue J, Meterissian S. Accuracy of axillary ultrasound in the diagnosis of nodal metastasis in invasive breast cancer: a review. World J Surg. 2012;36(1):46–54.
17. Rahbar H, Partridge SC, Javid SH, Lehman CD. Imaging axillary lymph nodes in patients with newly diagnosed breast cancer. Curr Probl Diagn Radiol. 2012;41(5):149–58.
18. Dietlein M, Dressler J, Grunwald F, Joseph K, Leisner B, Moser E, et al. [Guideline for in vivo- and in vitro procedures for thyroid diseases (version 2)]. Nuklearmedizin. 2003;42(3):109–15. Leitlinie zur Schilddrusendiagnostik (Version 2).
19. Freesmeyer M, Winkens T, Darr A. Diagnosis of small papillary thyroid cancer via sensor-navigated (124)

iodine PET/ultrasound ((124)I-PET/US) fusion. J Clin Endocrinol Metab. 2015;100(1):13–4.
20. Freesmeyer M, Opfermann T, Winkens T. Hybrid integration of real-time ultrasound and freehand-SPECT: proof of concept in patients with thyroid diseases. Radiology. 2014;271:851–61.
21. Singh AK, Kruecker J, Xu S, Glossop N, Guion P, Ullman K, et al. Initial clinical experience with real-time transrectal ultrasonography-magnetic resonance imaging fusion-guided prostate biopsy. BJU Int. 2008;101(7):841–5. Epub 2007/12/12.
22. Xu S, Kruecker J, Turkbey B, Glossop N, Singh AK, Choyke P, et al. Real-time MRI-TRUS fusion for guidance of targeted prostate biopsies. Comput Aided Surg. 2008;13(5):255–64. Epub 2008/09/30.
23. Minami Y, Kudo M, Chung H, Inoue T, Takahashi S, Hatanaka K, et al. Percutaneous radiofrequency ablation of sonographically unidentifiable liver tumors. Feasibility and usefulness of a novel guiding technique with an integrated system of computed tomography and sonographic images. Oncology. 2007;72 Suppl 1:111–6. Epub 2007/12/22.
24. Kaplan I, Oldenburg NE, Meskell P, Blake M, Church P, Holupka EJ. Real time MRI-ultrasound image guided stereotactic prostate biopsy. Magn Reson Imaging. 2002;20(3):295–9. Epub 2002/07/16.
25. Ewertsen C, Ellegaard K, Boesen M, Torp-Pedersen S, Bachmann Nielsen M. Comparison of two co-registration methods for real-time ultrasonography fused with MRI: a phantom study. Ultraschall Med. 2010;31(3):296–301. Epub 2010/06/03.
26. Ewertsen C, Grossjohann HS, Nielsen MB. Image fusion involving ultrasound. Ultraschall Med. 2006;27(2):128–9. Epub 2006/05/13.
27. Ewertsen C, Henriksen BM, Torp-Pedersen S, Bachmann Nielsen M. Characterization by biopsy or CEUS of liver lesions guided by image fusion between ultrasonography and CT, PET/CT or MRI. Ultraschall Med. 2011;32(2):191–7. Epub 2011/01/13.
28. Ewertsen C, Saftoiu A, Gruionu LG, Karstrup S, Nielsen MB. Real-time image fusion involving diagnostic ultrasound. AJR Am J Roentgenol. 2013;200(3):W249–55.
29. Freesmeyer M, Winkens T, Kuhnel C. Real-time handheld emission spot allocator (rthESA) for simultaneous fusion imaging with ultrasound. Nuklearmedizin. 2014;53(6):265–71.

Part XII

Examples (Conventional Techniques and Innovations)

Case Reports 29

Christina Bluemel, Francisco Campos, Angela Collarino, Andreas Cramer, Stephan Dik, Alessandro Giordano, Hanns-Jörg Grimminger, Niel Groen, Ken Herrmann, Martin Horn, Georg W. Kajdi, Dikra Lajaab, Stefan Paepke, Jaume Pahisa, Pilar Paredes, Germano Perotti, Sergi Vidal-Sicart, Erik M. Von Meyenfeldt, and Thomas Wendler

Contents

C. Bluemel (✉) • K. Herrmann • G.W. Kajdi
Department of Nuclear Medicine,
University of Würzburg, Würzburg, Germany

F. Campos • P. Paredes • S. Vidal-Sicart (✉)
Department of Nuclear Medicine,
Hospital Clínic Barcelona, Barcelona, Spain

A. Collarino (✉) • A. Giordano • G. Perotti
Institute of Nuclear Medicine,
University Cattolica del Sacro Cuore, Rome, Italy

A. Cramer • H.-J. Grimminger
Department of Obstetrics and Gynecolog,
Missionsärztliches Klinikum Würzburg,
Würzburg, Germany

S. Dik
Department of Respiratory Medicine,
Albert Schweitzer Hospital, Dordrecht, The Netherlands
e-mail: S.Dik@asz.nl

N. Groen
Department of Nuclear Medicine, Albert Schweitzer Hospital, Dordrecht, The Netherlands
e-mail: N.Groen@asz.nl

M. Horn
R&D Department, SurgicEye GmbH,
Munich, Germany

D. Lajaab • E.M. Von Meyenfeldt (✉)
Department of Surgery,
Albert Schweitzer Hospital,
Dordrecht, The Netherlands
e-mail: 325161dl@student.eur.nl;
e.m.von.meyenfeldt@asz.nl

S. Paepke
Department of Women's Health,
Klinikum rechts der Isar, Munich, Germany

J. Pahisa
Department of Gynaecology,
Hospital Clínic Barcelona, Barcelona, Spain

T. Wendler (✉)
R&D Department, SurgicEye GmbH,
Munich, Germany

Nuclear Medicine Department,
Klinikum rechts der Isar, Munich, Germany

K. Herrmann et al. (eds.), *Radioguided Surgery: Current Applications and Innovative Directions in Clinical Practice*, DOI 10.1007/978-3-319-26051-8_29

Abstract
Surgical resection comprises the standard of care in patients with early-stage breast cancer. For intraoperative detection of non-palpable breast cancer, commonly wire-guided localization is used (Hargreaves et al. J Surg Oncol 110:21–25, 2014). Alternatively, in experienced centers, a radioguided procedure (radioguided occult lesion localization, ROLL) is performed using either fluid radioactive tracers or seeds (Ahmed and Douek Breast Cancer Res Treat 140:435–446, 2013; Ahmed and Douek Breast 22:383–388, 2013). For intraoperative detection of the radioactive labeled tumor lesions, the surgeons employ an acoustical gamma probe. In this case we report on the feasibility and advantages of freehand SPECT-guided lesion localization providing additional intraoperative 3D imaging.

29.1 Radioguided Localization of Non-palpable Breast Cancer Using Intraoperative 3D Imaging

Christina Bluemel, Andreas Cramer, Georg W. Kajdi, Ken Herrmann, and Hanns-Jörg Grimminger

Surgical resection comprises the standard of care in patients with early-stage breast cancer. For intraoperative detection of non-palpable breast cancer, commonly wire-guided localization is used [1]. Alternatively, in experienced centers, a radioguided procedure is performed using either fluid radioactive tracers or radioactive seeds [2, 3]. For intraoperative detection of the radioactive labeled tumor lesions, the surgeons employ an acoustical handheld gamma detection probe. In this case, we report on the feasibility and advantages of freehand SPECT-guided lesion localization, providing additional intraoperative 3D imaging.

We report on a 66-year-old woman with diagnosis of a non-palpable breast cancer (T1, 6 mm; Fig. 29.1a). Distant and lymph node (LN) metastases were excluded by preoperative staging studies, including ultrasound of the axillary region and abdomen, bone scintigraphy, and chest radiography. According to the national guidelines, the patient was referred for sentinel lymph node (SLN) biopsy and resection of the primary tumor [4].

The radiotracer (20 MBq, ^{99m}Tc-nanocolloid) was injected in the center of the breast lesion under ultrasound guidance using a 20-gauge needle (Fig. 29.1b). No side effects or complications were observed. Scintigraphic imaging started 5 min after the injection, and ventral and lateral images were acquired (Fig. 29.2a, b). Consecutively, periareolar injection of 60 MBq ^{99m}Tc-nanocolloid was performed. Early static (Fig. 29.2c, d) and late static images were acquired (Fig. 29.2e ,f), showing a SLN in the right axillary region.

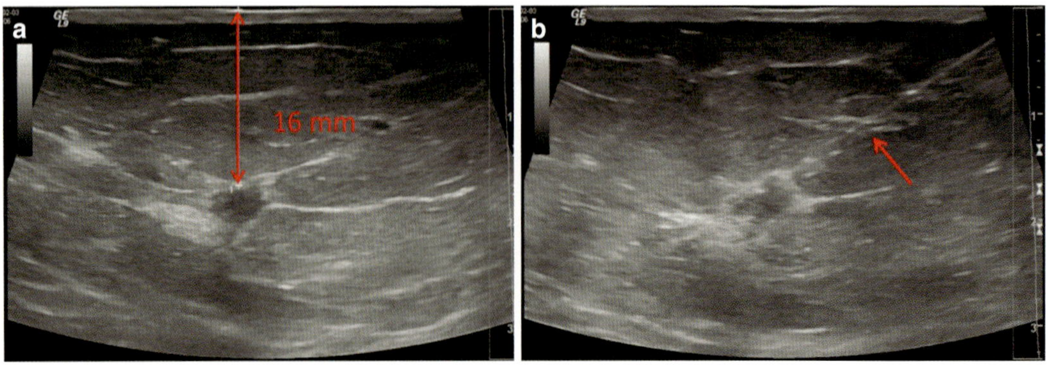

Fig. 29.1 Preinjection ultrasound showing the non-palpable tumor lesion in the right breast (upper quadrant, 2 o'clock). (**a**) The distance between the skin and the tumor was 16 mm; (**b**) Injection of ^{99m}Tc-nanocolloid in the ventral parts of the tumor lesion using a 20G needle (*arrow*)

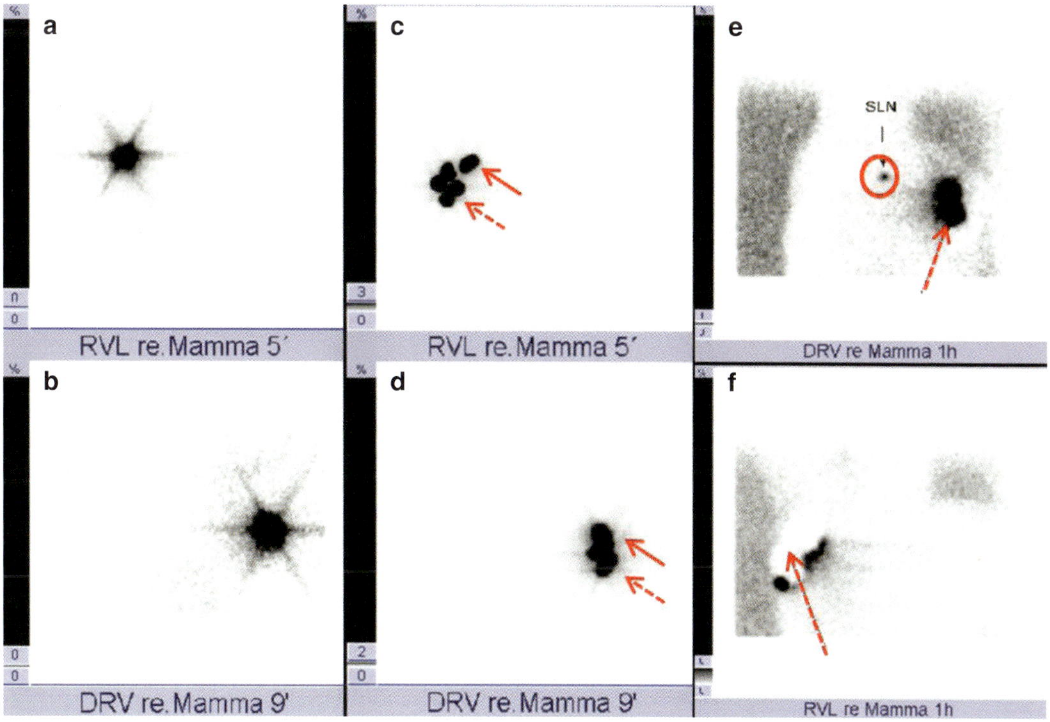

Fig. 29.2 Planar scintigraphy. (**a**, **b**) Ventral and lateral images showing the intratumoral injection; (**c**, **d**) ventral and lateral images showing the injection site (*dotted arrow*) and intratumoral injection (*arrow*); (**e**, **f**) late images showing the sentinel lymph node (*red circle*) and the injection site (*dotted arrow*).

On the next day, the SLN biopsy was performed and LNs were sent to frozen section. Concurrently, the primary breast tumor was resected using guidance from both the prior wire-guided localization and freehand SPECT. Before the incision, a scan with freehand SPECT (pre-incision) visualized the injection site and the primary tumor in the right breast. The depth measurement (Fig. 29.3b) correlated with the preoperative ultrasound images. This information can only be provided by imaging and 3D navigation. A conventional acoustical handheld gamma detection probe cannot assess the depth of the tumor within the breast. The surgical site was scanned again after the resection of the primary tumor to detect potential remaining activity, which was excluded (Fig. 29.3c).

Histopathological analysis revealed a breast cancer of non-special subtype with peritumoral and intratumoral ductal carcinoma in situ. The SLNs were negative, resulting in a tumor stage of pT1b (10 mm) N0 (0/2 SLNs), G3. The hormonal receptor status and expression of Her2/neu were negative. The margins were clear (R0), corresponding to the complete resection which was confirmed by the utilization of the freehand SPECT scan.

In summary, intraoperative imaging using freehand SPECT is feasible, and the depth measurement can help to guide the surgeon. Therefore, we conclude that freehand SPECT guidance is an alternative to wire-guided localization and provides the possibility for intraoperative imaging of the specimen and assessment of the tumor margins.

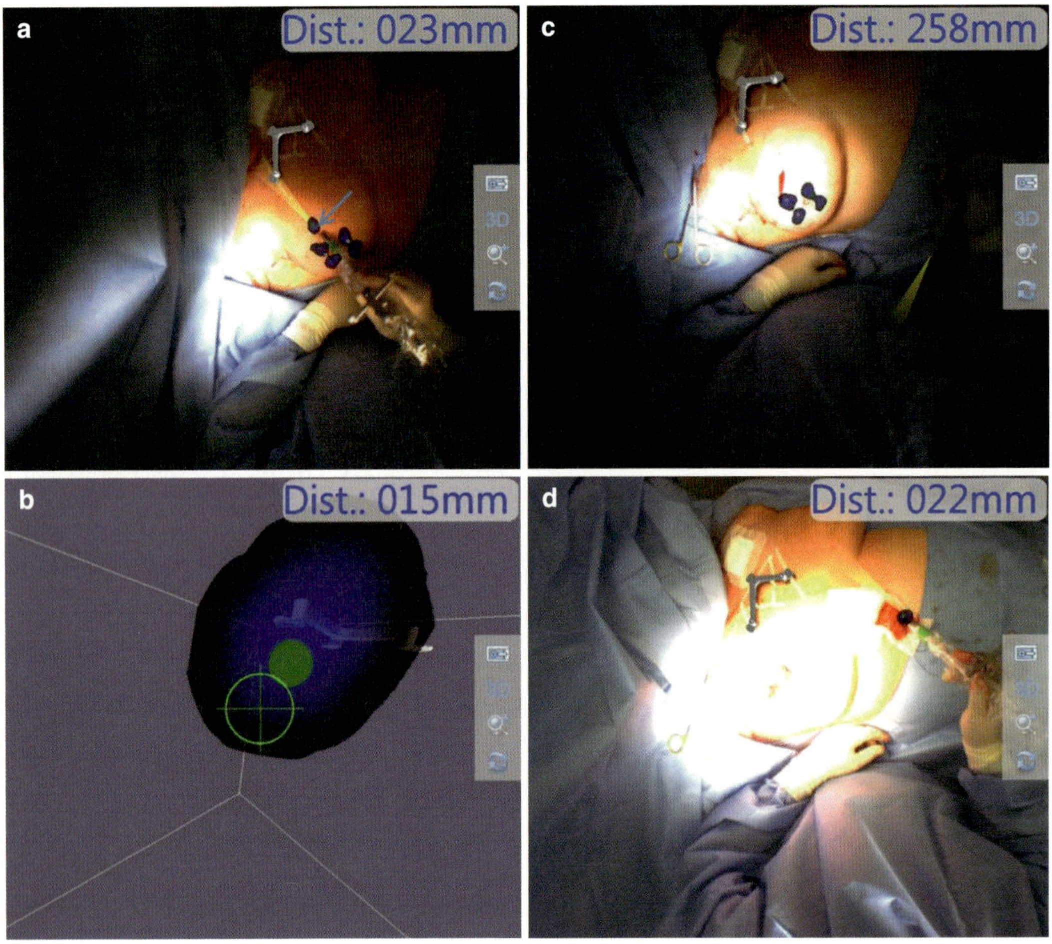

Fig. 29.3 Freehand SPECT scans. (**a**) pre-incision scan showing the injection site and the primary tumor (*arrow*); (**b**) distance measurement between the skin and the primary tumor; (**c**) post-excision scan showing only the injection deposits and a successful resection of the primary; (**d**) scan of the specimen showing the intratumoral injection deposit in a distance of 22 mm from the central specimen margin

29.2 Radionuclide-Guided Biopsy of a Rib Lesion in a Patient with Lung Cancer

Dikra Lajaab, Stephan Dik, Niel Groen, and Erik M. Von Meyenfeldt

A 62-year-old male was presented at the thoracic oncology multidisciplinary team meeting. He was diagnosed with lung cancer after being analyzed for dyspnea on exertion. Workup consisted of a thoracic CT (computed tomography), which showed a 10 cm lesion in the left upper lobe, but no hilar or mediastinal lymphadenopathy nor signs of distant metastases. CT-guided percutaneous biopsy confirmed the diagnosis of adenocarcinoma of the lung.

Further analysis using ^{18}F-fluorodeoxyglucose (^{18}F-FDG)-positron emission tomography (PET)/CT showed the FDG-avid primary lesion and no uptake in hilar or mediastinal lymph nodes. However, PET/CT did demonstrate an additional FDG-avid focus located in the anterolateral portion of the left 5th rib.

Since there was no recent history of chest trauma, a lung cancer bone metastasis was suspected (Fig. 29.4).

Confirmation of the histology of the rib lesion was of great importance. No bone metastasis would mean that treatment with curative intent was still feasible and induction therapy and surgical resection would be warranted. Confirmation of a bone metastasis would imply a worse prognosis despite aggressive treatment. This information would aid the patient and his treatment team in choosing between a surgical approach or a more restricted treatment plan with less morbidity.

On reexamination of the CT scan, still no bone abnormality was found. A subsequent technetium 99 m (^{99m}Tc) bone scan (SymbiaS, Siemens, Erlangen, Germany) and single-photon emission computed tomography (SPECT) showed high uptake in the left 5th rib region (Fig. 29.5). This made radionuclide-guided bone lesion biopsy possible (see Chapter 22).

On the day of operation, our patient received an intravenous dose of 590 MBq ^{99m}technetium-oxidronate (^{99m}Tc-HDP), followed by a second bone scan in the nuclear medicine department. During this bone scan, the location of the left 5th rib lesion was marked on the skin, using a cobalt (Co^{57}) marker (Fig. 29.6a, b).

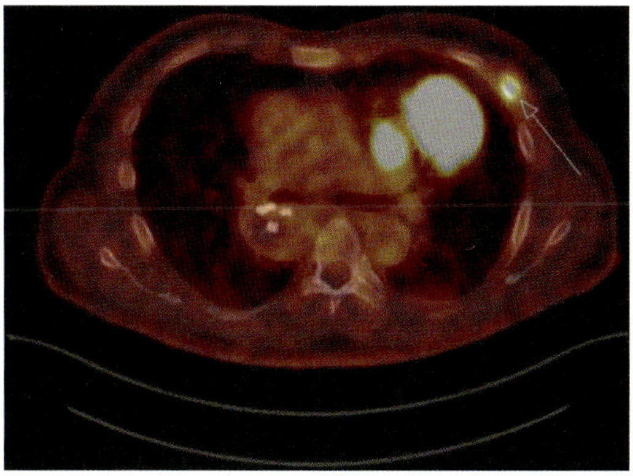

Fig. 29.4 PET/CT scan image with the large FDG-avid primary tumor in the left upper lobe and the left 5th rib bone lesion (*white arrow*)

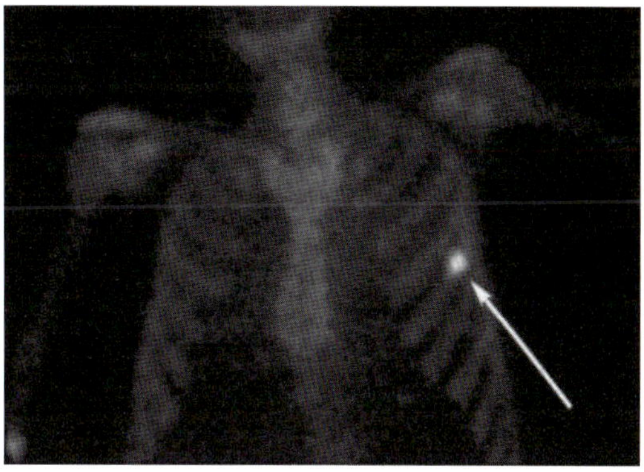

Fig. 29.5 ^{99m}Tc-bone scan image with high uptake in the left 5th rib bone lesion (*white arrow*)

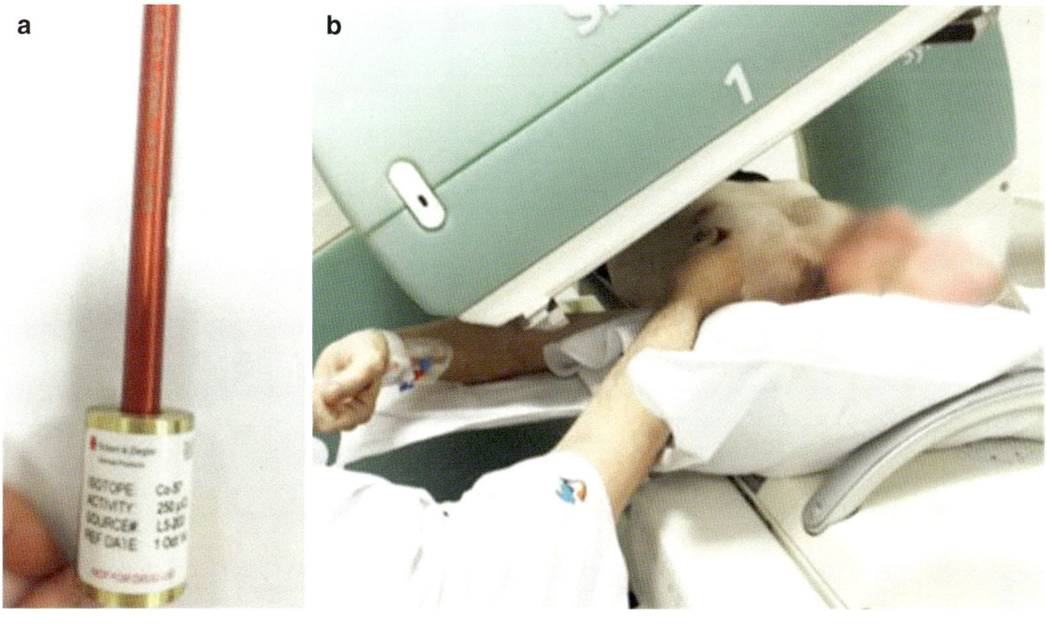

Fig. 29.6 (**a**) Cobalt source used for localization and skin marking. (**b**) Skin marking at the scanner

The patient was taken to the operating room approximately 4 hours after injection. After he was anesthetized and draped in supine position, the localization mark was checked with the 140 keV handheld gamma detection probe (Eurorad, Europrobe 2, Chennevières-sur-Marne, France). An incision was made over the skin mark. To find the exact location of the left 5th rib bone lesion, the 140 keV gamma detection probe was used on the rib surface (Fig. 29.7). The part of rib that showed the highest rate of radioactivity (1065 counts per second (cps) vs. background 250cps) was biopsied. The outer cortex was opened with a chisel, and the bone with high uptake was removed with a rongeur (Fig. 29.8). Decreased uptake at the biopsy site and high activity of the biopsy material confirmed the adequacy of the biopsy.

The postoperative chest X-ray showed no signs of complications. The patient was discharged from hospital on the same day. No complications occurred postoperatively.

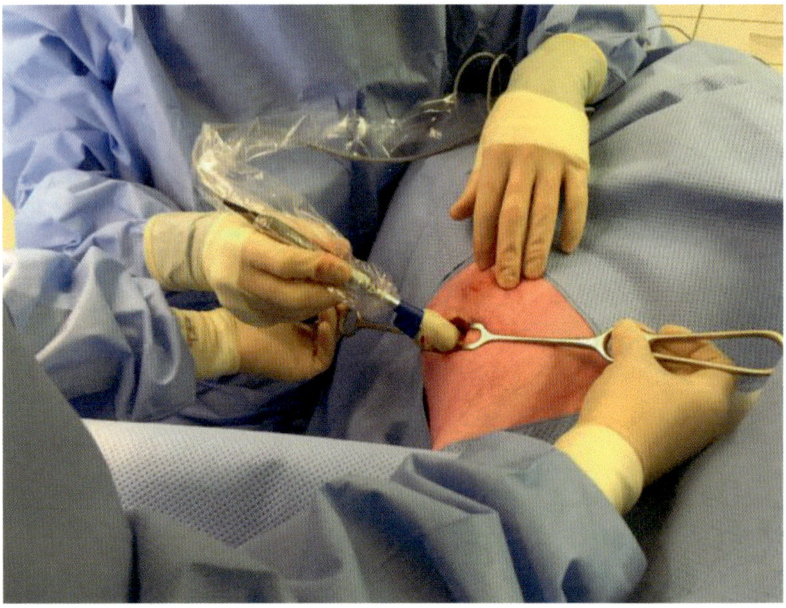

Fig. 29.7 140keV handheld probe localization of the left 5th rib area with the highest uptake

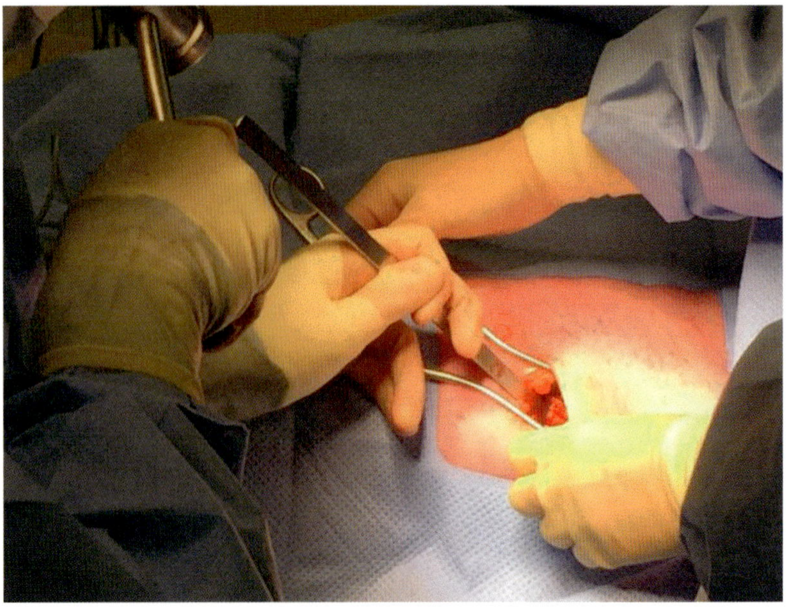

Fig. 29.8 Opening of the outer cortex of the left 5th rib with chisel

The pathologist concluded that there were no signs of malignancy in the biopsy. The bone tissue showed high remodeling activity, as seen in a posttraumatic reaction. The patient was sent for induction chemoradiotherapy, restaging, and subsequent surgical resection of his left upper lobe lung cancer.

Radionuclide-guided bone biopsy in this patient proved to be an accurate way to rule out a bone metastasis and fundamentally influence his treatment plan.

29.3 Added Value of SPECT/CT in Vulvar Cancer Sentinel Lymph Node Mapping and Biopsy

Angela Collarino, Germano Perotti, and Alessandro Giordano

A 70-year-old woman was referred to our center with bleeding ulcer, indicative of vulvar cancer, on the left labia majora (stage FIGO T1) and clinically node negative (cNO) by preoperative ultrasound of the groin. The patient was to undergo vulvectomy and sentinel lymph node biopsy (SLNB) to define the draining lymphatic basin at risk for metastatic disease and to identify the corresponding sentinel lymph node (SLN). After the application of lidocaine spray for local anesthesia, 74 MBq of ^{99m}Tc-nanocolloid (Nanocoll®) was injected intradermally in four peri-tumoral sites (total volume 0.8 mL). Dynamic images (15 frames 60 s each) were acquired immediately after injection in anterior projection with 64 × 64 matrix and zoom factor 1.33, followed by static images in anterior and lateral projection with a 256 × 256 matrix and zoom factor 1.33. Anterior planar image (a) showed the site of the injection (yellow arrow) and one SLN (blue arrow) in the left groin. Furthermore, left lateral planar image (b) revealed another focal area of uptake (red arrow) suggestive of another SLN (Fig. 29.9). A SPECT/CT scan (128 × 128 matrix, 20 s/frame, 3° angular steps) was performed to obtain better anatomical localization of the SLNs. The CT scan (c) and fused SPECT/CT image (d) showed only one SLN localized in the left groin (blue arrow) (Fig. 29.9). The other focal area of uptake seen on lateral planar image corresponded to a contamination area (red arrow) on CT scan (e) and fused SPECT/CT image (f) (Fig. 29.9). The contamination was determined by leakage of radiotracer from the bleeding vulvar lesion. This case underlines the utility of SPECT/CT in vulvar cancer. As reported in the current literature, SPECT/CT in women with vulvar cancer provides anatomical

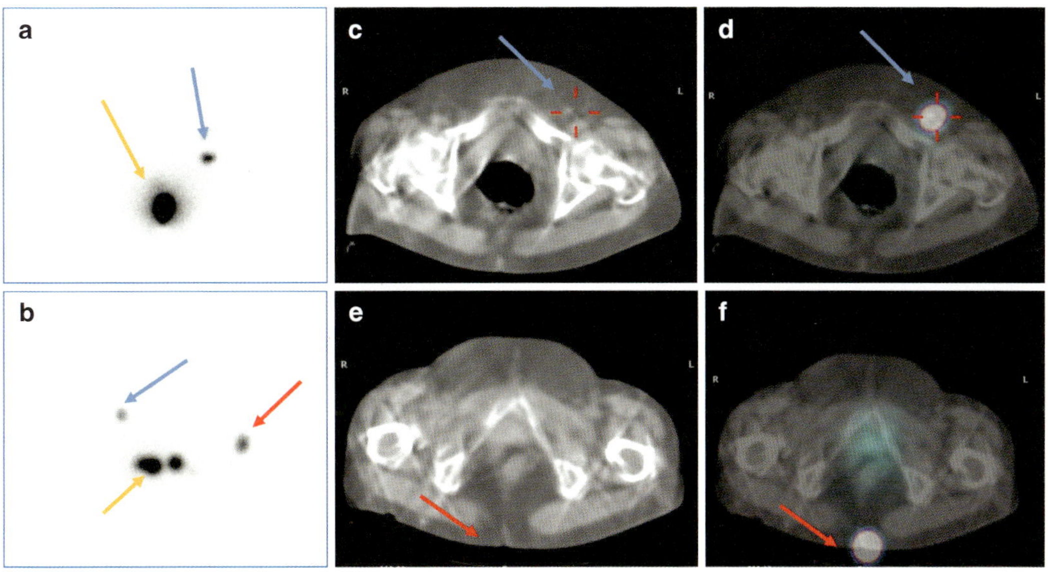

Fig. 29.9 (a–f) SPECT/CT in vulvar cancer sentinel lymph node mapping

and functional information useful to provide better localization of SLNs and to detect other possible SLNs with poor or without visualization seen at planar imaging [5–7]. As this case showed, SPECT/CT plays also an important role to reduce the false-positive rate, possibly due to external contamination or presence of radioactivity in enlarged lymphatic vessels. In conclusion, SPECT/CT represents a useful adjunct to planar imaging for SLN mapping in vulvar cancer.

29.4 Hybrid Tracer in Gynecology

Pilar Paredes, Jaume Pahisa, Francisco Campos, and Sergi Vidal-Sicart

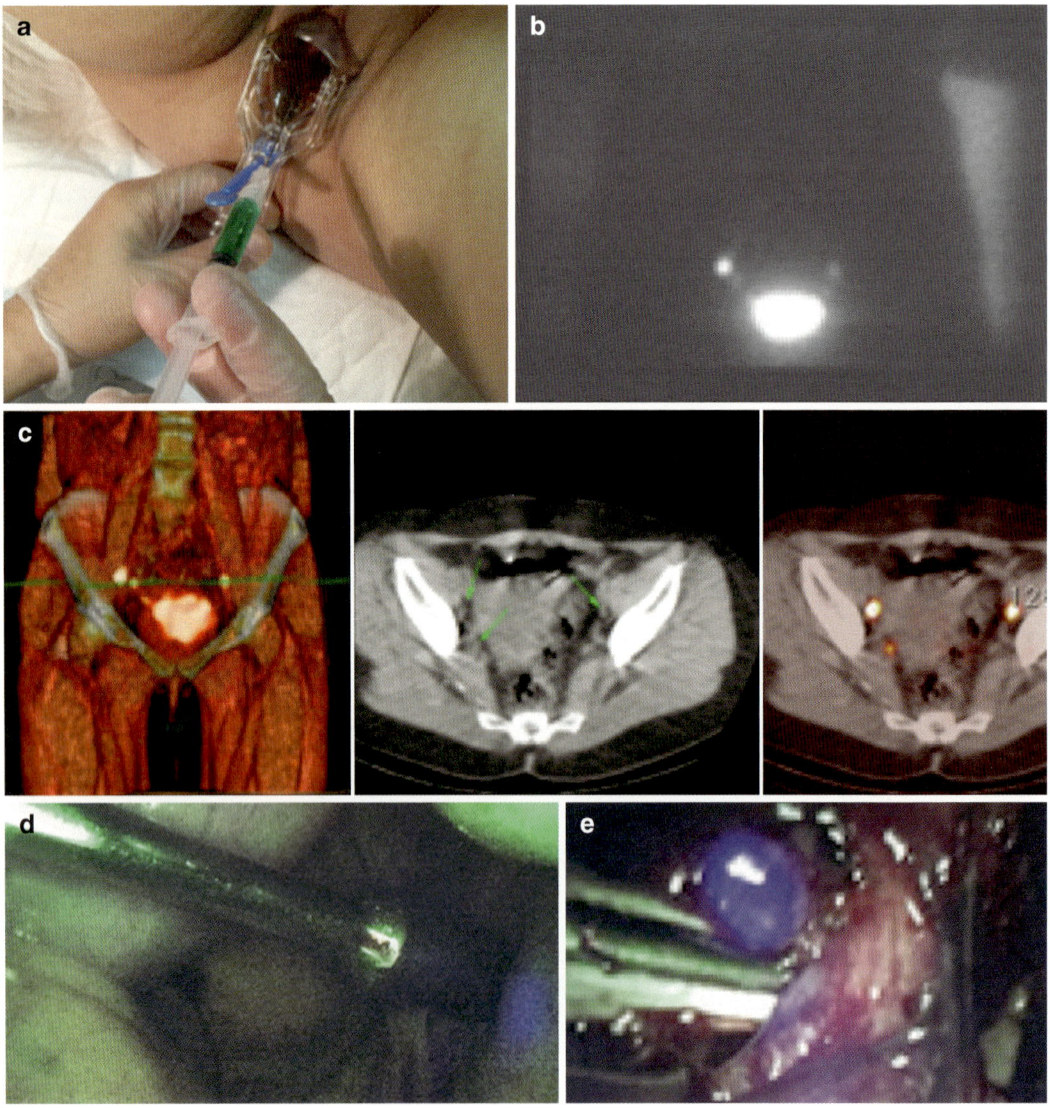

Fig. 29.10 Injection of ^{99m}Tc-albumin nanocolloid-ICG (**a**) the day before surgery. Planar lymphoscintigraphy showed bilateral drainage (**b**), confirmed on SPECT/CT images (**c**). MIP reconstruction (**c,** *left*) and axial CT and fusion images (**c**; *mid* and *right*) showed the SLN location on external iliac chains. During surgery, the laparoscopic gamma probe (**d**) allowed the identification of pelvic SLNs, which showed fluorescent emission detected by means of an optical camera (**e**)

A 53-year-old woman who presented with postmenopausal metrorrhagia was referred to the Gynecology Department for further study. Cone biopsy revealed squamous cervical carcinoma. Thoracoabdominal CT did not show lymph node involvement. MR showed no evidence of parametrial invasion. The patient was diagnosed of IB1 cervical cancer and was scheduled for lymphoscintigraphy, sentinel lymph node detection, and potential (eventual) hysterectomy.

Lymphoscintigraphy was performed the day before surgery to obtain a lymphatic map of the tumor. A dose of 111 MBq of a hybrid tracer ^{99m}Tc-albumin nanocolloid-indocyanine green (ICG) was injected around the modified external cervical os. Lymphoscintigraphy included planar images at 30 minutes and 2 hours after tracer injection and SPECT/CT images at 2 hours p.i.

At the onset of surgery, 2 ml of blue dye (50 % dilution) was administered with the same protocol as the hybrid tracer. Sentinel lymph node detection included visual inspection of blue lymph nodes and the use of a laparoscopic gamma detection probe and an optical camera suitable for fluorescence visualization (Fig. 29.10).

29.5 Minimally Invasive, Image-Guided Core Needle Biopsy of Sentinel Lymph Nodes as Nonsurgical Method to Detect Lymph Node Metastases

Stefan Paepke, Martin Horn, and Thomas Wendler

For over the past 20 years, sentinel lymph node (SLN) biopsy has become the widely accepted method for the diagnostic evaluation of the axillary lymph nodes in early-stage breast cancer patients [8, 9]. Recently, a commercial SPECT/ultrasound system (SentiGuide® by SurgicEye®, Munich, Germany) has been made available [10]. This system allows one to identify radioactive lymph nodes (i.e., SLNs) and distinguish them from non-radiative lymph nodes (i.e., non-SLNs) within the axilla. The addition of a core needle biopsy device to this system allows the performance of a minimally invasive, image-guided core needle biopsy procedure (i.e., nonsurgical SLN biopsy) which is specifically directed toward the SLNs (Fig. 29.11).

A 52-year-old female patient with a primary early-stage breast tumor and a clinically negative axilla was planned for a standard SLN biopsy procedure. The patient agreed to participate in the MinimalSNB study, which evaluates the feasibility of a minimally invasive, image-guided core needle biopsy to the SLNs (i.e., nonsurgical SLN biopsy) using SPECT/ultrasound.

The day before surgery, 132 MBq of ^{99m}Tc-nanocolloid was injected in a periareolar fashion into the ipsilateral breast. A single SLN was detected after 5 minutes using dynamic lymphoscintigraphy (ECAM by Siemens, Knoxville, TN, USA, LEHS collimator, 2-min integration time).

On the day of surgery, intraoperative SPECT/US imaging (1-min SPECT acquisition, 12 MHz transducer; using as detector the mini gamma camera CrystalCam by Crystal Photonics, Berlin, Germany) was acquired under general anesthesia and prior to the surgical incision. A single SLN, measuring 12.7mm × 5.3 mm, was identified at a depth of 19.9 mm. Seven core needle biopsy specimens were taken using a 14G HistoCore system (BIP Medical, Tuerkenfeld, Germany) in the semiautomatic mode to avoid damage of vital structures. The 7 harvested core needle biopsy specimens were radioactive, verifying that these specimens correctly targeted the SLN. Subsequently, a standard surgical SLN biopsy procedure was performed using a gamma probe (Gamma Finder by W.O.M. World of Medicine, Berlin, Germany), and 2 close radioactive lymph nodes were harvested (i.e., 2 SLNs). Intraoperative frozen section analysis of these 2 surgical excised SLNs was negative for metastatic disease (Figs. 29.12, and 29.13).

The resected breast tumor revealed to be invasive ductal carcinoma (pT1c, G2), measuring 15 mm in greatest dimension and which had negative surgical resection margins.

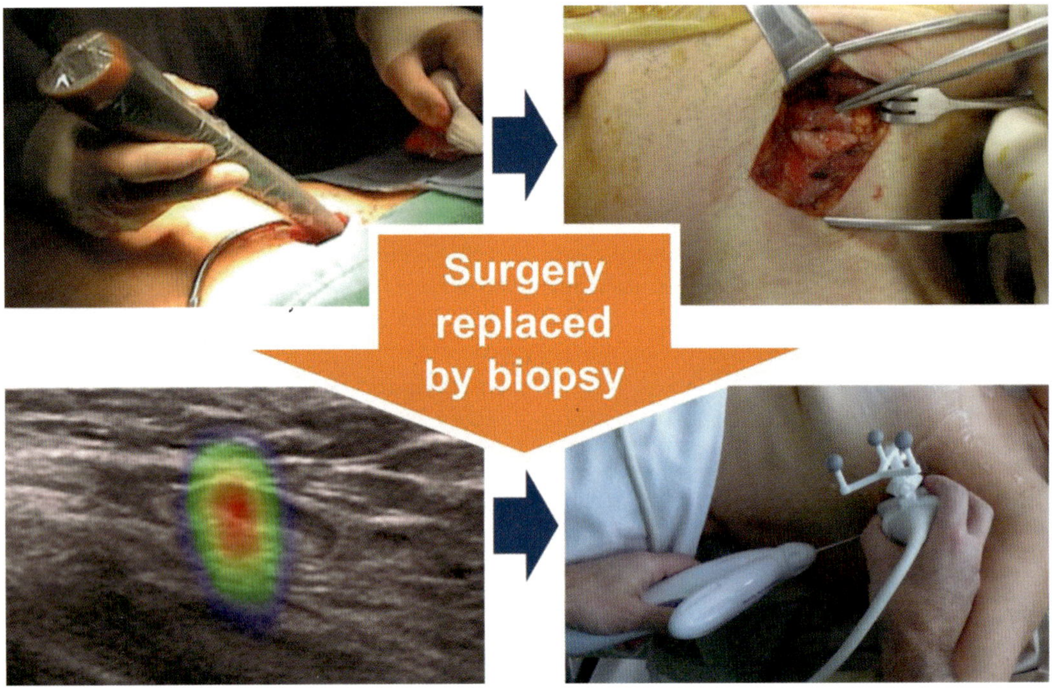

Fig. 29.11 *Top left*: intraoperative localization of SLN with gamma probe, *top right*: surgical resection of SLN, *bottom left*: SLN identification in ultrasound using SentiGuide® system, *bottom right*: needle biopsy of SLN

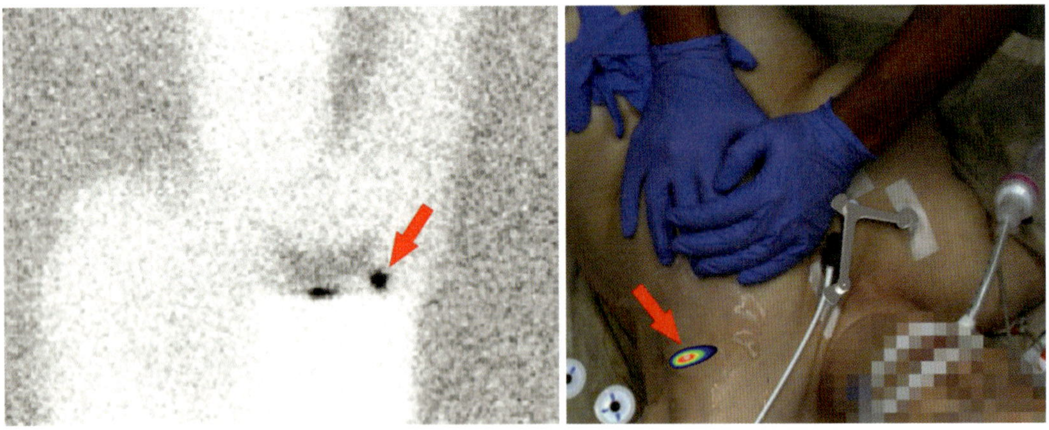

Fig. 29.12 *Left*: planar scintigraphy with lead covering of injection site with one identified SLN, *right*: 1 SLN confirmed by SentiGuide®

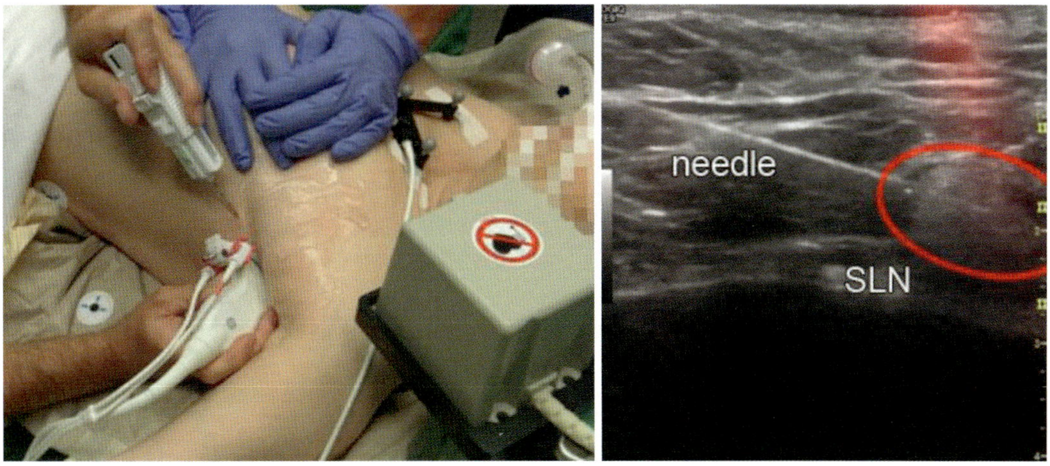

Fig. 29.13 *Left*: core needle biopsy of the SLN under ultrasound guidance, *right*: core needle inside the SLN overlaid by the SentiGuide® SPECT fusion

Subsequently, the initial permanent pathological examination (using H&E, step sectioning with 500 μm slices) of the 2 harvested SLNs was reported to show no evidence of metastatic disease, as was previously demonstrated on intraoperative frozen section analysis. However, permanent pathological examination of the 7 harvested core needle biopsy specimens from the minimally invasive, image-guided core needle biopsy procedure (i.e., nonsurgical SLN biopsy) of the single visualized SLN revealed micrometastatic disease within that SLN. As a result, a more thorough repeat permanent pathological examination of the 2 SLNs harvested at the time of the standard surgical SLN biopsy procedure revealed evidence of isolated tumor cells within one of the 2 surgically excised SLNs. Resultantly, the status of the SLNs was changed by the nonsurgical SLN biopsy procedure, representing a false-negative result from the standard surgical SLN biopsy procedure.

Minimally invasive, image-guided axillary lymph node core needle biopsy is an established diagnostic method for suspicious axillary lymph nodes seen on ultrasound. It is performed mainly by radiologists and breast surgeons [11]. Extending this technology to axillary SLNs using large-gauge core needle biopsy devices represent the next step in the evolution of the diagnostic evaluation of the axillary lymph nodes in breast cancer patients.

As demonstrated in this particular case, SPECT/US was shown to be a feasible and safe method for accomplishing percutaneous, minimally invasive, image-guided SLN core needle biopsy. However, this technology does require proper training and established expertise/experience with axillary lymph node core needle biopsy methods, including harvesting multiple cores using larger-gauge core needle biopsy devices for maximizing the diagnostic capabilities. These issues will be addressed within a running multicentric trial (MinimalSNB).

References

1. Hargreaves AC, Mohamed M, Audisio RA. Intraoperative guidance: methods for achieving negative margins in breast conserving surgery. J Surg Oncol. 2014;110:21–5. doi:10.1002/jso.23645.
2. Ahmed M, Douek M. Intra-operative ultrasound versus wire-guided localization in the surgical management of non-palpable breast cancers: systematic review and meta-analysis. Breast Cancer Res Treat. 2013;140:435–46. doi:10.1007/s10549-013-2639-2.
3. Ahmed M, Douek M. Radioactive seed localisation (RSL) in the treatment of non-palpable breast cancers: systematic review and meta-analysis. Breast. 2013;22:383–8. doi:10.1016/j.breast.2013.04.016.
4. Kreienberg R, Albert US, Follmann M, Kopp IB, Kuhn T, Wockel A. Interdisciplinary GoR level III guidelines for the diagnosis, therapy and follow-up care of breast cancer: short version – AWMF registry No.: 032–045OL AWMF-register-nummer: 032-045OL – kurzversion 3.0, Juli 2012. Geburtshilfe Frauenheilkd. 2013;73:556–83. doi:10.1055/s-0032-1328689.
5. Beneder C, Fuechsel FG, Krause T, Kuhn A, Mueller MD. The role of 3D fusion imaging in sentinel lymphadenectomy for vulvar cancer. Gynecol Oncol. 2008;109(1):76–80.
6. Kraft O, Havel M. Detection of sentinel lymph nodes in gynecologic tumours by planar scintigraphy and SPECT/CT. Mol Imaging Radionucl Ther. 2012;21(2):47–55.
7. Belhocine TZ, Prefontaine M, Lanvin D, Bertrand M, Rachinsky I, Ettler H, et al. Added-value of SPECT/CT to lymphatic mapping and sentinel lymphadenectomy in gynaecological cancers. Am J Nucl Med Mol Imaging. 2013;3(2):182–93.
8. Lyman GH, Temin S, Edge SB, Newman LA, Turner RR, Weaver DL, Benson AB, Bosserman LD, Burstein HJ, Cody H, Hayman J, Perkins CL, Podoloff DA, Giuliano AE. Sentinel lymph node biopsy for patients with early-stage breast cancer: american society of clinical oncology clinical practice guideline update. J Clin Oncol. 2014;32(13):1365–83.
9. Kuehn T, Bembenek A, Decker T, Munz DL, Sautter-Bihl ML, Untch M, Wallwiener D. A concept for the clinical implementation of sentinel lymph node biopsy in patients with breast carcinoma with special regard to quality assurance. Cancer. 2005;103(3):451–61.
10. Freesmeyer M, Winkens T, Opfermann T, Elsner P, Runnebaum I, Darr A. Real-time ultrasound and freehand-SPECT: experiences with sentinel lymph node mapping. Nuklearmedizin. 2014;53(6):259–64.
11. Paepke S, Ohlinger R, Blohmer J-U, Thill M, Gruber I, Hahn M, Kuehn T. Work Group on Minimally-Invasive Breast Interventions of the German Society of Senology. Survery on axillary lymph node biopsy in Germany. Annual meeting of the German Society of Senology, Leipzig, June 2015.

Index

K. Herrmann et al. (eds.), *Radioguided Surgery: Current Applications and Innovative Directions in Clinical Practice*, DOI 10.1007/978-3-319-26051-8

S

Printed by Printforce, the Netherlands